D1124505

Patients,
Physicians
and Illness

Patients, Physicians and Illness

A Sourcebook in Behavioral Science and Health

SECOND EDITION

Edited by

E. GARTLY JACO
University of California, Riverside

THE FREE PRESS
A Division of Macmillan Publishing Co., Inc.
NEW YORK

Collier Macmillan Publishers
LONDON

COPYRIGHT © 1972, 1958 BY THE FREE PRESS
A Division of Macmillan Publishing Co., Inc.

All rights reserved. No part of this book may be reproduced or transmitted in any form or by any means, electronic or mechanical, including photocopying, recording, or by any information storage and retrieval system, without permission in writing from the Publisher.

THE FREE PRESS
A Division of Macmillan Publishing Co., Inc.
866 Third Avenue, New York, N.Y. 10022

Collier–Macmillan Canada Ltd.

Library of Congress Catalog Card Number: 70–143526

Reprinted 1973 with corrections

Printed in the United States of America

printing number
3 4 5 6 7 8 9 10

To Adele, my wife,
whose healing powers far surpass
those of the greatest physician.

Contents

II. SOCIETAL COPING WITH ILLNESS AND INJURY

III. SOCIETY AND HEALTH CARE ADMINISTRATION 271

Preface

NEARLY A DECADE AND A HALF has gone by since the first edition of this anthology was compiled, during which time a tremendous growth and change in the developing specialty of medical sociology along with medical psychology and anthropology has occurred. It is my hope that this new edition will faithfully reflect these changes and developments in medical behavioral science, and particularly in medical sociology.

The reader who is familiar with the contents of the first edition may recall the wide array and divergence of sources, particularly of the reprinted articles, ranging from professional house-organs to scientific journals from many fields of health and medicine as well as from social and behavioral science. Some of the chapters were preliminary reports, others were so-called "thought pieces," and still others were observational treatises, whereas, of course, many were extensive research studies. These papers represented the varying levels of analysis and observations reflecting the field's rather embryonic state of development at that time.

In the past decade several journals devoted to social science and the health and medical fields have emerged along with several important reference and text books. An increasing number of social scientists have become actively engaged in teaching and research roles in medical schools, nursing schools, schools of public health, health care and hospital administration, and health research and action organizations, to mention a few. The rapid rise in membership of the Section on Medical Sociology in the American Sociological Association in recent years and increasingly frequent sessions on medical sociological topics at the national and regional meetings of sociological societies, along with the International Sociological Association, further indicate the remarkable expansion of interest and commitment especially to medical sociology. Medical sociology may no longer be regarded as a fad; the earlier courtship between the behavioral sciences and medicine is now a marriage with the honeymoon over.

The pressing need for a revised edition of this volume became obvious in light of these changes and advancements in medical sociology and behavioral science. Only two articles appearing in the first edition will be found in this revised edition, although several names are again represented either with revisions of their original chapters or with more recent contributions. The basic task of compiling this new edition changed from that of the first edition in having now to choose among so many excellent papers available. Consequently, many worthy studies and their talented authors could not be included within the space allotted to the new edition, much to our sincere regret.

This new edition has also been reorganized into what is hoped will be a more systematic and logical arrangement of the contents. Three major parts are presented. First, the existence of disease in human society as indicated by patterns of morbidity and mortality is presented as a contribution to the social epidemiology of illness and, it is hoped in time, to the social etiology of morbidity and disability.

Second, articles are included that deal with societal efforts to cope with illness and injury as reflected in health and illness behavior, the sick role and the patient role, and community responses. Part II comprises the largest section of this volume. Its emphasis is primarily on caring for the sick—the patient role, healers and healing practices, and health and the human community, all viewed as efforts to cope with the impact of disease and disability.

The third and final part is a major addition, dealing with society and the administration of health care facilities and services, including some current issues involving proposed changes in the health care system, a topic receiving increasing attention from social and behavioral scientists. Articles are presented on societal and community efforts to organize and manage health care services and on problems related to maintaining the total health care "system" in society. Many of these studies have implications for the development of public policy toward health care. Some current issues are examined to stimulate the discussion and further inquiry needed to evaluate the contemporary health care scene where improvements if not outright innovations may be indicated.

Nearly 40 per cent of the contents of this new edition are original articles and to their authors I give special thanks. The contributors and publishers of the other articles are also due our deepest thanks for kindly permitting their inclusion in this volume. We have shared a common goal to better understand disease and disability in their social and behavioral contexts. It is my hope that some of this knowledge will be communicated to the reader of this new edition, who may thus also share the enthusiasm, vitality, and excitement of these explorers into new arenas of knowledge that in turn may benefit all mankind.

E. GARTLY JACO
University of California, Riverside

The Contributors

Odin W. Anderson, Center for Health Administration Studies, University of Chicago.

Aaron Antonovsky, Israel Institute of Applied Social Research, Jerusalem.

Jay W. Artis, Department of Sociology, Michigan State University.

Barbara O. Baumann, Hunter College.

John Colombotos, School of Public Health & Administrative Medicine, Columbia University.

Ray H. Elling, Department of Medicine, University of Connecticut Health Center, Hartford.

Mark G. Field, Russian Research Center, Harvard University.

Walter E. Freeman, Division of Community Development, Pennsylvania State University.

Eliot Freidson, Department of Sociology, New York University.

Basil S. Georgopoulos, Institute for Social Research, University of Michigan.

Barney G. Glaser, San Francisco Medical Center, University of California.

Saxon Graham, Department of Sociology, State University of New York at Buffalo.

Robert M. Gray, Chief, Division of Behavioral Science, Department of Preventive Medicine, University of Utah Medical Center.

Elliott H. Grosof, Department of Sociology, State University of New York at Buffalo.

Llewellyn Gross, Department of Sociology, State University of New York at Buffalo.

Robert G. Holloway, Hospital Research Division, Industrial Relations Center, University of Chicago.

E. Gartly Jaco, Department of Sociology, University of California, Riverside.

Howard B. Kaplan, Department of Psychiatry, Baylor College of Medicine, Texas Medical Center.

Gene G. Kassebaum, Department of Sociology, University of Hawaii.

Ollie J. Lee, Department of Sociology, Lee College, Cleveland, Tennessee.

Sol Levine, Chairman, Department of Behavioral Science, School of Hygiene & Public Health, John Hopkins University.

Theodor J. Litman, Program in Hospital Administration, School of Public Health, and Department of Sociology, University of Minnesota.

Floyd C. Mann, Center for Research on Utilization of Scientific Knowledge, Institute for Social Research, University of Michigan.

Hans O. Mauksch, Department of Community Health & Medical Practice, School of Medicine, University of Missouri.

David Mechanic, Department of Sociology, University of Wisconsin.

Nahum Z. Medalia, Department of Sociology–Anthropology, Oakland University, Rochester, Michigan.

Jane R. Mercer, Department of Sociology, University of California, Riverside.

Philip M. Moody, Department of Behavioral Science, University of Kentucky Medical Center.

Talcott Parsons, Department of Social Relations, Harvard University.

Leo G. Reeder, School of Public Health, Center for the Health Sciences, University of California, Los Angeles.

William C. Richardson, Program in Hospital Administration, University of Washington.

Sam Schulman, Department of Sociology, University of Houston.

John D. Stoeckle, The Clinics, Massachusetts General Hospital, Boston.

Anselm L. Strauss, Graduate Program in Sociology, San Francisco Medical Center, University of California.

Edward A. Suchman, Graduate School of Public Health and Department of Sociology, University of Pittsburgh (deceased).

Daisy L. Tagliacozzo, Department of Sociology, Illinois Institute of Technology.

Albert F. Wessen, Department of Sociology, Brown University.

Paul E. White, Department of Behavioral Science, School of Hygiene & Public Health, Johns Hopkins University.

Constantine A. Yeracaris, Department of Sociology, State University of New York at Buffalo.

Irving K. Zola, Department of Sociology, Brandeis University.

Patients,
Physicians
and Illness

Society and Disease

THE EXISTENCE of disease, injury, and death is a universal fact of life in every human society; no society or individual is free from these conditions. What is perhaps not so well known or so widely recognized is the growing evidence that these unfortunate events do not necessarily occur by chance or randomly within human populations, groups, and societies. Increasingly, more studies are detecting certain uniformities and patterns of rates of illness (morbidity) and death (mortality) in specific populations and segments of society and social structures.

Social epidemiology, the study of the existence of disease and its possible causes in terms of social factors, is becoming an increasingly significant specialty in the traditionally important field of public health for which the medical sociologist, psychologist, and anthropologist are particularly prepared. The social and behavioral scientist's knowledge of differential modes of living, life styles, value systems, attitude sets, socialization processes, institutionalized ways of behaving, perceiving and coping with divergent demands in living, social interaction patterns and processes, normative components of social life, the enormous diversity in human behavior and personality, and the variability and pliability of human nature and conduct, to mention only a few factors of his subject matter, provide him with the analytic tools, perspective, and orientation forming a special expertise whose value to traditional medical epidemiology has only recently been recognized. Behavioral scientists are increasingly becoming full-fledged members of epidemiologic research teams and related endeavours, and they are making increasingly significant contributions to epidemiologic knowledge of disease and injury.

The determination of specified rates of disease for specific social components and groups of society contributes directly to *descriptive* social epidemiology, following MacMahon, Pugh, and Ipsen's definition.[1] Certain social groups of society—such as social classes, ethnic or racial groups, urban residents, rural residents, single persons, socially mobile persons, and the like—have been

[1]MacMahon, B., T. F. Pugh, and J. Ipsen, *Epidemiologic Methods.* Boston: Little, Brown & Co., 1960, Chapter 4.

found to have divergent rates of specific diseases or morbidity. An assessment of these results may well lead to the construction of hypotheses about potential social and behavioral etiology. The appropriate testing of hypotheses derived from descriptive epidemiological findings leads to the next stage of *analytic* social epidemiology and, if indicated, to *experimental* epidemiologic studies under highly controlled research conditions.

Admittedly, the bulk of social epidemiologic research to date has been largely confined to the more elementary, descriptive levels of determining morbidity in terms of social conditions, but it is a necessary first step in the long and tedious quest for specific social etiologic factors in disease. Some investigators have questioned the applicability of the traditional medical model of disease to social causation, suggesting other conceptual and empirical models as more appropriate to social causation. Whether or not social and behavioral conditions of human life will ever be fully determined as sufficient or necessary, primary or secondary, immediate or proximal, indogenous or exogenous causes of specific diseases in terms of medical or non-medical models is still a moot question.

Nevertheless, as the articles in this part represent, a small but definite beginning has been made in relating social factors to many forms of morbidity and mortality. These chapters are only a small portion of the many studies being conducted by social and behavioral scientists, but they illustrate the scope and variety of the inquiries that have established the validity and significance of the emerging specialty of social epidemiology, supplementing similar efforts from the more traditional epidemiologic areas of the biological, health, and medical disciplines.

The articles in this first part suggest the wide array of epidemiologic knowledge being contributed by behavioral scientists to a better understanding of the sociologic aspects of mortality and morbidity. An extensive survey and evaluation of social factors related to mortality is presented in the first chapter by Aaron Antonovsky, presenting widespread evidence of the relationship between differential social conditions and death rates.

A variety of studies relating social factors to specific aspects of morbidity or illness are presented in the next set of papers. Saxon Graham's penetrating analysis of certain types of cancer and their relation to cultural groups promises much future study of the social epidemiology of these major chronic diseases.

An area that until recently has received comparatively little attention is the relationship between pollution of the environment, especially the atmosphere, and social conditions. The chapter by Nahum Medalia, suggests the potentially significant contribution behavioral science can make to environmental health.

A unique and significantly new approach to the analysis of mild mental retardation by Jane Mercer is the product of extensive sociological research and may well supplant the more traditional medical and biostatistical perspectives on this little understood condition.

A new field may be emerging that could be tentatively termed *social physiology*. It may be regarded as a "basic science" approach to comprehending the basic connections between physiologic, bodily functioning or bio-processes and social interaction, as presented in the original article by Howard Kaplan. Rather than focus on pathologic conditions, Kaplan's studies demonstrate the linkages between so-called "normal" bodily or neuro-physiologic functions and types of social interaction in experimental groups of normal subjects. They are suggestive of considerable future potential research and theoretical formulations.

An appraisal of contemporary social epidemiologic research and some suggestions for the future in this emerging field are presented in an original contribution by Leo Reeder, which completes this first part.

. . . recalling what happened when an "unsinkable" trans-Atlantic luxury liner, the *Titanic*, rammed an iceberg on her maiden voyage in 1912. . . . The official casualty lists showed that only 4 first class female passengers (3 voluntarily chose to stay on the ship) of a total of 143 were lost. Among the second class passengers, 15 of 93 females drowned; and among the third class, 81 of 179 female passengers went down with the ship.[1]

1

Social Class, Life Expectancy and Overall Mortality

Aaron Antonovsky

DEATH IS THE FINAL LOT of all living beings. But, as the tragic experience of the *Titanic* passengers dramatically illustrates, the time at which one dies is related to one's class. The intent of this paper is to examine the evidence which bears upon the closeness of this relationship, ranging as far back as the data will allow. It will first focus on the question of life expectancy at birth, and subsequently turn to that of overall mortality.

Studies of Life Expectancy

The average infant born today in the Western world can look forward, barring unforeseen events and radical changes in present trends, to a life span of about 70 years. That this has not always been the case for the human infant—and still is not for by far most infants born today—is well known. Whatever the situation prior to the era of recorded history, for the greater part of this era, that is, until the nineteenth century, most men lived out less than half their Biblical span of years.

In what is probably the first study of a total population, Halley, using data for the city of Breslau, Germany, for 1687 to 1691, calculated an average life expectancy at birth of 33.5 years.[2] Henry's estimate for the expectation of life of Parisian children born at the beginning of the eighteenth century

was 23.5 years.[3] Half a century later, in the Vienna of 1752 to 1755, of every 1,000 infants born alive, only 590 survived their first year, 413 their fifth year, and 359 their fifteenth year.[4] Henry further cites an estimate, which he regards as "too pessimistic," of 28.8 years for the total French population toward the end of the Ancien Regime.[5]

In the nineteenth century, Villerme, in a careful first-hand study, reported a life expectancy at birth for the total population of the city of Mulhouse, France, of seven years and six months, based on the period 1823 to 1834. However, he also cites Penot's data for Mulhouse, from 1812 to 1827, which show an average life expectancy of 25 years.[6] Ansell found a life expectation at birth for the total British population in 1874 of about 43 years.[7] At about the same time, the reported figures for Italy were somewhat

[1] Hollingshead, A. B. and F. C. Redlich, *Social Class and Mental Illness*, New York: John Wiley, 1958, p. 6, citing W. Lord, *A Night to Remember*, New York: Henry Holt, 1955, p. 107.

[2] Cited in L. I. Dublin, A. J. Lotka and M. Spiegelman, *Length of Life*, rev. ed. New York: Ronald Press, 1949, pp. 34, 30–43. The book as a whole is one of the most detailed treatments of the subject of life expectancy.

[3] Henry, L. "The Population of France in the 18th Century," in D. V. Glass and D. E. C. Eversley (eds.), *Population in History*, London: Edward Arnold, 1965, p. 444.

[4] Peller, S., "Births and Deaths Among Europe's Ruling Families Since 1500," in Glass and Eversley, *op. cit.*, p. 94.

[5] Henry, *op. cit.*, pp. 445–446.

[6] Villerme, L. R., *Tableau de L'Etat Physique et Moral des Ouvriers*, vol. 2, Paris, Jules Renouard et Cie., 1840, pp. 249, 376–385.

[7] Ansell, C., "Vital Statistics of Families in the Upper and Professional Classes," *J. Royal Stat. Soc.*, 37:464, 1874, cited in R. Titmuss, *Birth, Poverty and Wealth*, London: Hamish Hamilton Medical Books, 1943, p. 19.

From *Milbank Memorial Fund Quarterly, Vol. 45: 31–73, April, 1967; by permission of the author and publisher.*

lower: 35 years (1871 to 1880); 36.2 years for males, 35.65 years for females (1881–1882).[8]

Whatever the discrepancies and unreliabilities of these various sets of data, they

A somewhat similar study, covering 1,908 individuals born between 1330 and 1954 as legitimate offspring of British kings, queens, dukes or duchesses, shows a corresponding increase in the eighteenth century, as can be seen in the following data:[11]

EXPECTATION OF LIFE AT BIRTH (YEARS)

Period of Birth	Males	Females
1330–1479	24	33
1480–1679	27	33
1680–1729	33	34
1730–1779	45	48
1780–1829	48	55
1830–1879	50	62
1880–1954	55	70

consistently paint a picture of the Western world up to recent centuries which is quite similar to that of the world of presently "developing" societies until the last decade or two. Moreover, in the period of recorded history prior to the eighteenth century, no sizable increment had been added to the average life span. But if, from Greco–Roman times through the eighteenth or perhaps even the nineteenth century, the mythical "average" infant could anticipate living some 20 to 30 years, does any evidence indicate that dramatic class differences existed? Though the evidence is perforce limited, the answer would seem to be no.

Two studies of male property owners in England of the generation born before 1276, and of a population born between 1426 and 1450, show average lengths of life being 35.3 and 33 years, respectively. Dublin, *et al.*, who report these studies, also cite a study by Peller of men in the "ruling classes of Europe" from 1480 to 1579 in which a life span of 30 years is given as the average.[9] In Peller's paper, the average life expectancy of males at birth in a population of "Europe's ruling families," which included a total of 8,500 individuals, was 32.2 years in the sixteenth century, declined to 28.1 in the seventeenth century, rose considerably to 36.1 in the next century and, from 1800 to 1885 was 45.8 years. (In each case the female figure was higher.)[10]

[8] Cipolla, C. M., "Four Centuries of Italian Demographic Development," in Glass and Eversley, *op. cit.*, pp. 578, 582.

[9] Dublin, Lotka and Spiegelman, *op. cit.*, pp. 31–32.

[10] Peller, *op. cit.*, p. 95.

At the opposite end of the social scale, the reported life expectancy at birth for a British Guiana slave population between 1820 and 1832 was 22.8 years.[12] A reasonable assumption, keeping in mind that the life expectancy at birth of countries such as India, Burma and Cambodia in the late 1950's ranged from 35 to 44 years,[13] is that class differences prior to the eighteenth century were relatively limited. In other words, given a society which, though it manages to survive, does so at or near what might be called a rock-bottom level of life expectancy, one is not likely to find great differences among the strata of that society.

The data suggest the possibility that the trend in the nineteenth century, and perhaps even earlier, was toward a substantial widening of class differences. No report is available comparing the life expectancies of social strata of the population prior to the nineteenth century. Titmuss quotes Milne as saying, in 1815, that "There can . . . be no doubt but that the mortality is greater among the higher than the middle classes of society."[14] Villerme's study of Mulhouse, which was based on an analysis of the

[11] Hollingsworth, T. H., "A Demographic Study of the British Ducal Families," in Glass and Eversley, *op. cit.*, p. 358.

[12] Roberts, G. W., "A Life Table for a West Indian Slave Population," *Pop. Stud.*, 5:242, March, 1952.

[13] United Nations Department of Economic and Social Affairs, *1963 Report on the World Social Situation*, New York, United Nations, 1963, p. 13.

[14] From Milne's *Treatise on Annuities*, quote in Titmuss, *op. cit.*, p. 17.

occupation of the head of household of 5,419 deceased out of a total of 6,085 registered deaths from 1823 to 1834, shows a life expectancy at birth which ranges from 28.2 years for "manufacturers, merchants, directors, etc." through 17.6 years for "factory workers, unspecified" and 9.4 years for day laborers, to 1.3–1.9 years for spinners, weavers and locksmiths. (Consideration of the life expectancy at age one of the same occupations indicates far smaller occupational differences.) Villerme concludes that "One sees here that most infants reach adulthood or die at a young age depending upon the condition or occupation to which they belong. . . ."[15] At about the same time (1832), an observer of the British scene remarked that members of the peerage had a lower expectation of life than the general population.[16]

Morris cites Gavin's analysis of the average age at death of 1,632 deceased in Bethnal Green (a suburb of London) in 1839 by social strata. "Gentlemen, professional men and their families" died, on the average, at age 45; "tradesmen and their families," at age 26; and "mechanics, servants, laborers and their families," at age 16. Very similar data are quoted by Titmuss for the years 1839 to 1841 for the city of York. For near-identical social groups, the average ages at death were: 48.6, 30.8 and 23.8. Morris also refers to Clay's report for the 1840's on chances of survival in the town of Preston, Lancashire, among 1,000 infants born into each of the families of gentry, tradesmen and operatives. Among the gentry, not until well past the fortieth year did more than one-half of those infants die. The average infant of families of tradesmen survived until just past his twentieth year. Among operatives' families, however, more than half of those born had died by their fifth year. Titmuss also reports, for this period, that a "gentleman" in London lived, on the average, twice as long as a "laborer." The corresponding figures for Leeds were 44 and 19 years, and for Liverpool 35 and 15.[17]

15 Villerme, op. cit., pp. 251, 376–385.
16 Farren, Observations on the Mortality Among the Members of the British Peerage, cited in Titmuss, op. cit., p. 17.
17 Morris, J. N., Uses of Epidemiology, 2d ed., Edinburgh and London: E. and S. Livingstone, 1964, pp. 161–162; Titmuss, op. cit., p. 18.

A study by Bailey and Day, published in 1861, is referred to in the same context by Titmuss, though their data are not cited. Collins, however, does cite the data, which show a narrower gap than the aforementioned studies. Bailey and Day studied the life tables of 7,743 members of families of British peers from 1800 to 1855, and compared them with deaths in the total population from 1838 to 1844. The mean duration of life for the two groups was 52 and 40.4 years, respectively.[18]

A further cautionary note on the class gap is sounded by William Farr, the great pioneer of English mortality statistics. In his discussion of the life expectancy of laborers employed by the East India Company compared with that of English peers over the course of centuries, using data for the latter published by Edmonds in 1838, Farr notes little difference in annual average mortality between the two groups, especially after age 50. "Are we," Farr comments, "to infer that the mortality among peers is now higher than among laborers, crowded within the metropolis? Should we not rather infer, that as the investigation extends far back into the centuries of bloodshed and pestilence, that the lives of peers were then shorter, and are now longer, than the lives of laborers? The plague, which was born in huts, and nursed by famine, rioted in luxurious halls, and smote the highborn."[19]

In the same cautionary direction, Ansell found that "the expectation of life at birth in the upper and professional classes was 53

18 Bailey, A. H. and A. Day, "On the Rate of Mortality Prevailing Amongst the Families of the Peerage During the 19th Century," J. Inst. Actuaries, 9: 305; cited in S. D. Collins, Economic Status and Health, Washington, U.S. Government Printing Office, 1927, p. 14.
19 Farr, W., Vital Statistics: A Memorial Volume of Selections from the Reports and Writings of William Farr, N. A. Humphreys (ed.), London, The Sanitary Institute, 1885, pp. 393–394. Also cited in Titmuss, op. cit., pp. 17–18. Titmuss notes that even when Farr excluded from the peer's mortality those deaths due to violence, the laborers had the lower mortality.

Table 1-1—Life expectancy at birth for selected populations, by sex and social class, in the twentieth century[21]

Population, Place and Time	I (Highest)	II	CLASS* III	IV	V (Lowest)	Differences between I and V (Years)
England and Wales, 1930–1932 All Males	63.1	60.8	60.0	57.3	55.7	7.4
Chicago, 1920 All Males	60.6	—	—	—	49.6	11.0
Chicago, 1930 All Males	63.0	—	—	—	49.5	13.5
White Males	63.0	—	—	—	51.3	11.7
Chicago, 1935 All Males	60.9	—	—	—	53.5	7.4
Chicago, 1940 All Males	65.4	—	—	—	56.5	8.9
White Males	65.4	—	—	—	57.8	7.6
Buffalo, 1939–1941 All Males	65.7	65.5	63.4	62.2	58.2	7.5
Baltimore, 1949–1951 White Males	68.5	66.4	65.4	63.9	61.4	7.1
Chicago, 1920 All Females	62.9	—	—	—	52.5	10.4
Chicago, 1930 All Females	67.1	—	—	—	54.5	12.6
White Females	67.1	—	—	—	56.2	10.9
Chicago, 1935 All Females	66.6	—	—	—	58.3	8.3
Chicago, 1940 All Females	70.3	—	—	—	61.0	9.3
White Females	70.3	—	—	—	62.7	7.6
Buffalo, 1939–1941 All Females	69.6	68.3	66.4	64.8	61.8	7.8
Baltimore, 1949–1951 White Females	73.1	72.4	71.2	69.8	68.4	4.7

* "Class" in the British data refers to the Registrar General's system of classification based on occupation, into which Tietze introduced a number of modifications. In the three American cities, "class" refers to the division of the city census tracts into quintiles based on the median rental in each tract.

years indicating an advantage of about 10 years over the expectation for the general population [in 1874]."[20]

Very few later investigators have dealt with class differences in life expectancy, preferring to concentrate on differences in mortality rates. A search of the literature has revealed only four such studies, whose data are presented in Table 1-1. The published data for Chicago refer only to the two extreme groups of census tracts with the highest and lowest median rentals. Because, after World War I, Chicago witnessed a tremend-

[20] Ansell, C., cited in Titmuss, *op. cit.*, p. 19.

ous influx of Negroes, most of whom were lower class, the available data for whites only has also been presented. From 1920 to 1940, the difference between the extreme groups seesawed, but did decline to a difference in life expectancy for whites, in both sexes, of 7.6 years. In England and Wales of about 1930, a direct gradient between class and life expectancy of males is evident, the extreme groups being separated by 7.4 years. Just about the same number of years separates the highest and lowest groups in Buffalo in 1939–1941. Although this is also true for white males in Baltimore in 1949–1951, the difference among white females in that city is only 4.7 years. In both cities, the direct gradient is clear.[21]

Can any conclusion be drawn from these data, most of which are admittedly tenuous and not overly reliable? A crude picture, as represented in Figure 1-1, could be inferred

FIGURE 1-1 *Model of class differences in life expectancy at birth in various populations*

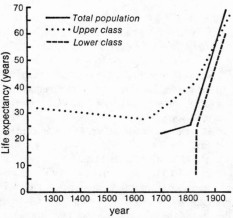

Data are derived from specific studies cited in the text and are plotted at the mid-year of each time period. The values for the last five years for the total United States population are from *The Facts of Life and Death*, Public Health Service publication no. 600, revised 1955, p. 21.

which indicates the following. The bulk of recorded history was one of high birth and high death rates, which offset each other and led to at most a very small increase in population. During the first 16 centuries of the Christian era, world population increased from about one-quarter to one-half billion people, an annual growth rate of about 0.005 per cent. Conceivably, throughout this period,

no substantial differentials in life expectancy could be found among different social strata of the population. From 1650 to 1850 world population again jumped, most of the increase being in the Western world, representing an average annual increase of 0.05 per cent. These two centuries would seem to mark the emergence of an increasing class gap in life expectancy, starting slowly but gathering increasing momentum and reaching its peak about the time Malthus made his observations. On the one hand, the life expectancy of the middle and upper strata of the population increased at a rapid rate. On the other, the lowest strata's life expectancy may have increased much more slowly or, conceivably, even declined as an industrial proletariat emerged. At some time during the nineteenth century, probably in the latter half, this trend was reversed, and the class gap began to diminish. This is reflected in the doubling of the world's population, again mostly in the West, this time in the 80 years from 1850 to 1930. In recent decades, the class gap has narrowed to what may be the smallest differential in history, but evidence of a linear gradient remains, with a considerable differential, given man's life span.

This supposition—not claimed to be more than that, since Figure 1-1 is no more than a very crude representation—seems to be of more than historical interest. It is, for two important reasons, most germane to the concern of this paper. In the first place, the scientist, no less than the lay person, often seems, in considering the question of the relationship between class and health, to be beset by a nineteenth century notion of perpetual progress. Ideologically committed in this area to the desirability of the disappearance of the class gap, he tends to assume, with or without data, that the historical picture is unilinear; the history of mankind, in his view, shows steady progress in this respect. The realization that this may well be an inaccurate image, that the relationship is more complex, suggests a more cautious orientation. Such an orientation would suggest various possibilities: a narrow-

[21] Mayer, A. J. and P. Hauser, "Class Differentiations in Expectation of Life at Birth," in R. Bendix and S. M. Lipset (eds.), *Class, Status and Power*, New York: Free Press, 1953, pp. 281–284; Tietze, C., "Life Tables for Social Classes in England," *Milbank Memorial Fund Quarterly*, 21: 182–187, April, 1943; C. A. Yeracaris, "Differential Mortality, General and Cause-Specific, in Buffalo, 1939–1941, *J. Amer. Stat. Assoc.*, 50: 1235–1247, December, 1955; M. Tayback, "The Relationship of Socioeconomic Status and Expectation of Life," *Baltimore Health News*, 34: 139–144, April, 1957.

ing gap being transformed into one which is widening; differing positions, on any given index of health, of different strata of the population at various times.

The second reason for stressing the possibility of a curvilinear relationship between class and life expectancy over time is that such a relationship may help in forming an adequate idea of the relationship between class and health, and, more broadly, an adequate theory of disease. Once the search begins for explanations of why, in a given period, one stratum seems to be making more health progress than another, and less so in another period, factors are uncovered which must be integrated into a theory of disease.

Thus, for example, McKeown and Brown, arguing that the increase in the population of England in the eighteenth century was overwhelmingly due to the decline in mortality, attribute that decline to improvements in the environment (housing, water supply, refuse disposal, nutrition) rather than to any advances in medical care.[22] Supposedly, such improvements first appeared in the upper strata of society, and only slowly percolated downward. This would explain the increasing class differences

in life expectancy. Once the environmental sanitation gap began to narrow, some reversal in the trend could be expected which, however, might soon be offset by other factors; e.g., the malnutrition of poverty. The point is that a very careful collection of data over time and the search for ups and downs may serve to pinpoint the various factors, and their modes of interaction, which influence overall mortality or the course of any specific disease.

Class Differences in Mortality before World War II

Twentieth century investigators have by and large focused on class differences in mortality rates. Chapin's study of Providence, Rhode Island, probably provides the earliest relevant information.[23] Using census and tax records of 1865, he located all but about 200 of the 2,000 taxpayers, covering a total of 10,515 individuals. Every deceased person in that year was assigned to either the taxpayer or non-taxpayer group. Chapin then calculated the death rates per thousand in each group. The crude annual death rate of the latter (24.8 per 1,000 living) was more than double that of the taxpayers (10.8). As seen in Table 1–2, this disparity is

Table 1–2—Annual death rates, taxpayers and non-taxpayers, Providence, Rhode Island, 1865[23]

Ages	DEATH RATES PER 1,000 Taxpayers	Non-taxpayers	Ratio of Taxpayers' to Non-taxpayers' Rates*
All Ages	10.8	24.8	230
Under 1	93.4	189.8	203
1 to 4	40.3	66.6	165
Under 5	50.5	94.0	186
5 to 9	15.9	15.7	99
10 to 19	3.0	8.2	273
20 to 29	6.0	11.8	197
30 to 39	4.5	15.5	344
40 to 49	1.4	14.5	1036
50 to 59	8.6	25.1	292
60 to 69	15.1	39.5	262
70 and Over	32.9	138.5	421
Population Size	10,515	44,080	
Number of Deaths	114	1,097	

* Taxpayers' rates = 100.

22 McKeown, T. and R. G. Brown, "Medical Evidence Related to English Population Changes in the Eighteenth Century," *Pop. Studies*, 9: 119–241, 1955 (reprinted in Glass and Eversley, *op. cit.*, pp. 285–307).

23 Chapin, C. V., "Deaths Among Taxpayers and Non–Taxpayers, Income Tax, Providence, 1865," in *Papers of Charles V. Chapin*, New York, Commonwealth Fund, 1934, pp. 217–228. (First published in *Amer. J. Pub. Health*, 14: 647–651, August, 1924.)

found in all but the five- to nine-years age cohort, and is greatest in the productive years (30 to 49) and in the 70 and over cohort. Since the non-taxpayer group includes more than 80 per cent of the population, had Chapin been able to make a finer class breakdown he presumably would have found even greater differences between the top and bottom strata.

Collins, in an early review of socio-economic mortality data, cites an 1887 paper by Humphreys on mortality in Dublin in 1883–1885, which shows a higher mortality among the poor, but presents no data. The earliest data presented by Collins refer to Danish mortality rates from 1865 to 1874, the 1870 census having been used to obtain denominator information.[24] Individuals were assigned to high, middle or poor classes on the basis of the head of household's occupation. The top category includes capitalists, professionals, wholesale dealers and higher officers. The middle group contains master mechanics, petty officers, teachers, clerks and small shopkeepers. The poor class is made up of workmen, servants and those in almshouses. The age-adjusted mean annual death rates, by sex, of the population aged 20 and over in Copenhagen and in other towns, is shown in Table 1–3. The data show that class differences are greater in Copenhagen than in provincial towns, and greater among males than among

and middle classes are relatively small compared to the gap between them and the poor class. The rates are based on 21,000 deaths in Copenhagen and 22,000 deaths in the other towns.

The first of many ecological studies was Rowntree's well-known survey of York, England, in 1899.[25] Rowntree divided the wage-earner areas of the city of York into three levels. The overall death rates per thousand persons (not age-standardized) he reports for 1899 are: highest, 13.5; middle, 20.7; poorest, 27.8 (ratios of 100:153:206). In this case, unlike the earlier Danish data, the inverse gradient is quite regular.

In a paper focusing on later data, Britten calculates overall death rates for 1900 in the nine states and the District of Columbia, which then comprised the death registration area.[26] He compared white-collar rates to those for the "laboring and servant" class in three age groups. Taking the white-collar death rate as 100, the ratios for the lower class group were: for ages 15–24, 151; for ages 25–44, 165; and for ages 45–64, 159.

As a prologue to her analysis of 1950 death rates, Guralnick presents, without analysis, the full set of data upon which Britten evidently based his calculations, as well as

Table 1–3—Mean annual death rates per thousand persons, age 20 and over, Denmark, 1865–1874, by sex and residence (age-adjusted) [24]

| Class | COPENHAGEN | | OTHER TOWNS | |
	Rate	Ratio	Rate	Ratio*
Males				
High	16.5	100	13.4	100
Middle	20.2	122	17.1	128
Poor	31.2	189	22.6	169
Females				
High	13.4	100	12.4	100
Middle	12.3	92	14.1	114
Poor	22.3	166	16.5	133

* High class rate in each group = 100.

females. More significantly, although the rates show primarily an inverse class gradient, the differences between the high

24 Collins, op. cit., p. 13.

25 Rowntree, S. B., Poverty and Progress: A Second Social Survey of York, London: Longmans, Green, 1941, p. 296.

26 Britten, R. H., "Mortality Rates by Occupational Class in the U.S.," Pub. Health Rep. 49: 1102, September, 1934.

similar data for 1890.[27] Table 1-4 presents the relevant data for mortality among roughly ranked occupational groups. For the employed male population as a whole, in both years, professionals have a somewhat higher mortality rate than do other white collar workers or those in industry, most of whom are presumably manual workers. Conceivably this may be explained by the fact that the rates are not age-standardized, and professionals might be an older group.

groups. In both 1890 and 1900, the ratio of this class is highest in ages 25–44 and 45–64, somewhat lower at ages 15–24, and lowest— though still relatively high—in the 65 and over category. An interesting pattern is shown by the clerical and official group: in the youngest age category its ratio is quite high, in 1900 approaching that of the lowest class; in each successive age category its ratio goes down, so that in the 65 and over category it has by far the lowest mortality rate.

Szabady,[28] reporting the data (non-age-

Table 1-4—Annual death rates per 1,000, and ratios, males, by age and major occupation group, United States, 1890 and 1900[27]

Major Occupation Group	ALL AGES Rate	ALL AGES Ratio**	15–24 Rate	15–24 Ratio	25–44 Rate	25–44 Ratio	45–64 Rate	45–64 Ratio	65 AND OVER Rate	65 AND OVER Ratio
1890										
Males in Specified Occupations*	13.8	100	5.6	100	9.3	100	18.4	100	70.1	100
Professionals	15.7	113	5.0	90	8.5	91	19.1	104	79.3	113
Mercantile and Trading	12.2	88	3.5	63	7.4	80	17.1	93	73.6	105
Clerical, Official	9.8	71	6.2	110	9.2	98	13.6	74	38.5	55
Manufacturing and Mechanical Industries	13.0	94	5.0	90	9.2	99	20.1	109	77.7	111
Laboring and Servant	22.6	163	9.7	174	17.0	182	33.2	180	114.9	164
1900										
All occupations	15.0	100	5.1	100	8.8	100	19.9	100	98.4	100
Professionals	15.3	102	4.8	94	7.6	86	20.7	104	105.6	107
Mercantile and Trading	12.1	81	2.6	51	6.7	76	19.9	100	93.8	95
Clerical, Official	13.5	90	7.2	141	11.1	126	19.9	100	55.9	57
Manufacturing and Mechanical Industries	13.8	92	4.4	86	8.4	95	20.2	102	105.4	107
Laboring and Servant	20.2	135	7.7	151	13.9	158	31.9	160	126.6	129

* Guralnick presents data for "all males" and for eight occupational categories. Only the five which can be reasonably ranked are selected here, though ratios are calculated on the basis of all eight categories.
** Rate for all occupations in each age category = 100.

The age-specific rates do show professionals as having a lower than average rate in the younger age groups and somewhat above average in the higher groups. The most striking fact about these data is the very sizable difference, at all ages, between the "laboring and servant" class and all other

[27] Guralnick, L., "Mortality by Occupation and Industry Among Men 20 to 64 Years of Age, U.S., 1950," *Vital Statistics, Special Reports*, 53: 56, September, 1962.

[28] Szabady, E., "Recent Changes in the Socio–Economic Factors of Hungary's Mortality," in *International Population Conference, Ottawa, 1963*, Liege, International Union for the Scientific Study of Population, 1964, p. 401. Szabady's paper presents mortality data for each decade from 1900 to 1960. Several other studies likewise give sets of data over periods of time. The present paper will disregard the within-study trend analysis, presenting the relevant data from all the studies consecutively. A separate section will be devoted to consideration of the trends over time within specific populations.

standardized) for the total population of pre-World War I Hungary, divides the non-agricultural population into non-manual and manual groups. For all persons, the death rates per thousand in 1900 were, respectively, 15.1 and 25.1; in 1910, the gap had narrowed, with both rates having fallen to 13.8 and 20.9. That differences in infant mortality contributed considerably to class differences in overall mortality is shown by considering only the rates of earners. In 1900, the non-manual death rate was 13.6, compared to 17.5 for manual earners. By 1910, the difference had nearly disappeared, the rates being 15.0 and 15.9 per thousand.

Huber[29] examined occupational mortality in France for 1907–1908, calculating death rates on the basis of the 1906 census. His figures are primarily for individual occupations, but he does give age-specific death rates for four broad groups, which are presented in Table 1–5. Managers and officials consistently show the lowest rates.

In another ecological study, Martin[31] calculated the correlations of the age-standardized mortality rates of the 28 boroughs of London in 1911–1912, with two measures of dwelling density: the percentage of population living in dwellings with two or more persons per room, and the average number of persons per room. The correlations were, respectively, 0.89 and 0.93. No change took place by the next decade (the correlations were 0.92 and 0.91). In 1920–1922, however, a third measure reflecting class was used—the percentage of the labor force in the Registrar General's classes IV and V—whose correlation with mortality was, though highly significant, much lower (0.69).

In a relatively early review of morbidity and mortality data, Sydenstricker, one of

Table 1–5—Age-specific annual death rates per 1,000 and ratios, by occupational groups, males, France, 1907–1908[29]

Age Group	MANAGERS, OFFICIALS		CLERKS		CRAFTSMEN, KINDRED WORKERS		PRIVATE HOUSEHOLD WORKERS	
	Rate	Ratio*	Rate	Ratio	Rate	Ratio	Rate	Ratio
25–34	6.4	100	8.8	138	8.2	128	7.2	112
35–44	8.2	100	12.0	146	13.6	166	9.6	117
45–54	12.7	100	20.3	160	23.2	183	16.2	128
55–64	24.4	100	40.0	164	42.3	173	32.1	132

* Rate of managers, officials in each age group = 100.

Clerical workers have, at ages 25–34, the highest rates, but thereafter craftsmen and kindred workers have higher rates. The rates of these two groups are, throughout, closer to each other than to those of the managerial group. Class differentials are greatest at ages 45–54. Private household workers, presumably a low status group, have relatively low rates. Since the data refer only to males, who presumably served primarily in well-to-do households, such rates need not be inexplicable.

[29] Huber, M., *Bulletin Statistique General de la France*, fasc IV, 1912, quoted in Daric, J. "Mortality, Occupation, and Socio–Economic Status," *Vital Statistics, Special Reports*, 33, 175–187, September, 1951.

[30] Collins, *op. cit.*, p. 14.

the pioneers in the field, cites Bruno's study of 22,600 deaths among 1.3 million wage-earners in 1915–1916, with life insurance in 12 American companies, showing a clear inverse occupational gradient.[32] The death rates per 1,000 policyholders were: professional and semiprofessionals, 3.3; skilled workmen, 3.7; semiskilled workmen, 4.5; unskilled workmen, 4.8. Using the rate of

[31] Martin, W. J., "Vital Statistics of the County of London in the Years 1901 to 1951," *British J. Prev. and Soc. Med.*, 9: 130, July, 1955.

[32] Bruno, F. J., "Illness and Dependency," *Miscellaneous Contributions*, no. 9. The Committee on the Costs of Medical Care, Washington, 1931, cited in E. Sydenstricker, *Health and Environment*, New York: McGraw-Hill, 1933, p. 94.

the professional class as 100, the ratios of the other three were 112, 136 and 145.

Dublin[33] reported the results of a similar series of studies of policyholders with the Metropolitan Life Insurance Company. He divided the population into those holding "industrial" policies and those with "ordinary" life insurance policies. Though the former are taken as representative of "the urban wage-earning population," an undue

the first of these studies, covering 1911 to 1913, no comparative data are presented for the two populations, though the "industrial" death rates are compared to those of the total population in the death registration area of the time. The study covering 1922 to 1924 is based on 112,364 deaths among the 3.25 million "industrial" white male policyholders aged 15 or over. The ratio of age-standardized death rates of "industrial:ordinary" white male policyholders aged 20 and over are given differently in two of

Table 1–6—Ratios of death rates of industrial : ordinary policyholders of the Metropolitan Life Insurance Company, white males, age 20 and over

Period	20 and Over (Age-adjusted)	AGE GROUP RATIOS*					65 and over
		20–24	25–34	35–44	45–54	55–64	
1922–1924**	255	157	207	224	218	181	135
1922–1924***	187	120	187	207	192	164	121
1937–1939***	144	129	166	162	158	136	126

* Ratio = Industrial rate/Ordinary rate × 100.
** See reference 33 (Dublin and Vane, 1930, p. 7).
*** See reference 33 (Dublin and Vane, 1947, p. 1009).

Table 1–7—Mean annual death rates per thousand persons, Chicago, 1928–1932, by census tract rental levels, nativity and sex (age-adjusted)[34]

Median Tract Rental	NATIVE-BORN, WHITE		FOREIGN-BORN, WHITE	
	Rate	Ratio*	Rate	Ratio*
Males				
$75 and over	8.7	100	9.4	100
$60–74.99	9.2	106	9.8	104
$45–59.99	10.2	117	10.8	115
$30–44.99	11.6	133	11.9	126
Less Than $30	15.1	174	14.8	157
Females				
$75 and Over	6.8	100	7.1	100
$60–74.99	7.9	116	9.3	131
$45–59.99	9.1	134	9.6	135
$30–44.99	10.2	150	10.2	144
Less Than $30	12.3	181	12.7	179

* Highest rental group rate in each group = 100.

proportion of skilled and unionized workers are probably included. "Ordinary" policyholders are "composed mainly of the clerical, professional, and commercial classes." In

33 Dublin, L. I., *Causes of Death by Occupation*, Washington, U.S. Government Printing Office, 1917 (Bureau of Labor Statistics Bulletin no. 207); L. I. Dublin, and R. J. Vane, *Causes of Death by Occupation*, Washington, U.S. Government Printing Office, 1930 (Bureau of Labor Statistics Bulletin no. 507), p. 7; ———, "Occupational Mortality Experience of Insured Male Wage Earners," *Monthly Lab. Rev.*, 64: 1009, June, 1947.

Dublin's publications. In the earlier report this ratio is given as 2.55:1, and in the later report as 1.87:1. The discrepancy results from elimination in the latter analysis of those "ordinary" policyholders who had obtained insurance between 1919 and 1923, thus largely eliminating the factor of better medical selection. Data shown in Table 1–6 on the death rate ratios by age groups show —whichever set of figures is taken—a rising ratio till age 35–44 and then a decline, the 65 and over group showing about the same or a lower ratio than the 20–24 group.

Calculating the percentage differences between the two policyholder groups at different ages, for life expectation, Dublin shows roughly a 20 per cent difference between them, the advantage being that of the "ordinary" insured. This difference is somewhat smaller in the younger groups, rises to a peak between the ages 45 and 50, and declines after that age, being lowest after age 70.

In one of the first American studies of mortality rates, Coombs used all deaths in the city of Chicago between 1928 and 1932.[34] Each death was assigned to the census tract of residence at time of death. The tracts were grouped into five levels on the basis of the 1930 median monthly rental in the tract, using rounded cutting points (e.g., $30.00–44.99). Age-standardized data are presented separately by nativity, sex and race. Each of the four categories presented in Table 1–7 (whites only) shows a relatively smooth inverse gradient of mortality rates and median rental. Interestingly enough, the spread is greater among females than among males. Some indication of a minimum differential, among males, may be seen between the two highest rental levels, and, among all four groups, the greatest differential appears between the two lowest levels.

Within these qualifications, class differentials show clearly all along the line.

Whitney's study using 1930 data was the first large-scale American study following the pattern which had been set by the British Registrar General.[35] Death certificate data were obtained from ten states: Alabama, Connecticut, Illinois, Kansas, Massachusetts, Minnesota, New Jersey, New York, Ohio and Wisconsin. These states contained 39 per cent of the gainfully employed. The 1930 census was used to obtain denominator information. Analysis was limited to males aged 15 to 64, in an attempt to limit the unreliability introduced by retirement. Age-standardized data are presented within the social–economic classification developed by Edwards and used standardly by the United States Census.

As can be seen in Table 1–8, mortality rates vary inversely with class in the total age group of 15–64. Only the proprietor group is out of line. If retail dealers, whose rate is 8.4, are excluded from this category, the rate would be 7.0, making a linear relationship. The curve, however, is not smooth,

Table 1–8—Annual death rates per 1,000 gainfully occupied males, aged 15 to 64 years (age-standardized) by age groups according to socio-economic class, 1930[36]

Socio–economic Class	Age Groups *							
	15–64		15–24		25–44		45–64	
	Rate	Ratio**	Rate	Ratio	Rate	Ratio	Rate	Ratio
All Gainfully Employed Males	9.1	100	3.2	100	5.5	100	17.9	100
Professional Men	6.7	74	2.3	72	3.5	64	16.2	90
Proprietors, Managers and Officials	7.9	87	3.1	97	4.2	76	15.8	88
Clerks and Kindred Workers	7.8	86	2.3	72	4.1	74	16.5	92
Skilled Workers and Foremen	8.3	91	3.0	94	4.9	89	17.1	96
Semiskilled Workers	10.1	111	3.2	100	6.1	111	20.8	116
Unskilled Workers	14.5	159	4.7	147	9.6	174	24.8	138

* The age-standardized figures for the age group 15–64 are based on the 53 occupational groups with 500 or more deaths (Whitney, Table 8, p. 32). These cover 79 per cent of the gainfully employed. This set of data was selected as more reliable than the figures for all deaths, given by Whitney in Table 1, p. 17. The trends in the two sets of data are very similar. The age-specific data are only available in Whitney's Table 1, and cover the entire surveyed population.
** Rate for all gainfully employed males = 100.

[34] Coombs, L. C., "Economic Differentials in Causes of Death," *Med. Care*, 1: 249, 250, 255, July, 1941.

[35] Whitney, J. S., *Death Rates by Occupation, Based on Data of the U.S. Census Bureau, 1930*, New York, National Tuberculosis Assoc., 1934, pp. 17, 32.

as can be seen clearly from the ratios presented in the table. The largest difference is found between unskilled and semiskilled workers, with a sizable difference between the latter and skilled workers. Beyond this level the differences, although existent, are relatively small.

The same general pattern appears in each of the three age-specific sets of data. The spread, however, is greatest in the 25–44 age group and least in the oldest group. In the latter, differences among the four occupational categories from skilled workers and up are almost nonexistent. This study indicates, then, that class is most intimately related to mortality rates among the unskilled and, secondarily among the semiskilled workers, and during middle age.[36]

Sheps and Watkins[37] sought to overcome the weakness of ecological studies by utilizing information obtained in careful sociological study which grouped areas in New Haven, Connecticut, into "natural areas." The boundary lines of these areas were such that information about census tracts could be used for purposes of setting denominators and standardizing for age. The seven resulting areas for which death rates for 1930 to 1934 were calculated contained from 10,000 to 51,000 people. A total of 8,201 deaths were recorded during this period. The seven areas were ranked from best to worst, based on a composite of factors including rental, delinquency rates, social standing and financial dependency. All data were age-adjusted.

Taking the average annual death rate over the five-year period of the best area (8.0 per 1,000 persons) as 100, the ratios of the other six areas, going down the socio–economic scale, were: 111, 110, 128, 136, 145, 148. Other than the fact that the rates for the second and third highest areas are almost identical, a clear inverse linear relationship is found. When the authors combined the seven areas into three, the range was substantially narrowed (100:114:134). The strongest relationship between mortality rates and economic level were found at ages 0–5 and 25–64.

Stocks[38] calculated the correlation of the 1934 mortality rates in the 83 county boroughs (cities of 50,000 or more, excluding London) of England and Wales, with the mean number of persons per room and a social class index, i.e., the percentages of males aged 14 and over in the labor force in the Registrar General's classes IV and V. He found a crude correlation coefficient of 0.77 between mortality and the housing measure, and 0.68 between mortality and the class measure. When both class and latitude are controlled, the partial coefficient for the housing measure is somewhat reduced to 0.51. Controlling for density and latitude, the partial coefficient for mortality and class is greatly reduced to 0.29. As noted earlier, Martin[39] used the same measures for the 28 London boroughs. The 1930 to 1932 age-standardized mortality rates correlated 0.80 with the mean number of persons per room and 0.62 with the percentage in classes IV and V. A somewhat higher correlation was found (0.87) with the percentage of persons living in dwelling units of two or more persons per room.

Szabady,[40] whose data for Hungary for earlier years showed almost no difference in the death rates between nonagricultural and manual and non-manual gainfully employed workers in 1910, also shows the same picture for 1930–1931. He then notes, however, that if correlations are made for the differential age-distribution, the picture changes considerably. The standardized death rates for 1930–1931 were 14.7 per 1,000 persons for manual workers compared with 11.3 for non-manual workers (130:100; earners only). Non-standardized rates for 1941 showed a reversed picture: 13.4 for non-manual as compared to 11.1 (83:100) for manual workers, for which Szabady offers no explanation.

In 1935, Rowntree returned to the city of

---

[36] Whitney's data are quoted and discussed by Britten, *op. cit.*, and Guralnick, *op. cit.*

[37] Sheps, C. and J. H. Watkins, "Mortality in the Socio–Economic Districts of New Haven," *Yale J. Biol. and Med.*, 20: 51–80, October, 1947.

[38] Stocks, P., "The Effects of Occupation and Its Accompanying Environment on Mortality," *J. Royal Stat. Soc.*, 101, part IV, 681, 1938.

[39] Martin, *op. cit.*, p. 130.

[40] Szabady, *op. cit.*, p. 402.

York to make his second well-known study of poverty.[41] He notes that York differs little from England as a whole and from other large cities in its overall and infant mortality rates. His study was based on a house-to-house survey of 16,362 families, including 55,206 persons out of the total city population of 90,000. Since his concern was primarily with poverty, he included only wage-earners. Thus the study includes some on the lower white-collar level, and excludes a few high-income manual workers and domestics working in well-to-do areas. The mortality spread between the top and bottom groups, therefore, is probably less than what it would be had the total population been included.

The surveyed population was divided into five levels, two of which are considered to be below the poverty line. The age-standardized death rates per thousand persons for 1935–1936 were: for the two highest levels, 8.4; for the middle level, 11.2; and, for the two poverty levels, 13.5 (ratios of 100:133:161).

Dublin and Vane's analysis of life insurance policyholder data, referred to

basis of per capita income. The mean incomes for the three groups of cities were $918, $789 and $668. The age-adjusted death rates per thousand people, using 1939–1940 data, were, respectively, 10.9, 11.0 and 12.1 (100:100:111). Thus, in what is probably the crudest kind of ecological comparison, in that the groupings are quite heterogeneous, the poorest third of the cities showed a higher death rate, though the magnitude of the difference hardly approaches that found in more detailed studies, while the other two-thirds, as groups, do not differ from each other.

Following the model set by Coombs in her earlier study of Chicago, Yeracaris[44] divided the 72 census tracts in the city of Buffalo into five levels on the basis of the 1940 median rentals. Death rates were calculated for each of the five levels, using 1939–1941 data. As Table 1–9 shows, an inverse gradient is found for both sexes.

Table 1–9—Age-standardized annual death rates per 1,000 persons, and ratios, Buffalo, 1939-1941, by census tracts grouped on basis of median rentals[44]

Rental Group	MALES		FEMALES	
	Death Rate	Ratio*	Death Rate	Ratio
1 (Highest)	9.4	100	7.2	100
2	9.9	105	8.1	112
3	11.4	121	9.0	125
4	12.2	130	10.0	139
5 (Lowest)	14.9	158	12.4	172

* Highest rental group = 100.

previously, presents data for 1937 to 1939, shown in Table 1-6.[42] The death rate ratios of "industrial" to "ordinary" policyholders are lowest at ages 20–24 and 65 and over (129 and 126) and highest at ages 25–34 and 35–44.

World War II to the Present

Altenderfer[43] divided the 92 United States cities with a population of 100,000 or more in 1940 into three equal-sized groups on the

Though female death rates are consistently below those for males, the actual spread between the tract groups is larger for females. With each successively lower step in the rental ladder, the differential between the tract groups increases, so that the largest gap appears between the lowest and next lowest groups, whereas a relatively small difference appears between the two top groups.

Yeracaris notes that, if the death rate of the highest tract group had prevailed throughout Buffalo, 19.1 per cent of the deaths would not have occurred. Had this rate prevailed in the second highest tract

[41] Rowntree, *op. cit.*, p. 296.

[42] Dublin and Vane, *op. cit.* (1947), p. 1009.

[43] Altenderfer, M. E., "Relationship Between Per Capita Income and Mortality, in the Cities of 100,000 or More Population," *Pub. Health Rep.*, 62: 1681–1691, November, 1947.

[44] Yeracaris, *op. cit.*, pp. 1235–1247.

group, 6.8 per cent of its deaths would have been avoided. This percentage increases to 17.3 in the intermediate level, 24.5 in the fourth level and 38.5 in the lowest level.

Patno's analysis of Pittsburgh mortality data followed the same pattern.[45] The 1940 census tracts were ranked by using either the median value of owner-occupied or the median monthly rental. The tracts were then grouped into three levels, each containing about one-third of the city's white population. Data for 1950 were also employed, using median family income in each tract as a third criterion for classification.

the economic levels. No indication is given that economic differentials are any greater among males than among females.

Mortality rates in the Netherlands are among the lowest in the world. In this context, determination of social class differences becomes of particular interest. DeWolff and Meerdink[46] studied the mortality rates of gainfully employed males, aged 15–64 in Amsterdam in 1947–1952, using the 1947 census to provide denominator information. The population was divided into six occupational levels. The annual, average, age-adjusted death rates per thousand persons were: liberal professions, civil service, etc., 3.6; independent businessmen, 3.9; clerical

Table 1–10—Mortality ratios* among white residents of Pittsburgh, by census tracts, age and sex[45]

				Economic Level		
		1940				1950
Age and Sex	High	Middle	Low	High	Middle	Low
Males						
All Ages**	93	97	111	88	99	113
Under 10	84	98	114	73	105	119
10–29	102	86	113	90	116	95
30–39	73	88	143	64	83	148
40–49	67	114	117	85	85	131
50–59	93	89	123	75	104	123
60–69	98	97	108	92	98	108
70 and Over	103	98	99	97	98	104
Females						
All Ages**	93	100	114	91	105	106
Under 10	107	103	91	116	85	101
10–29	80	114	107	87	112	100
30–39	88	102	113	77	96	127
40–49	81	101	127	68	121	118
50–59	79	92	165	84	99	123
60–69	93	99	120	87	103	113
70 and Over	100	100	103	95	109	97

* Rate in each age–sex category = 100.
** Age-standardized.

With few exceptions, the data, shown in Table 1–10, indicate an inverse gradient of mortality with economic level of the tract groupings in the age–sex categories. This is true for both 1940 and 1950. The largest differentials are found in the 30 to 59 age group, particularly in the first of these decades. For females under ten, the gradient is direct, and in both sexes the 70 and over category shows no clear difference among

workers, 5.1; managers, foremen, higher technical staff, 3.3; skilled workers, 4.2; unskilled labor, 4.2. The difference between the most favored group and the workers (117:100) barely reaches statistical significance. In contrast to the findings of all other studies, unskilled workers do not differ from skilled workers. Only the clerical group

[45] Patno, M. E., "Mortality and Economic Level in an Urban Area," *Pub. Health Rep.*, 75: 841–851, September, 1960.

[46] DeWolff, P. and J. Meerdink, "Mortality Rates in Amsterdam According to Profession," *Proceedings of the World Population Conference*, 1954, vol. I, New York, United Nations (E/Conf. 13/413), pp. 53–55.

is relatively high (though a death rate of 5.1 is, as such, quite low). The authors suggest two reasons for this rate. First, the clerical workers do not reach the standards of physical fitness required to obtain civil service employment, which would have placed them in the top level. Second, many are probably children of manual workers and are not sufficiently fit to work.

By the 1950's, the number of studies of socio–economic mortality differentials had increased considerably. Szabady's review of the Hungarian data,[47] which had pointed to a higher rate among non-manual earners in 1941, shows a relatively small difference, though in the direction to be expected, for 1948–1949. Manual workers had a rate of 10.4 per thousand compared to 8.6 for non-manual workers (not age-adjusted). By 1959–1960 the difference had narrowed slightly, with rates of 10.5 and 9.0, respectively. Age-standardization reduces this gap somewhat, to 11.7 and 10.9 (107:100).

Tayback[48] divided Baltimore's 168 census tracts on the basis of the 1950 median tract rentals, grouping them into equal-sized population quintiles. The 1949–1951 death rates for the socio–economic levels, excluding the nonwhite population, are shown in Table 1–11. In overall terms, a clear inverse class gradient is seen, the male slope being somewhat steeper than the female slope, with very few figures being out of line. The gap tends to be quite large in the younger age groups, where the death rate is low. Class differences in middle age (35–54) are very sizable. At this age, the major differences seem to be at the top and bottom, between the highest and next-highest and between the lowest and second-lowest economic levels. Differences remain considerable at ages 55–64, but tend to become much smaller thereafter.

Ellis conducted a very similar study in Houston.[49] The index used to rank census tracts was a modification of the index of

social rank developed by Shevky and Williams, which utilizes measures of education, occupation and median family income. Tracts were grouped into quintiles, each of which contained 12 or 13 tracts. The 1949–1951 age-standardized, annual, average death rates per thousand persons for the white population of Houston by socio–economic level are shown in Table 1–12. Although class differentials do appear, they differ from those in other studies. The range of differences is smaller, though still substantial. The two top groups of tracts, for males, and the three top, for females, are quite similar in their death rates. Most puzzling, perhaps, is the fact that males in the lowest tract level have a lower rate than do those in the adjacent level. Ellis suggests as a possible explanation the availability of free medical treatment for the lowest group. Group 4, not having such an advantage but having a limited income, may utilize funds for the females, who do have a lower rate than the females in group 5, whereas the males go on working and refrain from using such funds for themselves.

Stockwell, whose concern was methodological as well as substantive, presents data exactly parallel to the above. These data also appear in Table 1–12. He also used a modified form of the Shevky–Williams index, studied deaths in 1949–1951, and included about one-fifth of the number of tracts in each socio–economic level. Stockwell's data pertain to Providence and Hartford. The class differentials in these two cities are quite similar to those in Houston. In Providence, little difference is found among the top three levels of males or the top two levels of females. Hartford females do not differ among all five strata; levels 2 and 3 and levels 4 and 5 have almost identical rates.

Stockwell proceeded to compute rank order correlation coefficients between the census tracts in each city ranked by age–sex-standardized death rates and each of eight socio–economic variables (occupation, two education variables, two income variables, two rent variables, crowding). In all cases,

[47] Szabady, op. cit., pp. 401, 403.

[48] Tayback, op. cit., p. 142.

[49] Ellis, J. M., "Socio–Economic Differentials in Mortality from Chronic Diseases," Social Problems, 5: 30–36, July, 1957. In expanded form in E. G. Jaco (ed.), Patients, Physicians and Illness, 1st ed., New York: Free Press, 1958, p. 32.

Table 1–11—Annual death rates per 1,000 white population, by age and sex, in five economic levels, Baltimore City, 1949–1951[48]

Economic Level	15–24		25–34		35–44		45–54		55–64		65–74		75+	
	Rate	Ratio*	Rate	Ratio	Rate	Ratio	Rate	Ratio	Rate	Ratio	Rate	Ratio	Rate	Ratio
White Males														
Highest	0.8	100	0.8	100	3.2	100	6.8	100	24.1	100	57.0	100	128.2	100
2	1.0	125	1.5	188	4.3	134	10.9	160	26.6	110	57.2	100	135.2	105
3	1.3	162	1.6	200	4.1	128	12.7	187	29.5	122	56.5	99	124.1	97
4	1.3	162	1.7	212	4.8	150	13.8	203	32.9	136	61.9	108	137.3	107
Lowest	1.4	175	2.2	275	6.4	200	17.6	259	40.5	168	72.8	128	142.3	111
White Females														
Highest	0.4	100	1.1	100	1.8	100	4.8	100	13.4	100	34.2	100	110.2	100
2	0.4	100	0.8	73	2.7	150	5.7	119	13.4	100	36.8	108	106.7	97
3	0.4	100	1.2	109	2.6	144	6.3	131	16.8	125	38.3	112	118.5	108
4	0.7	175	1.3	118	3.1	172	7.6	158	16.1	120	42.4	124	132.8	120
Lowest	0.8	200	2.1	191	3.4	189	7.9	164	21.9	163	42.8	125	123.8	112

* Highest economic level in each group = 100.

the correlation coefficients were significant.[50]

Since the British Registrar General system of social classification is the richest source of data on mortality differences over time among different socio–economic levels, a number of attempts have been made to construct a comparable ranking in the United States. Breslow and Buell,[51] using the 1950 census for denominator data, classified all deaths of California males, aged 20–64, from 1949 to 1951, in one of five occupational classes. Class I includes pro-

fessionals and kindred workers; class II is an intermediate group; class III includes sales, clerical and skilled workers; class IV includes semiskilled workers; and class V includes unskilled workers. Data for farmers and farm laborers are presented separately, differing from the British system, because the data on death certificates for these men

Table 1–12—Age-standardized average, annual death rates per 1,000 population for five social rank areas, by sex, 1949–1951, in Houston,[49] Providence and Hartford[50]

Socio–economic Level	HOUSTON Rate	HOUSTON Ratio*	PROVIDENCE Rate	PROVIDENCE Ratio	HARTFORD Rate	HARTFORD Ratio
White Males						
1 (Highest)	7.5	100	10.8	100	9.3	100
2	7.9	105	11.8	109	10.3	111
3	9.1	121	11.2	104	11.2	120
4	11.1	148	12.7	118	11.8	127
5 (Lowest)	9.9	132	14.0	130	12.5	134
White Females						
1 (Highest)	5.4	100	7.3	100	6.6	100
2	5.3	98	7.6	104	7.5	114
3	5.6	104	8.9	122	7.5	114
4	7.1	131	9.4	129	8.2	124
5 (Lowest)	7.5	139	10.4	142	8.3	126

* Highest economic level in each group = 100.

[50] Stockwell, E. G., *Socio–Economic Mortality Differentials in Hartford, Conn. and Providence, R. 1.: A Methodological Critique*, unpublished doctoral dissertation, Brown University, 1960. Relevant papers published by Stockwell based on his dissertation include: ———, "A Critical Examination of the Relationship Between Socio–economic Status and Mortality," *Amer. J. Pub. Health*, 53: 956–964, June, 1963; ———, "Socio–economic Status and Mortality," *Connecticut Health Bull.*, 77: 10–13, December, 1963.

Stockwell investigated the difference made in the analysis of socio–economic mortality data when different indices of class are used. He notes that the precise conclusions one draws will "vary considerably with the methodological conditions characterizing a particular study," however, the overall patterns are sufficiently similar so that, for present purposes, it is adequate to refer to only one or two of his measures. Since many studies reported in the present paper used median rental, however, it is important to note that Stockwell's data indicate that, of all eight variables, this is the poorest predictor of mortality rates.

[51] Breslow, L. and P. Buell, "Mortality from Coronary Heart Disease and Physical Activity of Work in California," *J. Chronic Dis.*, 11: 421–444, April, 1960.

were thought to be unreliable. All data are presented in terms of the standardized mortality ratio which is a ratio of the observed deaths in an occupation to the age-standardized expected number of deaths, as determined by the age-specific rates for men in all occupations. The standardized mortality ratio for all men is equal to 100. The California data are presented in Table 1–13.

For the entire age group, a rough inverse gradient is seen between class and mortality. To all intents and purposes, however, classes I and II do not differ, nor do III and IV, though the latter two have a somewhat higher rate than the former. Class V has a strikingly higher rate. A smoother gradient appears at ages 20–34, and is most strikingly regular at ages 35–44, though in both cases class V is set off from the others by its high rate. Class differences begin to be attenuated at ages 45–54, with the exception of class V. This is even more true for the 55–59 group, and in the 60–64 group almost no class differences exist.

A more ambitious attempt along the same lines was conducted by Guralnick, who analyzed all male deaths in age group 20 to 64 in the United States in 1950.[52] In view of the fact that one primary purpose was to compare the United States data with the British, Guralnick collapsed classes II to IV to make this intermediate group comparable

Guralnick,[53] in which standard mortality ratios are given separately for the five classes, presents figures almost identical with the California figures. The standardized mortality ratios for all United States males aged 20–64, in 1950, from class I to class V, are: 83, 84, 96, 97, 120. These ratios are for whites only, except for class I, which contains a few nonwhites. Once again classes I and II do not differ, nor do classes III and IV.

Table 1–13—Mortality ratios, California men, ages 20 to 64, by social class, 1949 to 1951[51]

| | | | SOCIAL CLASS | | |
Age Group	I	II	III	IV	V
20–64 *	87	85	94	98	132
20–34 *	62	66	77	91	183
35–44	69	76	86	105	171
45–54	90	81	94	102	141
55–59	99	88	99	99	115
60–64	95	96	101	91	107

* Age-standardized.

Table 1–14—Annual death rates per 1,000, and ratios, males, by age and social class, United States, 1950[52]

| | | | | SOCIAL CLASS* | |
Age Group		All Occupations	I	II–IV	V**
20–64	Death rate	8.1	6.4	7.6	10.6
	Ratio***	100	79	94	131
20–24	Death rate	2.0	0.9	1.6	2.6
	Ratio	100	45	80	130
25–34	Death rate	2.2	1.1	1.8	3.2
	Ratio	100	50	82	145
35–44	Death rate	4.4	2.9	4.0	6.5
	Ratio	100	66	91	148
45–54	Death rate	10.9	9.3	10.5	14.2
	Ratio	100	85	96	130
55–64	Death rate	24.7	23.2	24.8	26.9
	Ratio	100	94	100	109

* See text for definition of class.
** White only.
*** Rate for all occupations in each age category = 100

in the two countries. The data are presented in Table 1–14. For the entire age group, the picture is quite similar to that presented in the California study: a linear inverse gradient, with the intermediate occupational level being closer to class I, and the major gap occurring between class V and the intermediate group. Another publication by

Examination of the age-specific rates in Table 1–14 shows the largest class gap to lie in the 25 to 44 age group, with classes II to

52 Guralnick, L., "Socio-economic Differences in Mortality by Cause of Death: United States, 1950 and England and Wales, 1949–1953," in *International Population Conference, Ottawa, 1963, op. cit.*, p. 298.

53 ——, "Mortality by Occupation Level and Cause of Death Among Men 20 to 64 Years of Age, U.S., 1950," *Vital Statistics, Special Reports*, 53, 452–481, September, 1963. For an earlier paper reporting provisional death rates in the same population by the five classes and seven age categories, see I. M. Moriyama and L. Guralnick, "Occupational and Social Class Differences in Mortality," in *Trends and Differentials in Mortality*, New York: Milbank Memorial Fund, 1956, p. 66.

IV being closer to class I than to class V. A considerable gap remains at ages 45–54, but it is substantially narrowed by ages 55–64.

Guralnick also analyzed the same 1950 data along more traditional American lines, using the occupational classification developed by Edwards for the United States Census.[54] This scheme seeks to rank occupations by socio–economic levels. The standardized mortality ratios presented in Table 1–15, for white males aged 25–59, show an inverse gradient, but one which does not distinguish among all of the eight occupational groups. The lowest ratios are found among the top three groups; they are followed closely by sales, skilled and semi-skilled workers, whose ratios are identical. Service workers fare substantially poorer, and, finally, laborers have a considerably higher mortality ratio.

This pattern does not hold in all age groups. Prior to age 30, only the roughest gradient, appears, though laborers fare markedly worst. A clear gradient appears in the 30–34 groups, which is maintained in the next ten year cohort. In both cases, the ratios of the top three occupational groups are nearly identical. This pattern holds in ages 45–54 and 55–59 in part. Three mortality levels can be distinguished in these groups, which do not conform to the socio–economic ranking: non-manual workers except sales workers; sales, skilled and semiskilled workers; and service and unskilled workers. In the oldest age category, only laborers continue to differ from all other groups.

A state-wide ecological study merits mention in passing. Hamilton[55] analyzed the age-adjusted 1950 death rates in the 100 counties of North Carolina. Three of the eight variables used in the multiple correlation analysis may be regarded as socio–economic measures: percentage of families owning own homes; percentage of homes with modern plumbing and not dilapidated; mean number of grades completed by adults.

Only the first of these, with a correlation of −0.69 with mortality, makes a statistically significant contribution toward explaining the intercounty mortality variation. Home condition and education measures have almost a zero correlation with mortality rates. Of far greater importance are variables such as percentage of whites and ratio of hospital beds to the population.

Despite the tremendous shifts in the London population and the overall decline of about one million persons during the two decades following 1930, Martin's data for 1950–1952, correlating age-standardized death rates with percentage of two or more persons per room, average number of persons per room and percentage of employed in classes IV and V in the 28 London boroughs, continue to show highly significant correlations. For these three variables, the correlations were: 0.36, 0.80 and 0.90.[56]

Hansluwka's review of Austrian mortality data[57] begins with reference to a number of early studies which were based upon workers covered by social insurance, reflecting only a very small part of the population. He does, however, present data for the entire employed population for 1951–1953. Table 1–16 presents these rates for males in different age groups. For the very gross categories of "middle and upper class" and "working class" occupations, few sizable differences emerge, though the latter's rates are higher. At ages 14–17, the former's rate is appreciably higher. At ages 60–64, however, the working class has a much higher death rate. Hansluwka also presents a bar chart showing mortality in Vienna in 1951–1953. The city's 23 districts were classified on the percentage of workers of the labor force in each district and grouped into four categories. The data, he concludes, show "a clearcut pattern of social grading of mortality."

[54] Guralnick, L., "Mortality by Occupation and Industry Among Men 20 to 64 Years of Age, U.S., 1950," *Vital Statistics, Special Reports*, 53, 59, 61, 84–86, September, 1962.
[55] Hamilton, H. C., "Ecological and Social Factors in Mortality Variation," *Eugenics Quart.*, 2: 212–223, December, 1955.

[56] Martin, *op. cit.*, p. 130.
[57] Hansluwka, H., "Social and Economic Factors in Mortality in Austria," in *International Population Conference, Ottawa, 1963, op. cit.*, pp. 315–344.

Table 1-15—Annual death rates per 1,000, and ratios, white males, by age and major occupation group, United States, 1950[54]

Major Occupation Group	25-29 SMR**	20-24		25-29		30-34		35-44		45-54		55-59		60-64	
		X	Y*	X	Y	X	Y	X	Y	X	Y	X	Y	X	Y
All Occupations	93	1.7	100	1.6	100	2.0	100	3.9	100	10.1	100	1.⌐	100	28.8	100
Professional, Technical, Kindred	82	1.2	73	1.2	70	1.5	76	3.2	81	9.4	93	18.9	98	29.2	101
Managers, Officials, Proprietors, Nonfarm	85	1.5	86	1.3	79	1.5	76	3.3	85	9.5	94	18.9	98	28.9	100
Clerical, Kindred	83	0.9	54	1.3	78	1.5	76	3.3	86	9.6	95	18.2	94	26.9	93
Sales	94	1.1	62	1.1	66	1.7	82	3.6	94	11.0	109	21.7	112	31.8	110
Craftsmen, Foremen, Kindred	94	1.8	103	1.6	97	2.0	99	4.0	102	10.1	100	20.8	107	32.1	111
Operatives, Kindred	94	1.8	106	1.8	108	2.2	107	4.1	106	10.3	102	19.4	100	28.6	99
Service, except Private Household	116	1.2	72	1.6	98	2.4	117	5.1	133	13.8	136	22.4	116	29.2	101
Laborers, except Farm and Mine	131	2.6	149	2.8	171	3.6	178	6.5	167	14.5	144	23.8	123	34.9	121

Age Group

* X = death rate per 1,000. Y = ratio, computed on the basis of rate for all occupations in each age category = 100.
** Standardized mortality ratios are computed on the basis of the entire population. Since non-whites are excluded in this table, SMRs can fall below 100.

A problem which has consistently bedeviled those who seek to study socioeconomic differentials on mortality by use of death certificates and census records is the frequent noncomparability of data in the two sources, which leads to overestimation of the denominator in some occupations and underestimation in others, or difficulty in making any calculations. The nature of the problem has been explored, theoretically and empirically, by several writers.[58] Among

levels of completed education by persons 25 and older, shows an inverse gradient of mortality rates by amount of education for both sexes in ages 25 to 64. Interestingly enough, this gradient disappears for males 65 and over, but remains quite strong for females of this age.

Table 1–16—Annual death rates per 1,000 employed males, by age and socio–economic category, Austria, 1951–1953[57]

Age Group	Middle and Upper Class Occupations (1)	Working Class Occupations (2)	Ratio of (2) to (1)*
14–17	2.0	1.3	68
18–29	1.7	1.8	110
30–49	3.4	3.8	112
50–59	12.6	13.4	106
60–64	15.8	24.4	154
65 and Over	65.1	73.9	114

* Rate of (1) = 100.

these, Kitagawa and Hauser have sought to overcome the difficulties by individual matching of 340,000 death certificates from deaths occurring in the United States from May through August, 1960, with census information recorded for these individuals in the 1960 census. In addition, personal interviews were conducted with individuals knowledgeable about 94 per cent of a sample of 9,500 of the descendents.

A preliminary analysis of the data using education and family income for white persons has been reported, though not yet published.[59] Consideration of the education variable, which is broken down into four

The latest mortality study available is Tsuchiya's presentation of standardized mortality ratios for an occupational–industrial categorization of Japanese males, age 15 and over, in 1962.[60] No clear occupational gradient emerges from the data. The ratios, ranked from low to high, are: "management," 58; "clerks," 67; "mechanics and simple," 88; "sales," 89; "professional and technical," 92; "transporting and communicating," 135.

Class Mortality Differentials in England and Wales

Since William Farr initiated the systematic study of occupational mortality statistics in 1851, the decennial reports of the British Registrar General for England and Wales have served as the outstanding source of information on the relationship of social class and mortality. For many years, the focus was on differential mortality risks of specific occupations. In the analysis of the 1910–1912 data, the various occupations were, for the first time, grouped together

[58] Buechley, R., J. E. Dunn, Jr., G. Linden and L. Breslow, "Death Certificate Statement of Occupation: Its Usefulness in Comparing Mortalities," *Pub. Health Reps.*, 71: 1105–1111, November, 1956; E. N. Kitagawa and P. M. Hauser, "Methods Used in a Current Study of Social and Economic Differentials in Mortality," in *Emerging Techniques of Population Research*, New York: Milbank Memorial Fund, pp. 250–266; and ———, "Social and Economic Differentials in Mortality in the U.S., 1960: A Report on Methods," in *International Population Conference, Ottawa, 1963, op. cit.*, pp. 355–367.

[59] Kitagawa, E. M. and P. M. Hauser, "Social and Economic Differentials in Mortality, United States, 1960." Paper presented at the 1966 annual meeting of the Population Assoc. of America.

[60] Tsuchiya, K., "The Relation of Occupation to Cancer, Especially Cancer of the Lung," *Cancer*, 18: 136–144, February, 1965.

into five social classes, which excluded textile workers, miners and agricultural laborers, for whom separate statistics were presented. This classification was, in large part, industrial. Substantial changes were introduced in the following decade, making the classification more properly occupational.

In 1930–1932 a further step was taken in moving from a concern with occupational hazards toward one with comparison of mortality risks of people sharing a given social environment: the mortality of married women classified according to husband's occupation was introduced as a systematic part of the data analysis. Since this time, despite reclassification of various occupations, the five-class scheme of the Registrar General has been maintained. During the war years, no census was taken. Moreover, a number of technical difficulties have arisen in the analysis of the data based on the 1961 census, hence nothing has yet been published for the latest period.

The Registrar General identifies 586 occupational unit groups to which every occupation in the country is assigned. Each of these groups is assigned as a whole to one of five social classes, on the basis of the predominant characteristics of the majority of persons in the unit group. "The basic common factor of all groups is the kind of work done and the nature of the operation performed. . . . The occupations included in each category [of the five social classes] have been selected so as to secure that, so far as is possible in practice, the category is homogeneous in relation to the basic criterion of *the general* standing within the community of the occupations concerned."[61]

[61] Quote is from the Registrar General's *Decennial Supplement, England and Wales, 1951, Occupational Mortality*, part II, vol. 1, *Commentary*, London, Her Majesty's Stationery Office, 1958, pp. 12–13. This system of classification is also described in W. P. D. Logan, "Social Class Variations in Mortality," in *Proceedings of the World Population Conference, op. cit.*, pp. 185–188; and F. C. Brockington, *The Health of the Community*, 3rd ed., London: J. & A. Churchill Ltd., 1965, pp. 325–334. The percentage distribution of the social classes is taken from Logan, p. 201. For further discussions of

The five social classes are described as follows (the proportion of occupied and retired men aged 15 and over in 1951 is given in brackets):

Class I. Higher administrative and professional occupations and business directorships (3.3 per cent).

Class II. Other administrative, professional and managerial, and shopkeepers: persons responsible for initiating policy and others without this responsibility, but with some responsibility over others (15 per cent).

Class III. Clerical workers, shop assistants, personal service, foremen, skilled workers: skilled workers with a special name, special responsibility and adaptability (52.7 per cent).

Class IV. Semiskilled workers: persons who are doing manual work which needs no great skill or training but who are doing it habitually and in association with a particular industry (16.2 per cent).

Class V. Unskilled workers: laborers, cleaners and other lowly occupations (12.8 per cent).

Farmers and farm managers are included in class II and agricultural workers in class IV. Also, class III, which includes more than half the population, is composed of both manual and non-manual workers.

From the great amount and variety of data available in the reports of the Registrar General and papers based on these reports, those that seem to be the most important have been selected for present purposes. These are presented in Table 1–17. Collins' analysis of the 1910–1912 data for occupied and retired males aged 15 and over, which refers to classes I, III and V and excludes textile workers, miners and agricultural laborers, shows a regular inverse gradient, with the largest gap being between class III and class V.[62] Stevenson's figures for the

[62] Collins, *op. cit.*, p. 15.

the antecedents and development of the Registrar General system of classification, see M. Greenwood, *Medical Statistics from Graunt to Farr*, Cambridge Univ. Press, 1948; and ———, "Occupational and Economic Factors of Mortality," *British Med. J.*, 1: 862–866, April, 1939.

Table 1–17—Standardized death rates per 1,000 and standardized mortality ratios, England and Wales, for selected age–sex groups and time periods, by social class

Time Period	I	II	III	IV	V	Population Group
1910–1912						
Death rate per 1,000	12.0	—	13.6	—	18.7	Occupied and retired males, age 15+, excludes textile workers, miners, agricultural laborers.[18]
Ratio (I = 100)	100	—	114	—	156	
Standardized Mortality Ratio	88	94	96	93	142	Males, age 25–64, excludes textile, miners, agricultural laborers.[63]
Standardized Mortality Ratio	88	94	96	107	128	As immediately above, modified by Stevenson.[63]
1921–1923						
Death Rate per 1,000	7.4	8.6	8.7	9.2	11.5	Males[64]
Ratio (I = 100)	100	116	117	124	155	
Standardized Mortality Ratio	82	94	95	101	125	Males, 20–64 *
1930–1932						
Standardized Mortality Ratio	90	94	97	102	111	Males, 20–64 *
	81	89	99	103	113	Married women, 20–64 *
1949–1953						
Standardized Mortality Ratio	98	86	101	94	118	Males, 20–64 *
	96	88	101	104	110	Married women, 20–64 *
	100	90	101	104	118	Occupied males, 20–64, adjusted to control for occupational changes since 1930–1932.
Death Rate per 1,000	6.6		6.4		9.5	Males, 20–64, excludes agricultural workers.[65]
Ratio (I = 100)	100		97		144	

* See reference 61 (Registrar General, page 20). Logan (ref. 61, p. 204) gives only figures for 1950.

same period,[63] which also exclude the same three occupational categories, but refer to males aged 25–64 in the five social classes, show a similar gradient. The ratios for classes II, III and IV, however, are nearly identical, and not very much higher than for class I. Stevenson argued that about 10 per cent of the laborers on the census are misclassified as class IV rather than class V, which tends to lower the rates for the former and increase those for the latter. Changing

[63] Stevenson, T. H. C., "The Social Distribution of Mortality from Different Causes in England and Wales, 1910–1912," *Biometrika*, 15: 384–388, 1923; Logan, *op. cit.*, p. 204. Logan's paper was also published, with variations, under the same title, in *British J. Prev. and Soc. Med.*, 8: 128–137, July, 1954, and in *Pub. Health Rep.*, 69: 1217–1223, December, 1954.

the denominators to this extent would, he notes, produce a smoother gradient, as shown in Table 1–17. Collins also took the 1900–1902 and 1890–1892 data for 100 specific occupations and classified them as they had been classified in 1910, adjusting the death rates for age. "The results," he comments, "need not be presented here since they merely confirm the findings for 1910–1912." Collins proceeded to analyze the age-specific rates, which show that class differentials were largest in the 25–54 age groups. This is supported by Stevenson's analysis.

A similar picture emerges from the data for 1921–1923, despite the significant changes in classification. The gap between classes I and II is somewhat greater than in the previous decade. Classes II and III have near-identical ratios and class IV a somewhat higher ratio, while class V is still widely distinct from the others. Britten's analysis[64] of the age-specific rates compares class I to class III and class III to class V. For the former comparison, the greatest gap is at ages 16–19, and declines with regularity at each succeeding age. The pattern of the class V:III ratio, however, is different. Here the greatest gap is at ages 35–44 and, though a bit less so, at 45–54.

By 1930, class differentials, though now presenting a regular inverse gradient, had narrowed, with standardized mortality ratios of 90 for class I and 111 for class V, for males, aged 20–64. The innovation introduced in the data analysis for these years shows that general socio–economic differences rather than specific occupational hazards were crucial in the relationship between class and mortality. This is seen in the data for married women classified by husband's occupation, in which the gradient is somewhat more steep than for the males.

The latest available data, for 1949–1953, show a rather different picture than that of previous decades. Class V still has a substantially higher ratio than the other classes; for the males, it is even higher than in 1930. Class II, however, now has the lowest ratio, followed by classes IV, I and III, in that order. For married women, the inverse gradient persists, except that here too, as among the males, class II has a lower ratio than class I. The relatively low ratio of class IV may well be an artifact of classificational changes from one social class to another. Adjustment of the data for occupied males to take account of these changes "has had the important effect of raising the SMR of Social Class IV from 94, where it was second lowest, to 104, where it occupies the second highest position, as it did in 1921–1923 and 1930–1932."[65] Guralnick's analysis of the British data,[66] excluding all gainfully employed in agriculture, and collapsing classes II–IV, shows that this latter group had a

very slightly lower death rate than class I, while class V remains very much higher.

Moriyama and Guralnick,[67] in their attempt to compare data for males from the United States and England and Wales, present age-specific ratios for the latter combining the three middle classes and excluding all engaged in agriculture, for 1950 only. For most age groups, little difference is seen between class I and classes II–IV; this is particularly true from age 45 upwards. Class V has consistently higher rates; but whereas this is the case to a moderate degree at ages 20–24, the differential increases thereafter, reaching a peak at ages 35–44, after which it declines again and nearly disappears at ages 60–64. (The respective ratios of the three class groups I, II–IV, taking the rate of all occupations as 100, are: at ages 20–24, 102, 94, 122; at ages 25–34, 90, 95, 138; at ages 35–44, 83, 96, 143; at ages 45–54, 98, 97, 129; at ages 55–59, 99, 99, 115; and at ages 60–64, 100, 101, 106.)

Viewing the data for England and Wales in overall terms, class differentials in mortality in the twentieth century both have and have not declined. On the one hand, the differentials between the middle levels (among whom mortality rates differed little even in the earlier years) and class I have more or less disappeared. On the other hand, class V is still strikingly worse off than the rest of the population. Though indications are that its relative position improved in the earlier decades of the century, this does not seem to be the case between 1930 and 1950.

Conclusions

This statistical examination clearly provides no basis to reject the inference drawn from the figures of the *Titanic* disaster. Despite the multiplicity of methods and indices used in the 30-odd studies cited, and despite the variegated populations surveyed, the inescapable conclusion is that class influences one's chance of staying alive. Almost without exception, the evidence shows that classes differ on mortality rates. Only three such exceptions were found, indicating no or almost no class difference.

[64] Britten, R. H., "Occupational Mortality Among Males in England and Wales, 1921–1923," *Pub. Health Rep.*, 43:1570, June, 1928.

[65] Registrar General, *op. cit.*, p. 20.

[66] Guralnick, *op. cit.* (International Population Conference), p. 298.

[67] Moriyama and Guralnick, *op. cit.*, p. 69.

Altenderfer, comparing 1939–1940 mortality rates of 92 United States cities classified into three mean income groups, shows a relatively small difference among them. Szabady, comparing nonagricultural manual and non-manual workers in Hungary in 1959–1960, shows the same. In both cases, the classification is so gross as to minimize differences which a finer analysis might reveal. Only DeWolff and Meerdink's study in Amsterdam in 1947–1952 can legitimately be regarded as strongly contradictory of the link between class and mortality. Their data, however, must be seen in the context of a population which has just about the lowest death rate ever recorded. This is not to dismiss the importance of their findings. On the contrary, it suggests the extremely important hypothesis that as the overall death rate of a population is lowered, class differentials may similarly decline.

This hypothesis finds support in an overall trend reflected in the studies reported. In the earlier studies, the differential between the mortality rates of extreme class groups is about a 2:1 ratio, but later studies show a narrowing of this differential, so that by the 1940's, a 1.4:1 or 1.3:1 ratio is much more typical. As can be seen from studying the death rates, these years witnessed a progressive decline in the overall death rate. At the same time, a cautionary note must be exercised. Despite an undoubted overall decline in mortality in the past three decades, the trend in the earlier decades of the century toward the closing of the class gap has been checked, if not halted.

This indication focuses on the differences between mortality rates of the lowest class and other classes. A more accurate picture of the overall pattern would be to suggest that what has happened is a blurring, if not a disappearance, of a clear class gradient, while class differences remain. On the basis of the existent data—using, for the sake of convenience, a five-fold class distinction, this being the most popular—it is difficult to conclude whether classes I to IV now no longer differ in their mortality rates, or whether classes I and II have the lowest rates, and II and IV have higher rates, though not necessarily substantially so. What seems to be beyond question is that,

whatever the index used and whatever the number of classes considered, almost always a lowest class appears with substantially higher mortality rates. Moreover, the differential between it and other classes evidently has not diminished over recent decades.

At this point discussion of the complex question of explanations for such patterns would not be appropriate. A possibility could be suggested, however. The truly magnificent triumphs over infectious diseases have been crucial in both narrowing the overall class differentials and in nearly eliminating differentials among all but the lowest class. In recent decades, however, access to good medical care, preventive medical action, health knowledge, and limitation of delay in seeking treatment have become increasingly important in combating mortality, as chronic diseases have become the chief health enemy in the developed world. In these areas, lower class people may well be at a disadvantage. As such factors become more and more important, as the historical supposition presented in the first pages of this paper suggests, increasing class differentiation may occur. This approach does not necessarily preclude consideration of genetic selection and what has commonly come to be called "the drift hypothesis."

The data reviewed lead to a further conclusion. With amazing consistency, the class differentials are largest in the middle years of life. This is no less true in the latest than in the earliest studies. Over and over again, the greatest gap is found in young and middle adulthood. The predominant pattern characterizing class differentials by age is that in which class differences are moderately high in the younger ages, rise to a peak at ages 30 to 44, begin to decline at that point and tend to disappear beyond age 65. Where a given set of data varies from this pattern, it is in one of two directions: in the former cases, class differentials are lowest in the younger and older groups; in the latter, the decline in class differentials only begins in late middle age.

This pattern of greatest class differences in middle adulthood may be linked to the two historical suppositions which have heretofore been presented. To hypothesize in more general terms, when mortality rates are extremely high or extremely low, class differences will tend to be small. In other words, when men are quite helpless before the threat of death, or when men have made great achievements in dealing with this threat, life chances will tend to be equitably distributed. On the other hand, when moderate progress is being made in dealing with this threat, differential consequences are to be expected. The crucial idea that may be involved here is that of preventable deaths, at any given level of knowledge, technique and social organization. Where and/or when such deaths are concentrated, class differentials will be greatest, unless appropriate social action is taken. This differential is not inevitable.

Much more, of course, could be said in summary, with reference to both substantive and methodological issues. Needless to say, consideration of patterns of class differences by cause of death is essential for a full understanding of this relationship. But this would have extended the paper into a book.

Acknowledgments

Work on this study was conducted while the writer was attached to the Social Science Unit of the Department of Public Health Practice, Harvard University School of Public Health, under a Special Research Fellowship from the National Institute of Mental Health, U.S. Public Health Service (1–F3–MH–29, 642–01, BEH). My gratitude is hereby expressed to my hosts and colleagues, Profs. Sol Levine, Norman Scotch, Sidney Croog and Lenin Baler.

TEN YEARS AGO, when the data linking tobacco and cancer were mainly based on animal studies, defenders of the tobacco companies' position remarked that the only thing the scientists had proved was that mice should not smoke. Today there are a large number of studies on humans, all of which show increased risk of lung cancer with increases in amount smoked. But as men who know tobacco know, such relations do not prove anything, they are only statistical, and statistics are not science.

Things have come to such a pass that in one of the suits brought by the families of lung cancer victims against tobacco companies, a jury has decided that one of the causes of the disease is smoking. Juries are less prone than scientists to philosophical nit-picking regarding cause, and the tobacco companies have perforce reacted in an equally pragmatic manner. Thus, there are those who say that they welcomed the legislation forcing them to label cigarettes as dangerous to health because by so doing they would no longer be liable to suit.

The data implicating cigarettes in cancer of various parts of the respiratory system are of several kinds: (1) studies in which tar from cigarettes is applied to animals, e.g., on the shaved skin of mice or in the pouches of hamsters; (2) retrospective studies in which human lung cancer cases and control patients are queried as to their former smoking habits; (3) prospective studies in which well persons are interviewed regarding their tobacco consumption—the investigator then examines death certificates and hospital records of his study group over the next several years and computes incidence of disease for each smoking category; (4) studies of cell changes in the respiratory tracts of individuals as related to their smoking behavior.

The findings of all these types of research are consistent. In all, cancer risk increases with increases in exposure to cigarette tar.[1] In the human studies, including our own, risk decreases with increases in length of time since ex-smokers abandoned the habit. Most recently, we have found variations

[1] Dorn, H. F., "Tobacco Consumption and Mortality from Cancer and Other Diseases," *Pub. Health Rep.*, 74: 581–593, July, 1959.

2

Cancer, Culture and Social Structure

Saxon Graham

(Figure 2–1) in human smoking behavior patterns, have simulated these on an analytic smoking machine and discovered that different patterns yield different amounts of tar.[2] We then found that lung cancer patients evince the high tar-yield patterns more than

FIGURE 2-1 Mean amounts of tar retrieved from taking puffs in three different smoking patterns

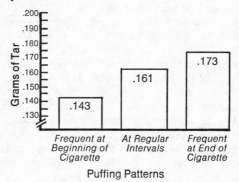

controls (Figure 2–2). This new means of comparing changes in risk with changes in exposure needs replication, but it is consistent with the earlier findings.[3]

The burden of this tale is that although scientists who typically do animal research

[2] Graham, S., S. Crouch, M. L. Levin and F. G. Bock, "Variations in Amounts of Tobacco Tar Retrieved from Selected Models of Smoking Behavior Simulated by Smoking Machine," *Cancer Res.*, 23:1025–1030, August, 1963.

[3] Graham, S., "Cancer of Lung Related to Smoking Behavior," *Cancer*, 21:523–530, March, 1968.

sometimes find it incredible that anyone interested in human cancer should want to study humans, it is the research on human behavior which has been most convincing in studying cancer of the lung. In spite of the fact that the biochemistry of human lung cancer is not understood, prevention could be effected with the human social epidemiological research at hand.

FIGURE 2-2   Lung cancer risk

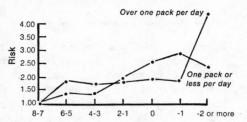

In the case of lung cancer, investigators in the earliest years were lucky in having ready at hand a logical culprit to investigate. Clinicians had noted that lung cancer rarely developed in a non-smoker, the chronic cough and bronchitis of smokers was a signal, and the time-trend of the disease showed an increase which corresponded to the adoption curve of cigarette smoking. People interested in other forms of cancer, however, have rarely had such a logical candidate available to them. Frequently, at the start of investigation of a disease of unknown etiology, a fruitful procedure has been to examine the incidence in various sub-groups of the population, beginning with demographic categories. If the different races, social classes, ethnic or religious or other groups show differences in distribution of the condition, a clue is provided as to where one should look further for behavioral or genetic relationships to the disease. Groups with unusually low incidence of the illness in question are just as interesting as those with very high incidence: In one case the investigator seeks possibly protective folkways; in the other, ones which could promote pathology.

Thus, as is shown in Figure 2–3, the demographic is only the first line of investigation. It serves to narrow the search area in which the crucial behavior pattern, if there is one, may be found. This strategy is based on the model of disease causation illustrated with cancer of the scrotum (Figure 2–3).

FIGURE 2-3   Etiological chain of events producing some disease

Specific Nationality, Social Class, Race, Etc.
(English Lower Class, Urban White)
▼
Occupation
(Chimney Sweeps)
▼
Behavior Pattern
(Working in Intimate Contact with Soot)
▼
Vehicle
(Product of Incomplete Combustion)
▼
Agent
(Unknown)
▼
Susceptible Host
▼
Tissue Change
(Cancer of Scrotum)

The train of events leading to contraction of scrotal cancer, as Sir Percival Pott found in studying the disease in 1775, was somewhat as follows: (1) an environmental need for heated dwellings (2) was met with a socio–cultural response in the form of widespread installation of home space-heaters, (3) the preferred fuel for which produced so much smoke and soot that (4) exhaust passages required frequent cleaning; (5) an occupation, chimney sweep, developed which put the worker into close and frequent contact with soot, which in individuals who were susceptible caused scrotal cancer.

Thus, the chain of events which may produce a disease may start with an occupational or other group, drawn typically from given social classes, who may display a pathogenic behavior pattern. The behavior pattern may act directly on the organism, as in the case of accidents, mental or sociosomatic disease, or it may put the individual into contact with an agent which can cause disease. In susceptible hosts, tissue change may result. Whether or not the host is susceptible may depend on his genetic makeup, his previous socio–environmental exposures and possible immunities and his general physical and mental state. The last two host factors, of course, may be strongly affected by the social situation. Thus, the ubiquitous tubercle bacillus is more likely to produce clinically recognizable disease in an individual from the lower classes. Non-behavioral environmental factors (e.g. sunlight) and genetically determined host characteristics may figure importantly in the chain, as in the case of skin cancer and diabetes, respectively. Even here, however, it is clear that social factors, in these cases occupations involving exposure to the sun, and diet, may significantly condition the effect of the non-social.

As Pott found when he prescribed baths as a preventive for cancer of the scrotum, the chain of events may be interrupted at almost any stage and incidence of the disease reduced. It is not even necessary to understand all elements in the chain to effect this reduction. In the case of scrotal and lung cancer the agent is still unknown, but incidence can be reduced by a change in behavior patterns. Occasionally, as in the case of lung and scrotal cancer, hints of a relation between a disease of a specific organ and a behavior pattern exist. For many diseases, however, no such hints exist, and it is necessary to examine demographic, occupational and other factors in the etiological chain to determine where the search for clues can continue.

Because of its special relation to disease, particularly childhood and degenerative disease, age has been a favorite demographic category. Because of the relation between time and incubation periods and spread of infectious disease, temporal and spatial relationships are also usually measured. Socio–economic status recently has been found to be related to as varied conditions as hypertension and poliomyelitis. In the case of cancer, incidence studies in Copenhagen, New Haven and Buffalo show increased risk of cancer, of the lung, stomach and cervix in the lower classes, and higher risks of cancer of the breast and uterine body in the

upper classes (Figure 2–4).[4-6]. Later inquiry has uncovered other factors, consistent with the socio–economic distributions, which shed additional light on the etiology of these diseases. Breast cancer, for example, has been found to be less frequent in women

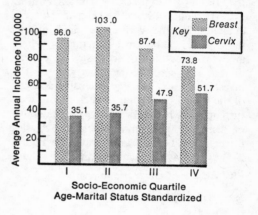

FIGURE 2-4   Cancer of reproductive organs, Buffalo, 1948-1952

with many pregnancies, who have nursed many children and who have had early menopause by virtue of hysterectomy or oophorectomy.[7] The evidence is good that all these are characteristic of lower, rather

[4] Clemmesen, J., and A. Nielson, "The Social Distribution of Cancer in Copenhagen, 1943–1947," *Danish Cancer Registry*, April 30, 1951.

[5] Cohart, E. M., "Socio–economic Distribution of Stomach Cancer in New Haven," *Cancer*, 7: 455–461, 1954; "Socio–economic Distribution of Cancer of Female Sex Organs in New Haven," *Cancer*, 8: 34–41, 1955; Cohart, and C. Muller, "Socio–economic Distribution of Cancer of the Gastrointestinal Tract in New Haven," *Cancer*, 8: 379–388, 1955.

[6] Graham, S., M. Levin and A. M. Lilienfeld, "The Socio–economic Distribution of Cancer of Various Sites in Buffalo, New York, 1948–1952," *Cancer*, 13: 180–191, January–February, 1960.

[7] Wynder, E., T. Kajitani, J. Kuno, J. Lucas, A. De Palo and J. Farrow, "A Comparison of Survival Rates Between American and Japanese Patients with Breast Cancer," *Surgery, Gyn. and Obs.*, 117: 196–200, August, 1963.

than higher, status women and may be related to their lower risk of breast cancer. These relationships suggested the hypothesis that decreased years of menstrual function, which is associated with early menopause and the other factors, might be associated with decreased risk of breast cancer. Data from Buffalo are consistent with the hypothesis.[8] Thus, it is possible that some factor associated with menstrual function, possibly hormonal, may figure in the etiology of some cases of breast cancer.

Certain of the distinctive behavior patterns exhibited by the various religious groups may have pathogenic potential. Where analyses show high or low rates of a given disease for specific religious groups, the investigator suspects that intensive analysis of the folkways peculiar to such groups may turn up one which is protective or productive of disease. For example, incidence studies in the United States and Israel (see Figure 2–5) as well as cross-cultural mortality data,

FIGURE 2-5 Cancer of the cervix

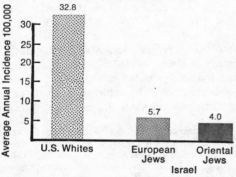

confirm that Jewish women are much less at risk of cancer of the cervix than non-Jews.[9] A number of Jewish folkways have been considered, including circumcision and abstinence from intercourse for the period after menses specified in Leviticus. Study

of the first factor has always been done by asking women about their husband's status. This has turned up a small relationship in one case and none in two others. Our inquiry as to the extent to which men know whether they are circumcised or not compared their statements with physical examination results. This showed that for our series, which is fairly representative in educational status, about 34 per cent of the men were in error in assessing their own condition.[10] Whether their wives would be less so is something to ponder on. With regard to the prescription in Leviticus, most American Jews stoutly assert that this is one rule which is rarely followed.

A number of pieces of research suggest other factors as being related to cervix cancer. These include experiencing multiple births, having first coitus early in life, frequent coitus and multiple sex partners either extra- or intra-maritally.[11]

Most of these findings have been reported several times in studies in the United States and abroad. Some interesting corroborative evidence includes the observations that nuns have very low incidence of cancer of the cervix, prostitutes excessively high risks and the lower classes and Negroes, with typically earlier marriage and more births, a higher risk than the rest of the population in general and Jews in particular. Just as it has been instructive to examine smokers who do and do not develop lung cancer, Clyde Martin searched into marital factors among a series of Jewish women with and without cancer of the cervix. It was difficult to assemble a sizable series because of the scarcity of such patients, but his findings suggested that there

[8] Levin, M. L., P. R. Sheehe, S. Graham and O. Glidewell, "Lactation and Menstrual Function as Related to Cancer of the Breast," *Amer. J. Pub. Hlth.*, 54: 580–587, 1964.

[9] Stewart, H., L. Dunham, J. Casper, H. Dorn, L. Thomas, J. Edgcomb and A. Symeonidis, "Epidemiology of Cancers of Uterine Cervix and Corpus, Breast and Ovary in Israel and NY City," *J. NCI*, vol. 37, no. 1, 1966.

[10] Lilienfeld, A., and S. Graham, "Validity of Determining Circumcision Status by Questionnaire As Related to Epidemiological Studies of Cancer of the Cervix," *J. NCI*, 21: 713–720, October, 1958.

[11] Dunn, J., and P. Buell, "Association of Cervical Cancer with Circumcision of Sexual Partner," *J. NCI*, 22: 749–764, 1959; M. Terris and M. C. Oalmann, "Carcinoma of the Cervix," *J. AMA*, 174: 1847–1851, Dec. 3, 1960; E. Wynder, J. Cornfield, M. B. Schroff and K. R. Doraiswami, "A Study of Environmental Factors in Carcinoma of the Cervix," *Amer. J. Obs. & Gyn.*, October, 1954, 1016–1052; E. Stern *et al*, "Cancer of the Uterine Cervix," *Cancer*, 20: 190–201, 1967.

is higher risk for Jewish women who have multiple sex partners, particularly if some are non-Jewish. Stressing that his research needs replication, Martin develops a theory embodying both sociological and virological elements. This is to the effect that the uncircumcised non-Jew is more apt to harbor a carcinogenic virus, that only certain males carry it, that as the number of men with whom a woman has sexual intercourse throughout her life increases, so does her probability of exposure to the virus and hence her risk of cervix cancer. Whether Martin's theory is ultimately justified or not and despite his inclinations to the contrary, the sociologist must admit the possibility that Jews in general may hold some genes in common which are protective against cervix cancer.[12] There is some genetic evidence of aggregation of certain other physical traits in Jews (e.g., fingerprint whorls), and there is no reason to exclude a cervix cancer protective factor as yet.[13] It is tantalizing to contemplate the possible results of research on other groups of similar gene heritage and circumcision folkways, such as people of North Africa and the eastern Mediterranean.

Brian MacMahon first suggested that Jews may have an unusual risk of another cancer, leukemia.[14] He did not examine the question by type of leukemia, but in upstate New York recently, we found that although the relationship did not hold for leukemia of children, there was a very strong association among adults. There is some evidence that irradiation with x-rays is related to the etiology of leukemia, and some have suggested that the Jewish risk may be related to the possibility of their getting better medical care and hence more x-rays; nevertheless, our finding holds regardless of irradiation. The Jewish relationship may partly be a product of nationality back-ground, but only partly. Thus, we find a higher risk for American foreign-born in general than the native born, and a higher risk for non-Jewish Eastern Europeans in general than other foreign-born, but Jews among the Eastern Europeans have much higher risks than non-Jews in the same nationality groups.[15]

Because of the potential of irradiation for altering cell structure (both germ and somatic cells), the relation of irradiation to leukemia is interesting. It has been found that irradiation after birth increases risk; but equally important, suggestions from studies in Buffalo and England are that irradiation of the pregnant mother raises risk in the child subsequently born.[16] And, equally interesting because of the pathogenic impact of irradiation on cell structure, is the New York State finding that irradiation of the patient prior to conception increases risk in offspring subsequently born. Irradiation, however, may account for only a part of the total leukemia; and it is significant that there is a higher Jewish risk regardless of irradiation history.

The finding of a higher risk of adult leukemia in the foreign-born than among the native-born was not unexpected. Indeed, even when factors such as age, occupation, socio–economic status, urban–rural residence, and smoking behavior are controlled (Figure 2–6), the foreign-born have higher risks of cancer of the stomach, lung and esophagus than the native-born. Although they have some experience in common, the foreign-born are a heterogeneous category, to say the least, and it is more useful in

[12] Martin, C., "Marital and Coital Factors in Cervical Cancer," *Amer. J. Publ Hlth*, 57: 803–814, 1967.

[13] Sachs, L., and M. Bat-Miriam, "The Genetics of Jewish Populations: I. Finger Print Patterns in Jewish Populations in Israel," *Amer. J. Human Genetics*, 9: 117–126, June, 1957.

[14] MacMahon, B., and E. K. Koller, "Ethnic Differences in the Incidence of Leukemia," *Blood*, 12:1–10, January, 1957.

[15] Graham, S., R. Gibson, A. Lilienfeld, L. Schuman and M. Levin, "Religion and Ethnicity in Leukemia," *Amer. J. Pub. Hlth* (in press).

[16] Graham, S., M. L. Levin, A. M. Lilienfeld, L. M. Schuman, R. Gibson, J. E. Dowd and L. Hempelmann, "Preconception, Intrauterine, and Postnatal Irradiation As Related to Leukemia," *J. NCI*, Monograph 19; R. W. Gibson, I. D. J. Bross, S. Graham, A. Lilienfeld, L. Schuman, M. L. Levin, and J. E. Dowd, "Leukemia in Children Exposed to Multiple Risk Factors," *New England J. Med.*, 279: 906–909, October 24, 1968.

FIGURE 2-6 *Relative risk of developing cancer*

Foreign Born Compared with American Born

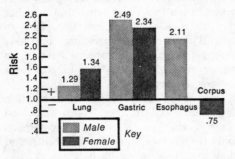

narrowing the search for behavioral factors to compare risks in the various nationality groups comprising the foreign-born. In Buffalo, the Irish, Germans, Italians and Poles bulk large in the foreign-born population. Controlling the factors noted above, we found (Figure 2–7) that the Polish-born

FIGURE 2-7 *Relative risk of developing cancer*

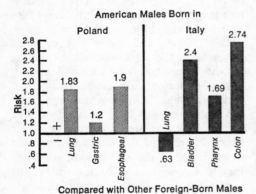

had risks of lung and esophageal cancer almost twice those of other foreign-born. The Germans and Irish showed little difference in risk from any type of cancer in comparisons with the remaining foreign-born population. The Italian-born, however, showed a significantly smaller risk of cancer of the lung as compared with other foreign-born, risks 2.4 and 2.7 times those of other

foreign-born for cancer of the bladder and colon, and an enhanced risk for cancer of the pharynx, as well. These findings are statistically significant and based on large numbers of well-diagnosed cases from one research hospital (in Roswell Park Memorial Institute).[17] With the exception of that regarding bladder cancer, these results have been replicated in national mortality studies using less accurate death certificate information as to diagnosis, but a much more representative population.[18]

Especially useful in ethnic investigation may be the analysis of international distributions of disease. There are two major sources of these for cancer, first, the World Health Organization collection, based on age-adjusted mortality statistics from 1952 to 1956,[19] and Mitsuo Segi's 1964 collation of age-adjusted mortality data from registrars of vital statistics in countries throughout the world.[20] Comparisons of mortality data from one country to another may be biased because of variations among countries in diagnostic habits, therapeutic effectiveness, survivorship and reporting systems. Nevertheless, where mortality differences among countries are large and where case-fatality rates are high, as with the cancers discussed below, comparisons of mortality rates are useful in suggesting areas for further research.

Figure 2–8 lists the three sites of cancer among males for which countries reported the largest differences in mortality. France, for example, reported about 9 deaths for cancer of the larynx per 100,000, whereas Norway reported 0.40. France's rate thus was 22.5 times that of Norway. It is noteworthy that the countries reporting the four highest rates of laryngeal cancer are all

17 Graham, S., M. Levin, A. Lilienfeld and P. Sheehe, "Ethnic Derivation As Related to Cancer at Various Sites," *Cancer*, 16: 13–27, January, 1963.
18 Haenzel, W., "Social Factors in Cancer Epidemiology," *J. NCI*, vol. 26, no. 1, January, 1961.
19 World Health Organization, *Epidemiological and Vital Statistics Report*, 12: 171–226, 1959.
20 Segi, M., and M. Kurihara, "Cancer Mortality for Selected Sites in 24 Countries," no. 3 (1960–1961), Sendai, Japan: Tohoku University School of Medicine, March, 1964.

Latinate: France, Portugal, Italy and Belgium. Among many other traits they have in common, they are all wine-drinking countries. Both Wynder in the United States and Schwartz in France found an increased risk for cancer of the larynx among heavy drinkers of alcohol, particularly wine, when adjusted for smoking.[21,22] This may suggest that wine-drinking patterns in these countries should be investigated to see whether they figure in the etiology of the disease. It is interesting, on the other hand, that three of the four countries with the lowest rates reported are Scandinavian: Denmark, Sweden and Norway. Explanations of the possible reason for such uniformly low rates in countries which are hardly abstemious might furnish clues as to the etiology of this disease.

pared with non-Jews. It is noteworthy that populations with high and low mortality from cancer of the prostate also have high and low mortality from cancer of another sexual site, the cervix.

We might speculate that the United States non-white population is exposed to a carcinogenic agent which is present in smaller degree in Japan and among Jews. Using the virus hypothesis described above, one might also speculate that this agent could be transferred from one sex to another and perhaps stimulate development of cancer in these sexually related sites. Smegma could be a vector carrying this agent to susceptible

FIGURE 2-8   International differences in mortality, males 1958-9

Site of Cancer	Highest Mortality	Rate/ 100,000	Lowest Mortality	Rate/ 100,000	Ratio
Larynx	France	8.98	Norway	0.40	22.45
Prostate	U.S. Non-White	22.80	Japan	1.39	16.40
Thyroid	Switzerland	1.52	Japan	0.17	8.94

The highest rate reported for cancer of the prostate, that of the United States non-white, is 16 times the Japanese rate. Quisenberry, studying Hawaii, also found low rates for the Japanese living there as compared to the Caucasoid populations.[23] The country with the third lowest rate is Israel; this is consistent with findings on Jews in the United States.

Figure 2–9 presents WHO data on cancer of the cervix and shows that the U.S. non-white population has the highest rate, whereas the Japanese and Israeli rate is low. Israel's low rate is reminiscent of the findings already presented on Jews as com-

[21] Wynder, E., I. Bross, and E. Day, "A Study of Environmental Factors in Cancer of the Srynx," *Cancer*, vol. 9, no. 1, January–February, 1956.

[22] Schwartz, D., J. Lellouch, R. Flamant, and P. F. Denoix, "Alcohol et Cancer Resultats d'Une Enquete Retrospective," *Revue Francaise d'Etudes Cliniques et Biologiques*, 7: 590–604, 1962.

[23] Quisenberry, W. B., "Sociocultural Factors in Cancer in Hawaii," *Ann. N.Y. Acad. Sci.*, 84: 795–806, December 8, 1960.

tissues. Associated with poor hygiene and lack of circumcision, smegma has been found carcinogenic to the cervices of some strains of mice, and it may also be oncogenic to the human cervix. Lack of circumcision, venereal infections, poor penile hygiene and smegma are also possibly related to cancer of the penis, and may partially explain the higher penile cancer rate among United States non-whites as compared with whites. One might well question whether these factors could be related to high rates of cancer of the prostate, penis and cervix

FIGURE 2-9   Mortality from cancer of cervix

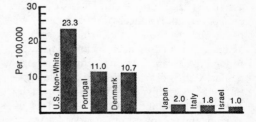

in non-whites. Nevertheless, it is clear that research is needed to examine further this coincidence of high and low rates for different, but sexually related, sites in the same national and religious populations.

Figure 2-10 shows that Denmark's rate

FIGURE 2-10   Mortality from cancer of breast, females

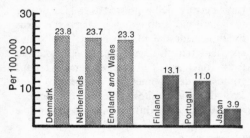

of mortality from breast cancer is six times that of the country reporting the lowest rate, Japan. The Netherlands and England and Wales have the second and third highest rates. Of the nine countries having highest mortality from this disease, six are of English derivation. It is interesting that Haenszel, studying mortality from the majority of states in the United States, also found a high rate for English-born Americans. As noted earlier, some of our research suggested that an increase in risk is associated with each year of menstruation experienced by females and a decrease with each month of nursing. Applying this model to the Japanese nursing and menstrual experience, as reported by Wynder and Segi, we developed an expected ratio of differences between the Japanese and the United States mortality from breast cancer which was very close to that actually observed.[8]

One of the most interesting sites, as far as ethnic and cross-cultural distributions are concerned, is cancer of the stomach. We have already noted that this disease is associated with low socio–economic status, foreign birth and, among females in particular, Polish birth. Figures show the highest male mortality rates to be reported by Japan, Finland and Austria, as well as by Poland, and the lowest by Canada, Australia, New Zealand the United States whites. The

fact that countries with lowest rates are English in origin suggests the possibility that their cultures possess a protective characteristic.

Japan's mortality, on the other hand, was five times higher than that of the country reporting lowest mortality, the United States, for both males and females. Smith, studying mortality among Japanese in Japan, Hawaii and the West Coast of the United States, found a lower rate in Hawaii than in Japan, and a lower rate on the West Coast of the United States than in Hawaii.[24] West Coast Japanese still had much higher rates than Caucasians. Inasmuch as all these groups are full-blooded Japanese and probably genetically similar, there may be some sociological factor which can explain the differences. Perhaps it is one which is abandoned in increasing degree as the Japanese move east and adopt American culture. It is possible, of course, that migrating Japanese are different genetically from non-migrating ones and that this difference may be related to gastric cancer. Nevertheless, several investigators have suggested sociological traits to explain the high rate of cancer among the Japanese.

For example, Segi, studying a number of factors among cases and controls in Japan, found that the ingestion of alcohol seemed to carry a higher risk of gastric cancer, as did eating at irregular intervals.[25] Research on Roswell Park patients reinforced the hypothesis regarding irregular eating and tentatively implicated two elements frequently found in Polish diets: cabbage and potatoes.[26] In addition, there is some evidence that high rates may occur in the Polynesian people, such as the Maori and Hawaiians, as compared with the whites of New Zealand and Hawaii, respectively.[27]

[24] Smith, R. L., "Recorded and Expected Mortality Among the Japanese of the United States and Hawaii with Special Reference to Cancer," *J. NCI*, vol. 17, no. 4, October, 1956.

[25] Segi, M., I. Fukushima, S. Fujisaku, M. Kurihara, S. Saito, K. Asano and M. Kamoi, "An Epidemiological Study of Cancer in Japan," *Gann*, vol. 48, supplement, April, 1957.

[26] Graham, S., A. Lilienfeld and J. Tidings, "Dietary and Purgation Factors in the Epidemiology of Gastric Cancer," *Cancer*, 20: 2224–2234, December, 1967.

[27] Richard Rose, personal communication.

More research into the diets of these groups is needed, but there is some evidence that they are low in ascorbic acid and very high in carbohydrates.

It is apparent that the variety of ethnic differences in gastric cancer mortality rates demands elucidation and that in doing so new suggestions about etiologic factors in this disease may be obtained. Dietary folkways and dental characteristics may have the greatest potentialities for this because of their influence on the kind of substances brought into contact with the gastric mucosa.

Investigations of the various other sociological relationships that were discussed earlier might shed light on the etiology of cancer of the larynx, bladder, mouth, esophagus, stomach, colon, breast, cervix and prostate. This work has only begun. The kinds of variables examined have been few and limited to the "obvious" ones. Even for the results reported above, the wary writer will have had to be careful to hedge almost all statements with cautions. Attempts to explain the socio–biological relationships which have been found most usually have not been made, and where they have, as in the case of gastric cancer, frequently have been only partially successful.

On the bright (but by no means roseate) side, suggestions exist that further investigation of some of the relationships reported here might elucidate the chain of events leading to these diseases. The process is exceedingly slow: The studies in Buffalo described above have required about ten years to complete. Nevertheless, parallel work on these diseases will proceed in the various laboratory approaches. Hopefully these will suggest new hypotheses which can be translated into sociological and epidemiological terms and then tested. Similarly, as has already happened in several instances, the human findings can suggest hypotheses of interest to bio-chemists, geneticists and others. The limited but significant progress in the knowledge of lung cancer etiology is the result in large part, but certainly not wholly, of sociological epidemiology. It implies that this approach may be able to contribute to enlightenment about other diseases as well.

3

IN ITS REPORT, "National Goals in Air Pollution Research," the Surgeon General's Ad Hoc Task Group on Air Pollution Research Goals states: "The aspects of air pollution which are most apparent and of greatest personal concern to the individual probably are irritation to the eyes, nose, and throat, malodors, and the reduction of visibility. The pollutants responsible for these effects are undesirable whether or not they cause long-range health effects or economic losses, because they constitute an annoyance to people. The nuisance aspects of these effects together with those related to soiling give rise to the greatest number of complaints received by air pollution control authorities. There is no doubt that a person's well-being is eventually affected by exposure to these sensory annoyances and that this may result in economic loss."[1]

By conceptualizing certain aspects of air pollution in terms of "sensory annoyances," and by postulating a relationship between these annoyances and "a person's well-being," this statement clearly introduces a behavioral variable, the individual's definition of his situation, into the standard organismic paradigm of physical stimulus leading to physiological response, that has traditionally guided research on environmental health problems. Here a study is reported, that made an attempt to explore the behavioral variables of situation-defining in relation to a specific environmental stress, sulfate malodors associated with kraft pulp mill operation. Because of the small size of sample and universe, the results of the study are presented less for their substantive than for their methodological and conceptual implications relative to social science research on environmental health problems. These implications will be discussed under the following heads: scale analysis of awareness, and of concern, with air pollution; community satisfaction, and the concern with air pollution; the analysis of action potential with reference to environmental stress; ecological and social status variables in air pollution awareness and concern; and air pollution as an eco-system variable.

[1] "National Goals in Air Pollution Research," USPHS, August 1960, pp. 20–21.

Air Pollution as a Socio-Environmental Health Problem: A Survey Report

Nahum Z. Medalia

The Problem and Its Setting

In response to long-standing complaints of poor ambient air quality in X-ville,[2] a state public health agency undertook an aerometric survey in the town between the months of November, 1961 and April, 1962. X-ville with 5,000 population, lies in a river valley, separated by a small tributary from Y-town, with approximately 25,000 population. The X-ville complaints centered on malodors attributed to the stack effluent of a kraft pulp mill located three miles upwind, just outside Y-town. This mill, the Z Company, was built in 1951, and it provided the single largest source of employment for Y-town, though not for X-ville. Random interviews by state health officials in X-ville disclosed that residents used "the mill" as a generic term for malodors in the area— thus they would say " 'the mill' is pretty bad," or "not so bad, today."

Since residents expressed annoyance, principally with sulfate-type malodors, continuous measures of the hydrogen-sulfide (H_2S) level were made in X-ville, over a six-month

[2] To comply with the request of one of the health agencies that sponsored this survey, actual names of the two communities affected by air pollution, as well as of the major source implicated, have been deleted.

From Journal of Health & Human Behavior, *Vol. 5: 154–165, Winter, 1964; by permission of the author and publisher.*

period. These measures, taken by standard open air sampling techniques, revealed only rarely H_2S concentrations in excess of odor thresholds established by controlled psychometric study. Such a result was not unexpected, since the odors most characteristic of wood pulping have their source in minute traces of complex sulfur compounds, or mercaptans, impossible to detect by continuous air sampling techniques.[3] Measurement of hydrogen-sulfide level can serve at best only as a rough index of the presence of mercaptans in ambient air. Under these circumstances, the opinions of X-ville residents became the single best indicator of the environmental stresses which they claimed to experience, presumably in the form of sulfate malodors.

Survey Objectives and Methods

In designing a survey to assess these opinions, the factor of environmental stress or annoyance was conceptualized along two dimensions of variation: "awareness" and "concern." The survey's primary objective thus became determination of the nature and extent of awareness and concern with air pollution, on the part of X-ville residents. Also included was an effort to determine the nature of actions taken, planned, or recommended as desirable, by members of the X-ville population, with reference to air pollution. A second objective was to determine what associations might exist between the dependent variables: awareness and concern with air pollution; and demographic and socio–economic characteristics of the X-ville population.

The most important procedural consideration in questionnaire design was to ensure that respondents would never be put into the position of having to say that air pollution was a problem, or even existed, in X-ville; secondly, by focusing the interview at the outset on general community health

problems, to give respondents an opportunity to bring up air pollution spontaneously as such a problem. These measures aimed at avoiding an over-estimation of awareness and concern with air pollution, in X-ville. To avoid bias in the opposite direction, semi-projective questions were employed, of the type, "what do you think 'most people' (or significant others—e.g., doctors, local newspapers, local industries) feel about air pollution in this area?"

Heads of households and their spouses constituted the sampling universe. A randomized cluster approach based on areal stratification yielded 104 households for the sample. Within households, interviewers contacted heads and spouses alternately. Interviewers identified themselves as working for the state health department in conducting "a survey of health conditions in X-ville."[4]

Awareness of Air Pollution

At the outset, the survey found widespread awareness of the existence of air pollution in X-ville: approximately 80 per cent of respondents agreed to the question, "do you think there is air pollution in X-ville at any time during the year?" To gain some idea of the cognitive dimensions of this awareness, interviewers asked, "what do you think the words 'air pollution' mean to most people in this area?" Five fixed responses were provided: Frequent bad smells in the air; too much dirt and dust in the air; frequent haze or fog in the air; frequent irritation of the eyes; frequent nose and throat irritation.

Distribution of the sample as between these responses led to the inference that in cognitive terms, X-ville residents structured air pollution primarily as an odor problem (91 per cent of sample); secondarily as a problem of visibility (74 per cent); thirdly as a problem of nose and throat irritation (62 per cent); while a minority perceived it as "frequent irritation of eyes" (40 per cent); and as dustfall (27 per cent).

A second inference was that more people

---

[3] Dallavalle, J. M., and H. C. Dudley, "Evaluation of Odor Nuisance in the Manufacture of Kraft Paper," *Pub. Health Reps.*, 54: 2, January, 1939.

[4] Sampling design, sample selection, and interviewer training and supervision were all under the direction of Dr. A. L. Finkner, Research Triangle Institute, North Carolina.

were aware of the existence of "frequent bad smells" in X-ville air, than of "air pollution"—91 per cent as against 79 per cent, to judge by the sample. More exactly, although 21 per cent of the sample reported air pollution non-existent in X-ville, only 9 per cent said "most people in the X-ville area" would fail to associate "frequent bad smells" with the words "air pollution."

A third inference was that to members of the sample, the five listed dimensions of air pollution stood in a systematic rather than random relationship to one another; and that the model for this relationship was given by a Guttman scale of the following pattern:[5]

"To most people in this area, air pollution means:*

to them were worked out from the survey data with the following results:[6]

Perfect Scale Pattern	Per Cent Respondents
5	11.5
4	17.3
3	14.4
2	15.3
1	12.5
0	0.9

Total – 71.9 per cent

Seventy-two per cent of respondents, in other words, fell into one or another of the six perfect scale types; of these (N = 75),

Dust in Air	Eye Irritation	Nose Irritation	Haze, Fog	Bad Smells	"Perfect" Scale Type
+	+	+	+	+	5
—	+	+	+	+	4
—	—	+	+	+	3
—	—	—	+	+	2
—	—	—	—	+	1
—	—	—	—	—	0

* " + " means " Yes ".
  " — " means " No ".

Existence of such a systematic relationship between these five dimensions of air pollution was believed to imply further that the significance ("meaning") of air pollution to X-ville residents would represent a response to some factor or complex of factors in their environment which operated in a systematic way upon them all; rather than a response to factors idiosyncratic or randomly variable in their effect upon X-ville residents. The survey made no attempt to specify the nature of this factor, or complex of factors. However, monotonically increasing sensitivity, physiological in origin, to irritants in X-ville ambient air would be one example of such a factor; institutionalized consensus among X-ville residents as to the meaning of air pollution, would be another.

To test the inference of scalability on the Guttman model, among these five dimensions of air pollution, the response patterns

45, or 60 per cent fell into types 3, 4, and 5 —i.e., said that to most people in the X-ville area, "air pollution" meant at least frequent nose and throat irritation; frequent haze or fog in the air; and frequent bad smells in the air. Only one person (0.9 per cent of the entire sample) said that the words "air pollution" meant none of the phenomena listed in item 20, to "most people" in the X-ville area.

Examination of the total array of responses disclosed that the largest number not conforming to the hypothesized scale pattern related to the item, "too much dust and dirt in the air"; the next largest, to "frequent haze or fog in the air." These facts indicate that to this sample of respondents, eye irritation, nose–throat irritation, and malodors stand in a more consistent or systematic relationship with each other as dimensions of air pollution, than they do with the

[5] See M. W. Riley, *et al.*, *Sociological Studies in Scale Analysis*, New Brunswick, N.J.: Rutgers University Press, 1954.

[6] For computation methods see Ake, J. N., "A Rapid Machine Procedure for Determining Scalability of Any Number of Questions," *Pub. Opin. Quart.*, Fall, 1947, pp. 412–423.

dimensions of low visibility and dustfall. Furthermore, the low frequency of association of air pollution with dustfall (27 per cent "Yes" to 20b), coupled with the fact that 11 per cent of responses to the dust-fall item are discrepant by Guttman scale criteria, leads to the inference that the response to air pollution as "dust-fall" is a relatively idiosyncratic one, among X-ville residents; or else is a response to some factor that operates selectively on some respondents but not on others.

Nevertheless, when the non-scale response patterns were converted to scale patterns by the conventional "least-error" technique, and "error" frequencies related to total response possibilities, the five items, even including that on dustfall, formed an acceptable Guttman Scale by the criterion of reproducibility, the coefficient for which was 0.94. The distribution of the entire sample among the six possible scale types, both "perfect" and "imperfect," was:

The previous section showed the use of Guttman object–scale analysis to clarify not only the level but also the cognitive dimensions of awareness of air pollution on the part of X-ville residents; the present section reports a similar approach towards clarifying the level and cathectic structure of their "concern" with air pollution.

Four questionnaire items served as basis for this analysis, each taken to represent a different aspect of "concern": item 3a, "spontaneous mention of air pollution as a disadvantage to living in X-ville," the aspect of salience of concern; item 11, belief or disbelief in existence of air pollution, the aspect of awareness as such; item 13, extent to which "bothered" by air pollution, the element of personal concern; item 21, "is air pollution now, or has it become a problem in this area," the aspect of concern with such pollution as a community problem.

To facilitate analysis, responses to these four items were dichotomized according to

"Perfect" and "Imperfect" Scale Type	N Respondents	Per Cent Respondents
5	16	15.3
4	22	21.2
3	25	24.1
2	23	22.2
1	14	13.4
0	4	3.8
Total	104	100.0

This analysis concluded that although 20 per cent of the sample claimed air pollution non-existent in X-ville, the term "air pollution" did represent a well-structured concept to most X-ville residents; and that the most salient features of this concept were malodors, low visibility and nose–throat irritation.

whether or not they indicated concern with air pollution. This dichotomization, and the resulting distribution of responses appears in Table 3–1, ordered by frequency of responses indicating "concern."

This ordering of items by response frequencies generates the following response patterns on the hypothesis of perfect scalability:

Item No.				"Perfect"
3A	21	13	11	Scale Type
+	+	+	+	4
—	+	+	+	3
—	—	+	+	2
—	—	—	+	1
—	—	—	—	0

(+ is response indicating awareness or concern with air pollution)

Turning to the actual data, 83 per cent of the sample gave responses which fell into one of the five perfect scale types. The total array of actual response patterns, both "perfect" and "imperfect," yielded a coefficient of reproducibility of 0.96, well above the conventionally established lower limit of 0.90 for accepting the hypothesis of scalability. The largest number of responses that did not conform to the hypothesized scale pattern related to the spontaneous mention of air pollution as a disadvantage (item 3a). This fact suggests the possibility that such mentions, however valid as an index of the *salience* of a concern, may be misleading if taken to indicate the *seriousness* of that concern to a respondent. In the present instance, over a fourth of those who mentioned air pollution spontaneously as a disadvantage to living in X-ville, said in answer to item 21, that air pollution either was not a serious problem or was becoming a less serious problem each year, in that area. Even so, this scale provides possibly the best single index of the proportion of X-ville residents disturbed by air pollution. According to the distribution, 20, or a fifth of the scalable subjects, fall in Scale Type 0: they show no, or practically no awareness of or concern with air pollution in X-ville. By contrast, 76, or four-fifths of the scalable subjects, are concerned to some degree by air pollution in X-ville. For the 12 subjects in Type 1 the level of such concern may be regarded as "low"; for the 18 in Type 2, "moderate"; while the 46 subjects in Types 3 and 4 can be called "very concerned" with air pollution in X-ville.

Community Satisfaction and Concern with Air Pollution

It is noteworthy that awareness and concern with air pollution were expressed in this survey, against a background of general satisfaction with X-ville as a community: 85 per cent of the sample said X-ville was an "excellent" or "good" place to live; 10 per cent claimed it was "fair"; only 4 per cent answered "poor" or "very poor." When asked "what are some of the things you like about living in X-ville," only 6 were unable to specify some reason for liking their community. Of the remaining 98 subjects, 38 mentioned first some attribute of the community (e.g., good schools, small size, churches, parks, good government, nice physical appearance). An almost equal number, 35, mentioned first the climate or weather of X-ville as an advantage. Of the remaining subjects, 18 listed first some attribute of the people in the community (e.g., their "friendliness" or "neighborliness"), 3 mentioned "recreational opportunities," 4 gave advantages not classified under any of the above categories. Taking account of advantages in addition to those mentioned first by respondents (i.e., second and third mentions), the picture of X-ville as a "good community" in the opinion of this sample, becomes even clearer. Of the total number of X-ville advantages that

Table 3–1—Responses indicating concern or lack of concern with air pollution

Item	Responses Indicating Concern with Air Pollution	N: Respondents	Responses Indicating Absence of Concern with Air Pollution	N: Respondents
3A	All spontaneous mention of air pollution as a "disadvantage"	34	No spontaneous mention, air pollution as a "disadvantage"	70
21	Air pollution has continuously been a serious problem for this area; air pollution has become a more serious problem each year for this area	53	Air pollution has not been a serious problem; air pollution has become a less serious problem each year, for this area	45
13	I have been somewhat bothered; I have been bothered quite a lot, by air pollution	66	I have not been bothered by air pollution	37
11	Yes (i.e., air pollution exists in X-ville)	81	No (i.e., air pollution does not exist in X-ville)	22

respondents mentioned spontaneously (N = 188) 71 or 38 per cent concern community attributes. "Climate and weather" remains in second place as an advantage with 26 per cent of total mentions; while 22 per cent of the mentions concern attributes of the people in X-ville.

Three analyses undertook to clarify the relation of X-ville residents' satisfaction with their community, to their concern with air pollution. The first of these furnished confirmation of results obtained in the 1956 California Health Survey, "Air Pollution Effects Reported by California Residents."[7]

According to that study, "those affected by air pollution were more prone to report dissatisfaction with their community. In Los Angeles County 21 per cent said they were not satisfied with the local area in which they lived. Among respondents bothered by air pollution, the proportion was 25 per cent but only 13 per cent among those not bothered by air pollution. The difference was even greater in the San Francisco Bay

A second study of the relation of concern with air pollution to community satisfaction produced negative results: the analysis of seriousness of concern with air pollution among those who spontaneously mentioned the X-ville climate as an advantage to living there, compared to those who did not. To account for this relationship, two alternate hypotheses seemed equally plausible: (1) persons who like X-ville because of its climate, are insensitive to, or not bothered by, the air pollution that may exist in the area; or (2) persons who like the X-ville climate are more concerned with air pollution than those who are indifferent, or negative to it, because such pollution may detract from the climatic advantages they prize.

In the present case, the data show that neither hypothesis is tenable, at the conventional 0.05 level of statistical significance (see Table 3–2). At most, one can say that the distribution by spontaneous mention of climate as an advantage, of persons at the extremes of air pollution concern (Scale Types 0 and 4) is suggestive of the second hypothesis.

Table 3–2—Concern with air pollution, by spontaneous mention of climate as advantage

| | GUTTMAN SCALE (a): CONCERN WITH AIR POLLUTION | | |
Spontaneous Mention, Climate as Advantage	None Type 0	Low to High Types 1–3	Very High Type 4
Yes	7	25	13
No	13	29	9

Statistical analysis: X^2 not significant.

area: 37—14 per cent; and in the rest of the State: 30 to 16 per cent."

Although the proportion dissatisfied with their community is only two-thirds in X-ville what it was in Los Angeles (14 per cent versus 21 per cent), the ratio, community dissatisfaction among those "concerned"* to community dissatisfaction among those not "concerned"† with air pollution, was found to be approximately the same for X-ville as for Los Angeles—i.e., 2 to 1.

[7] "Air Pollution Effects Reported by California Residents," from The California Health Survey, State of California Dept. of Public Health, 1956.
*Scale types 3 and 4.
†Scale types 0, 1 and 2.

The final approach to the "community satisfaction–concern with air pollution" relationship was through analysis of responses made to the opening question, "are there some things (or, what are some of the things) you don't like about living in X-ville?" This analysis disclosed first, that as one might expect, the proportion of respondents who list "no disadvantages" varies directly with their rating of X-ville: 44 per cent among those who rate X-ville "excellent"; 30 per cent among those who rate it "good"; 13 per cent who rate X-ville "fair," "poor," or "very poor," list no disadvantages to living there.

The data also show that a somewhat higher percentage of those who rate X-ville

"Fair," "Poor," or "Very Poor," mention air pollution spontaneously as a community disadvantage, than do those in the other two rating groups: 40 per cent compared to approximately a third among those who rate X-ville "Excellent" or "Good."

Of greater significance, however, is that the ratio of persons who spontaneously mention air pollution *only* as an X-ville disadvantage, to respondents who spontaneously mention *some other* disadvantage, either alone or in combination with air pollution, is much higher among those who rate X-ville "Excellent," than among those who rate it "Good" or "Fair, etc.": 8/7 compared to 2/7 and 4/9, respectively. This finding indicates that for persons who are highly identified with their community, in the sense that they express high satisfaction with it as a place to live, air pollution tends to be *salient* as a source of annoyance or disturbance; while persons less strongly tied to their community tend to think of air pollution as only one of a complex of disadvantages they sense with community living. On the other hand, this analysis points up again the need to distinguish the *salience* of a phenomenon from its *seriousness*, as a source of concern. Air pollution, that is, may be more salient as a source of disturbance to people who rate their community an "excellent" place to live, than to people who rate it as only "good," "fair," or "poor"—in the sense that air pollution is the only disadvantage such persons may openly associate with that community. This does not necessarily mean, however, that air pollution is a more serious source of concern to them, than to persons who are less identified with the community—in the sense that they feel there is a greater need to "do something" about it.

Potential for Action with Respect to Air Pollution

From the foregoing sections there emerges the outline of a problem situation of concern in some degree to four-fifths of the sample of X-ville household heads; as with any problem situation, action with reference to it may be classified broadly into two types:

situation–withdrawal, or redefining; and situation–altering. "Withdrawal" may be cognitive, cathectic, or physical conditional in nature: i.e., it may take the form of denial that the situation exists; denial of emotions which it arouses; or physical removal from the problem–situation. "Situation–altering," the second possibility, may also be considered along a variety of dimensions, such as individualistic-collectivistic; active–passive; problem–source oriented, problem–effect oriented. Of these possibilities, the X-ville survey considered chiefly the potential for situation–altering action that was source–oriented in nature.

The first step was to discover to what extent respondents felt the situation could be altered, from a technical point of view. For this reason they were asked: "Do you believe that air pollution in X-ville . . .

a) *Cannot* be reduced below its present level?
b) *Can* be reduced below its present level?
c) Can be *almost completely eliminated*?"

Replies to this item show that only 4 per cent of the subjects who believed air pollution existed in X-ville took the position that it could *not* be further reduced, while 14 per cent said they didn't know. By contrast, 58 per cent felt air pollution *could* be reduced, and 21 per cent felt it could be almost completely eliminated in X-ville.

Next, interviewers asked respondents, "Which one of these statements do you think *best* describes the effort (each of the pollution sources respondent mentioned) is making to control air pollution in this area?" Considering only figures for the Z-mill, nearly three-fourths of those who listed it as a pollution source said to varying degrees that it was "not doing as much as it should" to control air pollution in X-ville.

These two sets of data led to the inference that a relatively high potential for situation–altering actions existed in X-ville, with reference to the air pollution problem. Eighty per cent of respondents who recognize the existence of such a problem say it can be ameliorated; 75 per cent of those who consider the Z-mill as principal source of the problem say it is not doing as much as it should towards such amelioration.

To explore the ways in which this action–potential might take expression the sample was asked:

"What do you think is the *most important* thing people should do about air pollution where it exists?" One emotional withdrawal possibility was offered: "Put their minds on their work instead of on imagined or minor annoyances"; and one situation–defining or redefining alternative: "Try to get more information on the subject." The other two alternatives were more situation–altering in nature although differing on the dimension of activity–passivity: i.e., "Support the efforts which industry is making to eliminate air pollution" (passive); "Ask their elected officials for effective controls on air pollution" (active).

pondents in the "low concern" category; while the latter are five times as likely to favor situation–defining or withdrawal actions.

Awareness and Concern with Air Pollution, in Relation to Ecological and Social Status Characteristics

The present section attempts to relate the variations in awareness and concern with air pollution found among the sample to demographic characteristics of the respondents who express them. This attempt is not presented in any sense as an "explanation" of variations in the attitudes under scrutiny, but only as a necessary first step in arriving at such explanation.

The first set of respondents' characteristics examined is the ecological; i.e., respondents' geographic location with reference to presumed sources of pollution in X-ville, and to topographic features of

Table 3–3—Recommended action re air pollution, by concern with air pollution (scale type a)

Action Recommended	SCALE TYPE (a): CONCERN WITH AIR POLLUTION Low (Types 0–2)	High (Types 3–4)	Totals
Put mind on work	6	0	6
Support industry efforts	19	16	35
Ask for effective controls	9	25	34
Get more information	14	4	18
Totals	48 *	45†	93

Statistical analysis: X^2 significant at 0.05 level.
* 2—"other".
† 1—"other".

Distribution of respondents as among these possibilities shows that while the sample favors situation–altering actions over the other types by a ratio of 3 to 1, it is fairly evenly divided as between the active and passive choices for situation–altering. This equivalence, however, disappears when the various types of actions recommended are analyzed by Scale Type for Concern with Air Pollution (Table 3–3). According to Table 3–3, persons who show high concern over air pollution in X-ville, are three times as likely to recommend the alternative of asking for effective controls, as are res-

significance in the meteorological diffusion of pollutants.

Previous studies have documented an ecological component in levels of exposure, by residence, to different types of ambient air pollution.[8] That component follows roughly

[8] Smith, W. S., L. D. Zeidberg and J. J. Schueneman, "The Public Reaction to Air Pollution in Nashville, Tenn.," Cincinnati, Ohio, May 9, 1963 (unpublished); W. Winkelstein, Jr., and I. de Groot, "The Erie County Air Pollution–Pulmonary Function Study: Study Design and Selected Preliminary Findings"; (mimeo)— Table 1, Erie County Health Dept., Buffalo, N.Y. (no date).

the pattern one would expect, reasoning from the concentric zone model of urban development advanced by E. W. Burgess:[9] i.e., of decreasing levels of exposure with increasing radial distances from the center of the city, and increasing socio–economic levels of its inhabitants. Differential exposure to particulates appears to follow this pattern more closely than does exposure to gaseous pollutants such as sulfates.[10]

In view of these findings, it seemed reasonable to attempt to relate awareness and concern with air pollution, on the part of X-ville residents, with their differential residential location. Examination of the contour map of the X-ville area shows that with six minor exceptions, all of the 20 potential air pollution sources of an industrial nature are located North, Northeast, or Northwest of the city limits of X-ville. In addition, a rise in altitude of approximately 150 feet occurs from the northern to the southern boundaries of the city although this gradient is of a very gradual nature.

Based on these two facts, a North–South division seemed the most likely to provide differences in residential exposure to pollutants, on the one hand; and differences in awareness of and concern with such exposure, on the other, on the part of sample members.

Turning now to responses of sample members in these two geographical areas, the major finding is that they show no significant differences in recognition of the existence of air pollution, or in concern with it as a personal or community problem. Sample members in the northern sector are divided on a 50–50 basis as between scale types indicating high concern (3, 4) and low (0, 1, 2). In the southern sector there is a slight preponderance of respondents in the low concern over the high concern scale types, in the ratio of 13–11. So far as sheer awareness, or recognition of air pollution is concerned, 10 respondents in the northern, and 13 in the southern sections of X-ville say air pollution does not exist in the X-ville area.

[9] "The Growth of the City," in R. E. Park, ed., *The City*, Chicago: Univ. of Chicago Press, 1925.

[10] Winkelstein, *et al.*, *op. cit.*

This finding throws into relief the significance of factors other than exposure to pollutants "objectively" present in ambient air that may underlie variations in expressed concern with air pollution as a personal and community problem. These are the factors of personality, social status, and culture, approached through behavioral rather than physical science. The relatively small size of sample precluded detailed examination of these factors in the present case; an attempt, however, was made to analyze variations in "concern" with air pollution in relation to three social status variables: occupation of household head; sex of respondent; and respondent's status with respect to length of residence in X-ville.

Social Status Variables in Relation to Concern with Air Pollution

Before proceeding to the findings on relationship of these social status variables to concern with air pollution, some explanation is in order of the selection of the variables themselves.

"Occupation of household head," rather than occupation of respondent, was selected because of its strategic position as indicator and determinant of the general cultural outlook of a household or family, commonly associated with its social class position. "Length of residence" is regarded here primarily as a social status variable, in the sense that it differentiates "old-timers" or "old settlers," from the relative "newcomers" to an area. To an undetermined extent, however, it is possible that "length of residence" may also be an indicator of different types or degrees of physiological adaptation to environmental conditions such as air pollution. Sex also is regarded here primarily as a social status rather than as a physiological variable, although here again it is possible that physiological differences associated with sex may enter into differential sensitivity to environmental conditions.

such as air pollution, independently of the behavior and culture patterns associated with sex as a status. The general findings on the relation of these three variables to concern with air pollution may be stated very simply in four propositions: (1) The "higher" the occupational level of the household head, the greater is the concern with air pollution which is expressed by the head or his spouse. (2) The longer the respondent's period of residence in X-ville, the greater is his concern with air pollution in that city. (3) The differentiation in concern with air pollution by occupational group becomes more pronounced with length of residence in X-ville —i.e., occupational status and length of residence status interact positively in relation to concern with air pollution. (4) There is no difference in the degree of concern with air pollution expressed by men and by women in the sample. These propositions are elaborated in the succeeding sections of the report.

OCCUPATION OF HOUSEHOLD HEAD
AS FACTOR IN CONCERN WITH
AIR POLLUTION

Three categories graded by social status or prestige constituted the occupational variables:

a) Managers, proprietors, professionals
b) Clerical and skilled labor
c) Semi-skilled and unskilled workers

Twenty-four respondents were classified in the first category; 37 in the second; and 26 in the third. Seventeen members of the sample fall outside the range of the occupational variable, since they were not in the labor market (NILM): household heads so classified were for the most part retired. Very little difference appears between respondents in the three occupational categories, so far as sheer awareness, or recognition of air pollution in X-ville is concerned. Among professionals and managers, 22 say air pollution exists in X-ville; 2 say it does not. Corresponding figures for the clerical and labor categories are 29 to 8, and 21 to 4.

Only among NILM's does the ratio, recognition–non-recognition, approach equality, at 9 to 8.

Similar distributions in the three occupational categories are also observed in response to questionnaire item 13, how much bothered by air pollution. As between the responses, "not bothered," "somewhat bothered," "bothered quite a lot," professionals, etc., are distributed 2–16–4; clerical workers, etc., 7–16–6; semi-skilled and unskilled, 5–14–2.

With respect to all other indices of concern with air pollution, however, respondents in the professional–managerial categories distribute themselves in a markedly different way from those in the other two occupational classes. Professionals, managers and proprietors are found nearly 4 times as frequently in scale types indicating high phenomenal awareness, as in the low (19 to 5). Among clerical workers and laborers, this ratio is approximately equal (20–17, 13–13). Twice as many professionals, managers and proprietors are in the "high concern" types of Guttman Scale (a) as in the low; 15 to 7. Among clerical and skilled labor respondents, this ratio is 17 to 19; for laborers it is 9 to 13. Respondents in the professional–managerial group are much more apt to say that they worry about the effects of air pollution on health, and on property, than are respondents in the clerical, etc., and labor categories, as Tables 3–4 and 3–5 show. They are much more likely to have remembered reading news about air pollution in the local paper (Table 3–6). Finally, professional and managerial respondents are much more likely to rate air pollution as a "serious" problem for X-ville today, than are respondents in the other two categories (Table 3–7). While none of these differences in concern with air pollution by occupation of household head is significant at the 0.05 level, taken together they add up to a picture which is significant, in the writer's opinion: namely, that respondents in the professional and managerial category regard air pollution as a serious problem facing the X-ville community to a much greater extent than do respondents in the other occupational classes. That professional–managerial persons do not at the same time express them-

Table 3—4—Response to item 17: "Do you worry about the effects of air pollution on your health?" by occupation of household head

Occupation of Household Head	WORRY ABOUT AIR POLLUTION RE HEALTH		
	Yes	No	Not Applicable,* Other
Professional, etc.	9	11	4
Clerical, etc.	10	17	10
Labor	3	18	5

Statistical analysis: X^2 not significant.
* Answered "No" to item, "Does air pollution exist in X-ville?"

Table 3—5—Response to item 18: "Do you worry about the effects of air pollution on your property?" by occupation of household head

Occupation of Household Head	WORRY ABOUT AIR POLLUTION RE PROPERTY		
	Yes	No	Not Applicable,* Other
Professional, etc.	12	9	3
Clerical, etc.	12	15	10
Labor	7	11	8

Statistical analysis: X^2 not significant.
* Answered "No" to item, "Does air pollution exist in X-ville?"

Table 3—6—Recent exposure to news about air pollution, by occupation of household head

Occupation of Household Head	RECENT EXPOSURE TO AIR POLLUTION NEWS	
	Yes	No
Professional, etc.	11	13
Clerical, etc.	7	30
Labor	9	17

Statistical analysis: X^2 not significant.

Table 3—7—Concern with air pollution (Guttman Scale (a)) by occupation of household head

Occupation of Household Head	SCALE (a) TYPE: CONCERN WITH AIR POLLUTION	
	Low (Types 0–2)	High (Types 3–4)
Professionals, etc.	7	15
Clerical, etc.	19	17
Labor	13	9

Statistical analysis: X^2 not significant.

selves as being "bothered" to a greater extent by air pollution simply supports the findings of other studies, that such persons are better able to distinguish between "personal" and "community" problems than are members of other occupational classes.[11]

[11] Schatzman, L., and A. Strauss, "Social Class and Modes of Communication," *Amer. J. Sociology*, LX: 329–338, January, 1955.

LENGTH OF RESIDENCE IN X-VILLE AND CONCERN WITH AIR POLLUTION

Theories of adjustment to noxious environmental conditions may be divided roughly into two types, according to whether they posit habituation or exacerbation as the primary adjustive mechanisms. According to theories of the first type, as length of exposure to the noxious condition increases, the condition itself tends to recede into the background of conscious awareness until the individual takes no more notice of the condition than a fish may of water. By contrast, theories of the second type hold that exacerbation with the condition increases with length of exposure to it, to the point where the individual requires change of the environment, or withdrawal from it.

As test of these hypotheses, respondents were divided into two categories by length of residence in X-ville: those who had lived in X-ville in 1950 or before, (N = 40) and those who had moved to X-ville in 1951 or after (N = 64). The second category included 13 respondents who had moved from Y-town to X-ville in 1951 or later.*

On one dimension of the attitudes under consideration, salience of air pollution as a source of "disturbance," very little difference appears between the "old residents" and the "new-comers": 35 per cent of the former, compared to 31 per cent of the latter mentioned air pollution spontaneously as a disadvantage to living in X-ville. On all other dimensions of awareness and concern, however, the old residents distribute themselves very differently from the new. On the dimension, concern with X-ville health problems, the two distributions are significantly different at the 0.05 level; 55 per cent of the old residents compared to 22 per cent of the new, say X-ville has health problems that need correction; nearly two-thirds of the old residents who say X-ville has such problems mentioned either "the mill" or "bad air" spontaneously as a health problem, compared to only 14 per cent of the new-comers who said X-ville had health problems. Twenty-five per cent of the new-comers, compared to 15 per cent of the old residents, say air pollution does not exist at any time in X-ville.† Thirty-five per cent of the old, compared to 17 per cent of the new residents, say air pollution is a "serious" problem for X-ville today; although nearly identical proportions of the old and new residents say it is either a "serious" or a

"somewhat serious" problem—72 per cent versus 70 per cent. Fewer old than new residents think that air pollution is becoming a less serious problem—33 per cent compared to 54 per cent. A significantly larger number of the old residents say they are "somewhat bothered" or "bothered quite a lot" by air pollution in X-ville, than do the new: 74 per cent versus 57 per cent. Significantly more of the old residents fall in the "high concern" scale types than do the new: 63 per cent vs. 38 per cent. Finally, when asked what they think is the most important thing people should do about air pollution where it exists, 45 per cent of the old residents say "ask their elected officials for more effective controls" by comparison to only 28 per cent of the newcomers.

These facts seem to provide fairly solid support for the theory that increasing length of exposure to what is defined as a noxious environmental condition produces increasing exacerbation, rather than habituation to it. A Swedish study of hygienic nuisances from a sulfate pulp mill also provides support for this view. According to its report:

> In answer to the question as to whether the annoyance had changed during the last three months, 5 per cent of those who were annoyed by the odor said that the annoyance had lessened and 22 per cent that it had increased.[12]

However, the facts of the X-ville survey cast some doubt on the validity, if not the veracity, of a further finding of the Swedish study, namely that "among those annoyed, 57 per cent said that they believed they would get used to the malodor."[13]

The facts reported in this survey have nothing to do with differences in residential location, of the old versus the new-comers; actually, a somewhat larger proportion of the former than of the latter, live in the southern half of X-ville (old residents: 17 in north, 23 in south; new residents: 34 in north, 30 in south). However, the differences

*1951 was the date of establishment of Z-mill in Y-town.
†Difference not significant at 0.05 level.

12 "Studies of Hygienic Nuisances of Waste Gases from a Sulfate Pulp Mill (Part I): An Interview Investigation," translation of article by L. Friberg, E. Jousson and B. Cederlof, in *Norsk Hygienisk Tidskrift* (Scandinavian Hygiene Magazine), 41, nos. 3–4, 1960, pp. 41–62.
13 *Ibid.*

in concern with air pollution reported between old and new residents may derive to some extent from differences in their occupational distribution: inasmuch as disproportionately more new than old residents are classified, by occupation of household head, in the clerical–skilled worker and labor categories, although this difference is not significant at the 0.05 level.

To gain some idea of the nature of the interaction between the two variables, length of residence and occupation of household head, so far as this expresses itself in concern with air pollution, Table 3–8 shows the distribution of respondents by occupational categories on Guttman Scale (a), controlled by length of residence. From the distributions in Table 3–8, it appears that length of

difference appeared in both younger and older age groups.[14]

Although the X-ville survey did not analyze response by age, its finding with respect to sex differs markedly from the Swedish results. Briefly, sex of respondent alone does not bear any relationship to differences in concern with air pollution, among the X-ville sample. Among men, 22 fall in the "low concern" types (Types 0–2); 21 in the "high concern" types (3–4). Among women, the corresponding figures are 28 and 25. If anything, men appear to have a greater degree of phenomenal awareness of

Table 3–8—Occupation, household head, by concern with air pollution (Scale a), controlled on length of residence, X-ville

Residence, X-ville
1950 or Before
OCCUPATION OF HOUSEHOLD HEAD

Concern with Air Pollution	Professional, etc.	Clerical, etc.	Labor
Low (Types 0–2)	1	5	4
High (Types 3–4)	9	7	5

1951 or After
OCCUPATION OF HOUSEHOLD HEAD

Concern with Air Pollution	Professional, etc.	Clerical, etc.	Labor
Low	6	14	9
High	6	10	4

residence operates in the same way on all occupational categories: i.e., in the direction of "producing" greater concern with air pollution; although the operation of this factor appears most pronounced in the case of professionals, proprietors, and managers. This observation, however, also leads to the conclusion that the difference in concern with air pollution between old and new residents of X-ville is not simply an artifact of their differential occupational distribution.

Sex of respondents is the final social status variable considered in relation to concern with air pollution. The Swedish study found that more women than men reported annoyance with sulfate odors, and that this

air pollution in X-ville than do women; 64 per cent of men are in the high phenomenal awareness types (3–5), compared to 58 per cent of women (n.s.).

When response by sex is controlled by other social status variables, however, differences do show up in concern with air pollution on the part of men, compared to women. Table 3–9 introduces as control, length of residence in X-ville. These data show that while the length of residence factor operates in the same direction for both men and women, i.e., to "produce" more concern with air pollution, this effect is much greater for men than for women.

[14] *Ibid.*

Air Pollution as an Ecosystem Variable

In a recent article, G. A. Hansen stated: "Since the time the first kraft mill was built back in 1891, the men who operated these mills were well aware of the fact that they had an air pollution problem. . . . Today, even with all of the progress in recent years, most kraft pulp mills are still living with this problem".[15]

research on environmental health problems, this study may be of interest in that it took place under circumstances which dramatized the independence of psycho–social variables (e.g., awareness of environmental pollution, and definition of such pollution as an individual or social problem), from physically defined levels of pollution. The physical level of air pollution in X-ville appears to be roughly a constant for people who live in different areas of the city; and yet phenomenal awareness and concern with it as a problem vary markedly as between socially defined subgroups of the X-ville population.

Table 3–9—Respondent's sex by concern with air pollution, controlled on length of residence, X-ville

Residence, X-ville
1950 or Before

Concern with Air Pollution	RESPONDENT'S SEX	
	Male	Female
Low (0–2)	4 (27%)	10 (44%)
High (3–4)	11 (73%)	13 (56%)
Total	15 (100%)	23 (100%)

1951 or After

Concern with Air Pollution	RESPONDENT'S SEX	
	Male	Female
Low	18 (64%)	18 (60%)
High	10 (36%)	12 (40%)
Total	28 (100%)	30 (100%)

Results of this survey of public opinion concerning air quality in X-ville, taken in May 1962, demonstrate fairly conclusively that air pollution in X-ville constitutes a problem which is community-wide in its scope, both geographically and socially. In addition, the survey finds that the more involved or identified persons are with X-ville as a community, the more concern they tend to express with air pollution as a community problem. In other words, concern with air pollution in X-ville does not apparently stem from, lead to, or express, generalized negative feelings towards, or rejection of the community as a place to live; on the contrary, such concern appears to grow out of wide-spread feelings of civic pride and community identification, and leads to attempts to ameliorate the situation.

From the methodological standpoint of

[15] Hansen, G. A., "Odor and Fallout Control in a Kraft Pulp Mill," *J. Air Pollution Control Ass'n.*, 12:9, September, 1962.

In turn, this independence of the psycho–social from the physical variables of the environmental health complex in X-ville demonstrates the need to deal with each set of variables in terms that are conceptually appropriate or relevant, rather than to reduce the one set of variables to dependence on the other.

Awareness or definition of pollution as a problem in a society cannot be regarded therefore as a simple direct function of the society's capacity to produce pollution. Indeed, some of the same factors which lead to high capacity to pollute the air may lead to low awareness of air pollution as a social problem. The individualism and sensual repression characteristic of Victorian society contributed to that society's high capacity for material production, both of capital goods and of air pollution, and they also may have contributed to a low awareness of air pollution as a social problem. Victorians adapted themselves to air pollution as did

British moths—by melanism; or they coped with it individualistically, by moving to the country if they could. Today broad changes in the social structure and ideology of American society have given rise to a generally increased awareness and a generally lowered tolerance of air pollution as an environmental condition. Among such changes may be cited:

(1) The constantly declining proportion of blue collar as compared to white collar workers, with a corresponding increase in middle-class white-collar dirt and odor phobia; and emphasis on cleanliness as a status symbol.

(2) The increasing ideological emphasis on values relating to consumption by comparison to those relating to production. Consequent upon this new emphasis, industrial pollution may no longer be regarded as positive evidence of success in production so much as evidence of lack of success in consumption, or "good living."

Because of changes such as these in the socio–cultural system, a situation is entirely conceivable in which an increasing concern with air pollution as a social problem may occur in the very same place and period when physical levels of pollution are decreasing. In fact, this may well be the situation in X-ville. This writer knows of no grounds for doubting the statements of Z-mill officials that they have taken measures to reduce substantially the quantity of odor-bearing effluent from the mill in the period 1951 to May 1962; yet in May 1962, 52 per cent of respondents to the present survey said air pollution as malodor had either remained unchanged over these years as a serious problem for X-ville, or had increased in its gravity.

Examples of this kind make evident the need for a broad research attack on the relationship between the social system and physical system dynamics which together constitute the eco-sphere of Man.[16] If men define situations as real they will be real in their consequences. The reality of the X-ville residents' definition of their air environment is evidently no simple function of the reality of that environment as defined aerometrically. From increased understanding of the independence—and [the] interdependence—of these two orders of reality may come progress in achieving the goals of environmental health.

[16] See O. D. Duncan, "From Social System to Ecosystem," *Sociological Inquiry*, 31: 140–149, 1961.

4

Who Is Normal? Two Perspectives on Mild Mental Retardation

Jane R. Mercer

EACH DISCIPLINE is organized around a core of basic concepts and assumptions which form the frame of reference from which persons trained in that discipline view the world and set about solving problems in their field. The concepts and assumptions which make up the perspective of each discipline give each its distinctive character and are the intellectual tools used by its practitioners. These tools are incorporated in action and problem solving and appear self-evident to persons socialized in the discipline. As a result, little consideration is likely to be given to the social consequence of applying a particular conceptual framework to problem solving.

When the issues to be resolved are clearly in the area of competence of a single discipline, the automatic application of its conceptual tools is likely to go unchallenged. However, when the problems under consideration lie in the interstices between disciplines, the disciplines concerned are likely to define the situation differently and may arrive at differing conclusions which have dissimilar implications for social action.

Moderate and mild mental retardation are such interstitial phenomena. Although persons identified as severely and profoundly retarded usually show obvious evidence of organic damage and thus clearly come under the aegis of the biological sciences and the medical profession, persons identified as moderately and mildly retarded frequently show no evidence of somatic involvement. They fall into the interstitial region between medicine, psychology and sociology, each

with its own conceptual tools and its own set of operations for defining what is "normal." Thus, the appropriate discipline for dealing with the problems of those labeled as moderately or mildly retarded and the definitional framework to be used in conceptualizing the issues involved are ambiguous.

The discipline of medicine typically approaches problems using a pathological model and defines normal performance within that model. Psychology is more likely to use a statistical model for defining normal. Together, these two models comprise what we shall call the "clinical perspective," because both are designed to identify abnormalities in a fashion which will direct some type of diagnostic and treatment process. Sociologists define normal from a non-clinical, social system perspective which is not oriented toward treatment. Each model is a map for conceptualizing the empirical world and is designed to serve the needs of a particular discipline. Each model presents a slightly different picture of reality and each has identifiable social consequences when applied to borderline phenomena such as moderate or mild mental retardation.

The purpose of this discussion is to describe the three different definitions of "normal" and the assumptions underlying each definition. Some of the social consequences of adopting each model will be explored by examining the case of moderate and mild mental retardation drawing on findings from an epidemiological study of mental retardation for illustrative material.[1]

The Medical Definition of Normal–Abnormal

Historically, the medical perspective was developed as a conceptual tool to interpret

[1] This investigation was supported by Public Health Service Research Grant no. MH–08667; Socio–Behavioral Study Center for Mental Retardation, Pacific State Hospital, Pomona, Calif., and Public Health Service General Research Support Grant no. 1–S01–FR–05643–02, Pacific State Hospital, Pomona, Calif. Special appreciation is extended to George Tarjan, M.D., and Harvey F. Dingman, Ph.D., for their financial and intellectual support through their research grants, and Mrs. June F. Lewis for her critical comments and assistance.

the nature of biological disease processes and to guide research and social action directed toward preventing and/or curing those afflicted with such diseases. The medical perspective, therefore, is a model generated to comprehend organic malfunction.

Because medical concern is ordinarily initiated by the appearance of physiological conditions which interfere with the biological functioning of the organism, the focus of the medical perspective is upon pathology and the symptoms of pathology. It is a pathological model in which disease syndromes are defined by the biological symptoms that characterize them. The pathological model concentrates on defining the nature of "abnormal" functioning. "Normal" becomes a residual category containing those organisms which do not manifest "abnormal" symptoms; that is, "normal" = absence of pathological symptoms and "abnormal" = presence of pathological symptoms.

What is a pathological symptom? This question is answered primarily through functional analysis—a method highly developed in biological studies. The basic value premise of a biological functional analysis is that life is better than death. The health of any biological organism can be evaluated against a universally accepted standard which regards those processes that preserve the biological system as a living organism as "good," i.e., "healthy," and those processes which interfere with system preservation as "bad," i.e., "pathological." Because one biological organism of the same species functions much like all others of its kind, there are few problems of sampling. Although inductive logic is implied, it is much less highly developed than in the statistical model. Findings based on biological processes operating in one human organism can be generalized with a high level of validity to most other human organisms.

In conducting a functional analysis, the physiologist first establishes the requirements which must be met if the organism is to survive and to operate with some degree of effectiveness. Then he describes the organs, the biological structures, and the processes through which these requirements are met in

"normal" cases. Frequently, "normal" function is most readily grasped by studying its opposite—those situations in which the requirements of the organic system are not being fully met and life processes are not being adequately maintained. Changes in the organs and biological structures occurring in these situations are defined as symptoms of the pathology. Maintenance of life processes is the criterion of "normal"; conversely, interference with life processes is the criterion of "abnormal," i.e., pathological. Thus, a person diagnosing individuals in clinical practice using a medical model begins with an abstract construct of the nature of the symptoms which constitute a particular disease syndrome as determined in functional analyses and works from this abstract definition to the diagnosing of particular cases.

The pathological model is conceptually a bipolar construct. At one pole is "normal," which is equated with health and the absence of pathological symptoms. At the other pole is "abnormal," defined as the presence of pathological signs and equated with disease, sickness, illness, "unhealth." Persons may be ranged along the continuum. It is assumed that being located near the "normal" end of the continuum, i.e., being "healthy," is good and a condition to be fostered. On the other hand, to be "abnormal," i.e., unhealthy, is "bad" and a condition to be prevented or alleviated. This bipolar conceptual framework is essentially evaluative. The medical practitioner is constantly involved in making value judgments about the biological state of his clients in terms of a health–pathology dimension which is readily translated into a good–bad polarity. Because his clients share the same value frame as the medical practitioner and wish to preserve their biological organisms, there is a high level of agreement between the trained professional's value system and that of his clients.

The American Association on Mental Deficiency nomenclature is a detailed classification system categorizing various types of mental retardation by their biological symptoms and provides an excellent illustration of the application of a pathological model.[2] The medical contribution to that nomenclature clearly illustrates the perspective of the pathological model and its influence on the field of mental retardation.

SOME IMPLICATIONS OF THE PATHOLOGICAL MODEL

Each definition of "normal" produces its own set of dispositions to action which will be illustrated by referring to the field of mental retardation. When the pathological model is used as a framework, the following dispositions are likely to emerge.

First, there is likely to be a decided emphasis on identifying the characteristics of abnormality with a tendency to neglect examination of the "normal," more positive aspects of behavior. Persons are likely to be studied in terms of what is "wrong" with them and labeled in terms of their disabilities rather than their abilities. For example, hospital and public school diagnostic reports describing the characteristics of children labeled as "mentally retarded" are replete with detailed information on all the pathological symptoms manifested by each child, but tend to say little or nothing about those aspects of behavior which are non-pathological.

Second, the process of medical diagnosis focuses specifically on the individual being assessed. The pattern or syndrome of symptoms manifested by an individual is used to identify the nature of his pathology which, in turn, is treated as a characteristic of the individual. The pathological model says a person *is* tubercular or syphilitic or mentally retarded. The pathology is perceived as residing *in* the person who has been diagnosed, as belonging to him.

Third, the medical perspective operates in terms of the logic of cause-and-effect

reasoning. If a person manifests signs interpreted as symptomatic of pathology, etiological questions are immediately raised. What conditions in the biological organism have caused these symptoms? The pathological model fosters research focused on etiology. If the cause can be identified, then prevention and/or amelioration of the pathology may be possible.

Fourth, the pathological perspective is heavily biased toward biological explanations. Pathological symptoms are defined by functional analysis, and, in turn, the search for causes tends to be directed toward organic malfunctioning and possible disease processes. Social and cultural factors which may be related to etiology tend to be discounted, unless it can be demonstrated that such factors have produced organic damage which, in turn, has produced the symptoms of pathology. Biological malfunctioning is often posited even if it cannot be clearly demonstrated. Those wedded to the pathological model in the study of mental retardation frequently continue to postulate the presence of "minimal brain damage" resulting from dietary deficiencies, inadequate prenatal or postnatal care, unhygienic conditions and so forth in cases of so-called cultural–familial mental retardation even though such damage has not been conclusively established.[3]

Fifth, from a medical perspective, a pathological condition can exist in an individual even though no one in his circle of significant others is aware of its presence. One of the purposes of epidemiological studies is to search out unrecognized cases of pathology so that they can be included in the prevalence count and the "real" number of pathological cases in the population can be ascertained. Medically speaking, the perfectly executed epidemiological study would be one in which all cases of a pathology, both diagnosed and undiagnosed, have been included in the analysis. This approach has been extremely effective in the control of contagious diseases such as tuberculosis,

2 Heber, R., *A Manual on Terminology and Classification in Mental Retardation*, Monograph Supplement to the *American J. of Mental Deficiency*, 2d ed., 1961.

3 Tizard, J., "The Role of Social Institutions in the Causation, Prevention, and Alleviation of Mental Retardation." Paper delivered at the Inaugural Peabody–NIMH Conference on Sociocultural Aspects of Mental Retardation, Nashville, Tenn., June 9–12, 1968.

but its beneficence and validity is more obscure when the epidemiological study is concerned with conditions not always directly related to organic lesions, conditions such as mental retardation.

Because it concentrates on the biological organism, those who use the pathological model tend to think in universal, supra-societal terms. In general, the biological organism of the human species responds in similar fashion to physical trauma and disease processes regardless of its cultural milieu. Thus, biological findings are applicable across cultural boundaries and biological concepts and technology may transcend social systems. Cross-societal comparisons of prevalence and incidence rates are accepted as valid and differences in rates of pathology in various societies are treated as real differences in the characteristics of their populations.

To summarize the characteristics of the pathological model: It identifies pathology through functional analyses based on the value premise that the life system ought to be maintained; it defines "normal" as the absence of pathological symptoms; it is bipolar; its classifications are basically evaluative; it focuses on biological explanations; it is based on cause-and-effect logic; it assumes pathology may be present although undiagnosed; and it regards its findings and definitions as transcending particular social systems.

The Statistical Definition of Normal–Abnormal

The statistical definition of "normal" is familiar to anyone who has taken an elementary course in statistics and been introduced to the concept of the normal curve. Psychologists who specialize in tests and measurements and their counterparts in the field of education are the primary users of the concept of the statistical norm.

Unlike the pathological model which defines the symptoms of pathology in relationship to some type of functional analysis, the statistical model defines abnormality in terms of an individual's position on an assumed normal distribution relative

to others in the population being studied. Establishing the statistically normal is a straightforward process. The investigator specifies the population of persons on which the norms will be based and then either measures the entire population or a representative sample of the population on the characteristics of interest. Scores on the measure are organized into a frequency distribution and the average score, i.e., the statistical mean, is calculated. The mean is accepted as the norm. Customarily, persons with scores which deviate not more than one standard deviation above or below the mean are regarded as falling in the "normal range" and comprise approximately 68 per cent of the population. Therefore, in the statistical definition, "normal" = statistical mean plus or minus one standard deviation from the mean.

Those who fall more than one standard deviation above the mean, but less than two standard deviations above the mean, are classified as "high normals" (approximately 13.6 per cent of the population), and those whose scores fall more than one standard deviation below the mean, but less than two standard deviations, are labeled as "low normals" (also approximately 13.6 per cent of the population). Those whose scores are more than two standard deviations above the mean are "abnormally high" (approximately 2.3 per cent of the population) and those with scores more than two standard deviations below the mean are "abnormally low" (also approximately 2.3 per cent of the population).

In establishing a statistical norm, the investigator uses the characteristics of the particular population of people being studied to delineate the boundaries of "normal." A "normal" established in this fashion does not necessarily imply "healthy" or "good." To be statistically normal has no implicit value assumption because the measurements could concern matters of indifference to the social world or could concern matters about which the social world has no knowledge.

Unlike the bipolar pathological model, the statistical model defines the boundaries of *two* types of abnormalities: those who have an abnormally large amount of the characteristic in question, and those who have an abnormally small amount. The statistical model as an abstract construct does not necessarily imply an evaluative judgment on the part of the investigator. There is no value touchstone which universally defines a particular position on the normal curve as "good" or "bad" in all cases. Being located in either extreme of the normal distribution carries no built-in value-loading per se, for the statistical model, as a general construct, is evaluatively neutral.

However, when the statistical model is used to describe socially valued characteristics, assessments may acquire a judgmental quality depending upon the social values associated with the characteristic being studied. In measuring some characteristics, it is "bad" for an individual to be located at either extreme; e.g., it is "bad" to be extremely heavy or extremely thin. In other cases, it is judged "good" to be high, and "bad" to be low; e.g., "good" to have an abnormally high IQ, but "bad" to have an abnormally low IQ. In still other instances, the poles are reversed and it is "good" to be abnormally low and "bad" to be abnormally high. Thus, value judgments are not implicit in the statistical model itself, as with the pathological model. However, the model can be readily used to reach value-laden conclusions if the characteristics being studied carry a heavy evaluative charge in society, as in the case of measures of intellectual ability for Western societies.

The use of a statistical model to define normal–abnormal appears in near pure form in the American Association on Mental Deficiency definition of the various levels of mental retardation.[4] In this definition, IQ scores reported in standard deviation units are the major criteria for determining the level of mental retardation, and each level has its own diagnostic designation. An IQ of 100 is set as the statistical mean. A standard deviation on the Wechsler Intelli-

gence Scales and the Stanford–Binet LM Form has been established as 15 points. Therefore, a person plus or minus one standard deviation (15 IQ points) from the mean of 100 is "normal" (IQ 85–115). A person between one and two standard deviations below the mean (IQ 70–84) is "borderline;" those between one and two standard deviations below the mean are "mildly retarded (IQ 55–69);" those between two and three standard deviations below the mean are "moderately retarded" (IQ 40–54); those between four and five standard deviations below the mean are "severely retarded" (IQ 25–39); and those more than five standard deviations below the mean are "profoundly retarded" (IQ under 25).

In the American Association on Mental Deficiency nomenclature, this statistical definition parallels the pathological definition and no attempt is made to integrate the disparate conceptual models from which the two are generated. Together, the two models comprise what I have elsewhere called the "clinical perspective."[5,6] The clinical definition of mental retardation presented in the official nomenclature is based upon a dual standard of "normal"—a pathological model for biological manifestations and a statistical model for behavioral manifestations.[7]

The statistical model *may* be used to describe biological processes and establish norms for biological characteristics such as body temperature, height and weight, but, unlike the pathological model, it is not limited to the description of biological characteristics. It can just as readily be used to establish norms for behavior. This helps to explain the uneasy marriage of the two dissimilar definitions of "normal" which appear in the official nomenclature. The pathological model, with its definition of

[4] Heber, *op. cit.*

[5] Mercer, J. R., "Sociological Perspectives on Mild Mental Retardation." Paper presented at the Inaugural Peabody–NIMH Conference on Socio–cultural Aspects of Mental Retardation, Nashville, Tenn., June 9–12, 1968.
[6] Mercer, J. R., "Social System Perspective and Clinical Perspective: Frames of Reference for Understanding Career Patterns of Persons Labelled as Mental Retarded," *Social Problems* 1965, 13:18–34.
[7] Heber, *op. cit.*

"normal" based on functional analysis, is used to assess biological manifestations. The statistical model is used to assess behavioral manifestations not readily comprehended within a pathological model. If amount of space allotted to each model in the manual indicates priority, the pathological model is clearly preferred, except in those cases in which there are no biological signs. Then the statistical norm is used.

SOME IMPLICATIONS OF THE
STATISTICAL MODEL

Although a general statistical model based on a normal curve is not inherently evaluative, in practice, most applications of the statistical model *are* evaluative. When this evaluation is conducted in close conjunction with other evaluations using the pathological model— as is true in the case of mental retardation— there is a tendency to think in terms of one model while operating with another. The implicit logic which underlies this transformation of a behavioral pattern into a pathological sign proceeds as follows. Low IQ = "bad" in American society: a social evaluation. "Bad" = pathology in the pathological model. Therefore, low IQ = pathology. The IQ, which was initially nothing more than a score based on responses to a series of questions, becomes conceptually transposed into a pathological sign carrying all the implications of the pathological perspective, but without any evidence based on functional analysis that this pathological sign is related to the biology of the organism or that it has any functional relationship to system maintenance.

When a statistical model is used to define normal performance, the norms emerging from measurements taken on one population cannot be safely generalized beyond that population. Such definitions of "normal" are not trans-societal nor universal. Statistical norms even for biological characteristics such as skin color, head circumference, height or weight established on the population of the United States are obviously not valid for the population, say, of Nigeria. This is even more true of characteristics more influenced by social and cultural factors—characteristics such as manual dexterity, verbal ability, abstract reasoning or IQ.

Another characteristic of the statistical model is that it assumes that the distribution of the characteristic in the population being measured is "normal." If, instead, the characteristic is not normally distributed, a statistically defined "normal" is a misleading indicator. Should the distribution be skewed, the mean will tend to move in the direction of the skew. Even more serious, if the distribution is bimodal or trimodal, and this factor is overlooked and the distribution is treated as unimodal, distinct distortions appear.

Suppose, for example, we are interested in establishing "normal" body weight for the United States population, but ignore the fact that the distribution is bimodal and that the average body weight for females is much lower than that for males. Of course, we can calculate a "normal" body weight for the combined sexes—but what is its value? The average is too low to tell us much about males and too high to tell us much about females. When a population is split evenly into two different groups, as with sex, the bimodality is obvious and not likely to be ignored. However, when the sub-group is small relative to the total population, their impact on the total curve may be miniscule and easily overlooked. They remain in the combined distribution defined as "abnormals," just as a population consisting of 20 per cent females and 80 per cent males would define most of the females as "abnormally" light. These simple statistical propositions place severe restrictions on the statistical model as a frame of reference for defining normality, restrictions which, though obvious, are frequently ignored in practice. The social consequences of such disregard will be explored later.

Even within a single society, the normal range established on the basis of testing a representative sample of the entire society will reflect the characteristics of the most numerous group in that society and automatically will categorize the characteristics of less numerous groups as abnormal if they vary systematically from the general population in the characteristic being studied. For example, a normal curve of skin pigmentation based on the total population of the United States would classify the Negro minority as abnormal, just as a test of English-language usage would classify children of Mexican and Puerto Rican heritage from Spanish-speaking homes as abnormal. When a statistical model is used, small numbers with a particular characteristic = abnormality. With this model, there will *always* be abnormals in a population because there are always two extreme tails to any distribution. Abnormality is intrinsic to the model.

Some Social Consequences of the Clinical Perspective

Together, the pathological and statistical models of "normal" form what I am calling the clinical perspective. This perspective is the viewpoint commonly adopted by persons in the field of medicine, psychology, social work and education—fields concerned with the helping professions. Medical persons are more likely to adopt a pathological model, while psychologists and educators are more likely to think in terms of a statistical model. However, there is a free exchange of ideas and the two approaches to the definition of "normal" are frequently used interchangeably by clinicians themselves. As noted earlier, the American Association on Mental Deficiency nomenclature is an excellent example of a treatise which attempts to describe mental retardation from both pathological and statistical frames of reference and to mold the two outlooks into a single clinical definition.[8]

The pathological model has been very effective in bringing many of the major physiological ills of mankind under control and is clearly appropriate when dealing with organically damaged persons such as the severely and profoundly retarded. Indeed, it

[8] *Ibid.*

has been so effective in the biological realm that it is increasingly used as a model for conceptualizing other kinds of problems which are similar but not identical to those on which it first proved its power. In order for non-physiological problems to be treated within a medical framework, they must first be redefined in terms of the pathological model. This transformation requires a basic reformulation of the definition of the situation. Where deviant behavior may have been defined in moralistic terms (He is bad. He lacks will-power and character.) or in magical terms (An evil spirit has possessed him.), the pathological model restructures the definition of the behavior to fit the health–pathology model. Aberrant behavior is defined as a symptom of individual pathology. Habitual users of drugs or alcohol are evaluated as physically sick; persons who behave in bizarre and irresponsible ways are labeled as mentally "ill"; those who do not respond appropriately to the abstract intellectual stimuli of American society are categorized as mentally retarded. Behavior associated with each of these conditions is regarded as symptomatic of the pathology. These "symptoms" are treated as characteristics of the individual which should be modified and, if possible, eliminated.

Applying a clinical perspective to situations which may contain some physiological component but which also contain significant cultural factors has numerous social consequences. Four general areas of impact will be discussed and illustrated using data from the field of mental retardation: (1) types of research; (2) the social role of the person labeled; (3) locus of social power in decision making; and (4) the social characteristics of persons identified as "abnormal."

TYPES OF RESEARCH FOSTERED BY A
CLINICAL PERSPECTIVE

When a pathological model is used to define normal–abnormal, abnormal = presence of the symptoms of pathology. Thus, research studies using a clinical perspective tend to concentrate on persons with pathological signs. If "normals" are studied at all, they are typically treated as a contrast

Because cause-and-effect logic is central
to the pathological model of abnormal,
research questions posed by investigators
operating from a pathological viewpoint
tend to be causal, and research is organized
around causal hypotheses. Such etiological
emphasis tends to preclude consideration of
the possible influence of the diagnostic
instruments themselves in creating the very
categories they purport to measure. The
role of the diagnostician and his instrument
is assumed to be value neutral. The quest
focuses on ascertaining "causal" factors in
the individual or in his environment.

The clinical perspective has influenced the
types of research questions which have been
posed in mental retardation research. Typical
questions are: What is the etiology of
mental retardation? What can be done to
prevent this condition? What can be done
to cure this condition? How can we develop
more reliable and more valid diagnostic
instruments? How many people are afflicted
by mental retardation? All these questions
are identical to those which might be asked
about contagious diseases. They are
questions suggested by the very nature of
the clinical model and illustrate how the
frame of reference used in describing a
phenomenon will predispose an investigator
to explore certain kinds of research questions.

The pathological model encourages biological explanatory systems and research
tends to center around the study of individuals as isolated organisms rather than as
persons functioning in a social network.
The social context in which individuals live
is viewed as irrelevant, except when there
is some hypothesized relationship between
certain environmental factors and physiological changes in the organism.

Because the pathological model is particularly effective when dealing with biological
variables, those hypotheses most effectively
handled by the model are likely to be selected
for testing—hypotheses concerning biological
factors in etiology. The possible effect of
this biological bias on mental retardation
research was explored. All etiological studies
reported in papers abstracted in *Mental
Retardation Abstracts* for the four-year

period, 1964–1967,[9] were reviewed and
organized by etiological groupings following
the classifications of the American Association on Mental Deficiency nomenclature.[10]
Table 4–1 presents the percentage of
etiological papers in each year which were
focused on each of the major etiological
groupings.

Apparently, there has been little or no
interest in exploring etiological hypotheses
for those types of mental retardation which
have "functional reaction alone manifest,"
e.g., have no observable biological component. Although over half of the persons
labeled as mentally retarded would fall in
this category, only 1 per cent of the 3,013
etiological reports appearing during this four-
year period studied this group of individuals.
There were only three papers in 1964 and no
papers in subsequent years covering the etiology of mental retardation in normal-bodied
persons. Instead, etiological studies centered
almost exclusively on biological questions
which the pathological model can handle
readily. The most popular etiological research area was "disorders of metabolism,
growth or nutrition" with 34.2 per cent of
the total papers. This was followed by "infections or intoxications" having 22.8 per cent
of the papers and reports on "general
genetics" with 14.9 per cent of the papers.
Other etiological groupings received less
than 10 per cent of the coverage. Undoubtedly, research publications reflect the
direction of research support and funds are
more readily available for studies which
focus on organic factors in mental retardation.

IMPACT ON THE SOCIAL ROLES OF
PERSONS LABELED RETARDED

When a pathological model is used to
define a phenomenon, persons labeled as

[9] National Institute for Mental Health,
Mental Retardation Abstracts, Washington, D.C.:
National Clearing House for Mental Health
Information, U.S. Public Health Service, Dept.
H. E. W. 1964–1967.

[10] Heber, *op. cit.*

deviant are regarded as "sick" and play the role of "invalid." Thus, a person labeled as mentally retarded and viewed within the pathological model will be perceived as "handicapped" because of genetic or biological malfunctioning and will play the role of "patient" and/or "inmate." These roles are quite different from that of "child" or "pupil." The fact that the mental retardate plays the "sick" role has social consequences both for the individual and for the larger society.

in the traditional patient–doctor or patient–nurse context. In such dyads, the medical role requires maintenance of an attitude of objectivity toward the patient which precludes emotional involvement, physical fondling or overt displays of tenderness. The superordinate position of the medical professional *vis à vis* the patient in the patient–doctor social system assures preservation of social distance and feelings of superiority on the part of the physician and feelings of inferiority on the part of persons holding the status of patient. The focus of concern for the doctor–patient dyad is the patient's

Table 4–1—Tabulation of types of research variables explored in etiological reports abstracted in mental retardation abstracts, 1964–1967

Etiological Groupings	Vol. 1 (1964)	Vol. 2 (1965)	Vol. 3 (1966)	Vol. 4 (1967)	Total
	(N = 359) %	(N = 718) %	(N = 1,049) %	(N = 887) %	(N = 3,013) %
Infections or Intoxications	16.2	24.8	29.0	16.8	22.8
Trauma or Physical Agent	4.7	6.4	5.9	7.3	6.3
Disorders of Metabolism, Growth or Nutrition	41.8	36.9	33.7	29.4	34.2
New Growths	2.8	3.8	3.2	1.7	2.9
Unknown Prenatal Influence	8.6	6.7	8.2	11.7	8.9
Unknown Cause with Structural Reactions Manifest	8.1	12.1	11.2	7.1	9.8
Uncertain Cause, Functional Reaction Alone Manifest	0.8	0.0	0.0	0.0	0.1
Genetics (General)	17.0	9.3	8.8	26.0	14.9
Total	100.0	100.0	100.0	100.0	100.0

An individual labelled as "sick" is more likely to be placed in a social institution designed to care for "sick" persons—a hospital. It is more than a coincidence that, with the rise of the medical perspective in mental retardation, many institutions for their care and management are now designated as "hospitals" rather than as "homes," "colonies," or "schools." There are numerous implications for the mental retardate in being placed in a medical-type total institution known as a "hospital" rather than in a "home" or a "school."

First, those responsible for his care will be persons trained for medical roles: psychiatrists, physicians, nurses and psychiatric technicians. These professionals will tend to handle their interactions with the retardate

biological organism rather than the more usual type of social dyad based on mutual attraction, as in friendship groups, or pursuit of a common goal, as in task-oriented groups. In the patient–doctor social system, the medical professional is the primary actor and the patient is the one acted upon. The medical person takes the initiative while the patient is expected to comply and cooperate in his own cure.[11] This social system differs greatly from most other social systems in the society and from the kinds of social systems in which the individual

[11] Parsons, T., "Definitions of Health and Illness in the Light of American Values and Social Structure," in E. G. Jaco (ed.), *Patients, Physicians and Illness*, New York: Free Press, 1st ed., 1958, Chap. 20 (chap. 8 in this edition).

would be operating if he were not in a "hospital." Such experiences are unlikely to prepare him for life on the "outside."

Tizard, King and Raynes have conducted a series of investigations on the quality of care in English residential institutions for handicapped children.[12] For this research, they developed a rating scale of child management practices based on observations of the practices of personnel in an institution over a period of time. Scores ranged from 0 to 60, with a high score characterizing a ward or house with rigid rules, block treatment of children, large social distance between children and staff and little opportunity for children to express their individuality. These are all characteristics of the "total institution" as described by Goffman.[13]

In one study, five hospitals for the mentally retarded were rated and compared with eight hostels and three homes. All institutions served children between five and sixteen years of age who had IQs under 50. Although severely handicapped children required different management practices from those who were able-bodied, children with comparable handicaps were cared for very differently in hostels than in hospitals. Hostels had a mean score of 11 points, voluntary homes 27.7, and hospitals 33. In another study, scores for children's homes ranged from 0 through 7, but for hospitals ranged from 17 through 31. Differences could not be accounted for by the size of the unit. The investigators noted that "institutions with over three hundred children could have a child-oriented pattern of care" and "institutional size, as such, was not the main determinant of patterns of child management."[14] Similarly, there was no significant correlation between scores on the scale and staff–child ratios ($r = 0.03$). However, they did find marked differences in staff roles and staff performance when the two types of institutions were compared:

In the hostels, the person in charge spent a much greater proportion of her time in social

and physical child care, and in the supervision of the children, than did the sister in charge of the hospital wards. Heads of units in hospitals did proportionately more administrative and domestic work than did their counterparts in hostels. . . . When they were actually looking after the children, the sisters in charge of hospital wards spoke much less often to them, played with them less, and handled them physically much less frequently than did their counterparts in the hostels.

The authors noted that these patterns of management were related to the type of training which the staff had had, "those who had received nurse's training being the most institutionally oriented."[15]

The impersonality of the hospital-type social system is accentuated by the frequency with which staff and children are moved. In a "model ward" established with the intention of keeping staff constant, the investigators found that children were cared for by 246 different adults in a $3\frac{1}{2}$-year period, about 70 a year! Changes on other wards must have been even more frequent.

Some children are likely to be moved as many as eighteen times between the time they are admitted and the age of eleven, and all children are likely to be moved at least twice during that period. It is also known that once a child is transferred from one ward to another, he is unlikely ever to return to his former home or see any of the children in it except fortuitously.

By way of contrast, the children living in children's homes

. . . lived lives which were free and unregimented; they used gardens as they wished; they mostly had the run of the house; few places were out-of-bounds. The houses were full of their possessions, including paintings and handwork brought from school and displayed in the living rooms or in their bedrooms. Treatment was individual and personal, adapted to the child's age and maturity. . . . In sharp contrast, children in long stay hospitals lead drab and uninteresting lives compared with those led, not only by children in their own homes, but also by those in other children's homes.[16]

[12] Tizard, *op. cit.*
[13] Goffman, E., *Asylums*, Garden City, N.Y.: Anchor Books, 1961.
[14] Tizard, *op. cit.*, p. 42.

[15] *Ibid.*, p. 45.   [16] *Ibid.*, p. 48.

LOCUS OF SOCIAL POWER AND DECISION-MAKING

Not only does the medical model influence the roles a child will play but it also has implications for social power and decision-making. It influences the type of professional who will be assigned responsibility for the care of persons labeled as deviant. When a social problem is defined as biological pathology and is treated within a pathological frame of reference, this perspective implicitly assumes that the persons most qualified to direct and supervise the care and treatment of those who are "sick" are persons trained in the field of medicine. Thus, the medical model tends to enhance the claims of the medical professions to priority in program development and management. For example, the legislature of the state of California recently authorized the establishment of mental retardation diagnostic centers throughout the state. If mental retardation is viewed primarily as an educational problem, the Department of Education would be the logical agency to establish such centers. If mental retardation is seen as a subcultural phenomenon resulting from a disadvantaged background, the Department of Social Welfare might lay claim to direction. If viewed primarily as an emotional or psychiatric problem, the Department of Mental Hygiene would be a reasonable choice. Significantly, the Department of Public Health was given direction of the program, a logical decision if mental retardation is viewed from a pathological model. This implies that a medically trained director will be appointed for each center and medically trained persons will be recruited to administer medical-type treatment and counseling programs. Undoubtedly, the medical orientation of these centers will determine the type of mental retardate who will be served—those with manifest biological symptomatology. The retardate with "no manifest structural reaction" will probably receive proportionately less service because his problems are not readily conceptualized within a medical framework.

Because the pathological model is most useful when applied to biological deviations and less useful in dealing with behavior, persons adopting a clinical perspective are likely to shift to a statistical model when establishing norms for behavioral manifestations. Consequently, persons labeled as mentally retarded who have "no structural reactions manifest" are likely to be identified as abnormal on the statistically determined criterion of the IQ test.

A statistical definition of "normal" establishes the behavior of the most numerous group in the population as "normal behavior" and, therefore, tends to classify any minority group which differs culturally from the general population as "abnormal" because their performance is likely to fall into one of the tails of the distribution. This tendency for the culturally different minority to be labeled as "abnormal" when a statistical model is used can be illustrated in the following data.

As part of an epidemiological study of mental retardation in a southern California city (population 85,000), IQ scores for a representative sample of 480 children, seven months through 15 years of age, were secured through individual testing using the Stanford–Binet LM and from school records. Each child was assigned a weight to correspond to the number of persons of the same ethnic group, socio–economic level, and age he represented in the community. Using these weighted frequencies, it is possible to reconstruct an estimated distribution of IQ scores for the entire community in this age group and for three significant sub-groups in that population: English-speaking Caucasian children (Anglos) who comprise 80.2 per cent of the total population; children of Mexican–American heritage who comprise 11.6 per cent of the total; and children of Negro heritage who comprise 8.2 per cent of the total.

Figure 4–1 shows the distributions for these IQ scores. The solid line in Figure 4–1A shows the IQ distribution curve for the total community combining all three ethnic groups. The shape of the total community population curve is quite normal. The presence of Mexican–American and black children in the total is not visible because their combined numbers, about 20 per cent of the total population, are too small to have a noticeable effect on the curve. The distribution has a mean IQ of 107.0 and a standard deviation of 16.3. Using a statistical model to define "normal" in this community, we would say that the normal IQ is 107 (seven points higher than the national norms) and the normal range for the community extends from 90.7 to 123.3. "Low normals" have IQs between 74.4 and 90.7, while "high normals" would have IQs between 123.3 and 139.6. Persons with an IQ below 74.4 would be the subnormals, while those above 139.6 would be the supranormals.

The most numerous group in the community are English-speaking Caucasian children. A separate curve, using a broken line, has been drawn within the total population curve for this group. The frequency distribution for the Anglo children also looks relatively normal, although the mean (110.3) is higher than for the total population. The standard deviation is 14.0.

The area between the broken line and the solid line, indicated by dots in Figure 4–1, represents the minority children present in each section of the total population curve. Thus, we can visualize exactly where the minority children fall and what proportion of each category of "normality" is composed of minority children. Although minority children compose 19.8 per cent of the total population, only 8.2 per cent of the "high abnormals" are minority children. In the "high normals" category, minority children still are only half as numerous as would be expected (10.2 per cent). The percentage of minority children increases in the normal range (12.6 per cent), but is still below the proportion of minority children in the total population. However, the "low normals," as defined by the total population statistical model, consist of 68.4 per cent minority children. The "low subnormals" are almost entirely minority children (82.8 per cent), four times higher than would be expected from their proportion in the total population.

FIGURE 4-1 *Influence of statistical model of "normal" in defining population subgroups as "abnormal"*

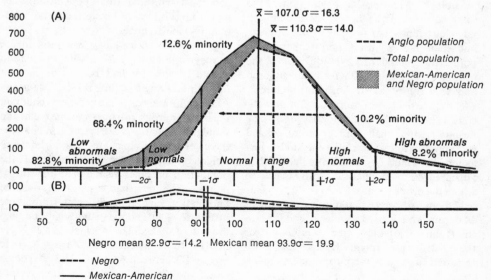

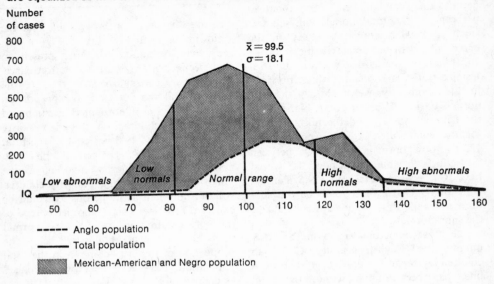

FIGURE 4-2 *Distribution of intelligence test scores when sizes of population subgroups are equalized so that there are one-third of each ethnic group*

Number of cases

$\bar{x} = 99.5$
$\sigma = 18.1$

Low abnormals   Low normals   Normal range   High normals   High abnormals

IQ

50 60 70 80 90 100 110 120 130 140 150 160

----- Anglo population

——— Total population

▨ Mexican-American and Negro population

The two curves in the lower part of Figure 4–1B show the frequency distributions for Mexican–American and black children. They were drawn separately because it was too confusing to insert them in Figure 4–1A. However, they are drawn to the same scale as Figure 4–1A and it is possible to visualize what proportion of the total curve is made up of these children. Each distribution is normal in appearance, but each has a mean approximately 16 points (one standard deviation) below the mean for the Anglos (92.9 for black children and 93.9 for Mexican–American children). Clearly, these three groups do not statistically belong to the same population.[17] The groups having small numbers were defined as "abnormal" by the statistical model, just as females would be abnormally light if they appeared in a population with males in which the proportions were 20 to 80 per cent.

If there had been equal numbers of Anglo, Mexican–American and black children in the total population, the bimodality of the distribution might have been more apparent and the inappropriateness of a

[17] Comparing Anglos and Mexicans, $t = 18.7$, $p < 0.0001$. Comparing Anglos and Negroes, $t = 18.0$, $p < 0.0001$.

statistical model which presumes a normal unimodal distribution would have been evident. However, the bimodality of the population was obscured by the fact that there are relatively few Mexican–American and black children in the community population, and when they are simply combined with the total population, they make no visible impression on the community-wide frequency distribution.

In Figure 4–2, we have drawn the curves as they would appear *if* the total population of the community had been composed of one-third Anglo, one-third Mexican–American, and one-third Negro children. Each ethnic group still has the same mean and standard deviation as before. When the three ethnic groups are combined and weighted equally, the bimodality of the population becomes visible. The IQ cutting points differentiating various levels of "normality" are quite different from those in Figure 4–1. The mean IQ would be 99.5 instead of 107.0. The normal range would be 81.4 to 117.6 and "low normal" would be any IQ between 63.3 and 81.3. A person would not be regarded as having a subnormal IQ unless it fell below 63.3.

Figure 4–2 illustrates graphically how the

statistical definition of "normal" is related to the composition of the population being normed and can be dramatically changed by giving "minority" groups equal weight in the determination of norms. Current practice, however, either excludes minority persons from normative samples or else includes them according to their proportion in the population.[18] Having established norms in this fashion, clinicians frequently proceed to operate as if the norms are universally applicable and the presence of subpopulations is irrelevant. In either case,

[18] In norming the Wechsler–Bellevue I and the Wechsler Adult Intelligence Scale (WAIS), the factors of subcultural differences in performance were not taken into account. Non-white subjects were not included in the original Wechsler–Bellevue standardization. In the 1955 WAIS standardization, some 10 per cent of the total sample of 1,686 were non-white, a percentage roughly representing the proportion of non-whites in the population of the United States in the 1950 census. According to Wechsler, "No attempt was made to establish separate norms for different racial (or national) groups in either the W–B 1 or the WAIS. The norms as they stand, particularly on the WAIS, seem to be reasonably representative of the country as a whole, and to this extent may be said to represent a fair cross-section of what may be called 'American intelligence' as of the time of standardization." D. Wechsler, *The Measurement and Appraisal of Adult Intelligence*, Baltimore: Williams & Wilkins Co., 4th ed., 1958, pp. 90–91. The final 1937 standardization group for the Stanford–Binet Intelligence Test "consisted of 3,184 native-born white subjects, including approximately 100 subjects at each half-year interval from $1\frac{1}{2}$ to $5\frac{1}{2}$ years, 200 at each age from 6 to 14, and 100 at each age from 15 to 18. Every age group was equally divided between sexes." Testing was done in 17 communities in 11 states distributed between urban, suburban and rural schools. The final sample contained no Negroes, was slightly higher in socio–economic level than the census population and had disproportionately more urban than rural subjects. The 1960 revision did not involve a restandardization. Over 4,000 subjects were used to determine the selection of items to be retained and to determine present item difficulty. These children "were not chosen to constitute a representative sample of American school children," although care was taken to avoid special, selective factors. Thus, the "native-born white subjects" of the 1937 standardization remain the basis for Stanford–Binet Intelligence Scale. (See L. M. Terman and M. A. Merrill, *Stanford–Binet Intelligence Scale, Manual for the Third Revision Form L–M*, Boston: Houghton–Mifflin Co., 1960, pp. 9–10.)

minority children coming from culturally different backgrounds frequently appear as "abnormals."

The social consequences of applying the clinical perspective, specifically the statistical model of normal, to a total population disregarding significant sub-groups in that population is that disproportionately large numbers of persons from culturally different homes will be labeled as abnormal. The performance of the most numerous population group will dominate the definition and smaller sub-groups will be regarded as deviant. The significance of this factor is best grasped by looking at the ethnic characteristics of mental retardates nominated by community agencies in our community epidemiology.

All agencies in the community who serve mental retardates and who systematically use clinically trained personnel in making diagnoses were contacted. Each agency was asked to report all mentally retarded persons known to them; duplicate nominations were identified; and a case register was developed containing all persons under 50 years of age certified as mentally retarded by one or more professionally competent clinicians.

Figure 4–3 compares the percentage of each ethnic group appearing in the register of 687 "retardates" nominated by these agencies with the percentage of each ethnic group in the general population of the community. When all socio–economic levels are combined, Anglos (English-speaking Caucasians) are underrepresented. Only 53 per cent of those diagnosed as mentally retarded are Anglo, although Anglos comprise 82 per cent of the population of the community studied. Both Mexicans and Negroes are overrepresented. Mexicans appear at a rate more than three times greater than would be expected, 32 per cent compared with 10 per cent in the general population. The Negro rate is approximately 50 per cent higher than would be expected: 12 per cent compared with 7 per cent in the population.

These disproportions are not as great as

FIGURE 4-3 *Comparison between the clinical case register of mental retardates and the community population (ages 0-49 years)*[a]

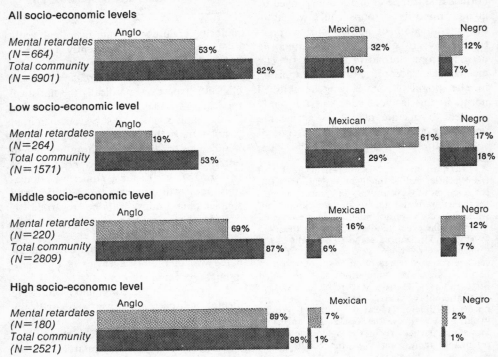

All socio-economic levels

	Anglo	Mexican	Negro
Mental retardates (N=664)	53%	32%	12%
Total community (N=6901)	82%	10%	7%

Low socio-economic level

	Anglo	Mexican	Negro
Mental retardates (N=264)	19%	61%	17%
Total community (N=1571)	53%	29%	18%

Middle socio-economic level

	Anglo	Mexican	Negro
Mental retardates (N=220)	69%	16%	12%
Total community (N=2809)	87%	6%	7%

High socio-economic level

	Anglo	Mexican	Negro
Mental retardates (N=180)	89%	7%	2%
Total community (N=2521)	98%	1%	1%

a Percentages do not add up to 100% because "other" ethnic groups are not shown on the chart.

would be anticipated from Figure 4–1. Whereas the two minority groups combined comprise 17 per cent of the community population and 43 per cent of those labeled as mentally retarded by community agencies, in Figure 4–1, they comprised 20 per cent of the population of children tested but 82.8 per cent of the population rated as "low abnormal" in IQ using community norms. We investigated to determine whether this discrepancy was due to the fact that agencies use national test norms rather than local community norms in evaluating IQ scores. By the national norms, an IQ of 100 is "normal" and an IQ of 69 or below places a person in the "low abnormal" group. Using national norms instead of local norms, we found that 81.2 per cent of the children who scored 69 or below were children of minority heritage. Thus, the overrepresentation of minority children in the "sub-normal" category was approximately the same whether national or local norms were used. We conclude, therefore, that community agencies identify as retarded only about half as many persons from ethnic minority groups as are retarded under a strict clinical definition. In spite of this underidentification, they label $2\frac{1}{2}$ times more persons from minority groups than would be expected from their percentage in the population. We will return to this point later.

Figure 4–3 also shows the ethnic comparisons within socio–economic levels.[19]

19 The socio–economic level of each case in the clinical register was rated by using the median value of housing on the census block of residence, 1960 census, as the measure. This was the one item of socio–economic information which was available for all cases. *U.S. Census of Housing: 1960*, Series HC (3)–62, City Blocks, Riverside, Calif., U.S. Department of Commerce, Washington, D.C.

Dividing the cases into three socio–economic levels and comparing ethnic groups within each level, we find that Anglos are under-represented in the mental retardation register on all three socio–economic levels, but the differential decreases as socio–economic level goes up. Mexican–Americans are over-represented on all social–economic levels, and differences remain sizable even in higher socio–economic categories where there are relatively few Mexican–Americans. Blacks appear in approximately the proportion which would be expected, when socio-economic level is held constant. Clearly, it is for the group for which cultural differences are greatest, the Mexican–Americans, that the discrepancies in rates of mental retardation based on a clinical perspective are also the greatest.[20]

The essential point of this discussion is that the statistical model, used on a heterogeneous population containing significantly different cultural sub-groups, tends to define the sub-groups as deviant. This bias is of more than theoretical interest because it appears in the community labeling process in agencies which adopt a clinical model and use statistical norms for establishing "normal" behavior.

We conclude that the use of a statistical model biases the definition of "normal" toward the behavioral expectations of the dominant core-culture and biases it against culturally different groups if they comprise a relatively small proportion of the total population. The American core-culture is thus elevated to the position of *the* standard normative system by which *all* persons are judged. There is a tendency for the norms which are codified in the diagnostic instruments to be regarded not only as the *official*

definition, but also as the *correct* definition of "healthy" behavior.

Thus, diagnostic instruments embodying the role-expectations and culture of Anglo–American society become endowed with the same degree of universality accorded diagnostic techniques developed by medical doctors for diagnosing physical malfunctioning.

These statistically established norms have broad social consequences for the individuals concerned. Persons defined as deficient are assigned to special education programs for the mentally retarded, programs with a limited curriculum which effectively excludes those enrolled from educational channels which lead to middle-class occupations and/or higher education. Those who are labeled by these norms may be placed in homes and hospitals for the mentally retarded or denied access to occupational opportunities which they might be able to fulfill.

The Social System Definition of Normal–Abnormal

The social system perspective deviates markedly from the clinical perspective in evaluating "normal–abnormal" behavior. It takes its beginning, not from the medical-disease tradition, functional analysis or statistical models, but rather from the sociological concept of the social system.

A social system consists of two interlocking structures: a patterned set of statuses and their associated roles and a normative structure. The statuses in a social system are the positions available to individuals participating in the system. Roles are the behaviors of persons filling particular statuses. For example, the social system of a state mental hospital is a complex organization with many statuses or positions—superintendent, clinical director, ward physician, ward nurse, physical therapist and so forth. Persons occupying a particular status behave in a certain manner and

[20] Based on a community survey of 10 per cent of the households of the city, it was established that 58 per cent of the heads of household of Mexican–American families have less than a ninth-grade education compared with 15 per cent of the majority families and 20 per cent of the black families; 56 per cent speak Spanish half the time or more compared with 1 per cent of the majority families who speak a language other than English and no black families; 28 per cent of the heads of household are foreign born compared with 4.5 per cent of the majority families and none of the black families.

perform certain duties and functions which comprise the role associated with that status. The acts performed by the superintendent differ from those of the clinical director, the ward physician or the ward nurse, and each of these other roles, in turn, differ from the rest.

Persons participating in any social system share certain common expectations about how persons occupying various statuses ought to act in performing their roles. These role expectations define the behaviors that are acceptable to other members of the system. Role expectations differ for different statuses. Collectively, they form the core of the normative structure of the social system. Norms define the behaviors which are obligatory for any person holding a particular status, the behaviors which are optional and the behaviors which are prohibited. The amount of leeway which an incumbent may take in fulfilling the normative expectations for his status varies from status to status and system to system, but there is always some flexibility in the application of sanctions.

The role expectations may be very explicit and formally written down or they may be informal, unwritten understandings. In either case, a person violating the norms of his status will receive negative sanctions, i.e., punishments from other members of the system. The most drastic negative sanction is removal from one's status in the system. Those fulfilling the expectations of their status in an exemplary fashion are positively sanctioned, i.e., rewarded.

In this context, "normal" is defined as that behavior which fulfills the expectations or norms of the social system while "abnormal" is behavior which either fails to meet role expectations or overfulfills role expectations. Behavior may overfulfill role expectations and be supernormal; it may meet role expectations and be normal; or it may fail to fulfill role expectations and be subnormal. Both supernormal and subnormal behavior is abnormal, or "deviant."

The social system defines what is "normal" for individuals holding various statuses in that system. In the social system model

"normal" = meeting the normative expectations of the social system for the status one is occupying. The norms of a social system operate at two levels—the general behavioral expectations for anyone holding any status in the system and the specific behavioral expectations unique to each status. Consequently, "normality" is both social system specific and status specific. It is not possible to speak of "normal" behavior without first specifying the social system which regards such behavior as "normal" and the status in that system for which the behavior is "normal." The reference point for evaluation is always the normative structure of the system in question and the perceptions of system members as to whether an individual's behavior is "normal" for one of his status. Comprehensive, supra–societal or cross-cultural epidemiologies of "normal" behavior are inconceivable from this viewpoint.

The extent to which any particular behavior is supernormal, normal or subnormal in a particular social system can be empirically determined by noting the direction and degree of positive and negative sanctions elicited in response to various types of behavior by other status incumbents. By noting the behaviors which are positively sanctioned and those which are negatively sanctioned, the investigator can map out the normative structure of a particular social system.

One of the more effective ways to study "subnormal" persons within a social system perspective is to note which persons have been assigned to disesteemed statuses reserved for those who have deviated sufficiently from role expectations as to be placed in a special "deviant" status. For example, the nature of mental retardation, from a social system perspective, is best studied by analysis of the characteristics of those who occupy the status of mental retardates, a study of how they were labeled and assigned to this deviant status and an investigation of the process by which some escape from this deviant status, i.e., become "normal" by being assigned to a "normal" status. Thus, the study of mental retardation, or any manifestation primarily behavioral, begins with close observation of the patterns of social system response rather than with some abstract construct about the nature of the symptoms which comprise an "illness." Unlike the statistical model, the social system model does not generate "abnormals" as part of the application of the model.

Differences between the clinical and social system perspectives can be illustrated with data secured as part of a study of desegregation of the public schools of a medium-sized California city.[21] A Wechsler Intelligence Scale for Children was individually administered to 1,298 elementary school children who were attending regular classes. The school system has a well-developed program for the mentally retarded. However, there were 121 of these children in the regular classes who had intelligence test scores ranging from 57 through 79. Being statistically subnormal, most of these children would probably be clinically evaluated as mentally retarded.

From a social system perspective, however, these 121 children are sociologically normal. They are holding the status of a regular student in a regular classroom. They have not been assigned the status of a mental retardate by any of the significant others in the social systems in which they participate nor are they playing the role of a mental retardate. Their IQ scores are irrelevant in a social system definition. So long as they occupy "normal" statuses in the social systems in which they participate, they are "normal." The critical sociological question is to determine how these children who are clinically eligible for the status of mental retardate have avoided becoming mentally retarded, i.e., placed in a special education class.

We have discovered many persons in our community epidemiology who play the role of a mental retardate in one community social system but do not play that role in other systems in which they participate. The most frequent pattern is for a child, usually of Mexican–American heritage, to hold the status of educable mental retardate in the public schools where he plays the

[21] The research in this paper was supported by the State of California, Department of Education, Office of Compensatory Education, McAteer Grant #M8–14 and the Public Health Service Grant #PH–43–67–756.

role of retardate for six hours a day. However, when he is at home he is normal. To his family, neighbors and peers he is no different than any other child his age, and he does not play the role of a retardate. When he is old enough to drop out of school, he can escape the status of retardate, marry, work, rear children and perform normal adult social roles. To say that this person was a retardate for six hours a day during 10 years of his life is a more precise description of the empirical world than to regard him as a chronically handicapped person who, on occasion, is able to pass as normal although he is "really" mentally retarded. Mild retardation, then, is like any other social status. Just as a woman may be a teacher at school but becomes a mother at home, a child may be a retardate at school and a normal at home.

We wish to reiterate that this discussion is not an indictment of the pathological–statistical model. That model has been a powerful tool in conceptualizing the nature of disease-processes. It is a useful frame of reference in conceptualizing severe and profound retardation, especially the organically damaged. In these cases, social system definitions and clinical diagnoses coincide because such persons would be classified as deviant in almost any human society. It is in the interstitial cases, such as moderate and mild retardation, that alternative models and definitions are needed.

Because the clinical perspective dominates most societal functions and the social system model has not been applied to any extent, we can only speculate about the possible social consequences which might result from its actual application. First, the social system perspective would shift the focus of interest, which has been primarily on the characteristics and behavior of the person labeled "abnormal," to simultaneous interest in the social system which is defining him as "abnormal" or "deviant." System processes would become as relevant to understanding the nature of abnormality as processes within the individual.

Second, perceiving "abnormality" as relative to the social context would allow those in the helping professions to think more flexibly and creatively about those whom they seek to serve. A person would not be labeled deviant on the basis of some diagnostic instrument if he is holding normal statuses and playing normal roles in the social systems in which he participates. His evaluation by his peers would be the critical determinant. Changes in an individual's social location could be manipulated imaginatively to facilitate his retaining a normal status.

Third, application of a social system perspective would eliminate the current practice of evaluating persons from minority subcultures by the standards, diagnostic tools and behavioral definitions of the majority culture. Instead, each subculture would be treated as a viable social system with a normative structure and status structure that varies from that of the dominant society. Such variation would be accepted as legitimate. Instead of classifying members of subgroups as "sick" because they fall into the extreme ends of a statistical distribution based on the majority culture and placing them in statuses reserved for deviants, society would accept the definitions of their behavior within the context of the social systems in which they have been socialized.

Fourth, research, instead of concentrating almost exclusively on etiological studies, might be more sensitive to the effects of differential socialization. Persons who, because of early socialization, are not socialized to play roles in an urban, industrial society, will not be regarded as "sick." Freed from the biological bias inherent in a medical model, researchers could experiment with varied re-socialization techniques and thus more creatively approach the task of assisting persons from ethnic sub-cultures to play new roles. This unburdening would be most salutary in the field of mental retardation. Historical beliefs in the biological root of all mental retardation and its essential incurability hover like a depressing cloud over the education and training of those labeled as mentally retarded.

Fifth, a social system perspective might sensitize professionals to the significance of the types of social systems which assume responsibility for the care of "abnormals." Long-term acting in the "sick" role, within a medical social system in which relationships with most significant other people are of a doctor–patient variety, is likely to hinder rather than facilitate eventual performance in "normal" roles such as those of student, employee or parent. How behavior is defined, the type of social system in which the individual lives and the roles which he plays in that social system are central concerns.

Instead of concentrating solely upon changing individual behavior, action taken from a social system perspective might more frequently concentrate on changing the normative structure of the system. Rather than always taking the behavioral norms of the majority group as the standard and attempting to change individuals to meet the demands of that normative structure, social action might focus on modifying the norms of the social system so that some behaviors now labeled as deviant would be evaluated as culturally different but normal.

Even when focusing on modifying the individual, helping professions aware of the social system perspective might provide more useful labels and more relevant programs for those identified as "abnormals." For example, when members of a sub-group are defined statistically as "abnormal" primarily because of characteristics acquired as a member of that sub-group, diagnosing them as abnormal by the norms of the dominant society provides little information relevant to the development of programs. It is simply quantifying what is obvious to anyone not blinded by diagnostic labels. Any child who has been reared in a Spanish-speaking home by parents who have little or no formal education is likely to fail an intelligence test requiring information about American middle-class society and facility in the English language.

If he is further labeled as mentally retarded, this placement may itself generate a self-fulfilling prophecy. The label "mentally retarded" obscures the fact that this child, reared in a different culture, has few

of the language skills and little of the information needed to pass an IQ test. His
educational needs are not in any way
similar to those of the middle-class, Anglo
child who achieves the same score on that
IQ test. The Spanish-speaking child needs a
program geared to acquainting him with the
American core-culture and its language,
while the Anglo child who fails the IQ test
at the same level is more likely to need the
kind of educational program usually offered
in special education classes. Anesthetized
by the clinical perspective and the magic of
the IQ score, however, public schools continue to label disproportionately large
numbers of children from cultural and ethnic
subgroups as mentally retarded and place
them in programs which compound rather
than ameliorate their problems. Hopefully,
a social system perspective would sharpen
professional insight into the bias inherent
in a clinical perspective and the diagnostic
labeling process as currently practiced.

Finally, recognizing that deviance is social
system specific may alert the helping professions to the possibility of alleviating
"abnormality," in some cases, by relocating
an individual in the social structure. If he
can find a place for himself in a sub-group
which does not regard his behavior as
"abnormal," he may be able to live out his
life as a "normal" person. Most "borderline" retardates, after leaving school, manage
this feat for themselves. Could more imagina-
tive placement efforts assist others who have
aberrant behavioral manifestations in one
system to find a place for themselves in
another system in which they could play
"normal" roles?

Summary and Conclusions

Three definitions of "normal" have been
identified: the medical model based on
functional analysis; the statistical model
based on the normal curve; and the social
system model based on an analysis of the
normative structure of each social system.
Definitions of abnormality generated by
these three models are likely to converge
when the behaviors being examined are
extreme and when they involve visible
biological irregularities. Thus, most children

with Down's syndrome (mongols) would
probably be labeled as "abnormal" by all
three models. That is, their biological deviations would be apparent in the pathological
model; most measurements taken on them
would place them in the extremes of the
normal distribution and thus make them
"abnormal" in the statistical model; and
most social systems would also regard them
as "abnormal." However, when there are no
biological signs and deviation is predominantly behavioral, the outcomes of the application of the three models are likely to
diverge. In interstitial cases, the pathological
model encounters difficulty because its
criterion for "normal" rests on a biological
functional analysis and there are few, if
any, biological "symptoms." The statistical
model is likely to label culturally different
sub-groups in the population as deviant
and this comes to be interpreted as pathological. A social system model, anchored in
the norms of individual subsystems, is likely
to reflect the social reality more accurately.

We conclude that each model has
strengths as well as limitations. When
organic damage and disease processes are
clearly involved, the pathological model is
the most powerful conceptual tool. When
there are behavioral components in the
phenomenon being studied which cannot be
directly related to physiological processes,
then a statistical model for "normal" may
be useful *if* the entire population being
studied has been exposed to essentially
similar socialization processes and has
internalized similar cultural norms and the
distributions on relevant characteristics are
"normal." However, when the entire population being studied is not culturally homogeneous and has not been exposed to similar
socialization processes nor internalized comparable values, then the social system model
for "normal" is to be preferred. Although
it is a more complex model which is cumber-
some to handle in empirical studies, it may
prove to be a more illuminating map with
which to explore culturally determined variations in human behavior.

5

Studies in
Sociophysiology

Howard B. Kaplan

Especially WITHIN the last decade a number of investigations have been reported concerning the relationship between patterns of human social interaction and physiological responses in laboratory situations. These investigations have been conceptualized as studies in "sociophysiology" or "interpersonal physiology"[1] and may properly be considered to fall within the realm of medical sociology. In the following pages we will attempt to review briefly the relevant literature which formed the empirical foundation for sociophysiological studies and describe in some detail certain investigations conducted by the author and his associates which were stimulated by consideration of this literature.

The Empirical Foundation of Sociophysiology

The initial impetus for these studies was derived from the numerous investigations of the effects of emotional distress upon the genesis of organic disorders. For example, several reports describe relationships between emotional factors and cardiovascular,

gastrointestinal and respiratory disorders.[2] However, the relevance of these studies for the medical sociological frame of reference was determined by the observation of associations between sociocultural patterns and emotional stresses (which in turn are related to the development of organic disorders).[3] Holmes and his associates[4] interpreted data collected from a tubercular population as indicating that culture conflict was contributory to the natural history of this disease. Spiegel and Bell[5] refer to other studies indicating relationships between family patterns and psychophysiological disorders. Kingsley and Reynolds[6] related patterns of psychosomatic illness to the subjects' ordinal position in the family. For example, only children tended to have gastrointestinal upsets, skin disorders, asthma, allergies and constipation. First-born children were characterized as having more constipation and feeding disorders. Second-born children were more likely to have respiratory and ear infections, tonsilitis, diarrhea, etc. Vincent[7] noted the association of loss of parents with the presence of diagnosed psychosomatic disorders. At

[1] Boyd, R. W., and A. DiMascio, "Social Behavior and Autonomic Physiology: A Sociophysiologic Study," *J. Nerv. & Ment. Dis.*, 120:207–212, 1954; A. DiMascio, R. W. Boyd and M. Greenblatt, "Physiological Correlates of Tension and Antagonism During Psychotherapy: A Study of 'Interpersonal Physiology'," *Psychosom. Med.*, 19:99–104, 1957.

[2] See, for example, M. F. Reiser and H. Bakst, "Psychology of Cardiovascular Disorders," in S. Arieti (ed.), *American Handbook of Psychiatry*, New York: Basic Books, 1959, pp. 659–677; T. Lidz and R. Rubenstein, "Psychology of Gastrointestinal Disorders," in Arieti, *op. cit.*, pp. 678–689; E. D. Wittkower, and K. L. White, "Psychophysiologic Aspects of Respiratory Disorders," in Arieti, *op. cit.*, pp. 690–707.

[3] Certain of these studies are reviewed by S. H. King, "Social Psychological Factors in Illness," in H. E. Freeman, S. Levine and L. G. Reeder (eds.), *Handbook of Medical Sociology*, Englewood Cliffs, N.J.: Prentice-Hall, 1963, pp. 99–121.

[4] Holmes, T. H., N. G. Hawkins, C. E. Bowerman, E. R. Clarke and J. R. Jaffe, "Psychosocial and Psychophysiologic Studies of Tuberculosis," *Psychosom. Med.* 19:134–143, 1957.

[5] Spiegel, J. P. and N. W. Bell, "The Family of the Psychiatric Patient," in Arieti, *op. cit.*, pp. 128–129.

[6] Kingsley, A., and E. L. Reynolds, "The Relation of Illness Patterns in Children to Ordinal Position in the Family," *J. Pediat.*, 35:17–23, 1949.

[7] Vincent, C. F., "The Loss of Parents and Psychosomatic Illness," *Sociol. & Soc. Res.*, 39:404–408, 1955.

another level of social organization, Ruesch and his associates discussed the relationship between psychosomatic conditions and social class-related variables, social change and social mobility.[8]

In general, these studies took the form of observing the relationship between demographic characteristics and the presence of psychosomatic disorders. Paralleling these studies were a number of *laboratory* investigations which might properly be termed psychophysiological in that they related physiological responses to intra-psychic processes, especially emotional responses. Usually, these studies took the form of observing the nature of physiological responses (heart rate, muscle tension, galvanic skin reflex, etc.) to standard stimuli such as emotionally significant words or pictures and were useful in demonstrating the sensitivity of physiological functions as indices of emotional conflict.[9]

Many of these studies, however, failed to demonstrate any *simple* positive relationships between emotional expression or presentation of affect-laden stimuli and physiological activation. Many of the findings could only be explained in terms of other aspects of the total situation.[10] Dittes,[11] for example, found that the association between a physiologic function and embarrassing sex statements was contingent upon the degree of permissiveness displayed by the therapist. Such findings as these led to assertions that personally relevant verbalizations and gener-

ally stressful situations were not the only, or even the most important, determinants of physiological responses. Very often the most potent variables appeared to be unanticipated aspects of the subject's interpersonal situation.[12] At one time physiological responses might be evoked by the subject's specific orientation to a social object in the interpersonal situation, and at another time to the subjective significance of the verbal content. In short, *the physiological responses of an individual had to be interpreted in terms of his total behavior within the context of the general situation.*

These conclusions prompted the review of several psychophysiological studies conducted in interpersonal laboratory situations to determine if the results were reinterpretable in terms of traditional sociological concepts.[13] For illustrative purposes, three such concepts will be discussed: social status, social sanction and definition of the situation.

SOCIAL STATUS

Social status is defined here as the social position that an individual occupies relative to other social positions, which serves as the focus for a complex of normative expectations incumbent upon the actor when interacting with specified relevant others. This concept has been employed as a variable in at least two sociophysiological studies.

In one study, Rankin and Campbell,[14] interested in studying the effects of aspects

[8] Ruesch, J., *et. al.*, "Acculturation and Illness," *Psychol. Monogr.*, 62 (5), 1958; *Chronic Disease and Psychological Invalidism*, Berkeley: Univ. California Press, 1948; "Chronic Disease and Psychosomatic Invalidism," *Psychosom. Med. Monogr.*, New York: Hoeber, 1946.

[9] McCurdy, H. G., "Consciousness and the Galvanometer," *Psychol. Rev.*, 57:322–327, 1950; J. W. L. Doust and R. A. Schneider, "Studies in the Physiology of Awareness: An Oximetrically Monitored Controlled Stress Test," *Canad. J. Psychol.*, 9:67–78, 1955.

[10] Lacey, J. I., "Psychophysiological Approaches to the Evaluation of Psychotherapeutic Process and Outcome," in American Psychological Association, *Research in Psychotherapy*, Washington, D.C., 1959, pp. 160–208.

[11] Dittes, J. E., "Extinction During Psychotherapy of GSR Accompanying 'Embarrassing Statements'," *J. Abnorm. Soc. Psychol.*, 54:187–191, 1957.

[12] Weiner, H., "Some Psychological Factors Related to Cardiovascular Responses: A Logical and Empirical Analysis," in R. Roessler and N. S. Greenfield (eds.), *Physiological Correlates of Psychological Disorder*, Madison: Univ. Wisconsin Press, 1962, pp. 115–141.

[13] Kaplan, H. B., and S. W. Bloom, "The Use of Sociological and Social–psychological Concepts in Physiological Research," *J. Nerv. & Ment. Dis.*, 130:128–134, 1960.

[14] Rankin, R. F., and D. T. Campbell, "Galvanic Skin Response to a Negro and White Experimenter," unpublished manuscript, 1954. Discussed in E. D. Lawson, *Attitude Shifts As Related to Palmer Sweating in Group Discussion*, doctoral dissertation, Univ. of Illinois, 1954, pp. 40–41.

of the experimental situation on physiological responses, used the psychogalvanometer to measure differential responses of subjects to physical contact with Negro and white experimenters. Two scales of attitudes toward Negroes were also administered. In general, the results demonstrated a positive relationship between the galvanic skin reflex (GSR) and attitude toward Negroes; that is, persons with greater prejudice toward Negroes showed increased GSR upon contact with a Negro.

The concept of social status, by implication, was also used by Reiser and associates[15] in their investigation of the effect of variations in laboratory procedure and experimenter upon physiological functions. In this connection, they suggested that the development of methods for the evaluation of the effects of such variations "might well make it possible to study some aspects of interpersonal relations (and their physiological concomitants) as they occur naturally, rather than through the use of artificial devices such as the superimposition of unusual and often incompletely understood 'stress'."[16] To this end, two experiments on comparable subjects (healthy young soldiers) were carried out. Half of the subjects were tested by a military captain–psychiatrist (Experiment 1), the other half by a military private–physiologist (Experiment 2). In each experiment, half of the subjects (control group) were immediately reassured that the experimental procedure was harmless, but half (experimental subgroup) were not given this information until later.

In the results of each experiment, there were significant differences between the control and experimental subgroups in the mean physiological response to the interview. However, in each experiment the differentiation between subgroups was related only to one of the several physiological functions; and the one function varied with the status

of the experimenter. In the first experiment, carried out by the military officer, the two subgroups were differentiated only by amplitude of the ballistocardiogram. In the second experiment, executed by the enlisted man, the two subgroups were distinguished from each other only by mean arterial blood pressure. Thus the nature of the physiological response of the subjects varied with the status of the person with whom they interacted. The interview data suggested that "the main emotional change during the experimental interviews in Experiment 1 was relief of uneasiness and tension, whereas the main emotional shift distinguishing the experimental subjects in Experiment 2 appeared to be the discharge or release of angry, resentful feelings"[17] which were presumably inhibited, in the first experiment, due to the presence of the military officer.

SOCIAL SANCTION

While the phenomenon of social sanction is present in all social interaction, it has been systematically studied as a variable in few experimental *psycho*physiological studies. Social sanction is defined here as behavior by the subject that serves, either by intent of subject and/or perception by the social object, as a reward or punishment for behavior by the social object.

Perhaps the clearest example of the utilization of this concept is a study of the interaction between interviewer and interviewee by physiological recording techniques conducted by Malmo, Boag and Smith.[18] While the experimenters did not employ the term "sanction," their operational definition clearly conforms to the requirements of our definition. Nineteen female psychoneurotic patients were asked to relate a story in response to a Thematic Apperception Test (TAT) card. The examiner then either praised or criticized the patients' stories. Among the results was the finding that, during the rest intervals following the praise or criticism, the speech muscle tension fell rapidly following praise in contrast to the non-

15 Reiser, M. F., R. B. Reeves and J. Armington, "Effects of Variations in Laboratory Procedure and Experimenter upon the Ballistocardiogram, Blood Pressure, and Heart Rate in Healthy Young Men," *Psychosom. Med.* 17:185–199, 1955.
16 *Ibid.*, p. 186.

17 *Ibid.*, p. 198.
18 Malmo, R. B., T. J. Boag and A. Smith, "Physiological Study of Personal Interaction," *Psychosom. Med.*, 19:105–119, 1957.

falling tension following criticism. Thus, differential sanctions were accompanied by differential physiological responses.

DEFINITION OF THE SITUATION

Other studies, either in the research design or in the interpretation of results, discussed phenomena that are closely related to the traditional sociological concept, "definition of the situation." This concept is defined here in terms of the relative clarity of the normative expectations that are applicable to the individuals in a social situation.

Boyd and DiMascio[19] found in their study of the psychotherapeutic interview that, as the particular interview under study proceeded, the heart rate became slower, sweating increased and face temperature increased. These findings suggested to the investigators that the interview produced an immediate increase in sympathetic nervous tension, but as time passed and the patient apparently *adapted socially* to the psychiatrist, sympathetic relaxation occurred. This investigation is based on the study of only one patient in therapy, but its results are suggestive especially in the light of other related studies.

It will be recalled that Reiser, *et al.*,[20] performed two experiments on healthy young soldiers, half of whom were tested by an officer (Experiment 1) and half of whom were tested by an enlisted man (Experiment 2). However, they also introduced another variable—relative uncertainty as *to the exact nature of the procedure.* In each of the two experiments, half of the subjects (control subgroup) were immediately "reassured as to the benign nature of the procedure "[21] and half (experimental subgroup) were not given this information until later. In each case, the subgroups were distinguished on the basis of a statistically significant difference in the mean physiological response, indicating that variation in the definition of the situation may lead to variation of physiological response.

The review of these and other studies clearly indicated that it is feasible to study directly the relationships between parameters of social interaction and variation in physiological functioning in experimental-laboratory situations, and prompted the initiation of a series of studies to determine the specific dimensions of group interaction which have consequences for variability in physiological functions.

Two Studies in Sociophysiology

Although a number of studies in the area of sociophysiology were accomplished between 1958 and the present by the author and his associates, only two will be described in some detail for purposes of illustrating the methodology and substantive findings of this area of investigation.[22]

STUDY I

The major purpose of this study was to investigate the effects of sociometric relationships (those characterized by attraction, repulsion or emotional indifference) upon physiological responses in small peer groups. It was hypothesized that, under conditions of intense emotional orientations

[22] These studies were accomplished in laboratories of the Department of Psychiatry, Baylor University College of Medicine and Houston State Psychiatric Institute. The methodology and results of these investigations are reported in greater detail in a series of publications including: H. B. Kaplan, "Social Interaction and GSR Activity During Group Psychotherapy," *Psychosom. Med.*, 25:140–145, 1963; H. B. Kaplan, N. R. Burch, S. W. Bloom and R. Edelberg, "Affective Orientation and Physiological Activity (GSR) in Small Peer Groups," *Psychosom. Med.*, 25:245–252, 1963; H. B. Kaplan, N. R. Burch and S. W. Bloom, "Physiological Covariation and Sociometric Relationships in Small Peer Groups," in P. H. Leiderman and D. Shapiro, *Psychobiological Approaches to Social Behavior*, Stanford: Stanford Univ. Press, 1964, pp. 92–109; H. B. Kaplan, N. R. Burch, T. D. Bedner and J. D. Trenda, "Physiologic (GSR) Activity and Perceptions of Social Behavior in Positive, Negative, and Neutral Pairs," *J. Nerv. Ment. Dis.*, 140:457–463, 1965; H. B. Kaplan, "Physiological Correlates of Affect in Small Groups," *J. Psychosom. Res.*, 2:173–179, 1967.

[19] Boyd and DiMascio, *op. cit.*
[20] Reiser, Reeves and Armington, *op. cit.*
[21] *Ibid.*, p. 198.

among group members, the affective response of these members to the pattern of interpersonal activity in the group would be reflected in unique physiological patterns.

Method—A class of medical students responded to a sociometric questionnaire requesting an indefinite number of names of their classmates that they "like" and "dislike." At the time of the administration the subjects had been classmates for approximately 18 months. On the basis of these data, 3 four-man groups were chosen that may be respectively termed positive, negative and mixed. The positive group consisted of four students each of whom was liked by every other member of the group. The most negative group available consisted of students each of whom was disliked by one other member of the group and none of whom was liked by any other member of the group. The mixed group was composed of two individuals who were liked by one other member of the group and one who was disliked by one other member of the group.

Each of the three groups met for five sessions, each of 45 minutes duration, to discuss one of five topics of interest to medical students. The topics were assigned at random. Sound film recordings were made of each of the 15 sessions from an observation room. The social responses of the subjects were characterized by coding the sound film recordings in terms of Bales' interaction process categories.[23] Each observed act was coded in one of the following 12 categories.

Positive socioemotional responses
1. Shows solidarity, raises other's status, gives help or reward.
2. Shows tension release, jokes, laughs, shows satisfaction.
3. Agrees, shows passive acceptance, understands, concurs, complies.

Instrumental responses: answers
4. Gives suggestion, direction, implying autonomy for the other.
5. Gives opinion, evaluation, analysis, expresses feeling, wish.

[23] Bales, R. F., *Interaction Process Analysis*, Cambridge, Mass.: Addison-Wesley, 1951.

6. Gives orientation, information, repeats, clarifies, confirms.

Instrumental responses: questions
7. Asks for orientation, information, repetition and confirmation.
8. Asks for opinion, evaluation, analysis, expression of feeling.
9. Asks for suggestion, direction, possible ways of action.

Negative socioemotional responses
10. Disagrees, shows passive rejection, formality, withholds resources.
11. Tension—asks for help, withdraws out of field.
12. Shows antagonism, deflates other's status, defends or asserts self.

The physiological function chosen to represent autonomic nervous system activation was the galvanic skin response (GSR), a measure of the changes in resistance of the skin to electrical conductance. The GSR is generally accepted variously as an index of emotional significance, physiological arousal or adaptive mobilization and is recognized to be extremely sensitive to sensory and ideational stimuli.[24] Continuous recordings of GSR activity were collected for each subject for all sessions.[25] By the nature of the method the GSR responses were synchronized with the social responses.

Analysis—With Spearman's rank–order coefficient as the measure of association and the minute as the varying time unit, the GSR responses of each subject were correlated with the number of his own responses in each of the 12 social categories, and his total social responses, regardless of the person to whom they were addressed; and the number of his responses in each of the

[24] Davis, R. C., "Physiological Responses As a Means of Evaluating Information," in A. D. Biderman and H. Zimmer (eds.), *The Manipulation of Human Behavior*, New York: Wiley, 1961, pp. 142–168; I. Mantin, "Somatic Reactivity," in H. J. Eysenck, *Handbook of Abnormal Psychology*, New York: Basic Books, 1961, pp. 417–456.

[25] The physiological recording techniques are described in more detail in the publications cited in footnote 22 and in R. Edelberg, and N. R. Burch, "Skin Resistance and Galvanic Skin Response (Influence of Surface Variables and Methodological Implications)," *A. M. A. Arch. Gen. Psychiat.*, 7:163–169, 1962.

categories, and his total responses, *directed toward each other person in the group*. The specific questions deriving from the general hypotheses were posed in terms of the relative probability of obtaining positive correlations of 0.29 or above in one sociometric grouping as opposed to another, using chi-square analysis to test the relationship.[26]

The subjects met in four-man groups but, for present purposes, the paired affective relationship was chosen as the unit of analysis. The positive group consisted of six pairs in reciprocal "liking" relationship. The negative group consisted of three negative pairs (at least one member of each pair disliked the other pair member) and three neutral pairs (the pair members indicated neither like nor dislike for each other). The mixed group consisted of one unilateral positive, one unilateral negative and four neutral pairs. Combining the similar relationships for the three groups, there were seven positive, four negative and seven neutral pairs for each of the five sessions (a total of 90 relationships).

Results—Among the major conclusions of the study were those relating to the associations between physiological activity and the subject's behavior depending upon the nature of his relationship with the group members and the nature of the social behavior.[27] Two of these findings will be discussed.

1. Subjects who were interacting with positive (liked) or negative (disliked) social objects were significantly more likely to manifest physiological responses along with

[26] It is of particular importance to appreciate that the use of Spearman's rank–order coefficient in Study I is not related to determining level of significance, but rather to establishing the nominal class "positive correlation" between various parameters of 1-minute sample durations. The chi-square test has been employed to determine level of significance of the difference between the class "positive correlation above 0.29 magnitude" as compared with the other class of this universe "correlation below 0.29 magnitude" as both classes are distributed in the three sociometric groups. It should be noted that events within a class are not ordered.

[27] A number of other findings, particularly those relating to physiological covariation, are reviewed in Kaplan, Burch and Bloom, *op. cit.*

their overt social responses than were subjects who were interacting with neutral (neither liked nor disliked) social objects. There was no difference in this regard between persons interacting with positive social objects and those interacting with negative social objects. This conclusion was derived by correlating the GSR responses of each subject for a given session with his own responses in each of the social categories, and with his own total responses that were directed toward each other person in the group.

Apparently it was the presence of affective involvement rather than the direction of the affect which was the main factor in determining physiological response, since no difference was observed with regard to the number of significant positive correlations between GSR and social responses directed toward positive as opposed to negative social objects. But significant differences were observed between each of these conditions and behavior directed toward neutral social objects (see Table 5–1). These findings are consistent with those reported above concerning the role of groups based on intense emotional relationships (such as families) and patterns of psychosomatic disorders.

A further question remained to be answered. Since the presence of an affective relationship tended to produce physiological concomitants of social responses, might we also expect that certain forms of social behavior would be more significant than others in this regard? Apparently this is the case as is indicated by the following conclusion:

2. Subjects who were interacting with positive or negative social objects were significantly more likely to manifest GSR responses in association with *socioemotional* responses than subjects who were interacting with neutral social objects. However, no significant differences were observed with regard to instrumental acts or total number of acts.

The third conclusion was derived in much the same way as the second but for the separate treatment of the socioemotional categories (1–3, 10–12), instrumental categories (4–9) and total number of acts. It

Table 5–1—Subjects' GSR correlations with own categorized and total social responses directed toward negative, positive and neutral objects

	NEGATIVE OBJECTS		POSITIVE OBJECTS		NEUTRAL OBJECTS	
	N	%	N	%	N	%
Significant Positive GSR Correlations with Own Categorized and Total Social Responses	46	22	86	22	59	14
No Significant Positive Correlations with Own Categorized and Total Social Responses	164	78	304	78	364	86
Total Correlations	210	100	390	100	423	100

Affective (positive and negative) vs. neutral: $x^2 = 10.6$, $P < 0.005$.
Negative vs. Neutral: $x^2 = 6.4$, $P < 0.02$.
Positive vs. Neutral: $x^2 = 9.1$, $P < 0.005$.
Negative vs. Positive: x^2 not significant.

Table 5–2—Correlations of GSR responses with own behavior toward positive or negative and toward neutral objects

	POSITIVE OR NEGATIVE OBJECTS		NEUTRAL OBJECTS	
	N	%	N	%
Socioemotional Behavior				
Significant Positive GSR Correlations with Own Behavior	52	16	22	9
No Significant Positive GSR Correlations with Own Behavior	281	84	218	91
Total Correlations	333	100	240	100
$x^2 = 5.2$, $P < 0.025$				
Instrumental Behavior				
Significant Positive GSR Correlations with Own Behavior	43	27	21	18
No Significant Positive GSR Correlations with Own Behavior	116	73	95	82
Total Correlations	159	100	116	100
x^2 not significant				
Total Acts				
Significant Positive GSR Correlations with Own Behavior	37	34	16	24
No Significant Positive GSR Correlations with Own Behavior	71	66	51	76
Total Correlations	108	100	67	100
x^2 not significant				

was reasoned that if the GSR as an affect indicator were more likely to be associated with social behavior in the context of affectively based relationships when compared to neutral relationships, then *a fortiori* this association should be even greater for primarily affective behavior.

As Table 5–2 indicates, the differences in the number of significant positive correlations between GSR and behavior directed toward positive or negative as opposed to neutral social objects was significant for socio-emotional behavior ($x^2 = 5.2$, $P < 0.025$), but was not significant for instrumental behavior and total acts, although the differences were in the same direction. This is not to imply that the GSR is associated only with socioemotional activity. Indeed, there are proportionately more significant positive correlations between GSR and social responses in the case of instrumental activity and total responses than for socioemotional behavior. The progressive increase in the proportion of such correlations for both positive and negative relationships combined and for neutral relationships as we proceed from socioemotional through instrumental to total acts suggests that the amount of activity is in part related to GSR response. Nevertheless, the neutral relationships were significantly differentiated from positive and negative social relationships on the basis of correlations of the GSR with socioemotional behavior, but such differentiation, although in the same direction, was not significant for either instrumental or total activity.

Thus, while the GSR may be associated with such factors as amount of activity, the data demonstrate that the GSR is also related to the kind of social activity and to the nature of the subject's interpersonal relationship with the person toward whom the behavior is directed.

STUDY 2

The results of Study 1 and other considerations derived from the sociological literature on small groups suggested that a variety of structured variables engender different interactional problems and patterns for group members and determine the differential satisfaction of a range of group and individual

"needs"; under certain conditions the probability of particular "needs" arising or being satisfied–unsatisfied is greater than under other conditions. One such variable or condition is the mutual affective orientation of the group members. It was expected therefore that social behaviors which are closely associated with specific interactional problems would have a meaning for members of one affective grouping that these behaviors would not have for members of another affective grouping. Thus, it might be expected that the management of interpersonal hostility would more likely be an interactional problem of negative-pair members than of positive- or neutral-pair members. If different problems are likely to arise under different affective conditions, those forms of perceived social behavior that are relevant to a given problem should have higher arousal value than perceived social behaviors which are not relevant to the dynamic interaction of the group process or to the "needs" of the individual members. Again taking the GSR as an index of arousal, it may be predicted that within each affective grouping, individuals with more GSR activity will be distinguishable from those with less GSR activity in relation to the extent to which they perceived different forms of social behavior as present and that, insofar as the interactional problems and "needs" vary among the affective groupings, the GSR activity of the group members should be differentially related to patterns of perceptions of social behavior as a function of the affective grouping.

Method—Each member of a class of female nursing students was asked to rate her degree and polarity of affect orientation for the other class members along a five-point scale (extreme liking to extreme disliking) and also to indicate how she thought other class members would respond to her along the same scale. From these data, 29 *pairs* of subjects (Ss) were chosen (10 positive, 11 neutral and 8 negative). Each negative pair member indicated extreme disliking for her partner and perceived her partner as having similar feelings toward her. Each positive pair member indicated extreme feelings of liking for her partner and perceived her partner as responding toward her in the same fashion. For the neutral pairs, each member indicated neither liking nor disliking toward her partner (midpoint on the scale) and perceived her partner as being similarly affectively neutral toward her.

Each pair met for two consecutive 20-minute sessions during which they discussed two topics previously determined to be of equally strong interest to both members. For each session GSR recordings were obtained using the same method as in Study 1. Following each session the pair members responded to a slightly modified version of an instrument reported by Stock and Thelen[28] consisting of 10 statements characterizing social behavior. These statements are presented in Table 5–3. Each S ranked the 10 statements according to the degree to which she perceived the statement to be characteristic of her own behavior during the preceding discussion (from most characteristic to least characteristic). She then ranked the same statements according to the degree to which she judged each was characteristic of her partner's behavior during the session.

Analysis—In order to test the general hypothesis, it was necessary to characterize each S with respect to her GSR activity and her perceptions of interpersonal activity. An S was described as "high" on a given behavioral dimension if she assigned a rank of 1 to 5 to the item, perceiving the behavior as being "most descriptive" of her own and her partner's behavior. An S was described as "low" on a given statement if she assigned a rank of 6 to 10 to the item, thus perceiving the behavior as being "least descriptive" of her own and her partner's behavior during a given discussion session.

Each S was characterized with respect to her GSR activity in terms of the total number of GSR deflections she manifested during a given session relative to the total population. In view of the tendency of the GSR to adapt

[28] Stock, D., and H. A. Thelen, *Emotional Dynamics and Group Culture*, New York: New York Univ. Press, 1958, pp. 265–266.

to stimuli over time, each S's GSR responses from the first session were treated separately from her responses from the second session. All S's were ranked according to GSR activity (total number of deflections) during the first session and characterized as "high" GSR responders if they fell above the median value and "low" if they fell below it. The same procedure was followed for the GSR responses during the second session. The two "high" and two "low" categories for the two distributions were then each combined. The next step in the analysis was to test the significance of the relationship between number of GSR responses and the S's rankings of social behavior in each affective grouping, using chi-square.

Results—It was hypothesized that, as a result of different interactional problems arising in different affective groupings, the same form of social behavior would have different "meanings" to the members of each of the affective groupings, and therefore the self–other descriptions of behavioral items would be differentially associated with GSR responses in the three affective groupings. To test the hypothesis, the rankings of each behavioral item were cross-tabulated against the GSR responses for the members of each of the three groupings separately. Table 6–3 presents the percentages of "high" and "low" GSR responders high on the rankings of the various behavioral items for each grouping.

In general, the hypothesis was supported. With one exception, the self–other items to which GSR activity was related and/or the direction of the relationship varied with the affective grouping.

Among *negative-pair members*, GSR was significantly related to three items, and all three referred to socioemotional responses. "High" GSR responders (compared with "low" responders) were significantly less likely to describe themselves as "warm and friendly" during the session and were more likely to characterize themselves as "irritated" and "eager and aggressive." This pattern of relationships suggests that a major need for members of the negative groups is the management of affect expression, and their concern with this dimension is reflected in the

Table 5-3—"High" ranks on behavioral descriptions of self and partner among high and low GSR responders by affective grouping

High Rank on:	NEGATIVE					Pair Members POSITIVE					NEUTRAL				
	High GSR N=15		Low GSR N=17		X²*	High GSR N=17		Low GSR N=23		X²*	High GSR N=26		Low GSR N=18		X²*
	N	%	N	%		N	%	N	%		N	%	N	%	
I was especially warm and friendly to my partner.	7	47	15	88	4.6†	13	76	22	95		21	81	13	72	
She was especially warm and friendly to me.	8	53	15	88		16	94	23	100		25	91	16	89	
I did not participate much.	3	20	2	12		4	24	1	04		8	31	6	33	
She did not participate much.	2	13	3	18		4	24	7	30		8	31	6	33	
I concentrated on the job.	9	60	16	94	4.4†	15	88	21	91		19	73	15	83	
She concentrated on the job.	8	53	15	88		9	53	19	82	4.1	22	84	9	50	6.1
I tried to get my partner in the discussion.	11	73	8	47		13	76	13	56		20	77	16	89	
She tried to get me in the discussion.	10	67	10	59		10	59	17	74		19	73	12	67	
I took over the leadership.	9	60	11	65		11	65	10	43		13	50	8	44	
She took over the leadership.	10	67	11	65		11	65	10	43		9	34	12	67	4.4
I was polite to my partner.	11	73	17	100		15	88	22	95		26	100	18	100	
She was polite to me.	12	80	16	94		16	84	19	92		22	84	18	100	
My suggestions were frequently off the point.	2	13	3	18		2	12	7	30		6	23	10	56	4.8
Her suggestions were frequently off the point.	3	20	3	18		8	47	4	17	4.1	2	08	5	28	
I was a follower.	4	27	6	35		7	41	9	39		9	34	4	22	
She was a follower.	6	40	4	24		4	24	5	22		11	42	6	33	
I was irritated.	5	33	0	00	7.0	2	12	0	00		0	00	0	00	
She was irritated.	5	33	1	06		1	06	0	00		1	04	0	00	
I was eager and aggressive.	13	86	7	41		3	18	10	43		7	27	0	00	3.9†
She was eager and aggressive.	11	73	7	41		6	35	10	43		10	38	6	33	

*All chi-square values presented are significant at the 0.05 level or better (one degree of freedom).
†Yates' correction applied.

association between GSR and descriptions relating to the socioemotional parameters.

Among *positive-pair members*, GSR activity was significantly associated with two items, neither of which duplicated the relationships described above. "High" GSR responders (when compared with "low" GSR responders) were significantly less likely to describe their partners as "concentrating on the job" and more likely to characterize their partners' suggestions as "frequently off the point." Apparently the management of negative emotional expression was not a serious problem for negative group members. Rather, the tensions aroused in these Ss related to task fulfillment. The following explanation for these relationships is suggested based upon the assumptions that positive pair members are more highly motivated to accomplish the task than negative or neutral pair members and that, in view of the existing close personal relationship, too much time spent in positive socioemotional activity might impede task fulfillment. Given a high task motivation it would be expected that disruption of the task process ("not concentrating on the job," "suggestions off the point") would be accompanied by greater GSR response.[29]

Among *neutral pair members*, GSR activity was significantly related to four items. "High" GSR responders (when compared with "low" GSR responders) were significantly more likely to describe their partners as "concentrating on the job" and less likely to describe them as "taking over the leadership." "High" GSR responders were also significantly less likely to characterize their own suggestions as "frequently off the point" and were more likely to describe themselves as "eager and aggressive" when compared with "low" GSR responders.

In view of the relatively low task involvement in such groups, one would expect that under a condition of withdrawal by mutual consent the pair members would experience a minimum of tension, but that when the members tried actively to influence each

[29] The interpretations of these findings as they relate to associated social–psychological studies are discussed at some length in Kaplan, Burch, Bedner and Trenda, *op. cit.*

other, the consequent resistance would engender high tension levels and that the latter would be reflected in higher GSR activity.

In summary, it would appear that groups characterized by different sociometric relationships experience different interactional problems and that perceptions relating to these problems generate physiological responses.

Interpretation of the results suggest that (1) among the *negative pairs*, high GSR activity was associated with the members' self–other descriptions relating to expression of negative (as opposed to positive) affect; (2) for the *positive pairs*, high GSR activity was associated with descriptions relating to disruption of the task process (presumably by expressive positive socioemotional activity); (3) for *neutral pairs*, high GSR levels were associated with descriptions relating to resistance to active attempts at interpersonal influence (as opposed to passive mutual withdrawal).

Conclusion

As we have stated above, numerous empirical studies have described relationships between emotional stress and the genesis of certain organic disorders. Several of these investigations have also discussed the role of social and cultural factors in generating emotional stress. However, many of these studies in a very gross way simply demonstrate association between certain life experiences and the presence of organic states. As useful as these investigations are, they do not permit a fine delineation of face-to-face social processes and small group characteristics which induce emotional stress and, subsequently, organic disorders.

The review of some *socio*physiological studies presented above should demonstrate the feasibility of studying in a laboratory situation specific characteristics of the *ongoing interpersonal process* which, mediated by psychological processes, evoke physiological responses. By thus detailing the characteristics of social interaction which are associated with a wide variety of physiological responses, research in *sociophysiology* promises to contribute greatly to the ultimate understanding of the sociogenesis and psychogenesis of organic illness.

6

Social Epidemiology: An Appraisal

Leo G. Reeder

THIS PAPER was originally prepared as part of an invited response to a thoughtful and provocative paper by Professor Edward Rogers.[1] In his stimulating paper Professor Rogers has put his finger on some crucial nerve centers—not only for medical sociology but for large segments of sociology—that have relevance to the complex social problems of our time. Not that we have been unaware of these vital areas, but a solid reminder is a useful thing. He asks the help of sociology in discovering underlying and guiding structures for planning effective health programs. Sociology is asked to reduce concepts and research findings to simple action terms, else we "force public health into a more anomalous situation." Sociology is also asked to determine why health is valued in virtually all societies and in relation to what? It is taken to task, along with public health in general, for failure to solve "the riddle of the major chronic diseases and of mental illness." Certainly, medical sociology must admit some dereliction in failing to provide appropriate answers for the above. This paper will address itself primarily to that portion of Professor Rogers' paper called "The Social Etiology and Ecology of Disease," or what is generally referred to as social epidemiology.

Time does not permit a full answer to each of the objections and issues raised by Rogers and my comments must be limited to a few salient points. The issues discussed here are: first, the critical role that theory and, more importantly, a frame of reference plays in sociological research; second, the practicality of social epidemiological research; and finally, some suggestions for substantive and methodological research in social epidemiology. But first I would like to very briefly review the nature of social epidemiology as a field of research in sociology and public health.

A common meeting ground of sociology and public health may be found in the epidemiological model. As you are well aware, when the objective of the research is to study the role of social factors in the etiology of disease we refer to this as social epidemiology. This merging of sociology and public health epidemiology for fundamental and significant research in the increasingly important arena of the chronic diseases and the behavioral disorders is exceedingly important and promising. As in all investigations typically called basic research, the practical consequences may take years to develop.

One of the features of social epidemiology is that it seeks to extend the scope of investigation to include variables and concepts drawn from theory, a set of propositions or a frame of reference. As Rogers observes, the sociological approach is dynamic and oriented toward process. But this does not mean, as Rogers suggests, that sociological research is not interested in the proximal end of the causative chain. The methodological procedure in this field is similar to that of the classical epidemiological approach, i.e., to design an observational study of either a special population group or an analytical survey of a representative sample population. Hence, *both* are seeking the most information possible about the etiological agents of disease. But, the social epidemiologist would tend to agree with Cornfield that:

> The appropriate question to ask about agents in such situations (disease) is whether they

[1] Rogers, E. S., "Public Health Asks of Sociology," *Science*, 159:506–508, February, 1968.

Revised version of a paper read at the annual meeting of the American Sociological Association, San Francisco, September, 1969.

alter the probability of an event's occurrence, and not whether they do or do not cause it.[2]

An adequate sociological theory of etiology of disease or disorder will require specification of the most relevant independent variables, their linkages through the intervening processes to varying dependent variable outcomes (coronary heart disease, rheumatoid arthritis, etc.) and the conditions under which such patterns hold. As Homans puts it, "the office of theory is to explain."[3] But we may be better served at this stage of development to use a frame of reference provided by theory.[4,5] The frame of reference is a pretheoretical formulation; its functions are to define the proper concepts to be used in a field and to establish a set of axes for the field, i.e., delimiting the universe of inquiry. (Parsons[6] cites the frame of reference provided by supply and demand in economics.)

> It is pretheoretical in that it does not specify propositions, i.e., it does not state relationships between concepts, but merely defines a coherent body of concepts. . . . The main advantage of a frame of reference is that it provides a context for the accumulation of research findings.[7]

Finally, a frame of reference is exhaustive rather than narrow in its scope; too often our theories are conceptually limited and the accumulation of scientific findings into a body of knowledge is difficult. A frame of reference is necessary to unify otherwise diverse factual data and thus develop the science. I have emphasized this element of sociological research because I consider it to be a unique contribution to classical epidemiological research.

Although much is still unclear with regard to etiological mechanisms involved, preventive health action can be taken based upon the contributions of social epidemiology to disease control. Two examples may be cited; in the 1968 statement of the American Heart Association,[8] the personal attribute of "certain personality–behavior patterns" and the environmental factor of "emotionally stressful situations" are given official recognition for the first time as risk factors in coronary heart disease. In that document to practicing physicians, the American Heart Association suggests that these risk factors be considered in education and management aimed at:

> *preventing or retarding* the development of atherosclerosis and its thrombotic complications. This can be said despite uncertainty concerning the exact role of many of the factors believed to contribute to the rate of which lesions develop in individual vessels.[9]

Another example of public health action based upon social epidemiological research is the current campaign to reduce cigarette smoking among our population as a measure of controlling lung cancer. Much of the basic research on smoking behavior has been and is currently undertaken by sociologists.[10] Obviously, much more needs to be done in the way of research, but it is not too early to design action programs based upon existing knowledge of smoking behavior.

Furthermore, although public health control measures can be initiated on the basis of incomplete knowledge it is still worthwhile to continue to search for additional clues to the disease process. For example, on the basis of current knowledge, measles today

[2] Cornfield, J., "Principles of Research," *Amer. J. Mental Deficiencies*, 64:240–252, September, 1959.

[3] Homans, G., "Bringing Men Back In," *Amer. Soc. Rev.*, 29:809–818, December, 1964.

[4] Parsons, T., *Structure of Social Action*, New York: Free Press, 1949.

[5] McKinney, J. C., *Constructive Typology and Social Theory*, New York: Appleton-Century-Crofts, 1966.

[6] Parsons, *op. cit.*, pp. 28–29.

[7] Bailey, K., "The Reconstruction of Controversial Theory: Human Ecology as a Case in Point," unpublished paper presented at Pacific Sociological Association meeting, Seattle, 1969.

[8] American Heart Association, *Risk Factors and Coronary Heart Disease: A Statement for Physicians*, 1968.

[9] *Ibid.*

[10] Graham, S., and D. B. Heller, "Acceptance and Rejection of a Decremental Innovation: Cessation of Smoking," paper read at American Sociological Assoc. meeting and B. J. Bergen and E. Olesen, "Some Evidence for a Peer Group Hypothesis About Adolescent Smoking," *Health Educ. J.*, vol. 21, September, 1963.

can be controlled and perhaps even eradicated. Although the epidemiology and the course of the disease has been well understood since the days of Peter Panum, no one yet knows why measles is seasonal, i.e., why there is such a high incidence in the spring and a low incidence in the fall.

Some Suggestions for a New Phase of Socio–Epidemiological Research

In the balance of this paper I wish to limit the discussion to some of the positive steps that research in social epidemiology might attempt in the future. Rogers articulates a critical problem in social epidemiology related to the basic tool of this field, the survey method. The typical or classical methods of survey research, much used in health studies, have often been limited by the nature of the forms it has used. It has, in the words of Barton, "been a sociological meatgrinder, tearing the individual from his social context and guaranteeing that nobody in the study interacts with anybody else."[11] It typically fails to provide data on social contexts, on the social structure within which behavior can be understood. The critical nature of this kind of phenomena for understanding and explaining complex relationships between social behavior and biological outcomes is fairly obvious.

In his address to the American Sociological Association back in 1967, Barton discussed the problem and suggested methods for including social structure in survey research. As he pointed out, over the last 20 years there have been many experiments, particularly those of Lazarsfeld and his collaborators, that have undertaken to do just this. These methods include:

1) Measurement of perceived interpersonal environment.
2) Use of cluster samples to measure objective social contexts.
3) Use of sociometric samples to measure objective interpersonal environments.
4) Obtaining survey data on institutional settings and interinstitutional environments.

[11] Barton, A. H., "Bringing Society Back In," *Amer. Behavioral Scientist*, November–December, 1968.

These methods have important implications for studies not only in social epidemiology but also for health administration and health education on an action-oriented level. Let us briefly mention some of the research issues involved in trying to utilize these procedures.

SOCIAL CONTEXT STUDIES

The difficulties of using respondent reports of their social context are fairly obvious. They may not actually perceive the context, or they may not be aware of the characteristics of the social contexts that really do influence them. However, it is important to know their perceptions as well as the objective reality. The use of *cluster samples* to measure objective group contexts is relatively easy when we deal with identifiable organizational units, like workshops, offices and schools;[12] in a similar vein, the use of sociometric samples to measure interpersonal environments is not difficult in rural areas or small communities. The problem is considerably more difficult and complex in large urban areas, but not impossible as was initially demonstrated with the snowball sample first introduced by Katz and Lazarsfeld,[13] and later by Coleman and his colleagues[14] in the adoption of a new drug by physicians.

Related to the above issue is the matter of coping with the problem of social class or social status, specifically in urban studies. One of the major areas of neglect in urban research, according to Lauman, "concerns the patterns of intimate social interaction and their distribution in the stratification system."[15] What is needed in urban research are the types of studies that social anthropologists and rural sociologists have

[12] Lipset, S. M., *et. al.*, *Union Democracy*, New York: Free Press, 1956.
[13] Katz, E., and P. Lazarsfeld, *Personal Influence*, New York: Free Press, 1945.
[14] Coleman, J., *et. al.*, *Medical Innovation—A Diffusion Study*, Indianapolis: Bobbs-Merrill, 1966.
[15] Lauman, E. O., *Prestige and Association in an Urban Community*, Indianapolis: Bobbs-Merrill, 1966.

done of rural and small town life in America. Lauman's own work is a significant substantive and methodological contribution to urban social life with implications for medical sociologists. This type of research is desperately needed if we are to advance our knowledge and understanding of processes involved in etiology and prevention of disease as well as understanding urban health behavior. Most sociologists would agree that the simple correlation of a person's objective status characteristics and his health attitudes, behavior and physical outcome is not sufficient by itself as a research enterprise. It is recognized that:

> we must move toward specification and elaboration of the way in which these objective characteristics are translated into individual attitudes and behavior.[16]

It might be pointed out, however, that social class and similar broad variables assist us in closing in on more limited, precise variables —the object is to have a frame of reference that will permit a process of branching to take place in a systematic search for causative phenomena.[17]

Finally, attention should be given to the potential usefulness of "social indicators" for medical sociology, and it is well to discuss this concept, albeit briefly. The need for such indicators arises from rapid technological change and the necessity of anticipating that change. Although Bauer and his associates are careful to point out that such (technological change) effects are not easily anticipated,[18] there are some developments under way in the health field with respect to indicators of health and the HEW publication called *Indicators* is a step in this direction. Indicators of health do not necessarily reflect technological change but rather the whole complex of socio–economic and structural change in society.

The health of a specific population has traditionally been measured by the rate at which they die: a decreasing death rate is taken as an indication of increasing health. As Linder[19] notes, this measure is no longer an adequate index of a population's health. With greater interest in the *quality* of life rather than its prolongation, the absence of disease and infirmity are insufficient conditions to measure quality of health.

Social indicators, of course, need not be cold, statistical data; they could as easily be "soft" and qualitative as "hard" and quantitative. With the advancing state of medical science, the application of knowledge and techniques in the population needs to be continually assessed. Just as Bauer and his colleagues[20] reassessed the reliability and validity of various sacrosanct statistics, e.g., the Uniform Crime Reports, perhaps all the vital statistics, not only the death rate, long collected by government agencies "no longer yield enough information on which to base a sound national policy."[21]

What is needed is a GNP-like health index, and there are some efforts underway toward this end. The great advantage that the economists enjoy is a common unit of measurement—money. Indicators such as the amount of illness or the impact of illness in a population, measured by "number of days of restricted activity," is an excellent indicator of disability. As we know, such statistical indicators and other measure of general health and health services can be studied in the context of major social problems, i.e., poverty, minority justice, health care for the aged, urbanization. But even such indicators as amount of illness or days of restricted activity need to be carefully assessed. Zola has called our attention to the observation that illness may be so prevalent as to be the statistical *norm*.[22] He suggests that a socially conditioned selective process may be operating to influence the data that gets counted or tabulated as illness. Here Zola takes specific account of the cultural frame of reference and the role of societal values in both the diagnosis of a

[16] *Ibid.*

[17] Platt, J. R., "Strong Inference," *Science*, 146:347–353, October, 1964.

[18] Bauer, R. A., *et. al.*, *Social Indicators*, Cambridge, Mass.: M.I.T. Press, 1966.

[19] Linder, F. E., "The Health of the American People," *Scientific American*, 214:21–29, 1966.

[20] Bauer, *op. cit.*

[21] Linder, *op. cit.*

[22] Zola, I. K., "Culture and Symptoms—An Analysis of Patients' Presenting Complaints," *Amer. Soc. Rev.*, 31:615–630, October, 1966.

symptom as illness and for the degree of attention given to the symptomatology. He postulates that it might be this selective process "and not an etiological one which accounts for the many unexplained or over-explained epidemiological differences observed between and within societies."[23] His study, by the way, is a valuable contribution to the role of values in health and specifically indicates the practical consequences of this in medical practice, public health and preventive medicine campaigns that are symptom-based.

Interest in social indicators stems from the resurgence of interest in social change, in its causes, and in its measurement, and perhaps prediction. Those concerned with evaluation of social and health outcomes as a result of health programs, or with the formulation of major policy and administrative action as well as legislation, can benefit substantially from further development of social indicators. The sociologist can assist in the clarification of various interrelationships and statistical associations and help provide the factual basis for the health actions.

It is especially for those who have undertaken responsibility for bringing about publicly approved changes that the notion of "social indicators" is appealing. Such indicators would give a reading both on the current state of some segment of the social universe and on past and future trends, whether progressive or regressive, according to some normative criteria. The notion of social indicators leads directly to the idea of

"monitoring" social change. If an indicator can be found that will stand for a set of correlated changes, and if intervention can be introduced (whether on the prime, indicative, variable or on one of its systemic components), then the program administrator may have been provided a powerful analytical and policy tool.[24]

Social indicators have the potential of reducing a relatively large number of complex variables to a smaller and simpler set of indicators that are highly correlated with the former. This is certainly a worthwhile effort in social diagnosis. But a note of caution is indicated. Most of my remarks in this paper have been intended to suggest that sociological investigations resulting in findings that can be operationalized into simple action programs tend to be complicated by the processes of intervening and interacting variables. The result is that even a simple hypothesis, involving relatively simple independent variables, usually has to be recast to consider the effects of such intervening and interacting variables in explaining a dependent variable.

In summary, most of us would agree that there are no simple answers to the complex problems that mutually concern us. With more sophisticated methodological and substantive approaches we can, perhaps, narrow the gap between what public health wants and what sociology can provide.

[23] *Ibid.*, p. 619.

[24] Sheldon, E. B., and W. B. Moore, *Indicators of Social Change*, New York: Russell Sage Foundation, 1968, p. 4.

Societal Coping with Illness and Injury

AFTER RECOGNIZING the differential existence of disease and death among the various components of human society, ways and means of coping with such assaults evolve. Disease itself is not perceived or responded to in the same manner by all individuals and societal groups but in terms of the value-systems and attitude-sets prevailing in the society and culture. Medicine and its definitions of illness comprise only one component of those value-systems and attitude sets.

Once it has been recognized as a threatening condition, illness may become institutionalized into a set of behavioral norms within a network of social relationships termed the *sick role*. Thus, when behavior related to illness is organized into a social role, the sick role becomes a meaningful mode of reacting to and coping with the existence and potential hazards of sickness by a society, and which may or may not be independent and at times strikingly different from the criteria and norms of the medical profession and other healers in the same society. In this manner, human societies and their sub-components do not leave to chance the existence and consequent threats of disease but react by establishing norms of conducts, sets of expectations, and organized relationships that define illness and health behavior for its members. Consequently, as society's criteria for health and illness vary and change, the definitions and nature of the sick role correspondingly change. *Health* then becomes essentially a social value, as defined in meaningful terms by society for its members, and thereby accounts for the tremendous variety of definitions of health among human societies around the world.

This section presents articles dealing with health and illness behavior—the sick role, caring for the ill, the patient role, healers and healing practices, and health and the human community. All are viewed as efforts by society to cope with the threats and hazards of disease and injury, as societal responses to the existence of disease are perceived and evaluated by different segments of society.

Health and Illness Behavior: The Sick Role

The first part of this section presents a set of papers dealing with social, psychological, and cultural responses to illness in terms of the sick role. Talcott

Parsons has pioneered this discussion with his classic description of the sick role, particularly in terms of American society, in the first chapter of the section. David Mechanic expands this topic with his discussion of illness behavior and its implications for caring for the sick in society.

A critique of Parsons' formulation of the sick role is presented by Gene Kassebaum and Barbara Baumann, suggesting that Parson's criteria apply essentially to the acutely ill and that other aspects are needed to explain the sick role for the chronically ill person.

An extension of Mechanic's formulations of illness behavior into the realm of social patterns related to the seeking, finding, and carrying out of medical care is presented in the chapter by the late Edward Suchman, offering five stages in the sequence of medical events related to illness behavior.

Caring for the Ill: The Patient Role

A specific effort to cope further with illness and injury is to establish social roles for the care of those persons who have assumed the sick role, namely, the patient role, which may be regarded as an extension of the sick role itself. The larger society defines the legitimate criteria for sickness for its members, whereas the therapeutic and organizational setting in which the sick person obtains care and treatment sets up the criteria for his role as patient in that social system. The expectant mother in the delivery room of a hospital has a different set of expectations and norms of conduct as a patient from that of a person receiving surgery or a medical regimen for a gastric ulcer. Patients in a children's hospital have different roles from that of the terminal cancer patient in a chronic disease facility, as does the schizophrenic patient in a large public mental hospital, the patient with a toothache in the dentist's chair, and the convalescing stroke patient in a nursing home. All are legitimate incumbents in the sick role, but they are also interacting very diversely as patients, the latter role derived from but still different from the sick role *per se.*

How patients view their roles is analyzed in an extensive study by Daisy Tagliacozzo and Hans Mauksch in a large metropolitan hospital.

The importance of patients' self-concept and of other social and psychological aspects of rehabilitative therapy of the chronically ill and handicapped is reviewed by Theodor Litman.

The special care needed but too often neglected for the dying patient in today's highly technical and scientific medical facilities and settings is analyzed in a significant contribution by Barney Glaser.

Healers and Healing Practices

All societies have sickness and thus are in need of healers to treat and care for those afflicted. Consequently, another means of coping with disease and injury by society is to devise social roles in which their healers may legitimately perform their ministrations. Society also establishes organizations and settings to train the healers and others caring for the sick.

The practice of medicine has become a subject of increasing interest to social and behavioral scientists. Medicine is a social system and institution, with its own established norms, role-sets, values, structured activities and relationships, and it has established a high degree of autonomy in the control of its own affairs. Some of the conflicts and consequences of practicing medicine in the current American fee-for-service system are analyzed in a penetrating article by Eliot Freidson.

The physician-patient relationship is examined in several divergent contexts and socio-economic systems in the United States, England and the Soviet Union by Mark Field, who illuminates the social forces operating on the practice of medicine in society.

The social role of the nurse and her important functions in caring for the sick has been a topic of considerable interest to behavioral scientists. Sam Schulman has revised his original article that appeared in the first edition of this volume with some commentary on more recent changes in the contemporary role of the nurse.

Health and the Community

Although societies make formal attempts to cope with illness by defining sick roles, caring for the afflicted in their patient roles by an array of healers in therapeutic settings, and devising systems and organizations in which the providers and recipients of health care services interact, there will remain those who fail to cope with illness in the community and who inadequately utilize the health care system itself.

The articles in this section of Part II present a larger picture of societal responses and efforts to cope with disease, going beyond the role-components into the human community and its larger segments of health and illness behavior. Conditions of human life in the community may affect modes of responding to illness and the efforts to do something about it.

The direct relationship between conditions of poverty and illness is presented in the chapter by William Richardson. He also shows that the poverty-stricken obtain less adequate medical care in the current American system of health economics.

A controlled study by Philip Moody and Robert Gray contributes a new dimension to understanding why those in the lower socio-economic statuses do not obtain as much adequate medical care as those in the higher levels, indicating that the feeling of "alienation" may be a stronger predictor of resistance to preventive health care behavior than social class.

This section is completed with the contribution by the late Edward Suchman of an extensive survey of illness behavior in a large metropolitan population, a major finding being the association between the health orientations of certain cultural groups and their organization.

THE AIM of the present paper is to try to consider the socio–cultural definition of health and illness in the United States in the light, in the first instance, of American values, but also in terms of the ways in which the relevant aspects of the value system have come to be institutionalized in the social structure. I shall give primary attention to mental health, but will also attempt to define its relation to somatic health and illness as carefully as possible. I shall also try to place the American case in comparative perspective.

First, it is important to try to define the respects in which health and illness can be considered to be universal categories applying to all human beings in all societies and to distinguish them from the respects in which they may be treated as socially and culturally relative. It will be possible here to say only a few rather general things, but the development of social science does, I think, permit us to be somewhat more definite than it has been possible to be until rather recently.

There is clearly a set of common human features of health and illness; indeed more broadly there is probably a set of components which apply perhaps to all mammalian species. There is no general reason to believe that these common components are confined to somatic illness; my view would be that there are also such components for mental illness. It does, however, seem to be a tenable view that there is a range, roughly, from the "purely somatic" to the "purely mental"— both of course, being limiting concepts— and that as one progresses along that range the prominence of the factors of relativity as a function of culture and social structure increases. The importance of the "interpenetration" between somatic and mental aspects is so great, however, that it would be a mistake to draw a rigid line, in any empirical term, between them.

One point is relatively clear. This is that the primary criteria for mental illness must be defined with reference to the social *role-performance* of the individual.[1] Since it is

7

Definitions of Health and Illness in the Light of American Values and Social Structure

Talcott Parsons

at the level of role-structure that the principal direct interpenetration of social systems and personalities come to focus, it is as an incapacity to meet the expectations of social roles, that mental illness becomes a problem in social relationships and that criteria of its presence or absence should be formulated. This is of course not at all to say that the state which we refer to as mental, as of somatic, illness is not a state of the individual; of course it is. But that state is manifest to and presents problems for both the sick person and others with whom he associates in the context of social relationships, and it is with reference to this problem that I am making the point about role-performance.

At the same time I would not like to treat mental health as involving a state of commitment to the performance of *particular* roles. Such a commitment would involve specific memberships in specific relational systems, i.e., collectivities. Mental health is rather concerned with *capacity* to enter into such relationships and to fulfill the expectations of such memberships. In terms of the organization of the motivational

---

[1] Both health and illness, in general, I would like to treat as states of the individual person; the "pathology" of social systems, real and important as it is, should not be called "illness" nor the absence of it, "health." Cf. Talcott Parsons, "The Mental Hospital as a Type of Organization," in *The Patient and the Mental Hospital*, edited by Milton Greenblatt, Daniel J. Levinson, and Richard H. Williams, New York: Free Press, 1957.

system of the individual, it therefore stands at a more "general level" than do the more specific social commitments.

There is a set of mechanisms in the operation of which social system and personality aspects are interwoven, which make possible the many complex adjustments to changing situations which always occur continually in the course of social processes. It is when the mechanisms involved in these adjustive processes break down ("adjustive" as between personalities involved in social interaction with each other) that mental illness becomes a possibility, that is, it constitutes one way in which the individual can react to the "strains" imposed upon him in the course of social process. This can, of course, occur at any point in his own life cycle from the earliest infancy on. Also, I take for granted that mental illness is only one of several alternative forms which "deviance" can take, again at every stage. Mental illness, then, including its therapies, is a kind of "second line of defense" of the social system vis-à-vis the problems of the "control" of the behavior of its members. It involves a set of mechanisms which take over when the primary ones prove inadequate. In this connection it can also be readily seen that there are two main aspects of the operation of the mechanisms involved. First, the individual who is incapacitated from performing his role-functions would be a disturbing element in the system if he still attempted to perform them. Hence we may say that it is important to have some way of preventing him from attempting to do so, both in his own interest and in that of the system itself. Secondly, however, there is the therapeutic problem, namely of how it is possible to restore him to full capacity and return him to role-performance after an interval.

So far, I have been speaking of mental health with special reference to its place in the articulation between social system and personality. Mental health—and illness— are states of the personality defined in terms of their relevance to the capacity of the personality to perform institutionalized roles. For analytical purposes, however, I have found it necessary to make a distinction, which a good many psychologists do not make, between the personality and the organism. They are, of course, not concretely separable entities, but they are analytically distinguishable systems. There would be various ways of making the distinction, but for present purposes I think it is best to put it that the personality is that part of the mechanisms involved in the control of concrete behavior which genetically goes back to the internalization of social objects and cultural patterns in the course of the process of socialization. The organism, as distinguished from this, consists of that part of the concrete living individual which is attributable to hereditary constitution and to the conditioning processes of the physical environment. Hence, from the point of view of its relation to the personality, it is that aspect of the mechanisms controlling behavior which is not attributable to the experience of socialization in and through processes of social interaction.[2]

It will be noted that I have been careful not to say that the mechanisms through which the personality component of the concrete individual functions are not "physiological." In my opinion, it is not the distinction between physiological and in some sense "mental" processes which is the significant one here. Indeed, I think that *all* processes of behavior on whatever level are mediated through physiological mechanisms. The physiological mechanisms which are most significant in relation to the more complex forms of behavior are, however, mainly of the nature of systems of "communication" where the physiological mechanisms are similar to the physical media and channels of communication.

[2] I have put forward this general type of view on two previous occasions. For the general conception of the relation of personality to the internationalization of social and cultural objects, see Parsons and Bales, *Family, Socialization and Interaction Process*, New York: Free Press, 1955. A more extended discussion of the relation of personality and organism will be found in Parsons, "An Approach to Psychological Theory in Terms of the Theory of Action," American Psychological Association, *Studies in General Theory*, ed. Sigmund Koch, New York: McGraw-Hill, 1958.

Definitions of Health and 99
Illness in the Light of
American Values and Social Structure

Hence, in both cases the content of "messages" cannot be deduced from the physical properties of the media. In the higher organisms, including man, it seems clear that the focus of these mechanisms rests in the central nervous system, particularly the brain, and that the next level down in the order of systems of control, has to do with the hormones which circulate through the blood stream.

It is important to stress this "interpenetration" of personality and organism, because, without it, the complex phenomena usually referred to as "psychosomatic" are not understandable. Correspondingly, I do not think that the way in which *both* somatic and mental health and illness can fit into a common sociological framework are understandable without both the distinction between personality and organism and the extreme intimacy of their interpenetrating relationship.

Coming back to the relation of both to the social system, I should like to introduce a distinction which has not been consistently made by sociologists either in this or in other connections, but which I think is very important for present purposes. This is the distinction between *role* and *task*. There are many different definitions of the concept role in the sociological literature. For my present purpose, however, I think one very simple one is adequate, namely a role is the organized system of participation of an individual in a social system, with special reference to the organization of that social system as a collectivity.[3] Roles, looked at in this way, constitute the primary focus of the articulation and hence interpenetration between personalities and social systems. Tasks, on the other hand, are both more differentiated and more highly specified than roles; one role is capable of being analyzed into a plurality of different tasks.

Seen in these terms I think it is legitimate to consider the task to define the level at which the action of the individual articulates with the *physical* world, i.e., the level at which the organism in the above analytical

sense is involved in interaction with its environment in the usual sense of biological theory. A task, then, may be regarded as that subsystem of a role which is defined by a definite set of *physical* operations which perform some function or functions in relation to a role and/or the personality of the individual performing it. It is very important that processes of communication, the *meanings* of which are by no means adequately defined by the physical processes involved at the task level, are not only included in the concept of task, but constitute at least one of the most important, if not *the* most important, categories of tasks, or of components of them.[4]

Coming back to the problem of health and illness, I should now like to suggest that somatic illness may be defined in terms of incapacity for relevant task-performance in a sense parallel to that in which mental illness was thought of as incapacity for role-performance. In the somatic case the reference is not to any particular task, but rather to categories of tasks, though of course, sudden illness may force abandonment of level rather than any particular task.[5] Put

[3] This definition clearly matches that put forward by Merton as the "role-set." See R. K. Merton "The Role-Set," *British Journal of Sociology*, June, 1957.

[4] Thus I am at present engaged in the task of "writing" a paper on the institutionalization of the patterns of health and illness in American society. The "technique" I have chosen for this task is manipulating the keyboard and other parts of a typewriter. This process clearly engages the hands and fingers, eyes, and other parts of the physical organism; internally above all, the brain. The physical result is the arrangement on a number of sheets of paper, previously blank, of a very large number of what we call linguistic symbols; letters arranged in words, sentences and paragraphs. I could have chosen alternative techniques, such as writing longhand with a pen, or possibly dictating to a machine. In these cases the physical result might well have been different. But in any case the "significance" of the task is only partly "physical"; it lies more in the "meanings" of what has been physically "written." Finally, the task of writing this paper is only one rather clearly defined subsystem of my *role* as sociologist.

[5] Referring to the writing task, a paralysis of both arms would obviously incapacitate me for writing this and other papers on the typewriter, and for all other manual tasks, but not necessarily for dictating them to a secretary.

the other way around, *somatic health is, sociologically defined, the state of optimum capacity for the effective performance of valued tasks.*

The relation between somatic and mental health, and correspondingly, illness, seen in this way, bears directly on the problem of levels of organization of the control of behavior. It implies that the "mind" is not a separate "substance" but essentially a level of organization, the components of which are "non-mental," in the same basic sense in which for example, the hypothetical isolated individual is "non-social." It further implies that the mental level "controls" the somatic, or in this sense, physical, aspect of the individual, the "organism." Somatic states are therefore necessary, but in general *not* sufficient conditions of effective mental functioning.[6]

The Problem of "Cultural Relativity" in Health and Illness

Our present concern is with the relation of personality and organism on the one hand, the social system and its culture on the other. It is now possible to say something on the question of the relations between the universal human elements and the socioculturally variable ones in health and illness on both levels. Clearly, by the above definition, *all* human groups have highly organized personalities which must be built up by complex processes of the sort we call socialization and which are subject to various sorts

of malfunctioning at the level of social adjustment which has been referred to. All human societies have language, a relatively complex social organization, complex systems of cultural symbols and the like. The individual in such a society, however "primitive," is always involved in a plurality of different roles which are the organizing matrix of the various tasks he performs.

Clearly this personality element of the structure of the individual person is closely interpenetrating and interdependent with the organic–somatic aspect. Hence, there are clearly "problems" of both somatic and mental illness and health for all human groups. Furthermore, all of them are deeply involved with the structures of the social system and the culture.

That there are uniformities in the constitutions of all human groups at the organic level goes without saying, and hence that many of the problems of somatic medicine are independent of social and cultural variability. Thus such things as the consequences and possibilities of control of infection by specific bacterial agents, the consequences of and liability to cancerous growths and many other things are clearly general across the board. This is not, however, to say that the *incidence* and probably degrees of severity of many somatic diseases are not functions of social and cultural conditions, through many different channels. But within considerable ranges, independent of the part played by such factors etiologically, the medical problems presented are essentially the same, though of course, how to implement medical techniques effectively is again partly a socio–cultural problem.

It follows from the conception of personality put forward here, that constancies in the field of mental health are intimately related to uniformities in the character of culture and social structure. Here it is particularly important that, after a period in which a rather undiscriminating version of the doctrine of "cultural relativity" was in the ascendant, much greater attention has recently come to be paid to the universals which are identifiable on these levels. It is not possible here to enter into any sort of detail in this field, but a few highlights may be mentioned.

[6] This view of the relation of mind and body and in turn, their relations to the two great categories of health and disease with which we are here concerned, does not imply that all "somatic" phenomena can be analyzed as standing on one level. For various reasons it seems to me that at least one comparably basic distinction needs to be made within the organism, as defined above, namely, between the "behavioral" system and what might be called the "homeostatic" system (what Franz Alexander calls the "vegetative" system—cf. his *Psychosomatic Medicine: Its Principles and Applications*, New York: W. W. Norton and Co., Inc., 1950). For present purposes, however, it is not necessary to go into these further refinements.

Definitions of Health and   101
Illness in the Light of
American Values and Social Structure

Most fundamental, I think, is the fact that every known human society possesses a culture which reaches quite high levels of generalization in terms of symbolic systems, including particularly values and cognitive patterns, and that its social structure is sufficiently complex so that it comprises collectivities at several different levels of scope and differentiation. Even though, as is the case with most of the more "primitive" societies known, there is scarcely any important social structure which is not, on a concrete level, a kinship structure, such kinship systems are clearly highly differentiated into a variety of subsystems which are functionally different from each other.

With minimal exceptions, the nuclear family of parents and still dependent children is a constant unit in all kinship systems, though structural emphases within it vary.[7] It is clearly the focal starting point for the process of socialization and the source of the primary bases of human personality organization. But the nuclear family *never* stands alone as a social structure, it is always articulated in complex ways with other structures which are both outside it and stand on a higher level of organization than it does. This involvement of the nuclear family with the wider social structure is, from the structural point of view, the primary basis of the importance of the incest taboo, which, as applying to the nuclear family, is known to be a near universal.[8] Put in psychological terms, this means that the internalization of the object systems and the values of the nuclear family and its subsystems, starting with the mother–child relation, constitutes the *foundation* of personality structure in all human societies. There are, of course, very important variations, but they are all variations on a single set of themes. Because the internalization of the nuclear family is the foundation of personality structure, I suggest that *all*

[7] Cf. M. Zelditch, Jr., "Role Differentiation in the Nuclear Family," Chapter VI of Parsons and Bales, *Family, Socialization and Interaction Process*, New York: Free Press, 1955.

[8] For a general discussion of the significance of the incest taboo, cf. Talcott Parsons, "The Incest Taboo in Relation to Social Structure and the Socialization of the Child," *British Journal of Sociology*, Vol. V:101–117, June, 1954.

mental pathology roots in disturbances of the relationship structure of the nuclear family as impinging on the child. This is not in the least to say that there are not somatic factors in mental pathology; some children may well be constitutionally impossible to socialize adequately. But the *structure* of pathological syndromes which can legitimately be called mental will always involve responses to family relationships.

It is, however, equally true and important that in no society is the socialization of an adult exhausted by his experience in the nuclear family, and hence is his personality *only* a function of the familial object systems he has internalized. Correspondingly, mental pathology will always involve elements in addition to disturbances of the nuclear family relations, especially perhaps those centering about peer-group relations in the latency period and in adolescence. These other factors involve his relations to social groups other than the nuclear family and to higher levels of cultural generalization and social responsibility than any of those involved in the family.

It is thus, I think, fully justified to think of both mental and somatic pathology as involving common elements for all human groups. But at the same time both of them would be expected to vary as a function of social and cultural conditions, in important ways, and probably the more so as one progresses from the more "vegetative" aspects of organic function and its disturbances to the more behavioral aspects and then from the "deeper" layers of personality structure to the "higher" more "ego-structured" layers. It is also probable that the lower in this range, the more the variation is one of incidence rather than character of pathology, the higher the more it penetrates into the "constitution" of the illness itself.

Health among the Problems of Social Control

Health and illness, however, are not only "conditions" or "states" of the human individual viewed on both personality and organic levels. They are also states evaluated and institutionally recognized in the culture and social structure of societies. Can anything be said about the ways in which the constancy–variability problem works out at these levels?

Clearly the institutionalization of expectations with respect both to role and to task performance is fundamental in all human societies. There must, therefore, always be standards of "adequacy" of such performance and of the "capacities" underlying it which must be taken into account, and hence, a corresponding set of distinctions between states of individuals which are and are not "satisfactory" from the point of view of these standards. But by no means all types of "conformity" with performance-standards can· be called "health" nor all types or modes of deviation from such conformity "illness." Are the categories health and illness, as we conceive them, altogether "culture-bound" or is there something about them which can be generalized on the social role-definition level? To answer this question, it will be necessary to enter a little more fully into the sociological problems presented by these definitions.

Since I am attempting to deal with illness in the context of "social control," I should like to approach the problem in terms of an attempt to classify ways in which individuals can deviate from the expectations for statuses and roles which have been institutionalized in the structure of their societies. In spite of the fact that it will complicate matters, it seems unavoidable to deal with the problem on two different levels.

The first of these two levels concerns the relation of the problem of health and illness to the whole range of categories of deviant behavior. In this connection, I shall attempt to assess the relative importance given to the health complex in different types of society and to show that it is particularly important in the American case. The second level will take up the problem of selectivity and variation *within* the health–illness complex itself. Here, I shall discuss how this relates to selective emphasis on the different components of the role of illness and of the therapeutic process, and will attempt to show that, not only does American society put greater stess on the problem of illness than do other societies, but that its emphases in defining the role and in therapy are also characteristically different.

I shall outline the classification I have in mind on the first level in terms of the way it looks in our own society and then raise the question of how universally it may be assumed that the relevant categories are in fact, differentiated from each other in different societies. The first category is that of the control of the capacities of units in the social structure in the sense in which this conception has been discussed above in connection with the definition of health and illness. Every society must have important concern for the level of these capacities. The present context, however, is that of social control, not socialization, so it is not a question of how these capacities come to be developed in the first place, but rather of how tendencies to their disturbance can be forestalled, or, once having occurred, can be rectified.

Though comparable considerations apply to collectivities as units, in the present context the relevant unit is the human individual, and with reference to him we must consider both of the two aspects which have been distinguished, namely, somatic and mental health. Capacity, it will be remembered, is thought of as standing on a more "general" level than commitment to any particular role or task obligations. It does, however, include the motivation to accept such obligations given suitable situation and opportunity.

There is a second category of problem of social control in relation to the individual which in another sense also stands on a more general level than any particular action-commitments. This may be called the problem of *morality*. This concerns the state of the individual person, but not with respect to his capacities in the same sense as these are involved in the problem of health, but with respect to his commitment to the *values* of the society. This is the area of social control which has traditionally been most closely associated with religion, especially

Definitions of Health and 103
Illness in the Light of
American Values and Social Structure

when the reference is to the person, rather than to any collective unit of the society. When I associate the problem with religion, I do not wish to imply that every attachment to a religion or religious movement automatically implies reinforcement of commitment to the values of a *society*. This is by no means necessarily the case. The point is, rather, that it is in the sphere of religious orientation, or its "functional equivalents" at the level of what Tillich calls "ultimate concern," that the individual must work out the problem of how far he is or is not committed to the values of his society.

There is, of course, a great deal of historical and cross-cultural variation in the ways in which individuals may be treated as standing in religious states which need to be remedied or rectified. It seems, however, to be sound to distinguish two very broad types, namely, those involving "ritual impurity" of some sort, and those involving the problem of "salvation" or "state of grace" in a sense comparable to the meanings of these terms within the Christian tradition. In speaking of religion in this connection, I also do not wish to rule out cases which do not include an explicitly "supernatural" reference in the meaning we would tend to give that term. Thus from a "humanistic" point of view the problem still exists of ensuring commitment to the humanistic values. Perhaps the best single example of this reference is the ritualistic aspect of classical Chinese culture with its "secular" ideal of the "superior man."

Both the above two contexts of the problem of social control of individuals refer to rather generalized states of individuals which may be conceived to "lie behind" their commitments to more differentiated and particularized role-obligations and norms. If both of these latter categories be interpreted in the context of social system involvement, then it is a problem in every society how far different elements in its population maintain operative commitments on both these levels which are compatible with the social interest.

The reference to norms, which I have in mind in the first instance in a society as a whole, focuses on the legal system. Any going society must cultivate a rather generalized

"respect for law," and this must be specified in several directions to come down to the level of particular legal obligations.

It is important to note that commitment to law-observance stands on a level more general than that involved in any particular role. Such principles as honesty in the sense of respect for the property rights of others, "responsibility" in the sense of the obligation to fulfill contractual obligations once entered into, or recognition of the general legitimacy of political authority; none of these is specific to any particular role in a particular collectivity. In a highly differentiated society like our own, the practicing legal profession may be said to carry out functions of social control in this field which are in some ways parallel to those of the medical profession in the field of health.[9]

Of course, commitment to norms is by no means confined to the norms which in a modern type of society are given the "force of law." But the law first may serve as a prototype, and second is, in a well-integrated society, necessarily the paramount system of norms with respect to the society as a system, though norms of "morality" may as noted above, take precedence on a religious or purely "ethical" level. "Below" the legal level, however, every collectivity in the society has some set of rules, more or less formalized, to which it is essential to secure some order of commitment on the part of its members.

The last of the four contexts in which the problem of social control in the present sense arises is that of commitment to role-obligations in particular collectivities. This also is a broad category running all the way from the obligations of marriage to a particular spouse, and of occupational commitment in a particular "job" to the obligations of the citizen of loyalty to his national government. One would expect mechanisms of social control to cluster

[9] Cf. Talcott Parsons, "A Sociologist Looks at the Legal Profession," in *Essays in Sociological Theory*, Revised Edition, New York: Free Press, 1954.

about this area. In our own society, this is the least differentiated of the four, but certain relatively specialized agencies have begun to emerge. On the "lower" levels, social work is one of the more prominent. "Industrial sociology," so far as it is oriented to the problem of the individual worker as a member of a formal organization, is another. This is the area of which Chester Barnard spoke[10] as that of "efficiency" in the technical meaning he gave to that term.

I have taken the space to review these four different contexts of the problem of social control, because I think it is essential to have such a classification as a basis for placing the treatment of any of these problems in a comparative setting. In a highly differentiated society like our own, these four functions have become relatively clearly differentiated from each other, and the operative processes of social control are, with certain indefinite borderlines, of course, to be found in the hands of different organizational agencies. The last of the four I outlined is by a good deal the least firmly institutionalized as a distinct function and it is probably significant that, in our society, it is most fully worked out, through social work, for the lower status-levels of the society.

The present situation with respect to differentiation cannot, however, be said to be typical of all societies; indeed, I doubt whether any case can be found where a comparatively close approach to completeness in this differentiation can be found.

Two major "axes" of differentiation were implicit in the classification I have just presented. Both need to be taken into account in placing the problem of health and illness relative to the others. The first of these may be called the differentiation in terms of orientation, on the one hand, to the exigencies of the *situation* in which the person must act; on the other hand, orientation to or through *normative patterns*. The second axis concerns not this problem, but that of whether the "problem" lies in

10 C. I. Barnard, *The Functions of the Executive*, Cambridge: Harvard University Press, 1938.

the state of the person as a whole, at a level deeper than the problem of his acceptance of particular obligations, or whether it lies in the question of his "willingness" to accept certain more specific obligations, to particular norms and classes of norms—and to particular roles in particular collectivities.

The first of these two axes differentiates the types of deviance involved in illness and disturbance of commitments to collectivities on the one hand from those involved in disturbance of commitments to norms and to values on the other. The second axis differentiates the problems of illness and of disturbance of commitment to values on the one hand from the problems of commitment to collectivities and to normative patterns (rules and law) on the other. The tabular arrangement opposite may be helpful to the reader.

It is in terms of the first axis that one fundamental type of differentiation involving health can be made, that which treats health as a "naturalistic" state which is not to be explained by or treated through religio-magical media. It is of course a commonplace that in all nonliterate societies, with relatively minor exceptions such as fractures, this differentiation has not yet taken place, and much the same can be said about the high civilizations of the Orient such as India and China until touched by Western medicine. This of course, is in no way to say that "therapies" which are couched in magico-religious terms are necessarily ineffective. On the contrary, there is much evidence that they have been very effective in certain cases. It would, however, hardly be denied that with the clear differentiation of roles in this area which has taken place in the modern world, much greater effectiveness has been made possible over at least a very large part of the range.

Though differentiation on the first axis discriminates the problem of health from that of the "ritual" state of the individual, or his state of grace or, more generally, commitment to values, it fails to discriminate between the more general level of his state "as a person" and his commitment to the more specific obligations of societal membership and activity. Here a problem which has been very central in the modern world in drawing the line between problems of mental health and of law seems to be a major one. This is the question of whether and how far the "deviance" of the individual from conformity with social expectations can be considered to be "intentional," i.e., the question of how far he may legitimately be held *responsible* for his actions. In one area, at least, this has in fact come to be accepted as a main differentiating criterion and, I think, rightly so.

Definitions of Health and   105
Illness in the Light of
American Values and Social Structure

"formal" obligations is not "blamed on" the individual. But the distinction is, on the whole, clear; if he is not "ill" (or in a state of ritual impurity, or "sin"), or willfully recalcitrant, it must be the fault of somebody else or of "the system." The essential basis of this possibility of "holding responsible" is the particularity of specific norms and role-

	Disturbance of Total Person	Disturbance of Particular Expectations
"Situational" Focus	Problem of "capacities" for task and role performance	Problem of commitments to collectivities (Barnard's "efficiency")
	Illness as deviance Health as "conformity"	Disloyalty as deviance Loyalty as conformity
"Normative" Focus	Problem of commitments to values, or of "morality" "Sin" and "immorality" as deviance	Problem of commitments to norms, or of "legality" "Crime" and "illegality" as deviance
	State of grace or "good character" as conformity	Law-observance as conformity

Let me try to elucidate a little some of its implications in the present context. It has long been one of the principal criteria of illness that the sick person "couldn't help it." Even though he may have become ill or disabled through some sort of carelessness or negligence, he cannot legitimately be expected to get well simply by deciding to be well, or by "pulling himself together." Some kind of underlying reorganizing process has to take place, biological or "mental," which can be guided or controlled in various ways, but cannot simply be eliminated by an "act of will." In this sense the state of illness is involuntary. On the other hand, both obedience to norms and fulfillment of obligations to collectivities in roles are ordinarily treated as involving "voluntary" decisions; the normal individual can legitimately be "held responsible."

Certainly both in fields such as law and in that of collectivity obligations, there are many cases where failure to live up fully to

obligations. A normal person has the capacity to accept or reject particular obligations without involving a reorganization of the major structures of his personality or of his body. It is only when there is a "disturbance" which goes beyond these particularities that we can speak of illness, or of disturbed commitment to values.[11]

This same problem occurs in the relation to the commitment to values as operating through religion and cognate mechanisms. It is very clear that among many nonliterate peoples, states of ritual impurity are treated as outside the control of the individual victim. They are states for which he may

[11] An interesting case of difficulty with respect to the line of discrimination discussed above is presented by Mark Field in his study of Soviet medical practice, where pressure has been put on physicians, more than in our own system, to provide excuses for avoiding extremely onerous and rigorously enforced role-obligations. Cf. his *Doctor and Patient in Soviet Russia*, Cambridge: Harvard University Press, 1957.

not legitimately be held responsible, except, and this is a most important exception which applies to illness as well, for subjecting himself to the proper treatment institutionally prescribed for those in such a state. In general, some ritual performance is called for, which may even sometimes be self-administered, to "rectify" his state.

Without attempting to discuss the situation in other major religions, it is a very important fact that the conception of original sin in the Christian tradition defines the situation in a cognate way. Though retroactively and mythologically Adam is held to have sinned "voluntarily," the burden of original sin on mankind is held not to be the responsibility of the individual, but something which is inherent in the human condition. Conversely, it cannot be escaped from without outside help.

Here it is important to distinguish original sin from the infraction of the norms and role-obligations of a religious collectivity. I think it can fairly be said that that aspect of "sin" which is treated by religious authorities as *within* the responsibility of the individual is strictly analogous to the civil responsibility for law-observance and/or the responsibility for living up to the obligations of a particular role, in this case church-membership. Christianity thus has institutionalized the differentiation of these two aspects of the problem of social control. Original sin belongs, with respect to *this* axis of differentiation, on the same side as does illness.

With respect to the major categories I have been discussing for the last few pages, societies may be expected to differ in two major respects. The first I have already been stressing, namely with respect to the *degree* to which these major types of deviance are *differentiated from each other* and the functions of social control with respect to them institutionalized in differentiated agencies. In an evolutionary sense (with societal, not organic reference) they may be said all to have originated in religion.[12] Priests and magicians have thus been the "original" agents of social control everywhere. The roles of physician, of lawyer and, if you will, of "administrator" and social worker have only gradually and unevenly differentiated off from the religious roles.

The second range of variation concerns the relative stress put on conformity with social expectations in each of these categories and hence the seriousness with which deviance in each is viewed, and the importance given to building up effective mechanisms of social control in the area in question as distinguished from others. Thus in a society like that of Hindu caste in India, the overwhelming emphasis seems to have been religious, with ritual purity on one level, the problem of control of and emancipation from the Hindu counterpart of Christian original sin on another as the primary preoccupations. The neglect of health as Westerners understand it in India (until very recently) is too well-known to need emphasizing. Soviet society may be said to be a type which puts primary emphasis on effective role-performance in the socialist state and hence to bend its primary efforts to controlling the commitments of the population (above all through "propaganda" and "agitation")[13] to exerting the utmost effort, especially in production. Finally, with differences, of course, it may be suggested that both classical Rome and modern England have laid more stress on law and integration through the legal system than any other of the major features with which this discussion has been concerned.

Seen in this perspective, contemporary American Society is, with respect to the institutionalization of mechanisms of social control, probably as highly differentiated as any known, certainly as any outside the modern Western world. But among those which are highly differentiated, it is also one which places a very heavy emphasis on the field and problems of health and illness relative to the others, probably as high as any. It is also clear that our concern with problems of health has increased greatly since about the turn of the present century,

---

[12] This is a major thesis of Durkheim in *The Elementary Forms of the Religious Life*, New York: Free Press, 1947.

[13] Cf. Alex Inkeles, *Public Opinion in Soviet Russia*, Cambridge: Harvard University Press, 1950.

and furthermore, that the emergence of the problem of mental health into a position of salience, on anything like the scale which has actually developed, is a new phenomenon.

A Restatement of the Criteria of Health and Illness

Before attempting to relate this emphasis systematically to American values and social structure, it would be well to attempt to state somewhat more precisely what seem to be the principal general characteristics of health and illness seen in the context of social role structure and social control.

Health may be defined as the state of optimum *capacity* of an individual for the effective performance of the roles and tasks for which he has been socialized. It is thus defined with reference to the individual's participation in the social system. It is also defined as *relative* to his "status" in the society, i.e., to differentiated type of role and corresponding task structure, e.g., by sex or age, and by level of education which he has attained and the like. Naturally, also there are qualitative ranges in the differentiation of capacities, within sex groups and at given levels of education. Finally, let me repeat that I am defining health as concerned with capacity, not with commitment to *particular* roles, tasks, norms or even values as such. The question of whether a man wants to remain with his wife or likes his particular job or even feels committed to refrain from highway robbery is not *as such* a health problem, though a health problem may underlie and be interwoven with problems of this sort.

Illness, then, is also a socially institutionalized role-type. It is most generally characterized by some imputed generalized disturbance of the capacity of the individual for normally expected task or role-performance, which is not specific to his commitments to any particular task, role, collectivity, norm or value. Under this general heading of the recognition of a state of disturbance of capacity, there are then the

Definitions of Health and 107
Illness in the Light of
American Values and Social Structure

following four more specific features of the *role* of the sick person: 1) This incapacity is interpreted as beyond his powers to overcome by the process of decision-making alone; in this sense he cannot be "held responsible" for the incapacity. Some kind of "therapeutic" process, spontaneous or aided, is conceived to be necessary to recovery. 2) Incapacity defined as illness is interpreted as a legitimate basis for the *exemption* of the sick individual, to varying degrees, in varying ways and for varying periods according to the nature of the illness, from his normal role and task obligations. 3) To be ill is thus to be in a partially and conditionally *legitimated* state. The essential condition of its legitimation, however, is the recognition by the sick person that to be ill is inherently *undesirable*, that he therefore has an obligation to try to "get well" and to cooperate with others to this end. 4) So far as spontaneous forces, the *vis medicatrix naturae*, cannot be expected to operate adequately and quickly, the sick person and those with responsibility for his welfare, above all, members of his family, have an obligation to *seek competent help* and to cooperate with competent agencies in their attempts to help him get well; in our society, of course, principally medical agencies. The valuation of health, of course, also implies that it is an obligation to try to *prevent* threatened illness where this is possible.

These criteria seem very nearly obvious on a common sense level in our society, but some aspects of their subtler significance become evident when we consider the way in which, through the channels of mental and psychosomatic illness, the balance of health and illness comes to be bound up with the balance of control of the motivation of individuals in their relation to the society as a system. This is what I had in mind in discussing illness in the context of the problems of deviance and social control in the first place. I shall not take space to go into this set of problems here, since they have been dealt with elsewhere, but will only call attention to them, and draw a few inferences.[14]

The most important inferences for present purposes concern the importance of *two* related but distinct functions for the society of the health–illness role structure. The first of these is the *insulation* of the sick person from certain types of mutual influence with those who are not sick, and from association with each other. The essential reason for this insulation being important in the present context is not the need of the sick person for special "care" so much as it is that, motivationally as well as bacteriologically, illness may well be "contagious." The motives which enter into illness as deviant behavior are partially identical with those entering into other types of deviance, such as crime and the breakdown of commitment to the values of the society, partly they are dynamically interrelated with these so that stimulation of one set of motives may tend to stimulate others as well.

In the light of the motivational problem the important feature of insulation is the deprivation, for the sick person, of any claim to a more general legitimacy for his pattern of deviance. As noted above, the conditional legitimation which he enjoys is bought at a "price," namely, the recognition that illness itself is an undesirable state, to be recovered from as expeditiously as possible. It is at this price that he is permitted to enjoy the often very powerful gratifications of secondary gain. But the importance of the institutionalization of the role of illness is not confined to its bearing on the motivational balance of the sick person. As Durkheim pointed out for the case of crime, the designation of illness as illegitimate is of the greatest importance to

[14] I have dealt with them primarily in the following places: *The Social System*, Chapter X, New York: Free Press, 1951; the paper "Illness and the Role of the Physician," *American Journal of Orthopsychiatry*, July 1951, pp. 452–460, also printed in Kluckhohn, Murray and Schneider, *Personality, in Nature, Society and Culture*, 2nd Edition, New York: Alfred A. Knopf, 1953, and in somewhat more specialized context in T. Parsons and R. Fox, "Illness, Therapy and the Modern Urban American Family," *Journal of Social Issues*, Vol. 8, pp. 31–44.

the healthy, in that it reinforces their own motivation *not* to fall ill, thus to avoid falling into a pattern of deviant behavior. The stigmatizing of illness as undesirable, and the mobilization of considerable resources of the community to combat illness is a reaffirmation of the valuation of health and a countervailing influence against the temptation for illness, and hence the various components which go into its motivation, to grow and spread. Thus, the sick person is prevented from setting an example which others might be tempted to follow.

The second important implication of institutionalization of the roles is that being categorized as ill puts the individual in the position of being defined as "needing help" and as obligated to accept help and to cooperate actively with the agency which proffers it. The role of illness, that is to say, channels those categorized as belonging in it into contact with therapeutic agencies. It is therefore involved in both negative and positive mechanisms of social control, negative in that the spread of certain types of deviance is inhibited, positive in that remedial processes are facilitated.

An interesting and important intermediate aspect may also be noted. By defining the sick person as in need of help and tending to bring him into relation to therapeutic agencies, the role of illness tends to place him in a position of *dependency on* persons who are *not* sick. The structural alignment, hence, is of each sick person with certain categories of nonsick, not of groups of sick persons with each other.[15]

American Values and the Health Problem

Now let us turn to the question of the way in which American values and social struc-

[15] The latter does of course happen in hospital situations. It has been clearly shown (Cf. Ivan Belknap, *Human Problems of a State Mental Hospital*, New York: McGraw-Hill Book Co., 1956, and Barbara Burt Arnason, unpublished Ph.D. Dissertation, Radcliffe College, 1958) that in mental hospital settings the social group of chronic patients, particularly in a kind of symbiosis with attendants, can, under certain circumstances, come to constitute a seriously *anti*-therapeutic social community.

Definitions of Health and 109
Illness in the Light of
American Values and Social Structure

ture may be said to operate selectively with reference both to the place of the health–illness complex among other mechanisms of social control and with respect to emphases within the health–illness complex itself. To start with it will be necessary to sketch the main outline of the American value system in the relevant respects.

I would like to suggest that even so complex and highly differentiated a society as our own can be said to have a relatively well-integrated system of institutionalized common values at the societal level. Ours I shall characterize as a pattern emphasizing "activism" in a certain particular sense, "worldliness" and "instrumentalism." Let me try, briefly, to explain these terms.

In the first place, a societal value system concerns the orientations of members to conceptions of what is desirable for the society itself and as a whole as a system or object of evaluation. Only derivatively, does it provide patterns of evaluation of the individual. When I refer to activism, I mean that in relation to *its* situation or environment, the society should be oriented to mastery over that environment in the name of ideals and goals which are transcendental with reference to it. The relevant environment may be either physical or social, but because of our relative isolation from other societies until the last generation or so, the physical environment has been particularly prominent in our case. The reference point for exerting "leverage" on the environment has been, historically, in the first instance religious. It will not be possible here to go into the question of the sense in which, or degree to which this is still the case; nevertheless, the main orientation clearly is one of maintaining the pattern of mastery, not of "adjustment" to the inevitable. In no field has this been more conspicuous than that of health where illness has presented a challenge to be met by mobilizing the resources of research, science, etc., to the full.

When I speak of the "worldliness" of the American value system, I mean that, in spite of its religious roots, the *field* of primarily valued activity is in practical secular pursuits, not in contemplation or devotions, or aesthetic gratifications. In its societal application this means a concep-

tion of an ideal *society*, originally the Kingdom of God *on Earth*, in a secularized version a good society in which such ideals as liberty, justice, welfare and equality of opportunity prevail.

Finally, when I speak of "instrumentalism," I refer to the fact that, in the first instance for the society as a system, there is no definitive "consummatory" state which is idealized, no definitive societal goal state which is either attained or not—as in the case of "communism." There is rather an indefinite perspective of possible improvement, of "progress" which fulfills by degrees the ideal by moving in the right *direction*.

The absence of a definitive goal for the system as a whole, places the primary active achievement emphasis on the level of the goals of *units* and measures their achievements in appropriate terms. There is a kind of "liberal" pluralism in that any unit in the society, individual or collective, has liberty to pursue goals which to it may seem worthwhile, but more importantly, there are standards of *contribution* to the progress of the society. Perhaps the most obvious (though not the only) field of such contribution is that of economic productivity, for it is the productivity of the economy which is the basis of the availability of facilities for attaining *whatever* goals may seem most worthwhile, since income as generalized purchasing power is non-specific with respect to particular uses. This is the most generalized basis of opportunity to do "good things." But equally important is the provision of the society with units which have the *capacity* for valued achievement.

I may note that collective units and their achievements are of the utmost importance in the American system, for example, the business firm. But their achievements are fundamentally dependent on the capacities and commitments of the human individuals who perform roles and tasks within them. It is in this connection that the relevance of the valuation of health appears. For the individual, the primary focus of evaluation is universalistically judged *achievement*. The possibility of achievement is, of course, a function of opportunity at any given point in his life cycle, which in turn is a function of the economic level of the community, because openings both for self-employment, e.g., in independent business, and for employment by others, are a function of markets and of funds available through whatever channels. But on a "deeper" and in a sense more generalized level, this achievement is dependent on two basic sets of prior conditions which underlie his capacities, namely, on education in the broadest sense, and on health. It is in the first instance as an essential condition of valued achievement, that the health of the individual is itself valued.

There is another very central strand in the pattern of our evaluation in both respects. This is the relation of both education and health to the valuation of *equality* of opportunity. For reasons which cannot be gone into here, but which bear above all on the high level of structural differentiation of our society, it is one which shows a great deal of mobility of resources. Ascribed status is relatively minimized. The "pluralism of goals" which has to do with the instrumental emphasis in our value system raises the problem of "justice" with great acuteness. One aspect of this is distributive justice with references to the allocation of rewards. But with the emphasis on active achievement, even more crucial than justice of reward distribution is that of *opportunity* for value achievement. But education and health are clearly more fundamental conditions of achievement than is access to investment funds or to employment, since they condition capacity to exploit opportunity in this narrower sense. Hence, *access* to education and to health services becomes, in a society like our own, a peculiarly central focus of the problem of justice in the society.

On technical grounds I do not classify education as a function of social control in a society.[16] Within the field of problems of social control, as discussed above, the problem of health clearly constitutes the

16 In my own technical terms, it is a "pattern-maintenance" function.

"rock bottom" of the series. There seem, when the problem is seen in this light, to be a number of reasons which I may review briefly, why it has emerged into a position of special prominence in contemporary America.

First, and of course a very important point, the development of medicine and of the health sciences underlying and associated with it, has made possible an entirely new level of control of illness, both preventive and therapeutic, far higher than has ever existed before in history. There is, of course, interdependence. American medicine did not just take over a medical science ready-made, but has developed the European beginnings with an energy and resourcefulness probably matched only in the field of industrial technology. There is, hence, interdependence between the development, on the one hand, of medical science and technology, and on the other, of interest in, and concern for, effective handling of health problems.

Secondly, the order of significance of the problems of social control, starting with commitment to paramount values themselves, running through commitment to norms, then to roles and tasks, is probably, in a very broad sense, of evolutionary significance. This is to say that there is a tendency for a problem area to emerge into salience only when, to a degree, the ones ahead of it in the priority list have in some sense been "solved." This is not to say that any of them ever are definitively solved, but in a relative sense one can speak of solution.

It is not possible to discuss this question here in detail. But it may be suggested that by the mid-nineteenth century, with the very important exception of the problem of the South, a certain national unity had been achieved in terms of values and norms.[17] It can then be further suggested that in the latter half of the nineteenth century there was concentration on the problems of setting up the new industrial system with the institutionalization of the principal role-categories which have to go into that, notably, of course, an occupational role system which was structurally quite different

17 Dr. R. N. Bellah, in an unpublished paper, has suggested the great importance of revivalist religion in the former of these contexts.

**Definitions of Health and 111
Illness in the Light of
American Values and Social Structure**

from that of the earlier society of "farmers and mechanics." Not least important in this connection was the institutionalization of the repercussions of these changes on the family, because of the drastic nature of the differentiation of occupational from familial roles. From the point of view of the individual, it may be said that the development of the industrial economy provided, in terms of a structural type congruent with American values, a new level of solution of the problem of opportunity.

From this point of view, one might say that after the turn of the century the stage was set for a new level of concern with the problems of education and health, which have indeed figured very prominently in this period, though not by any means to the exclusion of the others. Their importance is, I think, further accentuated by another feature of the development of the society. This is the fact that, with the development of industrialization, urbanism, high technology, mass communications and many other features of our society, there has been a general *upgrading* to higher levels of responsibility. Life has necessarily become more complex and has made greater demands on the typical individual, though different ones at different levels. The sheer problem of capacity to meet these demands has, therefore, become more urgent. The motivation to retreat into ill-health through mental or psychosomatic channels, has become accentuated and with it the importance of effective mechanisms for coping with those who do so retreat.

Seen in terms of this kind of historical perspective, it makes sense, I think, that *the first major wave of development of the health institutions was in the field of somatic illness and the techniques of dealing with it, and that this has been followed by a wave of interest in problems of mental health.* This is partly, but by no means wholly, because the scientific basis for handling somatic illness has developed earlier and farther. In addition to this, it is well known that the resistances to recognizing the existence of health problems are stronger in the field of mental than of somatic health. Furthermore, a larger component of the phenomena of mental illness presumably operates through motivation and is hence related to the problems and mechanisms of social control. Social changes, however, have not only increased the strain on individuals, thus accentuating the need for mechanisms in this area, but some of the older mechanisms have been destroyed or weakened and a restructuring has been necessary.

For one thing, levels of mental pathology which could be tolerated under pre-industrial conditions, have become intolerable under the more stringent pressures of modern life; this probably includes the pushing of many types of personality over the borderline into overt psychosis, who otherwise would have been able to "get along." Furthermore, the family, for example, has undertaken a greatly increased burden in the socialization and personality-management fields, and new institutional arrangements for dealing with the health problems of its members are required. This seems, for example, to be one major factor in the rapid spread of hospitalization.[18]

I may sum up this aspect of the discussion by saying that both by virtue of its value system, and by virtue of the high level of differentiation of its social structure, American society has been one in which it could be expected that the problem of health, and within this more particularly of mental health, would become particularly salient. Its "liberal" cast which militates against highly stringent integration with reference to a system goal tends to emphasize the problem of getting units to "come along." The human individual is the end of the series of units on which the functioning of the society depends, and is hence the "last resort" in this connection. At the same time, the activistic orientation of the society militates against any orientation which would be inclined to let individuals "rest on their oars," but puts very much of a premium on the protection and development of capacity in the sense in which I have discussed it here.

[18] Cf. Parsons and Fox, *op. cit.* for a further analysis of this problem.

The same factors, particularly seen in the context of the stage of development of the society, tend to prevent too strong an emphasis on any of the other primary problems and modes of social control. Generally, I think, contrary to much opinion, it can be said that the American society is very firmly attached to its primary values, so much so that they tend to be placed outside the field of serious concern. There is, to be sure, much controversy about what are alleged to be changes in values. But a careful analysis, which cannot be entered into here, will reveal that very much, at least, of this does not lie at this level, but rather at ideological levels.

A very good example of this is the amount of concern displayed over the developing salience of problems of mental health, and the scope given to the permissive and supportive elements in the orientation to the mentally ill. But people who show this concern often forget to emphasize the other side of the coin, namely, the equally prominent concern with therapy, with bringing the mentally ill back into full social participation, which above all, means into full capacity for achievement. Particularly revealing, I think, is the conception that the therapeutic process involves active *work* on the part of the patient, his seriously *trying* to get well. He is conceived of as anything but a passive object of the manipulations of the therapeutic personnel.

American Selectivity within the Patterns of Health and Illness

I have argued above, that among the problems and mechanisms of social control, both the values and the social structure of American society will tend to place emphasis on the problems of health and illness which concern commitment to roles, as compared with those of commitment to collectivities, to normative rules, or to the values themselves. This essentially is to say that it is *capacity* which is the primary focus of the problem of social control for us. With the increasing complexity and "maturity" of

the society in turn, the problem of motivation to adequate role-performance and hence, to mental health becomes a salient one.

The problem now arises of what kind of selectivity we may expect, on the basis of the above analysis, *within* the complex of illness, and the corresponding attitudes toward therapy, relative to other ways of treating the problem of illness as such. In order to approach this question, I would like to use the formulation of the main components of the definition of illness, as stated previously herein, as my main point of reference. The first point, namely, a disturbance of capacity, is general, and is the link with the foregoing discussion of selectivity among the problems of social control. This is to say that in the United States we are more likely to interpret a difficulty in an individual's fulfilling social role-expectations as a disturbance in capacity, i.e., as illness, than is true in other types of society with other types of value systems.

The other four criteria, it will be remembered, were exemption from role-obligations, holding the patient not responsible for his state, conditional legitimation of the state, and acceptance of the need for help and of the obligation to cooperate with the source of the help.

My suggestion is that, compared with other societies in which other value systems have been institutionalized, in the American case the heaviest emphasis among these tends to go to the last. Essentially, this derives from the element in the American value system which I have called "activism" above. The implication of that element, in the context of the others to which it relates, is for the personality of the individual, the valuation of *achievement*. This in turn, as was developed above, implies a strong valuation of the capacities which underlie achievement, capacities which are primarily developed through education or socialization and protected and restored through health services. But in the American case, this does not imply that the primary stress is on the dependency aspect of the "need for help"— I shall return to the question of the role of dependency presently. It is rather, from the point of view of the society, the attitude which asserts the desirability of *mastery* of the problems of health, and from that for the individual sick person, the obligation to cooperate fully with the therapeutic agency, that is to *work* to achieve his own recovery. The rationale of this is plainly that, if he is not motivated to work to attain the conditions of effective achievement, he cannot very well be considered to be motivated to the achievements which require good health as a condition.

It might then be said that the other three components of the role of illness are institutionalized as subsidiary to, and instrumental to, this one. With respect to legitimation there is a particularly strong emphasis on its *conditional* aspect, that illness is only legitimized so long as it is clearly recognized that it is intrinsically an undesirable state, to be recovered from as expeditiously as possible. Similarly, with the factor of exemption from role-performance and the "admission" that the patient cannot be held responsible in the sense discussed above. In this connection, there is a very important relation to the scientific aspect of our cultural tradition. That the patient "can't help it" is simply one of the facts of life, demonstrated by medical science. Where scientific evidence is not available, the tendency is to give the benefit of the doubt to the possibility that he can help it. Thus, we tend to be relatively suspicious of plans for "free" health care because of the readiness to impute malingering wherever objective possibility for it exists.

I shall wish to suggest very tentatively how this American emphasis on active therapy differs from emphases in other societies, but before taking this up, I would like to try broadly to answer two other sets of questions about the American case. The first of these is how the patterning of illness in our society relates to the problem of the *directions* of deviant behavior, the second to selective emphases among the social components involved in the therapeutic process.

In a previous publication, I attempted to classify the directions which deviant orientations might take in terms of three major dimensions, two of which were very close to, if not identical with, those set forth by Merton.[19] These were first the variation

Definitions of Health and 113
Illness in the Light of
American Values and Social Structure

between *alienation* from social expectations and *compulsive conformity* with them, second between *activity* and *passivity*, and third between *object*-primacy and *pattern*-primacy. The first two of these are the ones selected by Merton.

In terms of these first two dimensions, illness clearly belongs in the general category of a type of deviance categorized by alienation and by passivity. This general type I have designated as withdrawal whereas Merton calls it "retreatism." This tendency to withdrawal as the most prominent type of deviance is typical of American society generally. But some of the dynamics of it are relevant to the questions of selectivity within the components of the pattern of illness.

Before entering into these, however, it may be noted that with respect to the American pattern of illness, I think it can be said that the primary focus is object-oriented rather than pattern-oriented. This is above all because illness focuses at the level of capacity for role and task performance, not at the level of norms or values and conformity with them. This would also be true of illness generally but for reasons which will be discussed presently. I think it likely that it is more accentuated in the American case than others.[20]

What then, can be said to be some of the main patterns of motivational dynamics relevant to the problem of illness in American society and their relation in turn to these features of the role of illness as an institutionalized role? I may start by suggesting that all patterns of deviant behavior, as distinguished from creative alteration of

---

[19] Cf. *The Social System*, New York: Free Press, 1951, Chapter VII, and R. K. Merton, *Social Theory and Social Structure*, New York: Free Press, 1957, rev. ed., Chapter IV.

[20] By the three criteria, then, of alienation, passivity, and object-orientation, the pattern of illness should be considered a case of "compulsive independence" (*Social System, op. cit.*, p. 259). Compulsive independence in this case may be interpreted to involve reaction-formation against underlying needs, as I shall note.

the cultural or normative tradition, involves the primacy of elements of *regressive* motivational structure in the psychological sense.[21] But for different types of deviance and within the category of illness as a type of deviance there will be selective emphases on different phases of psychological regression.

It is not possible to enter into all the complications here, but I suggest that in the American case, the primary focus lies in the residues of the pre-oedipal mother–child relationship, that phase of which Freud spoke as involving the "first true object-attachment." The basis on which this develops goes back to the very great, and increasing prominence in socialization of the relatively *isolated* nuclear family. The "American dilemma" in this case is that the child is, typically, encouraged to form an extremely intense attachment to the mother at this time, while at the same time he is required later to break more radically with this early dependency because the process of emancipation from the family of orientation is pushed farther and faster than in other systems. Independence training, that is to say, forms a particularly prominent part of our socialization process and the strength of the mother attachment is an essential condition of its successful carrying out.

The alienation involved in the motivation to illness may then be interpreted to involve alienation from a set of expectations which put particular stress on independent achievement. Because of this complex, the importance of the passivity component of the deviance expressed in illness is particularly great, because the ambivalent motivational structure about the dependency–independence problem is particularly prominent. Therapy then focuses on the strengthening of the motivation to independence relative to dependency and on overcoming the alienation, focussing on the expectations of independence and, through it, achievement.[22]

I suggest, then, that the American pattern of illness is focussed on the problem of capacity for achievement for the individual person. Therapeutically, recovery is defined for him as a *job* to be done in cooperation with those who are technically qualified to help him. This focus then operates to polarize the components of the "problem" in such a way that *the primary threat to his achievement capacity which must be overcome is dependency.* The element of exemption from ordinary role-obligations may then be interpreted as permissiveness for temporary relief from the strains of trying hard to achieve. The patient is permitted to indulge his dependency needs under strictly regulated conditions, notably his recognition of the conditional nature of the legitimacy of his state, and exposure to the therapeutic task.[23]

These elements of the situation relate in turn to the components of the therapeutic process. I have elsewhere[24] designated these, in terms of role-pattern, as permissiveness, support, selective rewarding and reinforcement. An essential point is that the dependency component of the deviance of

_____

21 A fuller discussion of the nature of the "regression scale" will be found in *Family, Socialization and Interaction Process, op. cit.,* especially Chapter II.

22 In this light the motivation to illness may, with only apparent paradox, be characterized as a case of "compulsive independence from the requirement to be independent." It is a kind of "to hell with it all" pattern of withdrawal.

23 Unfortunately, there will be no opportunity in this paper to take up the empirical problem of how far the available data on illness bear out this interpretation of the central importance of the dependency-independency axis. Not only do I suggest that this is more important in the American case than in others but also that it applies to somatic as well as mental illness. The ulcer complex is widely believed to relate especially to this problem. It may also be suggested that the special concern with polio in America relates to our horror of the dependency which the permanent cripple must bear. Almost better death than not to be able to do one's part, but remain dependent on others.

24 Cf. *The Social System, op. cit.,* Chapter VII and Parsons, Bales and Shils, *Working Papers in the Theory of Action,* Chapter V. In earlier versions, what I am now calling selective rewarding was called "denial of reciprocity" (this term emphasized only the negative aspect) and what I now call reinforcement was called "manipulation of rewards." The new term for the latter emphasizes the continuity of a *pattern* of rewards over time.

Definitions of Health and 115
Illness in the Light of
American Values and Social Structure

illness is used constructively in the thera-peutic pattern, essentially through what is in certain respects a recapitulation of the socializing experience. This is to say that through permissiveness to express depen-dency, both in exemption from role-obliga-tions and in supportive relations to others, the patient is encouraged to form a depend-ent attachment to others. The permissive and supportive treatment of the sick person, by giving him what he wants, undercuts the alienative component of the motivational structure of his illness. He finds it much more difficult to feel alienated toward social objects who treat him with kindness and consideration than he would otherwise be disposed to feel—though, of course, there may be a problem, particularly with some types of mental illness of getting him to accept such kindness and consideration, even to accept his need for the exemptions permitted by virtue of illness.

At the same time the element of depen-dency, through "transference," is the basis of a strong attachment to therapeutic per-sonnel, which can then be used as a basis of leverage to motivate the therapeutic "work" which eventually should result in overcoming the dependency itself, or miti-gating it sufficiently so that it no longer interferes so seriously with his capacities. Building on this, then, the active work of therapy, adapting to the fundamental con-ditions of the biological and psychological states of the patient, can take hold and operate to propel toward recovery.[25]

25 In Parsons and Fox, *op. cit.*, it was suggested that the trend toward hospitalization, again in cases of both mental and somatic illness, was related to these factors. On the one hand, it is related to technological exigencies of modern medicine. Also it is a way of relieving the family of burdens of "care." But at the same time it is both a way of protecting the family from the patient, that is above all the impact of his dependency needs on other members, and the point of primary present importance, of pro-tecting the patient from his family. The family, that is to say, is very likely to be "over-protective" and over supportive. Because of the temptations of "seduction" of the patient into more or less permanent dependency, it lacks the basis of effective leverage which a more "impersonal" agency may be in a position to exert. Also, it was noted above, there is reason to believe that the acuteness of the

I should finally like to turn to a brief and very tentative suggestion of the main differences between the orientations to illness in the United States and in two other modern societies, namely Soviet Russia and Great Britain. Let us take the Soviet case first.[26]

Whereas in the American case I suggested that our concern with capacity for role-achievement put the primary emphasis on the restoration of that capacity through therapeutic work, the general orientation of Soviet society is different; it is to the attainment of a collective goal for the society as a whole, the "building of social-ism." With reference to the problem of illness this tends to shift the emphasis from the obligation to cooperate in therapy to the problem of responsibility and non-respon-sibility. This is most conspicuous in the field of mental illness where the Soviet attitude is an extreme antithesis of our own precisely on this point.[27] One very telling expression of it is the complete prohibition of psycho-analysis, whereas psychoanalysis has had greater success in the United States than in any other country. My interpretation of this would be that psychoanalysis is a threat from the Soviet point of view, because through the theory of the unconscious, it so strongly emphasizes the elements in the personality of the individual which are outside this voluntary control. It would give too plausible excuses for too many for the evasion of responsibility. In the American case, on the other hand, psychoanalysis is defined more as offering *opportunity* for constructive therapeutic work, to the patient as well as the therapist.[28]

dependency problem has been increasing with recent developments in family structure.

26 My most important sources on Soviet medicine are Field, *op. cit.*, and R. A. Bauer, *The New Man in Soviet Psychology.* I am also indebted to Dr. Field for suggestions made in personal discussion which go beyond his book.

27 Cf. Bauer, *op. cit.*

28 The extent to which the ego as distinct from the id has come to be emphasized in American versions of psychoanalysis seems to fit with this interpretation.

The same general strain seems to be conspicuous, from Field's account, in the field of somatic medicine. The attitude seems to be one of reluctant concession to human frailties. Of course, it is part of socialism to have a national medical service, but at the same time party and administrative personnel keep strict watch on the medical people to be sure that they do not connive in malingering which—because of the great severity of labor discipline—they have been under strong pressure to do. To American eyes the Soviet treatment of illness seems to be marked by a certain perfunctoriness, as if it were up to the patient to prove that he is "really" sick rather than it being the physician's role to investigate the possibilities on his own. I suggest that this may be more than a matter of scarcity of personnel and resources; it is probably at least in part an authentic expression of Soviet values.

Reinforcing this conclusion is the probability that illness is not the primary type of deviance for Soviet society in the sense that I have argued it is in the American case. I think it probable that what I have called "compulsive acquiescence in status-expectations" is the most prominent type. This, of course, very generally does not appear overtly as deviance at all and hence is difficult to detect.[29]

There is, however, another side of the Soviet picture, just as there is in the American case of polarity between the emphasis on active mastery and the problem of dependency. This is that in medical care, especially in the hospital, there seems to be a particularly strong supportive emphasis. This is to say that, once the status of being sick is granted, there is not nearly so strong an emphasis on the conditional character of its legitimacy as in the American case, and patients are encouraged to relax and to enjoy being taken care of.[30]

This suggests a permissiveness for regression, but one which is differently structured from the American. It is less the need

to express dependency on particular social objects which does not threaten essential acceptance or belongingness. Psychologically it suggests primacy of oral components rather than of the mother–child love-attachment.

Thus, on the one hand, the role of illness is not given nearly so wide a scope in Soviet Russia as in the United States, particularly in the direction of mental illness. At the same time, it is also differently structured in that the primary focus is the problem of the responsibility of the individual rather than his capacity in our sense to achieve and to cooperate in recovery. The permissive element is more for "rest", for relaxation from responsibility, than it is for the direct expression of object-oriented dependency.

The British case does not seem to be quite so clear, but I think it is different in important ways from either the American or the Soviet. By contrast, with the other two, British society has a particularly strong integrative emphasis. From this point of view, illness is not so much a threat to the achievement of the individual or to his responsibility as it is a threat to his *status* as an acceptable member of the society and its various relevant subgroupings. The main emphasis in treatment then would be on reintegration, an element which is always present, but is more strongly stressed in the British case than in others.

One important type of evidence is the particularly strong British feeling that the sick individual has a *right* to care in case of illness. The whole welfare state is related to the integrative emphasis in the society, but the particularly full coverage provided by the National Health Service for the whole population is one very salient aspect of this general orientation. On the part of the nation and its health agencies then, it is strongly declared that illness, far from jeopardizing the individual's status, gives him special claims on the collectivity. The burden of proof is not nearly so much on him that he is "really" sick as in either the American or the Soviet cases. One might speak of a scale of decreasing "tolerance of the possibility of malingering" in the order, British, American, Soviet.

Another interesting point is that, with

---

[29] Cf. *Social System. op. cit.,* This is Merton's "ritualism."

[30] On this point I am directly indebted to Dr. Field (personal discussion).

Definitions of Health and 117
Illness in the Light of
American Values and Social Structure

respect to the scope given to the recognition of mental illness, the British case is intermediate between the American and the Soviet; this includes the position of psychoanalysis. I suggest that this has to do with the very strong British emphasis on the importance of self-control in social relations. Somatic illness is generally clearly beyond the responsibility of the individual, and generally the legitimacy of illness is not made so highly conditional as in the American case. But capacity is not so highly valued and mental disturbance is not to the same extent seen as an opportunity for therapeutic achievement. The deliberately encouraged regression which, with all the differences, is shared by the Soviet and American cases, is substantially less conspicuous in the British.

The above are, as I have emphasized, extremely tentative and sketchy impressions of relatively systematic differences between American, Soviet, and British selectivities in the definition of health and illness, and in the roles of patient and of therapeutic agencies. I have introduced them and carried the analysis as far as I have, only to try to give some empirical substance to the general view of the nature of variability from one society to another in those respects that have been presented herein.

8

Response Factors in Illness: The Study of Illness Behavior

David Mechanic

MEDICINE HAS THREE principal tasks—to understand how particular symptoms, syndromes or disease entities arise either in individuals or among groups of individuals; to recognize and cure these or to shorten their course and minimize any residual impairment; and to promote living conditions in human populations which eliminate hazards to health and thus prevent the occurrence of disease. Each task can only be pursued with maximal effectiveness if the *integral* importance of social and psychological, as well as biological, factors is appreciated.

Much medical activity—whether in research, clinical practice, or preventive work—requires an understanding of the cultural and social pressures which influence an individual's recognition that he needs advice, his decision whether to seek it, his choice of counsellor, his cooperation in carrying out any measures that are suggested and his willingness to remain in contact should there be any recommendation that further supervision is needed. Unless our knowledge of these processes is taken into account in training doctors, dealing with patients and designing sociomedical services, we shall continue to make grave errors in all three fields.

In this paper, I shall consider only one aspect of these problems: that concerning response factors in illness. Although there is a good deal to learn in this area, considerable knowledge is already available.

Data about illness, whether clinical or epidemiological, usually contain two kinds of information: one on the state of the patient (for example, a description of symptoms or dysfunctions); and the other on his reactions to his condition. The physician's diagnosis is influenced by each of these kinds of information. He obtains data from physical examination and laboratory studies and also from a clinical history, which usually includes the patient's reactions to his condition. Within the traditional medical model, the patient lodges a complaint and the physician attempts to account for, explain, or find justification for it through his investigation. Logically, if not empirically, the diagnostic situation involves two sets of facts: historical data and symptoms reported by the patient or other informants about his condition, and data obtained by the physician through a systematic examination for abnormal signs and through laboratory investigation if necessary. Thus it is logically possible for physicians to hypothesize that some patients are hypochondriacs or malingerers if they note substantial discrepancies between the patient's complaints and other findings elicited through an independent investigation of the complaints.

However, it is often very difficult in the process of medical (and particularly of psychiatric) diagnosis to make an objective and independent examination of the patient's state of health. So much depends upon information provided and processed by the patient and other informants, and colored by their needs and reactions, that the study of these responses becomes a central concern of medicine itself. It is these "secondary" psychological and social processes, as contrasted with the "primary" biological ones usually considered by doctors, that I refer

From Social Psychiatry, *Vol. 1: 11–20, 1966; by permission of the author and publisher.*

This work was supported in part by a Public Health Service Special Fellowship (MH—8516) from the National Institute of Mental Health. During the period of the fellowship the author was affiliated with the Medical Research Council Social Psychiatry Research Unit, Maudsley Hospital. The author is indebted to Dr. John Wing for his helpful comments.

to under the heading of "illness behavior." The term "illness" has always been used in two ways in medicine. On the one hand it has referred to a limited scientific concept (with which I am not here specifically concerned) and, on the other, to any condition which causes, or might usefully cause, an individual to seek advice from a doctor. "Illness Behavior" is any behavior relevant to the second, more general, interpretation. It is therefore necessary to consider what goes on even before a person sees a doctor. I also wish, in this paper, to illustrate how the importance of "reaction" components in illness has been independently recognized and explored in a number of different areas of medical and sociomedical investigation.

On the most simple and obvious level, the extent to which symptoms are differentially perceived, evaluated and acted (or not acted) upon by different kinds of people and in different social situations is obvious. Whether because of earlier experiences with illness, because of differential training in respect to symptoms, or because of different biological sensitivities, some persons make light of symptoms, shrug them off, and avoid seeking medical care. Others will respond to little pain and discomfort by readily seeking care, by releasing themselves from work and other obligations, and by becoming dependent on others (Mechanic, 1962a). Thus, the study of illness behavior involves the study of attentiveness to pain and symptomatology, the examination of processes affecting how pain and symptoms are defined, accorded significance and socially labelled, and the consideration of the extent to which help is sought, change in life regimen affected, and claims on others made.

The study of illness behavior by its very nature requires an epidemiological model. Since illness behavior affects the utilization of medical care, choice of paths to possible advisers, and responses to illness in general, the selection of patients who seek help from general practitioners, from clinics, or even from hospitals is usually biased. Groups of patients with a particular disease, selected from such populations, will usually be biased compared with those in the general population with the same disease, but untreated, and this is particularly true for illness of high

prevalence which are easily recognized by the public and known to have a benign course (Mechanic, 1963a).

Approximately, only one in three persons who report illnesses in a household interview seek a physician's advice, and in any given month only nine of 750 persons who report illnesses will be hospitalized (White, *et al.*, 1961).

Different patterns of illness behavior may be viewed from at least three general perspectives. First such patterns of behavior may be seen as a product of cultural and social conditioning, since they may be experienced and enacted naturally in the social contexts within which they appear relevant. Secondly, illness behavior may be seen as part of a coping repertoire—as an attempt to make an unstable, challenging situation more manageable for the person who is encountering difficulty. Thirdly, illness behavior may be analyzed in terms of its advantages for the patient in seeking and obtaining attention, sympathy and material gain.

1a. *Illness Behavior as a Culturally and Socially Learned Response*

Cultures are so recognizably different that variations in illness behavior in different societies hardly need demonstration. The idea implicit in much of the anthropological work is that primitive conceptions of illness are part of a learned cultural complex, and are functionally associated with other aspects of cultural response to environmental threat. Some of the earlier investigations of illness behavior in America were based on the same idea—that different patterns of response to illness are culturally conditioned and functionally relevant. Thus Koos (1954) observed that upper class persons were more likely than lower class persons to view themselves as ill when they had particular symptoms and when they were questioned about specific symptoms, they reported more frequently than lower class persons that they would seek the doctor's advice. Illness responses were described in this study as part of a constellation of needs including those associated with work, family and finances. Saunders (1954) described in some detail the differences between "Anglos" and Spanish-speaking persons in the American southwest in attitudes and responses toward illness and in the use of medical facilities. Whereas the Anglos preferred modern medical science and hospitalization for many illnesses, the Spanish-speaking people were more likely to rely on folk medicine and family care and support which was more consistent with their cultural conceptions. More recently, Clark (1959) has described how Mexican–Americans view various life situations and symptoms as health problems in contrast to physicians who do not view these problems with similar seriousness and alarm. Other problems among these people which are ignored and undefined are seen by physicians as serious health problems. Similar observations have been made concerning various American Indian groups, and in a variety of other cultural contexts.

The role of cultural differences in illness behavior was nicely described by Zborowski (1952) who, in a study of ethnic reactions to pain in a New York City hospital, observed that while Jewish and Italian patients responded to pain in an emotional fashion, tending to exaggerate pain experiences, "Old Americans" tended to be more stoical and "objective," and Irish more frequently denied pain. Zborowski also noted a difference in the attitude underlying Italian and Jewish concern about pain. While the Italian subjects primarily sought relief from pain and were relatively satisfied when such relief was obtained, the Jewish subjects were mainly concerned with the meaning and significance of their pain, and the consequences of pain for their future welfare and health. In trying to explain these cultural differences, Zborowski reports that Jewish and Italian patients related how their mothers showed over-protective and over-concerned attitudes about the child's health, and participation in sports, and how they were constantly warned of the advisability of avoiding colds, fights, and other threaten-

ing situations. Zborowski reports that: "Crying in complaint is responded to by parents with sympathy, concern and help. By their over-protective and worried attitude they foster complaining and tears. The child learns to pay attention to each painful experience and to look for help and sympathy which are readily given to him. In Jewish families, where not only a slight sensation of pain but also each deviation from the child's normal behavior is looked on as a sign of illness, the child is prone to acquire anxieties with regard to the meaning and significance of these manifestations." Although Zborowski presents something of a caricature, it is clear that he views the etiology of these behavioral patterns and attitudes as inherent in the familial response to the child's health and illnesses.

Zborowski's observations concerning ethnic differences in illness behavior have been supported in a variety of other studies. Croog (1961) administered the Cornell Medical Index to 2,000 randomly chosen army inductees. He found that Italian and Jewish respondents reported the greatest number of symptoms of illness. He further found that although the Italian response was associated with low educational status, reports of symptoms among Jewish respondents were not affected by the educational variable. Mechanic (1963b), studying 1,300 students at two American universities, found that Jewish students reported higher illness behavior patterns than either Protestant or Catholic students. Since income was also found to be related to illness behavior reports, and since Jewish students were also more likely to be represented in the higher income groups, the analysis was repeated, controlling income. The differences in illness behavior reports between Jewish and other students were only significant for the high income group. Mechanic also attempted to test the hypothesis that use of medical services was an alternative among several possible modes of dealing with stress, and that the difference in reports of illness behavior between Jewish students and Catholic and Protestant students could be explained by the relatively limited involvement in religious activities among Jewish students. This hypothesis was not confirmed.

The observed differences in illness behavior patterns has persisted in other studies. Segal (unpublished paper), in a study of student clinic facilities, found that Jewish students used such facilities somewhat more than Catholic or Protestant students. Similarly, several studies of the use of psychiatric facilities have shown a higher receptivity and utilization rate among Jewish subjects (Scheff and Silverman, 1966; Segal, et al., 1965; Srole, et al., 1962; and Linn, unpublished paper).

Suchman (1964 and 1965) in a recent study of 5,340 persons in different ethnic groups in New York City found that the more ethnocentric and socially cohesive groups included more persons who knew little about disease, who were skeptical toward professional medical care, and who were dependent during illness. He found that the Jewish respondents were more likely to report a high or moderate pattern of "preventive medical behavior" and "acceptance of the sick role" as compared with respondents from the other groups studied, but that they were not particularly different from other groups on the scale dealing with dependency during illness.

The studies described above suggest considerable consistency in ethnic variations in illness behavior. Although such trends are clear, the variation within groups is much greater than it is between groups. In any case, it is important to note that illness behavior patterns can have both healthy and unhealthy consequences. For example, the traditional concern about health among Jewish persons—especially the health of children—can under some circumstances lead to over-concern and can encourage doubts and anxiety. Such concern and attention can also encourage a high standard of infant rearing and caring as suggested by an early study of infant mortality among immigrants to America which showed that although the Jewish group was foreign born, had just as many children, and had an income which was much lower than that of native-born whites, this group had the lowest rate of infant mortality of all of the groups studied, including the native-white population (Anderson, 1958).

Although it is fairly clear that culturally learned differences in illness behavior are important to some extent, such differences explain only a small proportion of the total variation in behavior. Moreover, the contribution of other factors is not well understood. Mechanic (1964), in a study of 350 mother–child pairs, attempted to investigate the relationship between maternal attitudes and maternal illness behavior, and between these and the illness behavior of their children. The sample chosen from a relatively homogeneous population in the Midwest of America did not include any substantial ethnic diversity. Data were obtained from both mother and child independently, as well as from teachers, school records, and a daily illness log maintained by the mother. Mechanic found that the mother's attitudes toward illness and illness behavior were rather poor predictors of the attitudes of their children. Maternal attitudes however played a more important role in determining whether medical aid would be sought for the child when ill.

In this study of the illness behavior of children, the two best predictors of children's reports of "fear of getting hurt" and "attention to pain" were the child's age and sex. Boys were more stoical than girls, and older children were more stoical than younger children. These findings support the idea that age and sex role learning is important in illness behavior and attitudes toward health risks. The results are consistent also with a number of other observations such as the higher utilization of medical facilities among women compared with men (Anderson, 1963), and the higher rate of accidents among boys compared with girls of the same age. Similarly, in another study of reported responses to illness, Mechanic (1965) found that respondents expected women to be less stoical than men when ill.

In summary, it seems fair to conclude that cultural and social conditioning play an important though not an exclusive role in patterns of illness behavior, and that ethnic membership, peer pressures, and age-sex role learning to some extent influence attitudes towards risks and towards the significance of common threats.

1b. *Links Between Reaction Pattern and Physiological Response*

It is interesting to note that, in general, observations from field studies concerning ethnic differences in the perception of pain have withstood not only repeated study, but also more detailed scrutiny under laboratory conditions. Sternbach and Tursky (1965), for example, brought Irish, Jewish, Italian and "Yankee" housewives into a psycho–physiological laboratory where they administered pain by electric shock, recording skin potential responses. Their findings tend to support some of the observations made by Zborowski. They found, for example, that Italian women showed significantly lower upper thresholds for shock, and fewer of them would accept the full range of shock stimulation used in the experiment. The investigators believe that this response is consistent with the Italian tendency to focus on the immediacy of the pain itself as compared with the future orientation of the Jewish response tendency. Similarly, they believe that the finding that "Yankee" housewives had faster and more complete adaptation of the diphasic palmar skin potential has an attitudinal correlate to their "matter of fact" orientation to pain. As they note: "This is illustrated by our Yankee subjects' modal attitude toward traumata, as they verbalized it in their interviews: 'You take things in your stride.' No such action-oriented, adapting phrase was used by the members of the other groups. The similarly undemonstrative Irish subjects may 'keep a tight upper lip' but 'fear the worst,' a noxious stimulus being a burden to be endured and suffered in silence."

However, we must be careful in generalizing conclusions from laboratory pain situations to pathological pain experiences. Henry Beecher (1959), an eminent researcher and Anesthetist-in-Chief at the Massachusetts General Hospital, has reported the failure of fifteen different research groups to establish any dependable effects of even large doses of morphine on pain of experimental origin in man, although the effect of morphine on pathological pain is substantial. He has found it necessary to distinguish between pain as an *original sensation* and pain as a *psychic reaction*. As Beecher notes, one of the difficulties with most forms of laboratory pain is that they minimize the psychic reaction which plays an essential role in pain associated with illness. For example, in a comparative study of pain, he asked a group of wounded soldiers and a group of male civilian patients undergoing major surgery the same questions about their desire for pain medication. While only one-third of the soldiers wanted medication to relieve their pain, 80 per cent of the civilians wanted such pain relief although they were suffering from far less tissue trauma. He explains the variation in terms of differing definitions of pain in the two circumstances. The soldier's wound, Beecher explains, was an escape from the battlefield and the possibility of being killed; to the civilian surgical pain was viewed as a depressing, calamitous event. Beecher reports that the civilian group reported strikingly more frequent and severe pain and he concludes that there is no simple, direct relationship between the wound *per se* and the pain experienced. He further concludes that morphine primarily acts on the reactive component of the pain experience, largely through a process of "mental clouding."

The reactive or definitional component in illness has long been recognized as a significant aspect not only in defining the condition but also in the patient's response to treatment. Physicians working with the severely ill are often impressed by the attitudinal component and its influence on the patient's condition. In its extreme form, physicians have commented on the importance of the patient's "will to live" although it has been difficult to quantify this phenomenon or to present clear evidence in support of its importance. At best, we have anecdotal reports of preparation for death and actual death following witchcraft, and some physiological explanations have been offered to explain the mechanisms involved in such impressive happenings (Frank, 1961). But if we are to integrate such events with our common conceptual schemes we require a better understanding of such phenomena as they occur in more subtle but more observable forms.

Models for the experimental study of the psycho–physiology of stress that more closely take into account the reactive or definitional components are beginning to be developed. It has long been recognized that difficult life circumstances or experimentally constructed "stress situations" lead to varied physiological and social responses. It is believed that these differences are due to subjects' differing definitions and capacities to cope with these stimuli, and genetic differences. Until recently, psychophysiological investigations have not taken into consideration differing definitions of experimental "stressors" and the differing capacities of subjects to deal with them. Recently, Lazarus and his colleagues (Speisman, 1964) have developed a method for inducing different psychological sets in subjects who are viewing the same threatening films, and they have demonstrated the importance of the definitional set in the reactions of subjects to the experimental films. They as well as others have also observed that, as subjects are exposed over many trials to the threatening films, they appear to develop orientations or adaptations which allow them to experience the same stimulus more calmly. In sum, the reactive component is obviously important and manipulation of "reactive sets" in experiments appear to affect physiological response.

The definitional components in response to difficult circumstances have also been observed in natural situations where physiological response has been studied. Friedman and his colleagues (1963a and 1963b) in making observations of parents anticipating the death of their children who were suffering from neoplastic diseases found that urinary 17-hydroxycorticosteroid levels in parents would vary from one parent to another, and from one period in the child's illness to another. The period of highest "distress" as measured physiologically occurred for most parents well before the death of the child, the most common situation being when the child was put on the critical list for the first time. For some of the parents the death of

the child seemed to be a relief, and it appears as if they had already worked through a substantial part of their grief prior to the death of the child. Other parents, however, who maintained hope despite evidence to the contrary, and who showed little marked acceleration in 17-hydroxycorticosteroid levels at crucial points during the illness, seemed to experience a marked acceleration after the child died. The study illustrates both the tremendous variability in response to difficult circumstances, and the probable link between coping reactions and physiological responses under "stress."

2. Illness Behavior as a Coping Response to Situational Difficulties

The idea that illness is "stressful" and that it may engender further life difficulties is sufficiently obvious to require no elaboration. What is interesting to the behavioral scientist, however, is the tremendous variability in response to what is presumably the same illness condition. While one person will hardly acknowledge a condition and refuse to allow it to alter his life, another with a more mild form of the same condition will display profound social and psychological disabilities.

An emotional component has often been seen in the etiology or precipitation of illness (Wolff, 1953; Hinkle and Wolff, 1957; Roessler and Greenfield, 1962; Graham, et al., 1962; Meyer and Haggerty, 1962). What is often less appreciated is the importance of life difficulties in influencing illness behavior. Indeed, it appears from a careful scrutiny of psychosomatic evidence that "distress" is often more influential in its effects on seeking help and on the expression of illness, than it is on the actual occurrence of the condition. Balint (1957) has argued, for example, that the presentation of somatic complaints often masks an underlying emotional problem which is frequently the major reason why the individual has sought advice.

Certainly, what little evidence we have on this point suggests that a complaint of trivial illness may be one way of seeking reassurance and support through a recognized and socially acceptable relationship when it is difficult for the patient to present the underlying problem in an undisguised form. In such circumstances the real problem may not even be consciously recognized. The emphasis Balint places on emotional factors in the utilization of the general practitioner appears, nevertheless, to be oversimplified since it fails to take into account the more complex relationship between life difficulties and social and cultural patterns.

Mechanic and Volkart (1961) have attempted to examine this problem through an investigation of more than 600 students at a major university. One of the major concerns of the study was the relationship between measures of "stress," and measures of illness behavior, and their joint effect on the use of medical facilities. Analysis of the data showed that perceived stress (as measured by indices of loneliness and nervousness) and illness behavior (as measured by several hypothetical items concerning the use of medical facilities) were clearly related to the use of a college health service during a one-year period. Among students with a high inclination to use medical facilities and high "stress," 73 per cent were frequent users of medical services (three or more times during the year), while among the low inclination-low "stress" group, only 30 per cent were frequent users of such services. Our attention, however, centered on the interaction between our measure of "stress" on the one hand, and illness behavior on the other, in encouraging a person to present a complaint. When illness behavior patterns were statistically controlled, we found that the influence of "stress" was somewhat different among persons with a high receptivity to medical services than among those who were less inclined to favor medical services. In the high inclination group, "stress" was a rather significant influence in bringing people to the physician. Thus among those with high "stress," 73 per cent used facilities fre-

quently, while only 46 per cent did so among those with low "stress." Although the same trend was observed among those who were less inclined to seek advice from a doctor, the relationship was substantially smaller, and not statistically significant. Thus our data support the interpretation that "stress" leads to an attempt to cope; those who are inclined to adopt the patient role tend to adopt this particular method of coping more frequently than those who are not so inclined.

As I have already noted, the reactive component in illness is clearly relevant to treatment response. Beecher (1959), for example, has collected considerable data to show that the effectiveness of a placebo is very much greater when the patient is distressed than when he is not. Placebos, for example, have very little effect on relieving pain inflicted in the laboratory but they are impressive in relieving pain following surgery. Beecher has accumulated data from several laboratories which show placebos effective in relieving pain of angina pectoris, seasickness, headache, cough and so on. In reviewing fifteen studies totalling 1,082 patients he found an average of 35.2 (plus or minus 2.2) per cent relieved by placebo. In contrast, Beecher calculates the effectiveness of placebos in relieving experimentally contrived pain as 3.2 per cent; thus the placebo is ten times as effective in relieving pain of pathological origin (where distress is an important factor) than it is in relieving pain of experimentally contrived origin.

Studies in social psychology have shown that under situations that are difficult, usual habits and problem-solving patterns may be disrupted and behavior may become disorganized. Under these conditions the directions which coping attempts take depend on the one hand on external influences and stimuli which serve to define circumstances and their meaning, and on the other on past experience and preparation. We will discuss each of these in turn.

In a recent ingenious experiment, Schachter and Singer (1962) have shown how external cues influence behavior and feeling states under conditions of altered physiology. They demonstrated that whether subjects experienced anger or euphoria when injected with epinephrine was dependent on whether they had (i) an *appropriate explanation* for their altered physiological state and (ii) *directive external cues.* When the individual had an appropriate explanation for his feelings, he had little need for evaluating himself in terms of environmental stimuli and was not very much affected by them. However, when individuals had no immediate explanation for their altered feelings, external cues became important and, in the experimental situation, determined the emotional state. The same type of altered physiological experience was variously interpreted as happiness or anger depending on cues determined by stooges of the experimenter who were playing the role of subjects. Thus we see that, when persons lose their bearings, environmental cues play an important part in helping the person make sense of his subjective state. Placebos may determine cues in a similar way during illness.

Several studies similarly reflect the importance of cultural and developmental experiences in reactions to threatening circumstances. Schachter (1959), in another set of impressive experimental studies, showed that first-born and only children were more likely to affiliate when threatened in adult life than other adults. Schachter believes that the attention given to the first child, and the inexperience of parents, is likely to instil a greater dependence on others in first and only born children as compared with later born children. Although birth order has not been studied directly in illness behavior studies, several other investigations support the idea that past experience, habits, and social values help define—consciously and unconsciously—the alternatives that will be utilized in challenging circumstances.

Phillips (1965), for example, in a recent study has shown that attitudes of self-reliance and health values both affect the willingness of people to report that they would seek help when ill. Many studies of delay in treatment reflect the same tendency for delay to be related to a constellation of ingrained sociomedical habits (Goldsen, 1963) which tend to be typical—at least in the United States—of the lower socio-economic groups. Suchman (1964 and 1965) found, for example, that both individual

medical orientation (an index based on knowledge about disease, on skepticism about medical care, and on dependency in illness) and social group organization (an index based on ethnic exclusiveness, friendship solidarity, and family orientation to tradition and authority) were related to socio-economic status. A "parochial" as compared with a "cosmopolitan" social structure and a "popular" as compared with a "scientific" orientation to medicine were both linked with lower socio-economic status. Similarly, persons of higher socio-economic status were more likely to buy health insurance, to get a periodic medical check-up, to receive polio immunization, to eat a balanced diet, and they more frequently had eye examinations and dental care.

Under conditions of manageable difficulties, persons have a tendency to normalize or ignore symptoms that do not become too severe. For example in our study discussed earlier (Mechanic and Volkart, 1960) we found that when illness is of a kind that is common and familiar, and the course of the illness is predictable, the presentation of the illness for medical scrutiny is substantially related to the inclination to use medical services as measured by hypothetical illness situations. As symptoms become more atypical, less familiar, and less predictable in their course, the role of social and situational factors in bringing a person for medical attention becomes less important. Similarly, Scheff and Silverman (1966), in a study of the use of a college psychiatric clinic, found social and demographic factors to be better predictors of the use of such facilities than the "seriousness" of the patient's condition. However, when they stratified their psychiatric cases into those more serious and those less serious, it became clear that while social and demographic factors were crucial in the presentation of "moderate psychiatric problems," they were relatively unimportant in predicting use of such facilities among those with "severe psychiatric problems."

If we are to make progress in the study of illness behavior, it becomes necessary to move beyond gross cultural and social differences in illness patterns toward the development of a social–psychological model which gives a clear conception of the processes involved when someone seeks help. From our various studies, we are able to suggest a working model which describes some of the contingencies relevant to illness behavior (Mechanic, 1962b and 1966a). Seven groups of variables appear to be particularly important: (I) the number and persistence of symptoms; (II) the individual's ability to recognize symptoms; (III) the perceived seriousness of symptoms; (IV) the extent of social and physical disability resulting from the symptoms; (V) the cultural background of the defining person, group or agency in terms of the emphasis on tolerance, stoicism, etc.; (VI) available information and medical knowledge, and (VII) the availability of sources of help and their social and physical accessibility. Here we include not only physical distance and costs of time money and effort, but also such costs as fear, stigma, social distance, feelings of humiliation, and the like.

When we inspect these seven groups of variables, it becomes clear that what may appear salient to the definer may not appear relevant to the physician. For example, the recognizability of symptoms is not necessarily correlated with medical views of their seriousness. Similarly, some symptoms which are, for example, disfiguring or disruptive or which bring about work disability may be self-limited and medically trivial while other symptoms (such as signs of cancer) may have no disruptive effects at all. Yet one of the major cues patients use in deciding to seek help is the disruption of their activities. Illness behavior and the decision to seek medical advice frequently involves, from the patient's point of view, a rational attempt to make sense of his problem and cope with it within the limits of his intelligence and his social and cultural understandings.

Zola (1964) has attempted to delineate five timing "triggers" in patient's decision to seek medical care. The first pattern he calls "interpersonal crisis" where the situation calls attention to the symptoms and causes the patient to dwell on them. The second "trigger" he calls "social interference"; in this situation the symptoms do not change, but come to threaten a valued social activity. The third "trigger"—"the presence of sanctioning"—involves others telling him to seek care. Fourthly, Zola discusses "perceived threat" and, finally, "nature and quality of the symptoms." The latter "trigger" involves similarity of symptoms to previous ones or to those of friends, and the like. Zola reports the impression that these "triggers" have different effects in various social strata and ethnic groups.

The difficulty in preventive medicine is that commonsense models of health and coping with disease do not necessarily conform to scientific models, yet it is usually commonsense models that determine the use of medical facilities. Similarly, a frequent problem faced by the physician in providing care is the failure of the patient to conform to medical advice and most typically this occurs when the patient fails to take his drugs or return for follow-up because, subjectively, he feels well. From the patient's commonsense perspective, to stop medication or cancel a follow-up visit when he is feeling well, is logical.

3. *Illness Behavior as an Attempt To Seek Secondary Advantages*

Since illness is recognized as an acceptable cause for withdrawing from certain role obligations, social responsibilities, and expectations, persons may be drawn to the patient role in order to obtain secondary advantages, to make claims on others for care and attention, and to provide an, acceptable reason for social failure. Thus individuals may be motivated to adopt the "sick role" (Parsons, 1951), and others may be anxious to accord people the status of sickness in order to avoid embarrassment and social difficulties. The interpenetration between medical and other social institutions is quite complex, and often these relationships are not fully appreciated.

In the final analysis, illness and social disability are socially defined and somewhat arbitrary (Mechanic, 1959). The problem of mental subnormality, for example, is a greater problem in a highly developed industrial nation requiring a high level of skills than it is in a communal agrarian community; and if we had no schools most of the mildly subnormal would be unrecognized and undefined. Similarly, the extent to which people are to be held accountable for fulfilling responsibilities regardless of health status involves a compromise between personal and community needs. The need to minimize the consequences of ill health as a practical or a humanitarian gesture is theoretically only one value to be weighed against other personal and social goals, and the limits and scope of the definition of illness may serve different needs and different agencies, depending on social, political, and historical contingencies.

Since a discussion of problems of the definition of "illness," as distinct from "illness behavior," will take us too far afield, I will not develop the topic here (see Mechanic, 1966b). It should, however, be noted that the concept of illness can be used to support humanitarian values in the face of moral and legal sanctions (Szasz, 1962). Thus, illness concepts are used to overcome restrictive laws on abortion, or on criminal responsibility, as an excuse for academic failure, and so on. On other occasions, the concept of illness may be used to discredit peoples' views and actions, and to undermine their integrity. The use of illness labels may differ depending on who controls medical institutions, and the goals they are meant to serve (Field, 1957). Medical independence of political control is of obvious importance here as is the necessity for medical decisions affecting the community to be reviewed by expert laymen. In a free society the value and functions of medicine have primary relevance from a social standpoint in that they can enhance or retard the ability of the individual to fulfil personal and social choices. Physicians, on the whole, have been very successful in protecting medical systems from external manipulation for non-medical purposes. For the most part, even in this complicated age, the doctor serves as the patient's agent, and often even as his advocate.

As society becomes more humanitarian, and as illness becomes not only an excuse for social failure and neglect of social responsibilities but also cause, in and of itself, for monetary and social compensation, the relationship between illness as a physical state and as a secondary coping technique becomes even more difficult, It is fairly obvious that under some circumstances desire for compensation for injury and disability may encourage persons to exaggerate their inabilities to perform routine tasks, and discourage attempts to cope with the disability.

Discussion: Implications of Illness Behavior for Medical Care

The value of a medical perspective which takes into account illness behavior can be illustrated by a study at the Massachusetts General Hospital (Zola, 1963). The hypothesis was that the patient's cultural background would influence how the patient presented his symptoms, and thus, how the doctor evaluated them. The analysis was undertaken because the investigator had the impression that more Italian than Irish or Anglo-Saxon patients were being labelled as psychiatric problems although there was no objective difference in the extent to which members in these groups reported psychosocial problems. Zola selected a group of 29 patients who presented themselves at the Medical and Ear, Nose and Throat clinics, but for whom no medical disease was found. There was good reason to believe that these groups of patients did not differ in the extent of their life difficulties. But it was clear that their mode of cultural expression was very different. Italians are more emotional in the presentation of symptoms, and give more attention and expression to pain. Zola found that psychogenesis was implied in the medical reports of 11 of the 12 Italian cases, and only in four of the thirteen remaining cases. Although this was not a well-controlled study, the results strongly suggest that the patient's cultural mode of expression affected how the doctor viewed him and how he was medically evaluated.

The place of illness behavior is particularly important in disorders that are largely diagnosed through behavioral manifestations and the patient's social history. For it is particularly difficult to separate symptoms from sub-cultural patterns of expression and affect, and different behavioral patterns among the various social strata. Similarly, it is in such disorders that symptoms and etiological factors are more frequently confused with factors which may differentially lead to social intervention and the seeking of care.

The provision of care depends to a considerable extent on the social and cultural processes that lead particular people to define themselves as requiring care, or that lead others to define them as targets for community action. Many factors unrelated to the severity of illness and incapacity may assist in the selection of patients for care, while other persons requiring attention to a greater extent go unnoticed.

We all recognize that there are many persons in the general population who require care and treatment and who can benefit by it but do not come to the attention of care facilities. Conversely, there are some who have developed an over-dependence on the physician, psychiatrist, or social agency who can be adversely affected by particular kinds of intensive care and attention. Although psychiatrists, especially those more dynamically oriented, often work under the assumption that all persons can benefit from therapy—or at least, that it will not harm them—and although the plea for help is usually taken on pragmatic grounds as proof for the need for psychiatric assistance, it is important to consider the counter-proposition—that certain kinds of assistance, however well-meaning, can be detrimental for certain patients. There are those, for example, for whom excessive focus on symptoms and life difficulties may reinforce an already hypochrondrial pattern, induce or encourage further displays of illness behavior, and bring about reduced coping effectiveness. As we have already noted, illness is one of the few widely recognized and acceptable reasons for failing to meet social responsibilities and obligations and thus the sick role often carries advantages for those who wish to escape the difficulties of meeting social expectations without incurring disapproval. The improper use of the sick role and the willingness to encourage persons to assume the role of the patient without careful consideration of its implications involves serious dangers. The improper use of the sick role under some circumstances can reinforce "immature" and "irresponsible" patterns of behavior. Military psychiatrists have learned—and this is consistent with the observations of Beecher we discussed earlier—that under military conditions where persons often wish to evade responsibilities and dangers, the sick role may offer clear advantages. This is one of the reasons military organizations often make it so difficult to be sick, and similarly totalitarian governments have done so during periods of labor shortage. During the second world war, it was observed that when troops became upset under combat stress and were evacuated for treatment it was extremely difficult to return these men as functioning soldiers. When these men were brought back to the hospital, and when their problems were defined as having roots in their early years, the men had an acceptable reason for failure which could be viewed as beyond their control and it was difficult to mobilize them (Glass, 1953). In contrast, during the Korean war, when such problems were defined as problems of mastery of common fears shared by many others, it was possible to encourage men to make instrumental efforts to cope with the extreme difficulties in their situation (Group for the Advancement of Psychiatry, 1960).

The issue is not, of course, whether we should adopt a permissive approach to illness or on the other hand subjugate health organizations to other social institutions. From the perspective of a free medical system (that is, one where the doctor acts primarily as the patient's agent and on his behalf), the doctor–patient relationship is one where the doctor has considerable influence in affecting the patient's feeling state and behavior. As we have noted, patients often seek care when they are distressed; and there is a large amount of evidence that distressed persons are highly suggestible and open to influence (Frank, 1961). Thus, the doctor's attitude toward the patient and his illness are important forces which can be used to support coping efforts, or they can encourage an elaboration of the disability.

There are factors which affect illness behavior perhaps less visibly but which strongly influence coping efforts and the nature of disability. It is now well recognized that particular hospital environments can have deleterious effects on the patient (Goffman, 1961; Wing, 1962). Patients who are cared for in environments which fail to stimulate them may deteriorate. Wing and Brown (Wing and Brown, 1961; Brown and Wing, 1962) showed that in the case of schizophrenia, in socially poor hospitals, patients are more withdrawn and have more symptoms such as poverty of speech. Similarly, Brown and his associates found that schizophrenic patients have poor outcome in family environments characterized by "high emotional involvement" (Brown, et al., 1962). Through well planned programs encompassing community care and "social treatment," the advantages of more limited medical treatments and procedures can be realized without incurring inactivity, separation from social ties, loss of confidence and skills, and other liabilities associated with long-term patient roles.

As we noted at the beginning of this discussion, the problems of separating out "primary" biological from "secondary" psychological and social factors in conditions such as "institutionalism" are enormously complex, though perhaps easier with some physical diseases than with psychiatric disorders (Wing, 1962; Brown, et al., 1966). In research efforts, attempts to reliably separate these components is an important and necessary endeavor. In the practice of clinical medicine and psychiatry, however, concern with social and psychological disabilities may achieve results comparable, and under some circumstances superior, to those gained by directing attention to the "primary" disorder.

We often tend to forget that our language and the professional stances we take have a moral as well as a scientific and practical importance. And since our orientation toward patients implies a vocabulary of motives, it is not surprising that it has effects on their future motives and efforts. Over the years there has been an increasing tendency to view problems of living within a deterministic model of illness, and there is no question but that this tendency has served a valuable social function in perpetuating the humanitarian perspective which it encompassed. But as we increasingly recognize the social influences of the labelling process and of environmental contexts, it is important to consider how iatrogenic disability may be avoided without abandoning the human values to which medicine and psychiatry have made so important a contribution.

Bibliography

Anderson, O., "Infant Mortality and Social and Cultural Factors: Historical Trends and Current Patterns," in E. G. Jaco (ed.), *Patients, Physicians and Illness*, 1st ed. New York: The Free Press, 1958, Chap. 2.

——— "The Utilization of Health Services," in H. Freeman, *et al.* (eds.), *Handbook of Medical Sociology*, Englewood Cliffs, N.J., Prentice Hall, 1963, Chap. 14.

Balint, M., *The Doctor, His Patient, and the Illness*, New York: International Universities Press, 1957.

Beecher, H., *Measurement of Subjective Responses*, New York: Oxford University Press, 1959.

Brown, G. W., and J. K. Wing, "A Comparative Clinical and Social Survey of Three Mental Hospitals," The Sociological Review Monograph, 5, *Sociology and Medicine*, Studies Within the Framework of the British National Health Service, Keele, 1962.

———, *et al.*, "Influence of Family Life on the Course of Schizophrenic Illness," *Brit. J. Prev. Soc. Med.*, 16:55–68, (1962).

———, *et al.*, *Schizophrenia and Social Care*, London: Oxford University Press, 1966.

Clark, M., *Health in the Mexican American Community*, Berkeley: University of California Press, 1959.

Croog, S. H., "Ethnic Origins, Educational Level, and Responses to a Health Questionnaire," *Hum. Org.*, 20: 65–69, 1961.

Field, M., *Doctor and Patient in Soviet Russia*, Cambridge: Harvard University Press, 1957.

Frank, J., *Persuasion and Healing*, Baltimore: John Hopkins Press, 1961.

Friedman, S. B., *et al.*: "Behavioral Observations on Parents Anticipating the Death of a Child," *Pediatrics*, 32: 610–625, 1963a.

Friedman, S. B., *et al.*: "Urinary 17-Hydroxycorticosteroid levels in Parents of Children with Neoplastic Disease," *Psychosom. Med.*, 25: 364–376, 1963b.

Glass, A. J., "Psychotherapy in the Combat Zone," in *Symposium on Stress*, Washington, D.C.: Army Medical Service Graduate School, Walter Reed Army Medical Hospital, 1953.

Goffman, E., *Asylums*, New York: Doubleday-Anchor, 1961.

Goldsen, R., "Patient Delay in Seeking Cancer Diagnosis: Behavioral Aspects," *J. Chron. Dis.*, 16: 427–436, 1963.

Graham, D., *et al.*: "Physiological Response to the Suggestion of Attitudes Specific for Hives and Hypertension," *Psychosom. Med.*, 24: 159–169, 1962.

Group for the Advancement of Psychiatry, "Preventive Psychiatry in the Armed Forces: With Some Implications for Civilian Use, Report no. 47, New York, 1960."

Hinkle, L. E., and H. G. Wolff: "Health and the Social Environment: Experimental Investigations," in A. H. Leighton, *et al.* (eds.), *Explorations in Social Psychiatry*, New York: Basic Books, 1957.

Koos, E., *The Health of Regionsville: What the People Thought and Did About It*, New York: Columbia University Press, 1954.

Linn, L., "Social Characteristics and Social Interaction in the Utilization of a Psychiatric Outpatient Clinic."

Mechanic, D.: "Illness and Social Disability: Some Problems in Analysis," *Pacific Soc. Rev.*, 2: 37–41, 1959.

——— "The Concept of Illness Behavior," *J. Chron. Dis.*, 15: 189–194, 1962a.

———"Some Factors in Identifying and Defining Mental Illness," *Ment. Hyg.*, 46:66–74, 1962b.

———"Some Implications of Illness Behavior for Medical Sampling," *New Engl. J. Med.*, 269:244–247, 1963a.

——— "Religion, Religiosity, and Illness Behavior," *Human Org.*, 22: 202–208, 1963b.

——— "The Influence of Mothers on Their Children's Health Attitudes and Behavior," *Pediatrics*, 33; 444–453, 1964.

——— "Perception of Parental Responses to Illness," *J. Hlth Hum. Behav.*, 6:253–257, 1965.

——— "The Sociology of Medicine, Viewpoints and Perspectives," *J. Hlth Hum. Behav.*, 7:237–248, Winter, 1966a.

———"Community Psychiatry: Some Sociological Perspectives and Implications," in L. Roberts, *et al.* (eds.) *Community Psychiatry*, Madison, Wisc.: University of Wisconsin Press, 1966b.

———, and E. H. Volkart, "Illness Behavior and Medical Diagnoses," *J. Hlth Hum. Behav.*, 1: 86–94, 1960.

——— ——— "Stress, Illness Behavior, and the Sick Role," *Amer. Sociol. Rev.*, 26:51–58, 1961.

Meyer, R. J., and R. J. Haggerty, "Streptococcal Infections in Families," *Pediatrics*, 29: 539–544, 1962.

Parsons, T., *The Social System*, New York: The Free Press, 1951, chap. VII.

Phillips, D., "Self-reliance and the Inclination to Adopt the Sick Role," *Social Forces*, 43: 555–563, 1965.

Roessler, R., and N. Greenfield (eds.), *Physiological Correlates of Psychological Disorders*, Madison, Wisc.: University of Wisconsin Press, 1962, pp. 257–267.

Saunders, L., *Cultural Differences and Medical Care*, New York: Russell Sage Foundation, 1954.

Schachter, S., *The Psychology of Affiliation*, Palo Alto: Stanford University Press, 1959.

———, and J. Singer, "Cognitive, Social, and Physiological Determinants of Emotional State," *Psychol. Rev.*, 69: 379–399, 1962.

Scheff, T. J., and A. Silverman, "Users and Non-users of a Student Psychiatric Clinic," *J. Hlth Hum. Behav.*, 7: 114–121, 1966.

Segal, B., "Scholars and Patients: Religion, Academic Performance, and the Use of Medical Facilities by Male Undergraduates," unpublished paper, Department of Sociology, Dartmouth College.

———, *et al.*, "Emotional Adjustment, Social Organization and Psychiatric Treatment Rates," *Amer. Sociol. Rev.*, 30: 548–556, 1965.

Speisman, J. C., *et al.*, "Experimental Reduction of Stress Based on Ego-defense Theory," *J. Abnorm. Soc. Psychol.* 68: 367–380, 1964.

Srole, L., *et al.*, *Mental Health in the Metropolis*, New York: McGraw-Hill, 1962.

Sternbach, R. A., and B. Tursky, "Ethnic Differences Among Housewives in Psychophysical and Skin Potential Responses to Electric Shock," *Psychophysiology*, 1: 241–246, 1965.

Suchman, E., "Sociomedical Variations Among Ethnic Groups," *Amer. J. Sociol.*, 70: 319–331, 1964.

——— "Social Patterns and Medical Care," *J. Hlth Hum. Behav.*, 6: 2–16, 1965.

Szasz, T. S., "Bootlegging Humanistic Values Through Psychiatry," *Antioch. Rev.*, 22: 341–349, 1962.

White, K. L., *et al.*, "The Ecology of Medical Care," *New Engl. J. Med.*, 265, 885–892, 1961.

Wing, J. K., "Institutionalism in Mental Hospitals," *Brit. J. Soc. Clin. Psychol.*, 1: 38–51, 1962.

———, and G. W. Brown: "Social Treatment of Chronic Schizophrenia: A Comparative Survey of Three Mental Hospitals," *J. Ment. Sci.*, 107: 847–861, 1961.

Wolff, H., *Stress and Disease*, Springfield, Ill.: Thomas, 1953.

Zborowski, M., "Cultural Components in Responses to Pain, *J. Soc. Issues*, 8: 16–30, 1952.

Zola, I., "Problems of Communication, Diagnosis and Patient Care," *J. Med. Educ.*, 10: 829–838, 1963.

——— "Illness Behavior of the Working Class," in A. Shostak and W. Gomberg (eds.), *Studies of the American Worker*, Englewood Cliffs, N.J., Prentice Hall, 1964.

THE WAY IN WHICH different kinds of people respond to the occurrence of illness has come to occupy an increasing amount of attention of both legislators and the general public.[1] Arguments pro and con different proposals for medical care programs have leaned heavily on assumptions regarding the norms concerning illness in our society, yet empirical data which would document such assumptions are often lacking. The study reported here represents an attempt to test the applicability of a set of propositions about normative expectations for sick people to a specific group of patients. Using the concept of the sick role as a point of departure, it attempts to investigate dimensions of the sick role as revealed by a factor analysis of questionnaire responses made by clinic patients. It then seeks to relate tendencies to emphasize different dimensions of the role to differences in age, sex, ethnic origin, socio–economic status, and clinical diagnosis.

The Concept of the Sick Role

Central to the concept of the sick role is the premise that although sickness represents a deviant status for the individual (in terms of deviance from the "well" population), it nevertheless evokes a set of patterned expectations which define the norms and behavior appropriate to his new status, both for the individual himself and for persons who interact with him. These expectations are sufficiently structured to warrant the term "sick role." The content of these expectations has been described by Parsons and by others[2] and may be briefly recapitulated.

9

Dimensions of the Sick Role in Chronic Illness

Gene G. Kassebaum
and
Barbara O. Baumann

According to Parsons, sickness produces a temporary disturbance in the individual's capacity to fulfill his usual roles. It is a conditionally legitimate state, which has the effect of insulating the individual from certain types of mutual influence with other persons, and of alienating him from certain norms obtaining in the "well" population; in particular, those which value independent achievement. He is regarded as not responsible for having incurred his condition, which is by definition undesirable, and therefore he is motivated to "get well." Since he is incapable of achieving this end through volition alone, he has an inherent right to receive care, and, indeed, is obligated to seek and accept professional help. For the duration of his illness, "the element of exemption from ordinary role-obligations may be interpreted as permissiveness for temporary relief from the strains of trying hard to achieve. The patient is permitted to indulge his dependency needs under strictly regulated conditions, notably his recognition of the conditional legitimacy of his state, and exposure to the therapeutic task."[3] Thus, the normative expectations do not

[1] See, for example, the Proceedings of the Special Committee on Aging of the U.S. Senate, Government Printing Office, no. 75660.
[2] Parsons, T., *The Social System*, New York: Free Press, 1951, chap. 10; T. Parsons, "Definitions of Health and Illness in the Light of American Values and Social Structure" in E. G. Jaco (ed.), *Patients, Physicians and Illness*, New York: Free Press, 1958 (see chap. 8 herein); D. Mechanic, and E. H. Volkart, "Stress, Illness, and the Sick Role," *Am. Soc. Rev.*, 26: 51–58; D. Schneider, "The Social Dynamics of Physical Disability in Army Basic Training," in Kluckhohn, Murray and Schneider (eds.), *Personality in Nature, Society and Culture*, New York, 1953, pp. 386–397.
[3] Parsons (1958), *op. cit.*, p. 183.

From Journal of Health & Human Behavior, Vol. 6: 16–27, Spring, 1965; by permission of the authors and publisher.

preclude the fact that a patient may enjoy various secondary gains due to illness, but these are purchased at a steep price, and accompanied by the obligation to cooperate actively toward his cure and subsequent resumption of usual role-obligations.

The foregoing observations emphasize general characteristics of the sick role in relation to elements in the value system and social structure of American society for purposes of comparison with possible alternative emphases. Without questioning their applicability, especially for the typical case of acute, temporary illness, one may nevertheless call attention to the way in which this "model" of sick role expectations requires respecification in order to serve as an empirical, as well as a conceptual, tool.

Granted that the set of sick role expectations described is indeed broadly normative in American society, it is a sociological commonplace that normative expectations pertaining to any role vary in divers ways. First, people who occupy different positions in the social structure may hold different norms pertaining to the same role. Second, people differ in the intensity with which different norms are held, and also differ in their evaluations of the norms. Applied to the concept of the sick role, these statements give rise to a number of questions. For example, one may ask to what extent the set of expectations described by Parsons is actually representative of different population groups. This is to ask whether people from different segments of the society view the sick role along the same dimensions, or whether that role may have different dimensions, viewed from different perspectives. Again, one may ask whether certain attributes of the sick role have greater saliency for some people than for others, and if so, what influences determine which dimensions of the sick role will receive more emphasis and which dimensions receive less. Further, one may seek to determine how the same normative expectations are viewed by people who differ in ways likely to affect sick role expectations.

Once an individual is defined as "sick" (leaving aside for the present the basis on which this status may be imputed), it may be assumed that sick role expectations applied to him during his illness will be closely related to the role expectations that operate for him when he is well. These, in turn, are affected by a variety of considerations: his existing social statuses and roles, the cultural traditions which he shares, and idiosyncratic factors having to do with his particular personality and life history. For example, one study has found that patients' judgments regarding their own state of health are related to age, social class, and ethnic group membership.[4] Another study indicates that behavior during illness varies considerably among patients with different cultural traditions.[5] Similarly, the very term "sick" may evoke a variety of associations on the part of different individuals, and, depending on their existing social roles, different individuals may experience quite different effects resulting from the same illness.

However, mere awareness of a patient's social roles and membership in groups prior to his illness is not a sufficient basis for predicting his response to illness, as a host of clinicians can testify. The reason for this is obvious: people do not simply "get sick" —they experience a specific form of illness. Thus, it is a reasonable presumption that attributes of the illness may be as important as attributes of the patient in accounting for sick role expectations.[6] The present study was confined to patients with chronic illness.

[4] Kutner, B., *Five Hundred over Sixty*, New York: Russell Sage Foundation, 1956, esp. pp. 147–152.

[5] Zborowski, M., "Cultural Components in Responses to Pain," *J. of Social Issues*, 8: 16–30, 1952.

[6] The term "role expectations" as used here refers to ". . . patterns of evaluation, . . . Role expectations organize (in accordance with general value-orientations) the reciprocities, expectations, and responses to those expectations in the specific interaction systems of ego and one or more of his alters." T. Parsons, and Shils (eds.), *Toward a General Theory of Action*, Cambridge, Mass.: Harvard Univ. Press, 1951, p. 190.

Viewing chronic illness as a variation or sub-type of the sick role, its distinguishing characteristics depart from the "model" in crucial respects. First, chronic illness by definition is *not* temporary, so that role-expectations predicated on the assumption of the temporary nature of illness (for example, "motivation to get well") are clearly inapplicable without respecification. Also, since many chronic patients are ambulatory, incapacity for the performance of other roles is more often partial than total. Indeed, while the Parsonian view of the sick role implies that it is the patient's dominant role for the duration of his illness, in the case of the ambulatory chronic patient, this assumption is often unwarranted.[7] Hence, the degree to which illness produces alienation or insulation from norms of the "well" population, is itself a problem for investigation. Similarly, norms prescribing permissive treatment and exemption from role obligations in the event of acute illness may require respecification when prolonged adherence to them becomes a threat to the role-performance of the patient's alters.[8]

Finally, chronic illness is not distributed randomly in the population, but rather is associated with advanced age.[9] Because of this, and owing to certain similarities between "typical" attributes of the sick role and attributes of what may be called the "aged" role, normative expectations applied to the older chronic patient are likely to be highly ambiguous. Expectations concerning aging may also involve impairment of capacity for certain types of role-performance, exemption from obligations, and other forms of permissiveness. Like the sick person, the aging individual is not held responsible for incurring his condition, nor can he arrest it by any act of volition. If aging, like illness, may be accompanied by secondary gains, these too are mitigated by the negative regard in which this condition is often held, and by the alienation and dependency which have traditionally been associated with it.[10] Moreover, those usual role-obligations from which exemption is temporarily granted, and to which return is anticipated for the young patient with acute illness are far from clearly defined for the older chronic patient.

Failure to distinguish between illness and old age as bases for role-expectations may have dysfunctional consequences both for the patient's therapy, and for the doctor-patient relationship. From the clinician's point of view, fulfillment of the sick role requires that the patient acknowledge his need for qualified help, and cooperate in his therapy. This implies that he must first define himself as sick. There is evidence, however, that certain older patients with chronic illness tend to tolerate functional impairments unnecessarily (since such impairments could be ameliorated with medical care) because they erroneously associate their symptoms with aging, rather than with illness.[11] Excluding such symptoms from the category of conditions for which medical care is deemed appropriate often results in failure to adhere to the medical regimen. Typically, it is not until their capacity to perform usual roles is severely impaired that

[7] Havighurst distinguished between first, second, and third-order roles in terms of the degree of internalization of their role-expectations; the greater the internalization, the more competently the role is fulfilled. See R. J. Havighurst, "The Social Competence of Middle-aged People," *Genetic Psychol. Monographs*, 56: 297–375.

[8] Schneider, *op. cit.*

[9] According to National Health Survey data, three-fourths of all aged persons not in institutions have one or more chronic conditions. See "Health and Economic Conditions of the American Aged," a chart book prepared for the use of The Special Committee on Aging of the U.S. Senate. U.S. Government Printing Office, no. 70521.

[10] Phillips, B., "A Role-theory Approach to Adjustment in Old Age," *Am. Soc. Rev.*, vol. 22, April, 1957. This article makes the point that the degree to which a role is rewarding to an individual determines his adjustment to that role. See also Mechanic and Volkart, *op. cit.*

[11] Di Cicco, L., and D. Apple, "Health Needs and Opinions of Older Adults" in D. Apple (ed.), *Sociological Studies of Health and Sickness*, New York: McGraw-Hill, 1960, pp. 26–40.

patients of this kind endow previously tolerated symptoms with medical significance. By this time, both the patient's condition and the doctor–patient relationship may have undergone considerable deterioration.

The Sample

The sample in the present study consisted of 201 persons, each with one or more primary diagnoses of chronic illness, who attended the General Medical Out-patient Clinic of an' urban teaching hospital, and who thus may be considered as incumbents of the sick role to that extent. Approximately equal proportions of the sample were drawn from each of the three most prevalent diagnostic categories represented in the clinic: arteriosclerotic heart disease (ASHD), diabetes, and psychoneurosis.[12] The remaining quarter of the sample was comprised of patients with more than one of the three diagnoses, who are hereafter called patients with Multiple Diagnoses. While age and educational attainment ranged widely (from 14 to 91 years, and from no formal schooling to college degrees) the average age was 56, and the average educational level attained was eighth grade. Patients in the ASHD and multiple diagnoses categories were older, on the average, than other patients; 65 and 62 years, respectively. Diabetics and Psychoneurotics both had an average age of 49.

Women in the sample outnumber men by three to one, and only a small proportion (12 per cent) of the patients were non-white. Slightly more than half of the patients (54 per cent) were native-born Americans. Since limited income is one criterion for eligibility

[12] Patients in this category were of a type familiar to clinicians working in similar settings. Rather than fulfilling an academic definition of a single psychoneurosis, they were patients with divers symptoms which their physicians attributed to psychogenic causes but which were not of sufficient severity to warrant treatment in the hospital's specialized psychiatric facilities.

as a clinic patient, all respondents had reported incomes of $5,200 or less.

Although the quota sampling was based on diagnosis, the distribution of age, sex, ethnic origin and education in the sample is roughly representative of the clinic population as a whole.

Method

Respondents were presented with twenty statements having stipulated response-alternatives ranging from "strongly disagree" to "strongly agree" on a seven-point Likert-type scale. The content of the items was in part derived from Parsons (see above) and in part from information gathered in unstructured interviews and pretests designed to elicit the salient concerns within the clinic population. An attempt was made to present the same norm in more than one context, on the premise that different patients might concur in designating an expectation as normative, and yet perceive the norm in different contexts or with different affect. For example, the expectation that illness produces dependence may be associated with the prospect of enjoying certain secondary gains and compensatory behavior from one's alters. A patient who feels this way might agree with item 2 that "people make allowances," etc. However, the expectation of dependence may also be associated with feelings of unworthiness or alienation from one's fellows, in which case a patient might strongly agree with item 9 that "illness makes a person a burden. . . ." Still another patient may not acknowledge any association whatever between illness and dependence, and deny that normative expectations for sick people differ from those for people in general. Such a patient might strongly disagree with the above-mentioned statements, but maintain with item 20 that "a person's health is his own responsibility just like any other part of his life." He may, in short, deny the existence of a sick role. (See below for list of items.)

The method of factor analysis[13] was

[13] See L. L. Thurstone, *Multiple Factor Analysis*, Chicago: Univ. of Chicago Press, 1946, for a detailed exposition of the methodology

selected for its advantage in permitting the cognitive "grouping" of items made by respondents themselves to appear, independently of any *a priori* grouping by the investigators. In the event that the respondents' grouping should diverge from that which the investigators might have anticipated, this finding itself may provide valuable information in the interpretation of a factor. Thus, for example, should an item designed to measure "exemptions" have a high loading on a factor containing no other "exemptions" items, inspection of the other highly loaded items on the factor would supply the context in which the item had actually been perceived.

A scale was constructed for each factor, using the factor's most highly loaded items.[14] Each respondent was given a sum score on each factor's scale. The distribution of scores for each factor scale was trichotomized into "high," "medium" and "low" categories. The scores in each category were then cross-tabulated against the demographic and medical attributes of the respondents which are discussed below.

Findings: Dimensions of the Sick Role

The factor analysis yielded four factors. While no two factors have their highest loadings supplied by the same items, nearly all items have some loading on each factor. Despite this "overlap," which is itself of some interest, inspection of the highly loaded items on each factor indicates that among this sample of respondents, four distinct dimensions underlying sick role expectations could be observed [see p. 146].

---

employed. The factor analysis used here followed Thurstone's complete centroid technique. Rotation of the centroids was done "blind" in terms of numerical criteria alone, without reference to item content, using the Quartimax Analytical Solution to Orthogonal Simple Structure. While overlap among loadings might have been reduced by using item content as a criterion for rotating the centroids, thus imposing a preconceived grouping on the items, this would have sacrificed the information provided by the patients' spontaneous associations.

[14] For technique of scale construction see G. Thomson, *The Factorial Analysis of Human Ability*, Boston: Houghton Mifflin, 1948.

The common element in the items on Factor I is the negative affect associated with sickness, and particularly with the dependence produced by sickness. No highly loaded items refer either to performance of other role-obligations, or to reciprocal expectations involving exemptions or other forms of permissiveness. Item 16 contributes an element of guilt, implying a repudiation of the norm that a sick person is not held responsible for having incurred his condition. This factor has been labeled *Dependence*.

Factor II is characterized by congruence between role-expectations of the patient and those of his alters. These mutual expectations involve exemption from role-obligations, and generally permissive behavior. Here, however, incapacity for role-performance is not itself the primary concern, and illness evokes no associations with guilt or with feelings of alienation. This factor is therefore labeled *Reciprocity*.

Factor III also contains items referring to the effect of illness on role-performance, and here the principal concern is precisely with inability to meet the demands of the environment. There is no corresponding concern with reciprocity in interpersonal relations, as was the case for Factor II. This factor has been called *Role-Performance*.

The interpretation of Factor IV is complicated by the high loading of item 13. Apart from this item, all highly loaded items on this factor are characterized by their lack of affect or sentiment, a strong emphasis on autonomy, individual responsibility for one's physical condition, and a repudiation of special concessions for sick people. Item 14 suggests that the legitimacy of sickness may itself be open to question. Together, the impression conveyed by these items is that of *Denial* of the sick role. The high loading of item 13, given this context, gives rise to the speculation that this dimension of the sick role may function as a defense mechanism, where adopting the role may for some reason be threatening.

The grouping of items on the various factors is neither the only one, nor even the

Item	Loading	
9	.557	Illness makes a person a burden on other folks around him.
10	.494	The trouble with being ill is that you have to depend on other people.
16	.445	There is some truth to the saying that illness is a punishment for sins.
6	.419	The most important thing for a sick person to understand is that he needs outside help because he cannot help himself.
12	.358	Sick people deserve more consideration than they usually get.
11	.340	Most sick people are difficult to get along with.

Factor II—Reciprocity

Item	Loading	
19	.529	People in general realize it is not the patient's fault that he is ill.
2	.484	In general, people make allowances for the fact that a sick person isn't able to carry out his normal social responsibilities.
1	.440	While a woman is sick, people don't blame her for not managing the home the way she normally does.
15	.425	People in general are usually very kind and considerate to a person who is ill.
17	.423	Most people do not blame a person for being sick.

Factor III—Role-performance
(This factor has been reverse-scored.)

Item	Loading	
7	.601	People who are sick have a right to expect that others will help them.
5	.588	In general, people demand too much from a person who is ill.
3	.363	Often the only rest a busy person gets is when he is sick.
4	.355	When a person is sick, he usually isn't expected to hold a job.

Factor IV—Denial

Item	Loading	
14	.524	Many people act sicker than they are just in order to get sympathy.
18	.440	Most sickness is due to careless and wrong living habits.
8	.397	How fast a sick person gets well is due more to his own efforts than to any particular medicine he is taking.
20	.373	A person's health is his own responsibility just like any other part of his life.
13	.369	Most people do not understand the problems a sick person has in his life.

most obvious one that might have occurred. A certain amount of "overlap" in terms of numerical loadings has been noted, and a similar overlap may be observed in the verbal content of the items. While use of another rotation technique might have reduced this overlap statistically, it is possible that the greater "purity" so obtained would have been at the price of obscuring a finding which itself warrants attention; namely, that respondents tend to associate items on the basis of *both* similarity in verbal content and similarity in context.

Dimensions of the Sick Role in Relation to Differences in Respondents' Attributes

Since all respondents received a score on each factor scale, it must be emphasized that the following tables do not indicate that respondents hold *either* one conception of the sick role *or* another, but rather, that respondents who vary according to a given attribute exhibit differential tendencies to emphasize each dimension of the sick role.

Many of the attributes dealt with below are associated in this clinic population (which is somewhat typical of similar settings). Because the limited sample size precluded controlling for such associations, it is not possible to compare the influence of each attribute independently on sick role conceptions. While this imposes obvious disadvantages, the effect to some extent is to make a virtue of necessity. For example, when respondents are compared by age groups, each group possesses a certain degree of internal homogeneity with regard to a cluster of related attributes such as education and ethnic origin. To illustrate:

the proportion of foreign-born patients over age 60 (60 per cent) is nearly double that of younger patients (33 per cent). Also, only 32 per cent of the patients over age 60 had completed more than eight grades of schooling, while among younger patients, 66 per cent had gone beyond eighth grade.

In Table 9–1 it may be seen that the difference between the proportions of male and female high scorers is greatest for Factor I. *Dependence* appears to be of greater

findings of other investigators.[15] (See Di Cicco and Apple, *op. cit.*) There is also some tendency for older patients to have proportionately more high scores on Factor IV, *Denial.* This may indicate either that these patients do not feel impaired in their capacities to perform usual roles, or, their

Table 9–1—Scores on sick role dimensions for each sex

Dimension	Sex	HIGH SCORERS No.	%	Base
Dependence				
	Male	24	46	52
	Female	51	34	149
Reciprocity				
	Male	16	31	52
	Female	45	38	149
Role-Performance				
	Male	18	35	52
	Female	45	30	149
Denial				
	Male	20	38	52
	Female	44	30	149

Table 9–2—Scores on sick role dimensions in different age groups

Dimension	Age Group	HIGH SCORERS No.	%	Base
Dependence				
	Under 60 yrs.	34	34	102
	60 and over	41	41	99
Reciprocity				
	Under 60 yrs.	39	38	102
	60 and over	34	34	99
Role-Performance				
	Under 60 yrs.	18	17	102
	60 and over	45	45	99
Denial				
	Under 60 yrs.	27	26	102
	60 and over	37	38	99

concern to men than to women. This is also true, although to a lesser degree, for Factors III and IV, *Role-Performance* and *Denial.* Conversely, women appear more concerned than men with the *Reciprocity* dimension.

In Table 9–2 it can be seen that age difference are more discriminating among high scorers on Factors III and IV than on Factors I or II. High scorers on the *Role-Performance* dimension occur in greater proportion among older patients than among younger ones. Concern with role-performance in this age group is consistent with the

rejection of the sick role may be defensive. In any case, the combination of chronic illness and advanced age *per se* does not appear to produce a uniform tendency to emphasize any single dimension of the sick role. Sizable proportions of older patients have high scores on both Factor I and Factor IV, whose contexts are in marked contrast to one another. While the data do not indicate whether or not the same individuals are represented in both cases, it is reasonable to infer that they are not. Findings by other

[15] Di Cicco and Apple, *op. cit.*

Table 9–3—Scores on sick role dimensions of patients born in the United States and of foreign-born patients

Dimension	Country of Birth	HIGH SCORERS No.	%	Base
Dependence				
	U.S.A.	35	32	108
	Other	40	43	93
Reciprocity				
	U.S.A.	42	39	108
	Other	31	33	93
Role-Performance				
	U.S.A.	30	28	108
	Other	33	35	93
Denial				
	U.S.A.	30	28	108
	Other	34	37	93

Table 9–4—Scores on sick role dimensions in different educational groups

Dimension	Education Level	HIGH SCORERS No.	%	Base
Dependence				
	8th grade or lower	50	47	107
	Above 8th grade	25	27	92
Reciprocity *				
	8th grade or lower	41	38	107
	Above 8th grade	30	33	92
Role-Performance				
	8th grade or lower	40	37	107
	Above 8th grade	23	25	92
Denial				
	8th grade or lower	42	39	107
	Above 8th grade	22	24	92

* Two respondents gave no answer on education, and have not been included in the tabulations. Neither had high scores on any Factor except Factor II, and this accounts for the difference between the total number of high scorers on that factor in this table and the total in other tables.

Table 9–5—Scores on sick role dimensions in different occupational groups

Dimension	Occupational Group	HIGH SCORERS No.	%	Base
Dependence				
	White collar	16	24	67
	Blue collar	47	47	101
	None	12	36	33
Reciprocity				
	White collar	21	31	67
	Blue collar	37	37	101
	None	15	45	33
Role-Performance				
	White collar	15	22	67
	Blue collar	35	35	101
	None	13	39	33
Denial				
	White collar	17	25	67
	Blue collar	32	32	101
	None	15	45	33

investigators indicate that the extent to which attitudes toward illness converge with attitudes toward dependency is related to a number of considerations; among them, socio–economic status and anomie.[16] It is not unlikely, therefore, that the older patients in the present sample who emphasize the *Dependence* dimension of the sick role would be found to differ in these attributes from those who emphasize the *Denial* dimension. The high proportion of foreign-born patients in the older age category permits the speculation that some of the high scores on Factor I may be contributed by patients who experience cultural alienation as their circle of contemporaries of their own ethnic group diminishes. Differences between the age groups on Factor II, *Reciprocity*, are small, but their direction is consistent with the inference that young persons are more likely to be involved in emotionally supportive role-relationships than are older persons.

Inspection of Table 9–3 indicates that differences between U.S.-born and foreign-born patients do indeed occur in the same directions as those observed between younger and older patients in Table 9–2. Foreign-born patients tend more than others to emphasize the *Dependence* dimension of the sick role, and also tend to have a slightly higher proportion of high scores on *Role-Performance* and on *Denial*. Patients who were born in the United States, however, tend to show greater concern with *Reciprocity*.

Because of the inverse relationship between age and education in the sample, it is not surprising that low education appears to influence sick role expectations in the same manner as old age. Differences between education categories are most pronounced on *Dependence*; patients with low education tend to have high scores on this dimension, while more education appears to counteract this tendency, as shown in Table 9–4. Since more education is usually accompanied by the acquisition of generalizable skills, these

presumably provide increased alternatives with which to adapt to the physical limitations imposed by illness. Like older patients, those with less education tend to score high also on *Role-Performance* and *Denial*, but do not differ greatly from more-educated patients on *Reciprocity*. (See Table 9–4.)

Although a certain degree of economic homogeneity may be said to characterize the sample as a whole, owing to limited income, there are nevertheless socio–economic differences among respondents.[17] If different positions in the social structure are associated with different sick role expectations, this should be ascertainable by a comparison of patients in different occupational categories. Assuming an association between occupation and education, one might anticipate that education differences will also be reflected in Table 9–5, where patients are categorized according to the occupation of the family's principal breadwinner.[18]

16 See M. Davis, "Aging, Illness and Dependency; A Study in the Convergence of Attitudes," unpublished M.A. thesis, Purdue University, 1961. This thesis contains preliminary findings of the Adult Life Study, going on at Purdue University.

17 An income limitation is one of the criteria of eligibility for treatment in this clinic. However, Clinic Payment Rate, which is based on reported income, number of dependents, employment status, etc., was not a discriminator of sick role expectations. Because of the variety of circumstances determining payment rate (full, partial, or none) this is not a useful indicator of socio–economic status. Since only 20 patients reported professional or managerial occupations, either for themselves or family heads, and a similarly low number were engaged in skilled labor, the categories "white-collar" and "blue-collar" were used to facilitate comparisons. The majority of the former category represent clerical work, and the majority of the latter, unskilled labor and domestic service.

18 In this sample, family breadwinner's occupation is a more valid indicator of socio–economic status than the patient's own occupation. This is attributable to the preponderance of women in the sample, of whom approximately half reported their occupation as housewife. Tabulations to determine whether housewives differed in their sick role expectations from women reporting an outside occupation showed no appreciable differences between the two groups. Further tabulations within each group yielded the following findings: among women with outside occupations, differences in sick role expectations between occupational categories, consistent with those reported in Table 9–5 occurred under

Given the traditional importance of the family head's occupation in determining the socio–economic status of the family as a whole, it is interesting to observe that sick role expectations appear consistent with this tradition.

The difference between occupational categories is greatest on Factor I. Patients in the blue-collar category have nearly double the proportion of the white-collar group with high scores on *Dependence*. Blue-collar patients also tend to be more concerned with *Role Performance*. Scores on *Reciprocity* and on *Denial*, however, do not show sizable differences based on occupation. The distribution of scores for patients reporting no occupation (either own or of principal breadwinner) is somewhat puzzling. Lack of this important status does not appear to produce any considerable tendency to score high on *Dependence*, as might have been anticipated; blue-collar patients have more high scores than no-occupation patients on this dimension. However, it is probable that the combining of patients in a single category who have different reasons for reporting no occupation has obscured the influence of lack of occupation on sick role expectations. Further investigation is warranted concerning the influence of the lack of one role on expectations pertaining to other roles.

---

two conditions. One case was where the woman herself was the family breadwinner, and the other where she was not, but had an occupation equivalent in status to that of the principal breadwinner. In cases where there was inconsistency between the patient's and the breadwinner's occupational status, the latter was the better predictor of sick role expectations. Unfortunately, the number of such cases was too small to warrant any but the most tentative inferences. Among the housewives, sick role expectations are consistent with the occupational categories of family breadwinner also. These findings illustrate the complexity of the relationship between occupation, socio–economic status, and sick role expectations. It would appear that where the individual's occupation is not a reliable indicator of socio–economic status, or where it is not the principal source of income, occupation *per se* is not the most important determinant of sick role expectations. It is hoped that this line of inquiry will be the object of further research.

The emphasis placed by blue-collar patients on *Dependence* and *Role-Performance* presumably reflects their greater vulnerability to economic repercussions of restrictions on physical activity. Clearly, the effect of any given restriction may differ considerably depending on whether an individual's occupation is primarily sedentary or primarily dependent on strenuous physical effort. The blue-collar patient, especially if he lacks generalizable skills, is likely to experience dependence both at an earlier stage of his illness and to a greater degree than that which his physical capacities alone would warrant, by being obliged to relinquish his occupational role without having an acceptable substitute. Persons engaged in domestic service are especially vulnerable in this respect, since they typically lack economic "cushions" available to workers with union membership or other resources to help provide for the costs of illness. Because of the different consequences that restriction of activity may have for different types of role-performance, and for incurring dependency, no discussion of sick role expectations which fails to take such differences into account can be complete.

Considered in terms of sex, age, ethnic origin, education and occupation, even within this highly selective sample of respondents, persons with different attributes tend to emphasize different dimensions of the sick role. Indeed, such a finding might even have been anticipated among a sample of non-patients. However, a major premise of the present investigation was that attributes of the illness as well as attributes of the patient influence sick role expectations, attention is now directed to the influence of different diagnoses on sick role expectations.

It has already been observed that the incidence of chronic illness in the population is highly concentrated in the upper age levels. Within the present sample, a still more specific relationship exists between diagnosis and age, which must be borne in mind in interpreting the data in Table 9–6. In two of the diagnostic categories, ASHD and Multiple Diagnoses, the average age of patients is above 60 years; more than ten years higher than that of Diabetics and of Psychoneurotics, who average 49 years of age. It is therefore of interest to observe, by comparing Table 9–6 with Table 9–2, the instances where the two influences, diagnosis and age, appear to operate in the same direction (in which case no inferences regarding independence can be drawn) and those where they appear to diverge. In the latter case, there is strong ground for presuming that diagnosis has an influence on sick role expectations independent of that of age.

There are marked differences among the diagnostic groups in their tendencies to score high on the *Dependence* dimension. Patients in the two categories where average

played attitudes unwarranted by either their physical condition or their age. More interesting, perhaps, is that ASHD patients and those with Multiple Diagnoses, despite greater age and, in the latter case, more numerous impairments, do not show a greater tendency to emphasize this dimension. Patients with ASHD are distinguished from others by their greater proportion of high scores on Factor II, *Reciprocity*. The particular significance of the heart in com-

Table 9–6—Scores on sick role dimensions in different diagnostic groups

Dimension	Diagnostic Group	HIGH SCORERS No.	%	Base
Dependence				
	ASHD	21	37	57
	Diabetes	11	24	46
	Psychoneurosis	25	53	47
	Multiple Dx	18	35	51
Reciprocity				
	ASHD	25	44	57
	Diabetes	16	35	46
	Psychoneurosis	16	34	47
	Multiple Dx	16	32	51
Role-Performance				
	ASHD	21	37	57
	Diabetes	11	24	46
	Psychoneurosis	12	25	47
	Multiple Dx	19	37	51
Denial				
	ASHD	19	33	57
	Diabetes	7	15	46
	Psychoneurosis	17	36	47
	Multiple Dx	21	41	51

is highest, ASHD and Multiple Diagnoses, have roughly the same proportions of high scores on Factor I. This proportion, however, is greater than that of one of the "younger" diagnostic groups, but smaller than that of the psychoneurotics, indicating that diagnosis alone does indeed influence sick role expectations, apart from the influence of age. Since excessive feelings of dependence and alienation are themselves frequently symptoms of psychoneurosis, it is scarcely surprising that psychoneurotics tend to score high on Factor I. Indeed, it is possible that some of these patients received this diagnosis partially because they dis-

parison with other portions of the anatomy, according to cultural traditions, may account for an especially high degree of supportive interpersonal relations among these patients and their alters. However, many of the patients with Multiple Diagnoses include ASHD among their illnesses, yet they tend to have fewer high scores on this factor. Possibly, ASHD is not the most salient feature of their condition, and thus they are not defined as "heart patients" by themselves or others. One may also speculate that the norm of permissiveness for the sick has a threshold, beyond which the strain on interaction produced by illness outweighs the norm. Put differently, a patient's alters may not find it difficult to be supportive where a single illness is involved, but their tolerance may be overstrained by a variety of symptoms and diffuse illness.

On the *Role-Performance* dimension differences between diagnostic categories resemble those between age levels. Both "older" categories, ASHD and Multiple Diagnoses, score high on this dimension more often than the two younger ones. Here again, it would be desirable to have further data in order to determine the relative influence of age and diagnosis in accounting for this orientation.

On Factor IV, *Denial*, diabetics are distinguished by their low proportion of high scores. Since their medical regimen actually permits them considerable autonomy in the management of their disease, as well as in their activities of daily living, their apparently low degree of concern with this dimension is of interest. Unlike the other patients in the sample, diabetics have visible quantitative indicators with which to maintain surveillance over their own conditions, and exercise considerable discretionary power over their own medication, etc. Presumably, then, neither the legitimacy of the illness nor the patient's capacity for autonomy is called into question sufficiently to require a defensive reaffirmation. For diabetics, the sick role appears to be less threatening than for other patients, perhaps because it interferes less with performance of other roles than does ASHD or psychoneurosis, and is less likely to dominate the individual's role-set. Their denial of the sick role may thus be taken at face value.

Summary and Interpretation

The responses of 201 chronically ill patients to twenty items pertaining to sick role expectations were factor-analyzed. Four factors were isolated, which are interpreted as representing four dimensions of the sick role. These have been called: (1) *Dependence*, (2) *Reciprocity*, (3) *Role-Performance* and

(4) *Denial*. Inspection of the highly loaded items defining each factor indicated that association of items was based on common contextual properties as well as on similarity of verbal content. Scores on scales measuring each factor were computed for each respondent and cross-tabulated with other attributes. Findings indicated that the tendency to score high on different dimensions of the sick role varies with age, sex, ethnic origin, education, occupational category and diagnosis.

The tendency to score high on *Dependence* was most characteristic of older respondents, of men, of foreign-born patients, of those with low educational attainment, of those in blue-collar occupations, and of patients with psychoneurosis. Female patients, those who were under 60, the U.S.-born, those who had completed more than 8 grades of school, those with white-collar occupations, and those with diabetes tended to have fewer high scores on this factor.

The tendency to score high on *Reciprocity* was not more characteristic of any one particular age, education, or occupational category than another. There was, however, some tendency for women to have more high scores on this dimension than men, and for patients reporting no occupation to emphasize this dimension more than other patients. Among the diagnostic categories, ASHD patients are more likely than others to have high scores on this factor.

The *Role-Performance* dimension appeared to be of greater concern for older patients, for foreign-born patients, for less-educated patients, and for those who reported either no occupation, or one in the blue-collar category. Patients with ASHD and those with Multiple Diagnoses were more concerned with *Role-Performance* than were Diabetics or Psychoneurotics.

Denial was more often emphasized by men than by women, by older and by less-educated patients than by younger or by better-educated ones, and by foreign-born patients. Patients who reported no occupation were more concerned in this area than others, while patients with white-collar occupations showed fewest high scores. Diabetics were distinguished from other patients by their low proportion of high scores on this factor, while patients with Multiple Diagnoses had somewhat more high scores than ASHD or Psychoneurotic patients.

As stated earlier, the study proceeded on the premise that the sick role, as described by Parsons, although a useful conceptual model for organizing normative expectations, may vary among different types of *patients*, that is, among persons occupying different positions in the social structure. Second, sick role expectations may vary among patients with different types of illnesses. Chronic illness, then, may be regarded as one sub-type of sick role, having special characteristics. Because of these characteristics, patients with chronic illness are likely to perceive the structure of the sick role along dimensions which differ from those perceived by patients with acute, temporary illness.

The dimensions of the sick role perceived in this sample clearly reflect various conditions especially characteristic of chronic illness: the impossibility of resuming full role-participation at pre-illness capacity, the necessity for adjusting to a permanent condition rather than overcoming a temporary one, and the emphasis on retaining, rather than regaining an optimal level of role-performance and autonomy. Possibly, too, the dimensions identified here also reflect the relatively low socio-economic status of the sample as a whole, in the emphasis on maintaining autonomy and denying illness, and in the view of dependency as a real threat rather than as an opportunity for enjoying secondary gains. From a more favored socio-economic perspective, it is possible that the view of the sick role has different dimensions. Nevertheless, the findings indicate that within this limited sample, given the four dimensions identified, different types of patients, viewed in terms of their demographic or socio-economic attributes, emphasize different dimensions of the sick role.

However, demographic and socio-economic differences by themselves are insufficient to account for differences in sick role expectations, as any clinician can testify from experience. The reason for this should be obvious; sick role expectations are

influenced not only by the patients' accustomed roles, but by *the effects of his particular diagnosis on his capacity for performing them.*

Thus, if most people with chronic illness tend to see the sick role in terms of certain dimensions, they may nevertheless not attribute equal importance to each dimension. Clearly, within the broad classification of chronic illness, different diagnoses have different consequences for different kinds of people. The different effects of restriction on strenuous activity for people with different occupations has already been cited as an illustration. Similarly, exemption from reporting to work is of a different order from that of fulfilling a social obligation. While the maximum degree of exemption a patient receives may be determined by the norms of his social groups, the minimum requisite degree of exemption is often determined by the attributes of his illness. For this reason, any attempt to describe sick role expectations in terms of behavior alone, without specifying a context, is necessarily inadequate. Again, while the structure of the sick role may be seen in terms of a set of dimensions by a broad category of patients, the emphasis placed on each dimension will probably be determined by the way in which the specific diagnosis affects the specific roles of the individuals involved.

Implications for Future Research

Further research is required to specify what dimensions of the sick role are perceived in different social settings. This involves investigation of the distribution of normative expectations pertaining to illness in different segments of the population, and ascertaining the conditions under which different dimensions of the sick role are given different hierarchical order. A correlative task is the identification of sick role expectations pertaining to different diagnoses, and to different types and degrees of impairment. This involves such problems as: what specific exemptions, and to what degree, are associated with different types of illness? For which illnesses, and to what degree, are people likely to consider themselves responsible? Which reference groups have the greatest influence on sick role expectations? Do different illnesses evoke different styles of interpersonal behavior? Do different illnesses have differential probabilities for eliciting acceptance or rejection of the sick role? Finally, a systematic investigation of the relationship between sick role expectations and response to different types of therapeutic programs would be of considerable utility to persons engaged in providing medical care for special population groups, of which the chronically ill are only one example.

THE CONCEPT OF "illness behavior" has been proposed by Mechanic and Volkart to refer to "the way in which symptoms are perceived, evaluated, and acted upon by a person who recognizes some pain, discomfort, or other signs of organic malfunction."[1] The present study attempts to analyze this behavior in terms of social patterns accompanying the seeking, finding and carrying out of medical care. We distinguish four principal elements in these patterns: (a) the content, (b) the sequence, (c) the spacing, and (d) the variability of behavior during different phases of medical care. Combinations of type of content and arrangement of content furnish us with such useful concepts as "shopping" (trying multiple sources of medical care); "fragmentation of care" (treated by a variety of medical practitioners at a single source of medical care); "procrastination" (delay in seeking care following recognition of symptoms); "self-medication" (repeated attempts at self-treatment and home remedies); "discontinuity" (lapses in treatment or interruption of care); and others.

To study these patterns, we have divided the sequence of medical events into five stages representing major transition points involving new decisions about the future course of medical care. These stages are:[2]

1. The Symptom Experience Stage
2. The Assumption of the Sick Role Stage
3. The Medical Care Contact Stage
4. The Dependent-Patient Role Stage
5. The Recovery or Rehabilitation Stage

[1] Mechanic, D., and E. H. Volkart, "Stress, Illness Behavior, and the Sick Role," *Amer. Sociological Rev.*, 25:62, February, 1961; "Illness Behavior and Medical Diagnoses," *J. Health and Human Behavior*, 1:86–91, Summer, 1960.

[2] All these stages do not have to be present in every case of illness, but they will usually be

10

Stages of Illness and Medical Care

Edward A. Suchman

We will briefly describe each of the stages in turn indicating the general focus of our research interests as well as specific hypotheses relating to medical care.

1. *The Symptom Experience Stage*—(The decision that something is wrong). There are three analytically distinguishable aspects of the symptom experience: (a) the physical experience, by which we mean the pain,

found, even if in a condensed form. Kadushin found the following five stages to be present in a depth decision to undertake psychotherapy: (1) recognition of an emotional problem, (2) exposure to the existence of a problem within the circle of friends and relatives, (3) decision to seek professional help, (4) selection of a professional area of help, and (5) selection of a specific practitioner. These correspond roughly to the first three stages in our formulation of the process. C. Kadushin, "Individual Decisions to Undertake Psychotherapy," *Admin. Science Quart.*, 3:379–411, December, 1958. Goldstein and Dommermuth propose a sick role "cycle" from health–illness–health as a framework for medical sociology. Goldstein, B. and P. Dommermuth, "The Sick Role Cycle: An Approach to Medical Sociology," *Sociology and Social Res.*, 46:36–47, October, 1961.

From Journal of Health & Human Behavior, *Vol. 6: 114–128, Fall, 1965; by permission of the author and publisher.*

This investigation was supported in part by Public Health Service Grant CH 00010–05 from the Division of Community Health Services, Dr. George James, principal investigator. Respondents for this study were selected from the Washington Heights Master Sample Survey, supported by the Health Research Council of the City of New York, Contract No. U-1053 to Columbia University, School of Public Health and Administrative Medicine, Dr. Jack Elinson, principal investigator. Dr. Sylvia Gilliam (deceased) and Margaret C. Klem were in charge of the study. John Marx and Ido de Groot aided in the initial project formulation, while Marvin Belkin, Raymond Maurice and Daniel Rosenblatt assisted in the analysis. Field work was directed by Dr. John Colombotos and Annette Perrin O'Hare with Regina Loewenstein in charge of sampling and data-processing.

discomfort, change of appearance, or debility actually felt, (b) the cognitive aspect, by which we refer to the interpretation and derived meaning for the individual experiencing the symptoms, and (c) the emotional response of fear or anxiety that accompanies both the physical experience and the cognitive interpretation. Basic to the initiation of the medical care process is the perception and interpretation of symptoms of discomfort, pain, or abnormality—the "meaning of symptoms" for the individual.[3] These symptoms, for the most part, will be recognized and defined not in medically diagnostic categories, but in terms of their interference with normal social functioning. Two aspects of the illness decision-making process during this stage with particular relevance for medical care are the denial of illness or "flight to health" and delay in seeking and securing treatment.[4] Also of interest for the parsimonious use of medical care is the other extreme related to hypochondriasis or the recourse to symptoms of illness for social or psychological reasons. In some cases a real dilemma is created for the individual who may wish to avoid "bothering" his family, friends, and doctor too early in the symptom experience stage but who fears the harmful consequences of waiting too long.

2. *Assumption of the Sick Role Stage—*(The decision that one is sick and needs professional care). During this stage, the potential patient begins to seek symptom alleviation, information and advice, and temporary acceptance of his condition by his family and friends. The lay referral structure of the individual assumes greatest importance at this time. How the individual's lay con-

[3] A great deal of anthropological and social research has been devoted to the varying meanings of symptoms and illness for different cultural groups. See, for example, W. Caudill, *Effects of Social and Cultural Systems in Reactions to Stress*, Social Science Research Council, Pamphlet 14, 1958; S. H. King, *Perceptions of Illness and Medical Practice*, New York: Russell Sage, 1962, pp. 120–130.

[4] Kutner, B., and G. Gordon, "Seeking Care for Cancer," *J. Health and Human Behavior*, II:171–178, Fall, 1961.

sultants react to his symptoms and their acceptance of any interference with his social functioning will do much to determine the individual's ability to enter the sick role. The ill person will seek confirmation, advice, reassurance, and, finally, a form of "provisional validation" which temporarily excuses him from his normal obligations and activities.

We hypothesize that for most people there will be some kind of discussion with significant others. These discussions will not be merely for the sake of seeking information and advice, but also, and perhaps more importantly, for seeking consent and confirmation to suspend normal obligations and activities. The giving up of duties and responsibilities and the violations of expected behavior, together with the demand for care and assistance from others, must be done in ways prescribed by the group as appropriate and acceptable.

3. *The Medical Care Contact Stage—*(The decision to seek professional medical care). At this stage of illness, the sick individual seeks a medical diagnosis and a prescribed course of treatment from a "scientific" rather than "lay" source. In consulting a physician, he seeks authoritative sanctioning to become "legitimately" ill or to return to his normal activities should such sanction be denied. In some cases, this stage may be prolonged if the sick individual refuses to accept the initial diagnosis or course of treatment and begins a "lay search" for another source of medical care more in keeping with his needs and preconceptions.

This stage is of fundamental importance to an understanding of the utilization of medical care facilities and services. We hypothesize that the selection of the source of care will reflect the knowledge, availability, and convenience of such services and social group influences upon the individual. We further hypothesize that the initial medical diagnosis and treatment will set the stage for subsequent medical care and play a crucial role in the sick individual's future medical behavior and progress towards health.

4. *The Dependent-Patient Role Stage—*

(The decision to transfer control to the physician and to accept and follow prescribed treatment). Not until this stage is reached does the sick individual become a "patient." However, contacting a physician does not necessarily mean that a person is willing to accept the recommendations of the doctor and to surrender certain of his decision-making prerogatives, that is, to assume a dependency upon medical care. The potential patient usually looks on the dependent-patient role with ambivalence. While he may wish to avoid it, he is also likely to see it eventually as the only possible way of achieving reentry into his normal roles and a return to health.

The significant factors during this phase are those which affect the individual's adjustment to being a patient—the physical, administrative, social, or psychological barriers that interfere with the course of treatment. Particularly important is the patient–physician relationship as it affects communication and interaction. We hypothesize that, in many cases, differing points of view regarding the meaning of illness and differing conceptions concerning medical care will produce conflicts between physician and patient which will interfere with the treatment process.[5]

5. *The Recovery or Rehabilitation Stage—* (The decision to relinquish the patient role). The course of medical treatment comes to a close when the patient is dismissed or withdraws from active medical care and is expected either to resume his old role of a healthy individual again, or to adopt a new role of chronic invalid or long term rehabilitee. During the stage of convalescence or rehabilitation, the ex-patient must learn to live once more in the world of the well. In the case of an acute illness the return may present no particular difficulties, but, for many chronic illnesses and physical impairments, this process is a slow and demanding one and may involve recurring episodes of illness. The returning patient may be given a period of grace during which inadequate

social functioning is acceptable, somewhat as in adolescence.[6] In the case of rehabilitation, a process of resocialization may be necessary through which the incapacitated individual must learn to establish new relationships with those around him.[7]

This stage contains some highly significant problems for medical care, especially in view of the increasing ascendance of the chronic diseases with little hope of definitive cures. The provision of home care for the aged, of rehabilitation for the handicapped, of long term care for the chronically ill are paramount concerns of public health and medicine today.[8]

These five stages, then, represent the content and sequence of illness behavior which constitute our major focus of interest. We will attempt to analyze this behavior within a framework of individual decision-making in relation to the seeking, finding, and carrying out of medical care.[9] Understanding which decisions have to be made, by whom, and when should prove helpful to the development of a more effective medical care system.[10]

[5] Wilson, R. N., "Patient–Practitioner Relationships," in H. E. Freeman, *et al.* (eds.), *Handbook of Medical Sociology*, Englewood Cliffs, N.J., Prentice-Hall, 1963, pp. 273–295.

[6] King, S. H., "Social Psychological Factors in Illness," in H. E. Freeman, *et al.* (eds.), *Handbook of Medical Sociology, op. cit.*, pp. 116–117.

[7] Landy, D., "Rehabilitation as a Sociocultural Process", *J. Social Issues*, 16:3–7, 1960.

[8] Davis, M. M., *Medical Care for Tomorrow*, New York: Harper and Bros., 1955.

[9] A similar approach which relates the decision to undertake psychotherapy to the general analysis of decisional acts, such as voting and buying, is developed by Kadushin. He draws a distinction between casual and depth decisions —illness usually requiring a depth decision. Kadushin, *op. cit.* A general review of the literature dealing with the seeking of medical care will be found in J. D. Stoeckle, I. K. Zola, G. E. Davidson, "On Going to See the Doctor, the Contributions of the Patient to the Decision to Seek Medical Aid," *J. Chronic Dis.*, 16:975–989, September, 1963.

[10] The decision-making process in the present instance must take into consideration a factor of great importance that is often omitted in the construction of theories of decision-making; the individual in our case cannot leave the decision field. As long as the symptoms last, he must consider them. He may decide to take no action but he cannot simply withdraw from the situa-

Method of Procedure

This analysis is based upon data obtained from a large scale community survey of health status and medical care. The major emphasis of this study was upon determining broad patterns of response to illness in general.[11] For this purpose, an area probability sample of 5,340 persons comprising 2,215 families residing in the Washington Heights community of New York City was selected for personal household interviews conducted from November, 1960, through April, 1961.[12]

While the above sampling procedure was satisfactory for relating broad social factors to general responses to illness, it did not provide detailed information concerning an individual's behavior during a single specific case of illness. This type of "natural history" of a specific illness episode, it was felt would be helpful in describing the decision-making process during the various stages of an illness. Consequently, the cross-section sample of household interviews was utilized as a preliminary screening procedure for the selection of a sub-sample of individuals

currently experiencing a relatively serious illness. All adults 21 years of age or older who satisfied the following criteria were selected for a detailed, follow-up interview on the specific illness episode: an illness occurring during the past two months which either (1) required three or more physician visits and incapacitated the individual for five or more consecutive days, or (2) required hospitalization for one or more days.

Using the above criteria, a sample of 137 cases was obtained. These cases constitute a 100 per cent sample of all individuals in the population survey satisfying these criteria and they may be viewed as representative of all such illness cases within the community.[13] For the purposes of this exploratory study, it was deemed advisable to eliminate minor ailments requiring little or no medical care. We might predict that many of the differences observed for the major illnesses would be even more pronounced for minor ailments where the response to the illness would be even more likely to be governed by social rather than medical considerations.[14]

These illness cases tended to be somewhat older and of lower socio–economic status than the cross-section but of the same sex composition. The comparisons are as follows:

	Illness Cases	Cross-section
Per cent Male	40%	43%
Per cent Over 44 Years	66%	54%
Per cent Low SES	66%	50%

tion, as he may in the case of voting or buying. Furthermore, the sick person and his lay referral group rarely surrender all their power to make decisions. Perhaps the decision most difficult for the lay referral group to surrender is an evaluative one: is the patient showing sufficient improvement, rapidly enough? The degree to which this decision (or others) is retained by the individual or his group will do much to determine the degree of conflict between the patient and his physician.

[11] A more complete description of this broader study is given in E. A. Suchman, "Social Patterns of Illness and Medical Care," *J. Health and Human Behavior*, 6:2–15, Spring, 1965 (see chap. 19 herein).

[12] For a detailed description of sampling procedures, completion rate and a comparison with Census data, see J. Elinson and R. Loewenstein, *Community Fact Book for Washington Heights*, New York: Columbia Univ. School of Public Health and Administrative Medicine, 1963.

[13] This sampling procedure eliminates several groups from our study which would be worth additional research. Although we gain the advantage of dealing with a group for whom the illness experience and medical care are more significant, we do lose the cases of minor illness and insidious symptoms not requiring medical care. We also miss those individuals who decided *not* to seek medical care and those ex-patients who are in the convalescent or rehabilitative stage but did not require the prescribed degree of medical care during the previous two month period. Of course, those cases which resulted in death are also not included.

[14] Mechanic makes the same point. "Illness behavior seemed to play a more important part in medical visits for symptoms usually regarded as not very serious." Mechanic, D. "Some Implications of Illness Behavior for Medical Sampling," *N. E. J. Med.*, 269:244, August 1, 1963.

While the number of illness cases is too small to permit extensive statistical comparisons, it does offer the possibility of a meaningful exploratory analysis of a single illness episode. It is hoped that this primarily descriptive analysis will provide the perspective for more detailed research intended to test specific hypotheses concerning decision-making in illness.

Findings

We present our main findings according to the five stages of illness described above. The questionnaire itself was divided into these stages and the interview followed in order the general time sequence from the first symptom experience stage to the final recovery stage, or as far as medical care had progressed at the time of the interview.

Stage 1. The Symptom Experience—First, in regard to the physical aspects of the initial challenge of illness, we have to consider what the symptoms were, their severity, the course they took, and the individual's knowledge about and previous experiences with such symptoms. Pain was by far the most important initial warning sign that something was wrong (66 per cent), followed by fever or chills (17 per cent) and shortness of breath (10 per cent). A wide variety of different symptoms was mentioned by less than 5 per cent of the respondents for each symptom.

These symptoms were first noticed by 2 out of 5 respondents (40 per cent) during the day (20 per cent during the evening, 14 per cent first thing in the morning, and 12 per cent during the night), usually while at home (63 per cent, 22 per cent while at work or school), and more often while the individual was engaged in some activity (44 per cent working or playing, 22 per cent in bed or resting). From the very beginning the symptoms were continuous (70 per cent) rather than intermittent or accompanying only certain physical movements. Most respondents report the first symptoms as "severe" (47 per cent) or "extremely severe" (24 per cent) and as resulting in "complete" (41 per cent) or "a great deal"

(19 per cent) of immediate incapacitation. In only about 20 per cent of the cases did the symptoms get better, disappear, or become less frequent before seeking medical care.

Thus, in terms of symptomatology, we find that, for the type of fairly serious illness case included in this sample, the initial symptoms were not easily to be denied. They were usually severe, continuous, incapacitating, and unalleviated. In most cases, the appearance of the symptoms created "very much" (46 per cent) or "quite a bit" (19 per cent) of concern. About half (55 per cent) had never had the symptoms before and only a small minority (16 per cent) thought the symptoms would last only a few hours or less.

How did most respondents interpret these symptoms? About 3 out of 4 (73 per cent) immediately saw the symptoms as indicative of an illness. It is not surprising therefore that a large majority (75 per cent) thought of contacting a doctor immediately with only about one out of 4 feeling that patent medicines or home remedies might help. About one-third of the respondents did try to disregard their symptoms (31 per cent), but in 50 per cent of these cases the symptoms worsened, in 30 per cent they persisted, and in 14 per cent new symptoms appeared. Despite their attempt to postpone making a decision about what to do about these symptoms, 63 per cent of these individuals were forced to make a decision within a week with only 14 per cent succeeding in delaying the decision for as much as one month. Three out of 5 (59 per cent) of these delayers tried to meet the problem by cutting down on their activities but to no avail. Only 16 per cent succeeded in convincing themselves that the symptoms did not indicate an illness. Finally, all but a small minority of this group (18 per cent) conceded the need for medical care and contacted a physician.[15] These findings indicate that most respondents when faced with frightening symptoms think

[15] Ultimately, of course, all of our respondents did end up with medical care or they would not have been included in our sample.

almost at once in terms of seeking professional medical care.

It is interesting to note briefly the respondent's interpretation of the cause of his illness. The most frequently given explanation refers to the weather or climate (13 per cent) with nervous tension or aggravation coming second in importance (9 per cent). It would appear that etiology is viewed largely in terms of those factors increasing exposure or lowering resistance rather than in terms of direct causal agents or processes.

What effect does the kind of symptoms the individual experiences have upon his illness behavior? As can be seen from Table 10–1, the more severe the individual's symptoms, the more serious they appear to be,

When we relate severity of symptoms, incapacitation, and the belief that the symptoms indicated an illness to the degree of seriousness with which the individual viewed the presence of the symptoms, we find that the sick individual is more likely to take his symptoms seriously if they are severe (high severity = 79 per cent serious vs. low severity = 21 per cent serious), incapacitating (high incapacitation = 81 per cent serious vs. low incapacitation = 40 per cent serious), and indicative to him of some disease (an illness = 75 per cent serious vs. no illness = 24 per cent serious).

It is obvious from these findings that one of the problems in educating the public to behave "rationally" in the face of symptoms of illness relates to the individual's natural tendency to under-emphasize symptoms

Table 10–1—Relationship Between Symptomatology and Illness Responses

	Degree of Concern (% High Concern)	Interpretation of Symptoms (% Symptoms As Illness)	Contact with Physician (% Contacting a Physician)
Symptomatology:			
Degree of Severity			
High (33) *	67%	85%	76%
Medium (65)	45	79	71
Low (31)	36	52	48
Degree of Seriousness			
High (25)	76%	93%	83%
Medium (54)	64	84	72
Low (48)	17	51	43
Degree of Incapacitation			
High (54)	56%	87%	84%
Medium (33)	45	76	58
Low (42)	38	60	50

* In all tables, the number of cases upon which percentages are based will be given in parentheses. These bases may vary slightly depending upon the number of "no answers."

and the more they interfere with the individual's ability to carry on his usual activities, the more likely is it that the individual experiencing these symptoms will become concerned about their presence, will fear that they probably signify the beginnings of an illness, and will think about and then actually get in touch with a physician. These differences are all quite pronounced, underscoring the importance of symptom severity in initiating medical action.[16]

[16] All relationships are statistically significant at or beyond the 0.01 level of probability, using chi-square measures (upper-tail test) as obtained from the 7090 electronic computer based upon all answer categories.

which are neither severe nor incapacitating. The increased importance of the chronic, degenerative diseases today, however, with their long period of pre-clinical development and their rather insidious beginnings, create a special problem for early diagnosis and treatment. Since many of these chronic diseases do not have serious and incapacitating initial symptoms, it is difficult to induce the public to seek early medical care.

Demographic Comparisons—In general, we find that women were about twice as likely as men to report severe symptoms (31 per cent vs. 17 per cent), to view these symptoms seriously (25 per cent vs. 12 per cent), and to become concerned about their importance (51 per cent vs. 42 per cent). Both women and men were about equally likely, however, to interpret these symptoms as indicative of some illness (73 per cent vs. 78 per cent).

Older respondents (over 44 years of age) as compared to younger (44 years or under) reported greater incapacity as a result of their symptoms (45 per cent vs. 35 per cent) and, perhaps as a result of this, were more than twice as likely to take the symptoms seriously (24 per cent vs. 11 per cent), and to view them as symptomatic of illness (81 per cent vs. 64 per cent). However, both old and young reported an equal degree of concern with the symptoms (48 per cent vs. 47 per cent).

Only minor differences appear according to socio–economic status.[17] The lower socio-economic groups reported somewhat more incapacitation (46 per cent vs. 35 per cent) but both lower and higher social groups reported the same amount of severity and concern, and both groups were equally likely to interpret the symptoms as illness.

We cannot in this analysis determine the degree to which these varying responses to illness by sex, age, and socio–economic status reflect different kinds and degrees of illness among these groups. In general, though, women and older people are more likely to take symptoms of illness with greater seriousness. Given the type of illness case upon which the present sample is based, however, the most significant finding perhaps is the equal alacrity with which all groups become concerned about their symptoms

and immediately view them as indicative of an illness requiring medical care.

Stage 2. The Assumption of the Sick Role— Of primary importance at this stage is the discussion process whereby the individual experiencing symptoms presents his problem to other members of his social group and seeks their "approval to be ill." Almost all of our respondents (74 per cent) report discussing their symptoms with someone before seeking medical care. Most of these discussions were limited to one other person (48 per cent) with only 5 per cent speaking to three or more individuals. Thus, it would appear that, contrary to popular stereotypes, the sick individual as defined by this study does not go around discussing his symptoms with all who are willing to listen.

Overwhelmingly, this discussion was apt to take place as soon as the initial symptoms appeared (91 per cent). The discussant was most likely to be a relative (84 per cent), usually the spouse of the ill person (53 per cent). The usual picture was for the respondent actively to seek out the discussant for his opinion and to tell him about the symptoms (57 per cent). A content analysis of the discussion between the individual experiencing symptoms of illness and the person he had sought out to discuss these symptoms indicates that most discussion results in "provisional validation" for the sick individual to relinquish his responsibilities and to seek medical care. The largest majority of discussants interpreted the symptoms as indicative of illness (66 per cent) and recommended that a doctor be seen (54 per cent). Most discussants emphasized the seriousness of the symptoms (44 per cent "serious" vs. 13 per cent "not serious") and one out of 4 (24 per cent) actually offered a diagnosis of the symptoms as indicative of a specific illness.

The respondents were asked to characterize their discussants and overwhelmingly these discussants were described in positive terms. Sixty-one per cent found them "sympathetic," "helpful" (59 per cent), and "concerned" (44 per cent). Four out of 5 had

---

[17] The Socio–Economic Status index was formed from the person's education, occupation and total family income as follows: education was divided into five categories: some college, high school graduate, some high school, grammar school graduate, and some grammar school. Occupation was divided into four categories: professional and managerial, clerical and sales, craftsmen, and household, service workers, etc. Total family income was divided into four categories: $7,500 plus, $5,000 to $7,500, $3,000 to $5,000 and less than $3,000. These were scored and distributed on an index which ranged from a score of 13 for highest SES to 3 for the lowest SES. Where information was not ascertained for one of the three index components, the score was based upon a linear interpolation of the remaining two components.

"a great deal" (59 per cent) or "quite a bit" (32 per cent) of respect for the discussant's judgment. It is probable, of course, that discussants were chosen partly because the respondent would naturally seek a sympathetic listener, but it is a favorable commentary upon the role of the family in illness to remember that 84 per cent of these discussants were relatives, most of them being husbands or wives (53 per cent).

In almost all cases, the sick individual followed the advice and recommendations of their discussants whether it was to see a specific doctor (87 per cent followed up), go to a clinic (70 per cent followed up), begin self-medication (75 per cent followed up), or wait further symptoms development (60 per cent followed up). The net result of the discussion was to leave most respondents with a fairly clear plan of action as to what should be done next (78 per cent).

This analysis of the lay discussion phase of illness prior to the seeking of professional diagnosis and treatment, in general, supports the positive contribution of such discussion to the medical care process. Few individuals, it would appear, are confident enough of their own knowledge to make the judgment that they need medical care by themselves. Even more important, most individuals appear to need the support and reassurance of others in their family before they can recognize and accept illness, relinquish their social responsibilities, and seek medical care. In most of our cases, discussion did succeed in providing the individual experiencing symptoms with the necessary support and in guiding him into professional medical channels.

Demographic Comparison—Discussion of one's symptoms with others varies according to sex, age, and socio–economic status. Women were much more likely than men to have discussed their symptoms with several other individuals (24 per cent vs. 13 per cent for two or more discussants). Younger people were also more likely than older to turn to others when experiencing symptoms (28 per cent vs. 15 per cent) while the upper socio–economic group was more likely than the lower to have discussed their symptoms

with several others before seeking medical care (25 per cent vs. 14 per cent).

As for the results of these discussions, the symptoms were more likely to be interpreted as indicative of a serious illness among the men as compared to the women (62 per cent vs. 42 per cent), among the older as compared to the younger (55 per cent vs. 41 per cent), and among the upper as compared to the lower socio–economic groups (57 per cent vs. 46 per cent). As in the case of symptom interpretation by the respondent himself, we do not know to what extent these interpretations by others reflect actual differences in the seriousness of the illness or social variations in the perception of seriousness.

Stage 3. *Medical Care Contact*—As was noted previously, overwhelmingly, the initial response to illness was to turn to a physician for aid. The immediate reaction of 75 per cent of the sample was to think of a physician and 65 per cent both thought and contacted a physician almost at once. The reasons most frequently mentioned by those who did delay were the feeling that the symptoms were not serious (48 per cent) or the inability to relinquish one's work or social responsibilities (24 per cent). Financial or economic problems were mentioned by only a small minority (8 per cent), as was fear of medical treatment (2 per cent). In any case, even among those who were inclined to delay, 3 out of 4 (75 per cent) were unable to postpone seeing a doctor for more than two weeks with 4 out of 5 (80 per cent) reporting new or worsening symptoms. These findings support our previous conclusion concerning the importance of painful or worrisome symptoms in motivating the individual to contact a physician and indicate the relative unimportance of financial considerations as a deterrent to seeking medical care in the face of serious symptomatology.[18]

[18] It is probable that economic factors would play a greater role in the case of minor ailments where medical care was more a matter of alleviating symptoms and speeding recovery rather than meeting a serious threat to one's health. To some extent the lack of any significant differences by socio–economic status may also reflect the currently wide-spread health insurance coverage of all economic groups.

The intensity of the initial impact of illness on the individual is a prime determinant of his subsequent behavior. Among those whose initial concern was ranked either high or medium, 90 per cent thought immediately of contacting a physician. Among those with a low degree of concern regarding their condition, only half as many (45 per cent) thought of contacting a physician. In place of a medical practitioner, less concerned persons were more likely to choose self-treatment, to turn to the use of a patent medicine, or to a change of activity.

Moreover, not only were the lower concerned less likely to think of contacting a physician but once having thought of such a contact they were less likely to act upon it. The Physician-Contact Ratio (i.e., the ratio of actual contact to considered contact) decreases as the level of concern decreases from 0.90 for the high and medium group to 0.76 for the low group.

In general, similar relationships were noted when reactions to initial symptoms were analyzed by other measures of illness impact such as perceived seriousness of illness, the severity of symptoms, or the interpretation of the symptoms as indicative of an illness. That is, the more seriously an illness was perceived (or the more severe the first symptoms), the more likely was the individual to think of contacting a physician and to actually make this immediate contact. Where illness was deemed less serious (or first symptoms less severe), other alternative self-medication procedures such as the use of patent medicines suggested themselves. Similarly, if the symptoms were interpreted as indicative of an illness, the individual was almost twice as likely to have thought of contacting a physician and to have actually made such a contact.

The respondents were asked a series of questions concerning the nature of their first medical contacts. Altogether the 137 respondents reported 215 visits to physicians in connection with the initial appearance of their symptoms. The following analysis is based upon these 215 physician visits.

Most of the physicians seen were general practitioners (63 per cent), with about one out of 4 (28 per cent) being a specialist who was not a surgeon (7 per cent being a surgeon). These doctors were seen at their offices (35 per cent), at home (27 per cent), at a hospital (21 per cent), or at a clinic or OPD (13 per cent). Most of these physician contacts were with a medical practitioner whom the patient had never seen before (57 per cent), with only about one out of 3 (30 per cent) being the person's family doctor. By and large, the non-family doctor contact was the result of a referral or recommendation (53 per cent), with a small proportion being assigned to the patient by the clinic or OPD (14 per cent) or being made available through some health insurance plan (9 per cent). Most frequently the non-home visits (40 per cent) were made by the patient alone, with the spouse accompanying the individual in one out of 3 cases (34 per cent) and some other relative in the remainder of the cases.

This description of the initial medical contact supports the general picture of a mixture of personalized and non-personalized medical care in the United States. The doctors an individual chooses to visit are either known personally to him or are referred to him by someone who does know the doctor personally. However, it is worth noting that in the majority of cases the physician seen was a complete stranger to the patient. This may reflect the fact that for the present sample which excluded minor ailments about one out of 3 initial contacts were, from the beginning, with a specialist or surgeon. Despite the seriousness of the illnesses, however, only one out of 4 physician visits were made in the patient's home. These findings underscore some of the current problems in the provision of continuous, comprehensive medical care.

More than a third (40 per cent) of the respondents had to see the doctor more than six times and for a period of time extending over more than one month (39 per cent). When we examine the diagnoses made, as reported by the respondents, we note that 3 out of 5 (61 per cent) of the visits produced a diagnosis after the first visit with only 7 per cent requiring more than three visits before a diagnosis was forthcoming. One out of 5 (20 per cent) of the respondents state that, to their knowledge, the physician never did make a diagnosis. In only one per cent of the cases does the respondent report a subsequent change in the doctor's diagnosis of the illness. The most frequent patient reaction to a diagnosis was one of resignation and relief (48 per cent), with only 18 per cent reporting that they became worried or frightened and 15 per cent that they became depressed. We must remember, of course, that these patient reports are undoubtedly colored by subjective factors.

One out of 3 (37 per cent) of the respondents report that the doctor did not tell them what to expect from the illness. Only 2 out of 5 (41 per cent) were given any indication of how long the illness might last, the majority of these (78 per cent) being estimated at less than one month. (We may assume that in the case of chronic disease, this estimate referred to the current episode of illness rather than to the disease itself.) Ninety-two per cent of the respondents report that the time estimate on the doctor's part proved to be correct.

The most frequent physician's recommendations for medical care reported by the respondents were medication (46 per cent), bed rest (37 per cent), hospitalization (23 per cent), surgery (13 per cent), and referral to another physician (12 per cent). One out of 5 respondents (20 per cent) report that the prescribed treatment called for a change in eating, drinking, or smoking habits. In very few cases (about 20 per cent for household duties and work, and 10 per cent for social activities) were the respondents asked to restrict their activities. In most cases (76 per cent), the respondents talked over the doctor's recommendations with someone, usually their spouse (50 per

cent) or some other relative (28 per cent). Invariably, they were encouraged to follow these recommendations, only 1 per cent reporting being discouraged. Overwhelmingly, the respondents report that they followed the doctor's orders (97 per cent), and without too much difficulty (80 per cent). Insofar as the individual's self-evaluation is concerned, it would appear that most people see themselves as obedient and conscientious patients.

Demographic Comparisons—Sex and age appear to be related to contacting a doctor with the following percentages both thinking of and actually contacting a doctor immediately upon experiencing symptoms of illness:

	Per Cent Thinking of and Contacting Doctor
Males	
Under 44 Years	81% (26)
44 Years and Over	61% (28)
Females	
Under 44 Years	63% (52)
44 Years and Over	58% (31)

Men and younger people were more likely than women and older people to think and act in terms of seeking professional medical care upon feeling ill. There did not seem to be any differences by socio–economic status with the lower income groups being just as likely as the upper income groups to think of and to seek medical care in the face of the relatively serious symptoms involved in the illnesses under study. The upper income groups, however, were more likely to have seen more than two physicians in their search for medical care (21 per cent vs. 8 per cent). As for the amount of delay, very few individuals altogether delayed more than one week, but the older respondents were somewhat more likely than the younger respondents to have delayed that long (13 per cent vs. 9 per cent).[19]

The physician to whom the ill person turned for care was more likely to be the

[19] For a detailed analysis of the utilization of medical services among all respondents, see M. C. Klem, *Health Status and Medical Care in an Urban Community*, New York City Department of Health, October, 1963.

individual's family doctor in the case of the older as compared to the younger (54 per cent vs. 30 per cent) and the higher as compared to the lower socio-economic groups (51 per cent vs. 44 per cent). The older (22 per cent vs. 16 per cent) and lower income groups (22 per cent vs. 12 per cent) were more likely to have seen their physician more than ten times, probably indicative of the more serious illnesses among these groups.

Stage 4. The Dependent-Patient Role— By and large, we find that most respondents expressed favorable attitudes towards doctors, with the majority (62 per cent) agreeing that "most doctors are more interested in the welfare of their patients than in anything else" and disagreeing (52 per cent) with the statement, "I have my doubts about some things doctors say they can do for you." In relation to their specific illness and its treatment, most of the patients felt that the doctor was able to help them "a great deal" (56 per cent), with only one out of 5 (19 per cent) saying "not much" or "not at all."

The acceptance of patient status does not come easily to most people. Three out of 4 of our respondents (74 per cent) agreed with the statement. "I find it very hard to give in and go to bed when I am sick," and a majority (58 per cent) stated, "I find it hard to turn over my responsibilities to someone else when I get sick." While almost all respondents (90 per cent) agreed with the statement, "I am willing to do absolutely everything the doctor advises when I get sick," almost as many (81 per cent) stated that, "When I am ill I demand to know all the details of what is being done to me." It would seem that, at least insofar as expressed wishes are concerned, patients are willing to do whatever a doctor advises but they do want to be kept informed about what is going to happen.[20]

Additional evidence on the reluctance of sick individuals to relinquish their responsibilities can be seen from the fact that only 2 out of 5 respondents (39 per cent) reported

20 A more complete analysis of these and other statements concerning medical care is given in Suchman, "Social Patterns of Illness and Medical Care," *op. cit.*

that they tried to get someone to take over their responsibilities during their illness. Most often the person assuming the responsibilities was the respondent's spouse (41 per cent) or some other relative (46 per cent) and only rarely a friend (7 per cent). Once more we see the extremely important role played by the individual's family during illness. A large majority (82 per cent) of those who sought to turn over their responsibilities to others report that the arrangements they made worked out satisfactorily.

The limitations imposed on activities by the illness were largely those that required the performance of work or school (80 per cent) or household tasks (70 per cent). Very few respondents (12 per cent) report that their social relationships were affected.

The respondents were asked a series of questions dealing with various economic, social, family, and health concerns that they may have had during their illness. They were also asked to specify at which point of the illness episode—before, during, or after—they felt the greatest concern. Table 11-2 gives the percentage of respondents reporting each type of concern and the point at which this concern was at its peak.

The most frequently mentioned concern was related to the illness itself—what the symptoms signified (59 per cent), whether or not there would be recovery (49 per cent), and the possible after-effects of the illness (40 per cent). The peak points of these concerns varied, in general, with concern over the meaning of symptoms occurring relatively more frequently before treatment, the concern with recovery during illness, and the worry about after-effects at the end of the illness.

Second in importance were social concerns—about being able to carry on or resume one's usual activities (50 per cent—mostly during and after the illness episode), the loss of one's independence (22 per cent—mostly during illness), and the interruption of important plans (15 per cent—mostly during and after illness). Economic worries came next in order—concerns about the costs of treatment (37 per cent), the loss of work time (30 per cent), and the loss of wages (18 per cent). Most of these economic concerns occurred during and after the illness episode.

The low percentage of respondents mentioning family concerns again testifies to the stability of family ties during illness for out study population. While one out of four (25 per cent) were concerned about their ability to carry out family obligations, only small minorities were worried about the loss of their place in the family (3 per cent), the loss of their children's affection (3 per cent), or the loss of their spouse's affection (2 per cent). Of course, these latter concerns would be difficult for a person to admit to himself as well as to an interviewer.

Continuity of Care—One of the goals of modern medicine is to provide continuity of care for the patient during an illness episode. By and large, most of our respondents (58 per cent) did remain with the same doctor during the entire course of treatment. While one out of four patients (25 per cent) was

referred to another doctor for specialist treatment (53 per cent of the referrals), hospitalization (44 per cent) or consultation (11 per cent), most of these patients receiving referrals still kept in contact with the referring physician (56 per cent). However, one out of four (23 per cent) respondents did report that they independently, and presumably against their doctor's wishes, changed physicians during the course of treatment. Three out of four of these independent changers (75 per cent) did not inform the attending physician that they were going to consult another doctor and only 9 per cent returned to their original doctor. Most of these changers (66 per cent) discussed the proposed move with someone, most often their spouse (47 per cent), before making it. These discussants were described almost unanimously as supportive of the respondent's desire to change doctors.

The major reason given for changing physicians was that the individual felt that his condition was not improving (38 per cent). The most frequently mentioned reason for seeking a different physician was to secure another medical opinion (25 per cent)

Table 10–2—Concerns felt over illness and point of greatest concern

Type of Concern	Total*	POINT OF GREATEST CONCERN		
		Before	During	After
Disease:				
Disease Symptoms—Meaning	59%	21%	37%	1%
Whether or Not There Would Be Recovery	49	5	29	15
After-Effects of Illness	40	4	18	18
Possible Hospitalization	22	11	10	1
Possible Surgery	19	7	11	1
Social:				
Inability to carry on or resume usual activities	50	7	25	18
Loss of independence	22	2	12	8
Interruption of important plans	15	2	6	7
Changes in appearance	10	2	4	4
Loss of social contacts	6	–	3	3
Inability to perform sexual functions	6	1	3	2
Economic:				
Treatment cost	37	9	17	11
Loss of work time	30	4	14	12
Temporary loss of salary or wages	18	2	7	9
Loss of job	7	1	2	4
Family:				
Inability to carry out family obligations	25	4	14	7
Loss of children's affection	3	–	3	–
Loss of place in family	3	–	3	–
Loss of spouse's affection	2	1	1	–

* Percentages add to more than 100 since respondents felt more than one concern.

or what the respondent felt was a more complete examination (22 per cent). The doctor–patient relationship did not figure prominently in either leaving one's old doctor (mentioned by 13 per cent) or in choosing a new doctor (16 per cent). It is interesting to note that, in the opinion of most of the changers (72 per cent), the new doctor did not continue the treatment of the previous doctor.

Hospitalization—A separate series of questions were asked of the 65 individuals in our sample who had undergone hospitalization. The average length of stay was about 10 days with 8 per cent staying only one or two days and 12 per cent more than one month. About half the cases (45 per cent) involved some form of surgery. Most patients stayed in semi-private rooms (63 per cent), with 31 per cent going into wards and 6 per cent taking a private room. Only 6 per cent engaged a special nurse.

One out of three patients (34 per cent) report no days of complete confinement to bed with 13 per cent being confined for more than two weeks. Most of the patients (71 per cent) had experienced previous hospitalization, one out of 4 (23 per cent) having been in the hospital 5 or more times. Previous hospitalization appears to act as a form of reassurance, with 41 per cent of those who had been in a hospital previously reporting that this previous experience made them feel better about going again, with only 4 per cent reporting feeling worse about it.

Hospitalization did not create any great concern about what was going on at home for most patients. Only one out of 5 worried "a great deal" (11 per cent) or "quite a bit" (8 per cent) about this. Almost all patients (91 per cent) were visited by relatives, the average number of visits being about 10. Visits by friends were less frequent, 2 out of 5 (39 per cent) reporting none, with the average being about 4 for those who did have visits by non-relatives.

Interaction with other patients at the hospital was not very great. Half the patients (51 per cent) report making no friends while at the hospital. Only a small proportion (6 per cent) of the patients report making friends with someone on the hospital staff.

Almost all patients who did strike up friendships with other patients discussed their case with them (82 per cent), received reciprocal help or comfort from them (78 per cent), and discussed personal matters with them (57 per cent). These patient friendships, however, were largely confined to the hospital, with only one out of 4 (24 per cent) continuing after the individuals had left the hospital.

In general, the respondents report that they were eager to leave the hospital (69 per cent), only 2 per cent feeling that they were not ready to leave when they were finally discharged. However, despite this eagerness, only 11 per cent asked the attending physician to let them go home, with only 17 per cent stating that anyone ever urged them to leave the hospital sooner (half of these requests coming from the attending physician himself).

Attitudes toward the hospital experience were in general favorable, with only 3 per cent agreeing with the statement, "They didn't pay enough attention to me," 5 per cent with the statement, "They made too much fuss over me," and 6 per cent with, "I was treated like a child." The majority (56 per cent) agreed that, "I felt comforted to be taken care of this way," although only one out of five (20 per cent) went so far as to say, "I was glad to have someone else take responsibility for me." It is interesting to note these generally favorable attitudes despite the fact that in nine out of ten cases (89 per cent) the respondents report that no one at any time bothered to explain the hospital routine to them. It may be that hospital patients are not concerned with hospital routines or that they have a low level of expectation and therefore do not feel disappointed when no one explains these routines to them.

Demographic Comparison—We find only minor sex, age, and socio–economic differences in general acceptance of the sick role and adjustment to illness. All groups are equally likely to feel that they were helped "a great deal" by their physicians and to have favorable attitudes toward their hospital experience. In general, men were more likely than women, older groups more than younger groups, and lower socio-economic groups more than upper socio-economic groups to have been hospitalized at all, or, if hospitalized, to have had a longer stay with greater confinement to bed.

These differences in hospitalization rates probably reflect a combination of physical need and social influences. While older and lower income patients may have more serious ailments which require hospitalization, it is probably also the case that these two groups are also likely to be at least able to provide for their own care at home. These are also the groups which are more likely to report that they were dependent upon their families to take care of them while ill: males (40 per cent) vs. females (22 per cent); young (22 per cent) vs. old (33 per cent); and low socio-economic status (32 per cent) vs. high socio-economic status (25 per cent). Possibly reflecting this more serious state of illness and greater dependency upon others, we find that men were more likely than women to report feeling depressed during their illness (75 per cent vs. 51 per cent), older people more than younger (66 per cent vs. 52 per cent), and the lower socio-economic group more than the upper socio-economic group (67 per cent vs. 51 per cent).

We find a number of interesting comparisons according to social factors in relation to referrals to other physicians for medical care as opposed to independent patient changes in physician. As can be seen from Table 10–3, these tend to go in opposite directions—referrals from one physician to another were more likely to take place among the women, the younger age groups, and the upper socio-economic status groups while independent changes from one physician to another were more likely to occur among the males and older age groups (no difference by socio-economic status). Both types of changes in physician—the physician-inspired and the patient-inspired—were more likely to occur in the case of hospitalized as compared to non-hospitalized cases.

Stage 5.   The Recovery or Rehabilitation Stage—At the time of the interview, most of the respondents were no longer seeing a doctor (72 per cent). Two out of 5 respondents (39 per cent) said they were feeling completely well, 47 per cent said they were improved, 13 per cent felt about the same, and almost none (1 per cent) described their condition as worse. More than half the respondents (58 per cent) had resumed all their usual activities, with only 12 per cent being completely restricted and 28 per cent partially restricted.

Almost all respondents (94 per cent) convalesced in their own homes. Half of them (55 per cent) were able to take care of themselves, the other half being looked after by some member of the household. During convalescence, half the respondents (47 per cent) were confined to their beds for an average of about eight days, with only 5 per cent being in bed for more than a month. Most of the patients who were confined to bed decided by themselves without asking the doctor that they were well enough to get out of bed (66 per cent)—only 2 per cent had to ask before the doctor told the respondent without his asking that he was

Table 10–3—*Social characteristics of referrals and independent changers*

	Per Cent Referrals	Per Cent Independent Changers
Male (52)	19%	42%
Female (77)	23	23
Under 44 Years (44)	30	27
44 Years and Over (85)	18	33
Low Socio–Economic (79)	20	33
High Socio–Economic (41)	29	34
Hospitalized (54)	31	42
Not Hospitalized (75)	15	24

well enough to get up (32 per cent being told by the doctor before they asked).

As far as most patients are concerned, the timing of their discharge from medical care was just right—neither too soon nor too late. Most patients (79 per cent) felt that they could not have gone back to their usual activities any sooner or that they went back too soon (71 per cent). In general, respondents disagreed with the statement that, "Nowadays doctors tend to get their patients back to work too soon" (80 per cent), although a large majority felt that they themselves were likely to try to resume their usual activities too soon, with three out of four (75 per cent) agreeing to the statement, "I usually try to get up too soon after I have been sick." Our respondents are split about 50–50 when it comes to the statement, "When a person starts getting well, it is hard to give up having people do things for him" (48 per cent agreeing and 52 per cent disagreeing).

How did the ex-patient feel about his convalescence? As in the case of hospital care, most convalescents expressed satisfaction with their care at home. Seventy-six per cent of those under care during convalescence agreed that they "felt comforted to be taken care of," while 52 per cent stated that they were "glad to have someone else take responsibility for them." No one agreed that they "didn't get enough attention," only small percentages that they were "made too much fuss over" (5 per cent), that they were "treated like a child" (15 per cent), or that

image of the complaining patient. Most patients and ex-patients appear pleased and grateful for the care they receive from both professional and lay sources.

The time of recovery from an illness is, however, a period of readjustment. Many of the respondents who state that they experienced anxiety about their illness pinpoint this recovery stage as the peak period of their concern over such economic matters as "loss of job" (57 per cent of such concerns occurring after the illness episode), "loss of wages" (50 per cent), "loss of work time" (40 per cent), or "cost of treatment" (30 per cent). The peak of social concerns also often occurs during this period, such as "interruption of important plans" (47 per cent) and "inability to carry on or resume usual activities" (36 per cent). This recovery period furthermore witnesses doubts as to "the after-effects of illness" (45 per cent) and "whether or not there would be recovery" (31 per cent). It would appear that as immediate involvement with one's illness declines, one becomes increasingly concerned with the consequences of such illness.

The ex-patients were asked the following question: "I'm going to read you some statements about how you felt during the time of your recovery. With which ones do you agree?" The statements and the per cent of respondents agreeing to each are given below:

	Per Cent Agreeing
"You enjoyed taking it easy during this period."	26
"You could hardly wait to get back to your normal routine."	25
"You were concerned about your ability to pick up where you had left off."	23
"You felt that the recovery period didn't need to be so long."	9
"You dreaded getting back to your normal routine."	7
"The days passed all too quickly."	7
"You were worried about what people might think about you when you returned to your usual activities."	7
"Too much attention began to annoy you and you wanted to be on your own."	5

they were "a burden to someone" (11 per cent). Either patients are a particularly satisfied group or else they feel that they have no right to complain. These overwhelmingly positive findings raise some question as to the validity of the popular

These responses support our previous conclusion about the relatively favorable state of mind of patients during their period of convalescence. While there was some concern about one's ability to pick up where one had left off before the illness episode (23 per cent), few respondents dreaded getting back to their normal routine (7 per cent) or were worried about what people might think when they did return (7 per cent). Similarly, while few people felt that the time passed quickly (7 per cent), only a small percentage (9 per cent) thought that the recovery period lasted too long.

Demographic Comparisons—The convalescent period was more likely to be enjoyed by younger people as compared to older (34 per cent vs. 20 per cent), possibly reflecting the much more successful return of the younger group to a good state of health following the illness episode (68 per cent vs. 24 per cent). However, while individuals belonging to the upper socio–economic group were somewhat more likely than lower socio–economic groups members to say that their health following the illness was good (46 per cent vs. 36 per cent), they were less likely to say they enjoyed their convalescence (18 per cent vs. 27 per cent). This lower level of enjoyment during recovery by the upper socio–economic groups may have been the result of the much higher level of concern which this group had over their ability to return to their usual activities following the illness (73 per cent vs. 51 per cent)—a concern which was shared more by men than by women (73 per cent vs. 50 per cent), and more by the younger ex-patients than by the older (72 per cent vs. 53 per cent). Finally, even though men were more likely than women to say that they were in good health following the illness (49 per cent vs. 33 per cent), they did worry more about their ability to recover during the actual illness period (56 per cent vs. 45 per cent).

Summary

The division of the illness episode into five different phases involving a transition on the part of the sick individual from experiencing symptoms to assuming the sick role, to contacting a doctor, to being a patient and, finally, to relinquishing the sick role does appear to provide a meaningful separation of the sequence of events surrounding the illness experience. Each of these stages does seem to give rise to different kinds of problems and to involve different types of decisions and actions concerning medical care. In this concluding section, we can only point to what we feel are some of the most significant aspects of each stage.

1.   *The Symptom-Experience Stage*— Severity of symptoms exerts an extremely important influence upon the decision to seek medical care. The success with which "denial of illness" can take place will depend largely upon the degree of pain or incapacitation produced by the symptoms of the illness. Thus, in the case of the chronic diseases, the insidious nature of the onset of illness will often mitigate against early medical care.

2.   *The Assumption of the Sick Role Stage*— Discussion of one's symptoms with family or friends plays a highly significant role in determining subsequent medical action. In most cases, such discussion provides "provisional validation" for the individual to relinquish his normal social responsibilities, but does urge him to seek professional advice. Thus, "lay" discussion seems to provide a functional and positive force toward the seeking of medical care.

3.   *The Medical Care Contact Stage*—Most people experiencing alarming symptoms do not delay contacting a doctor. Few individuals seem to have any difficulty finding a doctor, although in many cases this may be the individual's first contact with the particular doctor. This medical contact almost always produces a fairly clear-cut diagnosis, prescribed course of treatment, and prognosis of future developments. These are usually accepted without difficulty by the patient and secure his cooperation. Thus, it would seem that, once the decision to seek care is made, the initial medical contact is fairly well routinized and offers little difficulty to the patient.

4.   *The Dependent-Patient Role Stage*— The acceptance of patient-status is not easy for most people in our society. During ill-

ness, the major concerns are focussed upon the illness itself and upon its effect on the individual's future ability to resume his previous social and economic activities. For the most part, satisfaction is expressed with the medical care received and the physician-patient relationship. Insofar as the patient can himself judge, therefore, once he has turned himself over to the care of the physician, treatment and recovery proceed without too much difficulty—as a rule.

5. *The Recovery or Rehabilitation Stage*— Relinquishing the sick role appears to provide most people with less difficulty than assuming it. Convalescence, while not enjoyable, proceeds smoothly in most cases and ends with the patient's return to his former well status. While there may be some concern about picking up where one had left off, this is not a problem for most people.

In general, this description of the "natural history" of illness in our society would support a positive appraisal of the pathways and routines established by the medical system for the care of the ill. While we cannot, of course, say anything about the "quality" of such care, insofar as our present sample is concerned—and it must be remembered that these are all cases which did ultimately receive medical care—the seeking and finding of medical care appears to take place without too much difficulty. We do not know about those cases in the community which may require but are not receiving medical care, but for those that are receiving medical care, the mechanics of the current medical care system appear to function rather smoothly.

11

The Patient's View of the Patient's Role

Daisy L. Tagliacozzo
and
Hans O. Mauksch

Every society grants to the sick person special privileges and every society also imposes on the sick person certain obligations.[1] An understanding of such general norms can provide an effective guide to the study of the behavior and attitudes of the sick in our society. However, general norms gain meaning in a specific social setting, or may be modified by intra–institutional expectations. The extent to which a sick person may feel free to seek satisfaction for his emotional needs and to assume the "rights and privileges of the sick role" may thus depend on the social context within which behavior unfolds. Even if general rules for behavior remain the same, the patient may be influenced by considerations which involve efforts to accommodate to real or imagined expectations of significant others.

The experience of being hospitalized adds another dimension to the experience of being ill. This dimension consists of the rights and obligations which are legitimated by organizational forces and which are based on the fact that admission to the hospital is tanta-

[1] Parsons, T., "Definitions of Health and Illness in the Light of American Values and Social Structure," in E. G. Jaco (ed.), *Patients, Physicians and Illness*, New York: Free Press, 1958, pp. 165–187 (chap. 7 in this volume).

mount to assuming an organizational position with all the implications for normative compliance and sanctions. This discussion is based on a study which sought to ascertain to what extent the attitudes and needs which are organized around these two experiences, being ill and being hospitalized, may differ or even come into conflict with each other. The attitudes and reactions of patients were viewed within the context of a system of roles and as a consequence of the patient's efforts to conform to perceived systems of expectations. The study concentrated on the implications of hospitalization, with less concern for the illness role *per se*. It explored to what extent the role of the hospitalized patient may be lacking clear definitions of rights and easily definable criteria for legitimate claims. The question was raised whether the position and the attitudes of patients deprive them of genuine means to control others in the system and thus limit their readiness to express their claims and desires without fear of sanction.

Throughout the study the patient is shown to be aware of the degree to which he is dependent on those who care for him. This dependency is based largely on the power to heal and to cure. It is also based on the power ascribed to hospital functionaries to give or to withhold those daily services which, for the hospitalized patient, can embrace some basic survival needs. The single or double rooms and the rapid patient turnover in the modern hospital do not foster an effective patient community which could serve as interpreter and modifier of hospital rules. The patient, therefore, is much more dependent on his previous learning, be it from direct or indirect experiences with the patient role. More importantly, the absence of adequate interpretations by the patient community makes the patient more dependent on hospital functionaries for clues about the appropriateness of his behavior, demands and expectations.

The fact that patients frequently remain strangers in the hospital community tends to add to the power of those who, as

Based on a study conducted by the authors through the Department of Patient Care Research, Presbyterian–St. Luke's Hospital, Chicago, Ill. This study was supported by a grant from the Commonwealth Fund.

functionaries, are intimately familiar with the rules and expectations of the organization. The power which is vested in them can inhibit the patient to seek clarification and guidance. Also, those who are informed tend to become oblivious to the needs of their clients to be initiated into the "rules of the game."

The study was conducted in a metropolitan voluntary hospital with a capacity of 850 beds. The hospital is part of a large Midwest medical center. It is a teaching hospital for nurses and physicians. Patients occupy predominantly two-bed or private rooms.[2] This discussion rests on the analysis of 132 interviews which were administered to 86 patients. The sample was limited to patients who were admitted with cardio–vascular or gastro–intestinal diagnoses. All patients in the sample were Caucasian, American–born males or females between 40 and 60 years of age. All patients had been previously hospitalized and all were married. They paid for their hospitalization in part with private or industrial insurance. During the semi-structured interview, the patient was asked to express himself freely on present and previous hospital experiences. The interviews averaged one hour and were recorded and transcribed. The average day of interviewing was the fifth day of hospitalization. When possible, second interviews were conducted.

PHYSICIANS AND NURSES:
THEIR SIGNIFICANCE

Physicians and nurses are among the significant others in the network of role relationships in which the hospitalized patient becomes involved. Their significance is derived from different sources. The physician represents authority and prestige. His orders legitimize the patient's demands on others and justify otherwise deviant aspects of illness behavior. The physician is not only the "court of appeal" for exemption from normal role responsibilities,[3] he also

[2] Thirty-two per cent of the patients in this sample occupied a private room; 61 per cent occupied a two-bed room and 7 per cent shared a room with two other patients.

[3] Parsons, T., *The Social System*, New York: Free Press, 1951, pp. 433–477.

functions as the major legitimizing agent for the patient's demands during hospitalization. Yet his orders generally do not constitute guides to behavior in specific situations and they do not consider or modify the patient's understanding of the formal and informal expectations of nurses. Although the physician's authority ranks supreme in the eyes of most patients, they are also aware that he is only intermittently present and thus not in a position to evaluate the behavior of both patients and nurses and to sanction this behavior during the everyday procedures of hospital care.

The significance of the nurse stems not only from her authority in interpreting, applying and enforcing the orders of the physician but, in addition, from the fact that she can judge and react to the patient's behavior more continuously than the physician. From the patient's point of view, he also depends upon the nurse as an intermediary in the provision of many other institutional services.

For most patients it is of greatest importance to feel that they adjust to the expectations of the nurse and of the physician. To accommodate themselves to what they feel is expected of them, patients must be able to perceive these expectations as congruent or they must cope with the strains involved in efforts to adjust to what may appear to them as conflicting demands. Conflict is thus likely to arise if the nurse executes a plan of care which, from the point of view of the patient, deviates in detail or emphasis from the patient's interpretation of the physician's orders.

Close adherence to the orders of the physician was not equally important for all patients and not all patients appear to be equally intense in their sensitivity to congruence in the plan of care and cure. Those patients who expressed concern for complete adherence to the physician's word and expected strictest observance and literal interpretation of medical orders typically expressed distrust in the reliability and efficiency of anyone except the physician. These patients frequently feared that even minor deviations may result in further physical harm. For some patients, close adherence to medical orders appeared congruent with their conceptions of themselves; as did some patients, who resisted following certain medical orders, they used this area of conformity to convey something essential about themselves.

Demands for rigid adherence to medical orders were associated with the desire for "reliable" nursing care and "efficiency." The eagerly co-operative patient not only emphasized that he followed all orders willingly, he also expected the nurse to "co-operate" with him in his efforts to carry out the orders of the physician as he understood them. The patient's concern typically expressed itself in close observations of hospital personnel, in emphasis on observance of punctuality and in worry whether "orders have been written" and "charts double-checked." Such efforts to "co-operate with the physician" by seeing that "things get done" may become a source of stress. The patient who is ready to act on behalf of medical orders may have to call for services from the nurse and impose demands on her time or ask her to alter behavior. Thus, if the patient hears from the physician that the "specimen should be warm," he may feel obligated to insist that a "cooling-off" delay be avoided. If the physician has told him that he may "stay in bed another day," the patient's interpretation may lead him to actively resist a nurse's urging that he do some things for himself: "My doctor said that I can stay in bed another day." Patients' insistence on rigid adherence to the orders of the physician were frequently defended in the light of one implication of the sick role—the obligation to make efforts towards the restoration of health. Thus, patients who were critical of deviations from medical orders justified their criticisms by pointing out that they did not want to be "complainers" or "troublemakers"—but that they, after all, "want to get well."

When a patient's efforts to co-operate fully and to observe the details of medical orders expressed themselves in more frequent demands, he also reacted to the risks involved in violating his obligation not to be demanding of nurses. Those patients who reported that they had expressed their desire for compliance with medical orders in active demands or complaints also tended to be very observant of the reactions of members of the nursing staff. Praise and criticism of "good" and "bad" nurses revealed that these patients rejected the nurse who "grumbled" and that they praised enthusiastically the nurse who responded "willingly" and who "smiled" when she was asked to do things for the patient. Patients also praised the nurse who "helped the patient to co-operate" and who "did not mind" when she was reminded of an order.

Those patients for whom co-operation with a physician's order became the guiding principle during hospitalization tended to be very sensitized to the reactions of others. They appeared to be "on the alert" and reacted quickly to facial expression, a tone of voice and the general manner in which a request was received. If they felt that their demands were not well received, they frequently became angered and, when given an opportunity, expressed their antagonism in attacks on those members of the nursing staff who "do not treat you like a person," who "make you feel that you are at their mercy" and "who consider you just a case."

The conflict between the felt obligation to insist on precise implementation of medical orders and efforts not to appear demanding or inconsiderate *vis à vis* the nursing staff was often resolved in favor of striving for approval by nurses. The data indicate that many patients prefer not to risk appearing too demanding or too dependent. They accept what appears to them to be deviations from the physician's orders, and even violate what they believe is expected of them by the physician. They anxiously watch a medication being late, rather than object to the delay, and they watch the specimen get cold rather than pointing this out to a nurse. Frequently this endeavor to "please" the nurse may backfire. Patients who disobey the physician's orders and get up to do "small things" for themselves rather than call the nurse may find themselves reprimanded by her because she may view this as lack of co-operation or even protest. She also may consider such behavior an incident which could incur the anger of the physician.

Thus, patients may pay for the security of "being liked" by nurses and of having them "know that I am not demanding" with concerns over arousing the physician's criticism or harming their own recovery. But even where the obligation to be co-operative with the physician is not immediately at stake, patients may somewhat reluctantly forego the privileges which they could claim as a result of being sick. As one patient expressed it:

> If it is a hotel you won't hesitate to pick up a phone or to complain; in a hospital you think twice about it—you figure maybe they are busy or shorthanded. . . . It's a much more human thing, the hospital. . . it's more personal.

EXPECTATIONS AND CONSTRAINTS

When patients were asked what was expected of them by their physicians and by nurses, they responded with considerable consistency, indicating that several rules for "proper" conduct of patients were well defined and widely shared. The physician was seen as expecting "co-operation" and "trust and confidence." A large group of patients felt that the nurse, too, expected "co-operation." On the other hand, many patients were convinced that nurses expected them "not to be demanding," to be "respectful" and to be "considerate." Only very few patients listed these latter three categories for physicians.

Self-descriptions which patients introjected into the interviews followed a similar pattern. It was most important to patients that the interviewer saw them as having "trust and confidence" in those who took care of them. This was particularly true of those patients who also admitted to some negative reactions toward nurses or physicians. Many patients were eager to mention that they were not demanding, co-operative, not dependent and considerate. In spontaneous discussions of the obligations of the hospitalized patient, the pattern did not change significantly.

One of the factors underlying the patient's

hesitation to impose demands on hospital personnel is his awareness of the presence of other, often sicker patients. Observation of other patients introduces restraints. Comparisons of "my illness" with the illness of the roommate appeared to intensify the moral obligation to "leave them free to take care of the seriously ill" and comparisons of one's own claims or criticisms with the behavior of a very ill person seemed to intensify restrained behavior: "After I observed him I felt kind of bad. I felt that I should be grateful and not ask for anything." It is well nigh impossible and a latent source of difficulty for the patient to judge his comparative status relative to patients in other rooms. The nurse summoned to give him a glass of water may have been called away from "a critical case." The isolation of the patient and the ensuing inability to establish relative claims serve as restraining forces on the expression of needs,[4] even though this concern is counterbalanced with an occasionally voiced concern about "getting one's share."

The patient's perceived entitlement for service is also linked to his definition of the severity of his illness. Patients apparently feel more secure in ascertaining their rights if their understanding of their condition permits them to rank themselves in the upper strata of a "hierarchy of illness." However, a secure assessment of "my case" may be difficult. Communications from the physician are general and understanding of the relative severity of the illness does not appear to be facilitated by his explanations. In many cases, a statement such as "I want you to stay in bed" does not legitimize the demand for a glass of water—the patient gets up to avoid being considered "too demanding."

Patients thereforefore seem to link the

---

[4] This phenomenon suggests a parallel to the concept of "relative deprivation" described by R. K. Merton and P. Lazarsfeld (eds.), *Continuities in Social Research*, New York: Free Press, 1950. Just as deprivation is experienced in relation to relative norms, legitimacy of claims rests on a relative basis. If this basis is not ascertainable, uncertainty functions as restraining force.

extent of their claims on service to readily perceived and objectively visible indices. Thus, being in traction, having tubes attached or being restrained by dressings are highly ranked legitimators for patients' demands. Fever also serves as a criterion for claims; the patient who asks the nurse what his temperature might be not only may inquire about the severity of his illness but indirectly may also ask: "To what services am I entitled today?" Hospital rules which prevent the nurse from giving such information may deny the patient guidelines for the rules applicable to his behavior.

Two-thirds of all patients in the sample indicated that they had refrained from expressing their needs and criticisms at least once. The observation that nurses are too busy, rushed and overworked was given as the most frequent reason for this reluctance. Beliefs about the conditions under which hospital personnel work serve thus as another limiting factor in the patient's expression of demands. One has to keep in mind the admiration for nurses and for "all those who do such difficult work" to understand why some patients may spend a night helping another patient when being told "that there is a shortage on the nightshift." Some patients did not engage in these activities without some conflict. They admitted that they were concerned with the physician's reactions "if he finds out," and that they were fearful of the consequences of such activity for their health. Even though they never admitted it directly, many responses revealed indirectly their desire to take more advantage of the privileges of the sick.

Constraint in voicing demands was also reinforced by the patient's assessment of the power of hospital personnel and physicians relative to his own. Over one-fourth of those patients who admitted to restraint of their demands also expressed their often resentful assessment of their own helplessness. Efforts to be "considerate" of the conditions which limit services may thus be convenient rationalizations of the patient's fears of offending others and of endangering his good relationship with them. "Being on

good terms" was seen by these patients not only as a convenient but as an essential factor for their welfare. They directly expressed their awareness of their inability to control those who are in charge of their care. Patients felt that they were subject to rewards and punishment and that essential services can be withheld unless they make themselves acceptable. Some of these patients were dependent upon intimate forms of physical assistance, and their points of view reflected their awareness of this dependence upon others.

Feelings of helplessness were directly expressed in observations that "one is at their mercy," that "trying to change things is futile" and "won't get you anywhere" and that patients feel "helpless." The recognition of the power of others to withhold services also found expression in fears that one does not want to be considered a "complainer," or "trouble-maker" or a "demanding patient," and in such apprehensions as "they can refuse to answer your bell, you know," or "they can refuse to make your bed." The same fears were expressed in efforts "to save that button so they come when I really need them" or in enthusiastic reactions to nurses who "come in to inquire why you never call for them" or who "do not mind if you ring once too often."

Patients very rarely expressed openly a concern that their physician may impose sanctions on inappropriate behavior. They tried to be intensely considerate toward him, since he, too, is considered "very busy" and "on his way" to other sick patients. Attempts to accommodate demands to these pressures on the physician serve as a considerable restraint on the patient's willingness to ask questions.

The admiration for the physician was in most cases tied to a very personal and emotionally charged attachment to the man who is "so kind and understanding." Gratitude intensified efforts to "make things easy" for him. Although hostility or annoyances toward nurses was often directly expressed, patients actively resisted direct verbalization of any negative feelings toward "the physician." Typically, complaints were expressed reluctantly and in terms of "I wish he could" coupled with quick modifications such as "I know he can't—he is too busy."

Patients may also be concretely limited by the observation that the physician is "on the go." Thus, a patient may want to ask questions and feel that "taking his time" is legitimate, but may feel that the time is simply not made available:

> He'll say well, we'll talk about it next time. And next time he'll talk fast, he out-talks you —and rushes out of the room and then when he's out of the room you think, well, I was supposed to ask him what he's going to do about my medicine . . . you run in the hall and he has disappeared that fast.

A patient who was impressed with the fact that his physician was "overburdened and rushed" tried to describe how the resulting pressure of his own tensions and anxiety prevented him from fully comprehending what he was told:

> All I know is that your mind sort of runs ahead. You sort of anticipate what they are going to say, and you finish what they are going to say in your mind. I guess it's because perhaps sometimes you have trouble following them or maybe you would want them to say certain things, and you are listening—well, I don't know . . . you try to think what they are going to say, because otherwise, you have difficulty understanding them, but then, when they are out of the room, you don't remember a thing about what they have said.

In view of the above, it is not surprising that patients who were asked directly what they "considered their rights" had some difficulties responding. One-fourth of the respondents admitted that they did not know what their rights were; some patients stated outright that they had no rights. The majority of respondents limited themselves to general answers such as "good care," followed by the modification that specific claims depended upon the "seriousness of the illness." The belief that claims for service had to be justified in terms of immediate physical needs over-shadowed any inclination to voice the rights of paying consumers. Few patients justified their demands in relation to their monetary payment and many of those who introduced the criteria of a paying consumer quickly

added to their demands other legitimizing factors, such as the nature of their illness or the fact that they had been considerate in other respects. Conceptions of rights and obligations provide guidelines for alternative actions. They are used and "fitted" in accordance with the exigencies of situations and the developing meanings which individuals and groups bring to bear upon them. The general patterns which have been discussed should not conceal that differences in the characteristics of patients may contribute to significant variations in the more general theme. The following observations will illustrate the importance of further research in this area.

Patients who do not experience active and well-defined symptoms and whose activities are not visibly impaired may hesitate to present themselves to others as seriously ill and may find "co-operation" at times more difficult. Patients with cardio-vascular illness tended to focus more frequently on behavior involving co-operation with physicians and nurses; particularly in relation to the physician, this obligation appeared to preoccupy these patients. They were also more intent on presenting themselves as co-operative to the interviewer. Some of these patients were severely ill from the medical point of view, requiring complete bed rest and its concomitant extensive services. However, they seemed to have a difficult time accepting this state without concern that they may be considered "too dependent" or overly "demanding." At times, these difficulties appeared enhanced by social and economic pressures to leave the hospital, and by psychological needs for denial which also seemed to find expression in the insistence that they "really did not need any special attention" and that they were "not worried about their illness."

Some of the subtle difficulties of these patients are not easily verbalized. Only rarely can a patient formulate as forcefully the aftermath of a heart attack as did the patient quoted below. His statement sums up the allusions and hints dropped by other patients with a cardiac problem:

Well, you know, a heart patient is a peculiar animal. That heart attack has done something to him, not only physically but mentally. I can tell you this because I have been through it. It brings up something which you don't want to let go of. If he tells you you must stay in bed, well, how come this sudden change? I don't want to stay in bed, and if he tells you that you cannot walk upstairs, he is telling you that you are weak, that you are no longer strong. He has taken something away from you—ah, your pride. You suddenly want to do what you are not supposed to do, what you have been doing all your life and that you have every right to do. Besides, a heart patient has an excitability built up in him.

Patients with cardio–vascular conditions verbalized criticisms less frequently than other patients. On the other hand, they stressed the importance of "dedication and interest" when discussing their ideal expectations of nurses and physicians.

One explanation for these tendencies may be found in some common fears which occur among patients who suffer from a type of illness in which the onset of a crisis can be sudden and unpredictable. For a patient with a cardio–vascular illness, as probably for all patients who fear a sudden turn for the worse, it is of utmost importance to know that someone will be there when the patient really needs help. The need for this type of security is revealed in the following responses of cardio–vascular patients:

I think that there should be somebody out in front there all the time. I think the hospital would back me up on that. . . . If the patient was really ill, rang the buzzer and nobody was there to get it—no telling what would happen.

Well, as I said, some patients may need more care because they have a more serious illness and when you have a heart disease then you need to be watched much more, also you are more frightened and it is important that somebody is around to watch your pulse.

Patients with non-specific gastro–intestinal conditions were more likely to be pre-occupied with cancer. At times this was accompanied by the suspicion that the physician "really knows but will not tell me." Such apprehensions seemed to make it more difficult for the patient to sustain trust and confidence in personnel, particularly the physician.

Openly anxious and critical patients were found more frequently within the gastro–intestinal category. While patients with cardio–vascular conditions appeared to focus attention on concrete services which assured their safety, gastro–intestinal patients seemed more inclined to focus on the qualitative nature of their interactions with nurses and physicians. They were more easily threatened by the attitudes of others, more responsive to "personalized care" and more openly critical when these areas of expectations were not satisfied.

In each culture there is the recognition that it is legitimate to deviate from normal behavior under certain extreme conditions. For these conditions most societies develop differential standards for men and women. In our society men and women are generally not expected to respond in an identical fashion to pain nor are they expected to react identically to illness. We expect that expressive behavior (complaining or moaning) should be more controlled by men, and we frown less when women appear to exploit the illness role through passive and dependent behavior. All patients generally agreed that it was more difficult for men to be patients.

The data indicate that the sex of a patient may substantially affect orientations, needs and reactions to physicians and nurses. Evidence for such differences can be found in many areas. Women were considerably more critical of nursing care than were men, and more frequently expressed fear of negative sanctions from nurses. Women, more than men, emphasized personalized relationships when they discussed the needs of patients. Women were less concerned with problems of co-operation. On the other hand, they tended to focus on nurses' expectations for consideration and respect. When describing their expectations of nurses or when evaluating them, women focused more on personality attributes than men and also gave more emphasis to efficient and prompt care. Women were more critical when a quick response was not forthcoming and they were generally more concerned with efficiency. It is compatible with the male role to receive care and to have someone else maintain the physical surroundings. Women, however, are typically the managers of the home and the performers of major housekeeping tasks. They "know" from experience the standards of personal care and housekeeping, and thus tend to apply them to their judgment of the nursing team. The female patient's concern that the nurse may be critical of her may be indirectly an expression of her awareness that she tends to be demanding.

The more intense emphasis of women on "personality" and "personalized care" may also stem from a relationship which tends to be less personal and less informal than the relationship between nurses and male patients. Unlike his female counterpart, the male patient is probably not too critical of the technical aspect of those functions of the nurse which are reminiscent of the homemaker and mother. He may also derive satisfaction from his relationship to a member of the opposite sex. All this may not only contribute to tolerance of nursing care in general but may give the appearance of more "personalized" relationships. These conjectures may also help to explain the well-known preference nurses have for male patients.

FEARS AND APPREHENSIONS

Apprehensions and fears are the frequent companions of illness. The nature of the patient's concern springs, on the one hand, from his intense preoccupations with himself, with *his* body and with *his* state of mind. His dependence on others, on the other hand, prompts simultaneous concern with the meaning and consequences of their activities. Once the patient enters the hospital his attention may shift back and forth from himself to others. He is sensitive to any physical changes and watchful of any new and unexplained symptoms. He wonders about the outcome of an examination and about the effectiveness of his treatment. He ponders the reliability of those who are responsible for the many procedures and activities which to the patient remain unknown or unknowable, albeit essential.

Patients are preoccupied with safety in the hospital. This is revealed in the preoccupation with protection from mistakes and neglect which prevails when patients talk about their own needs or the needs of other patients. It is expressed in the nature of their recall of past experiences. Not only do patients concentrate on negative experiences, but they select those occurrences which signify the dangers of neglect and lack of attention. Although patients generally deny that they, themselves, are fearful, they have a tendency to ascribe such feelings to other patients.

These apprehensions cannot be entirely alleviated by admiration for the professional groups who are responsible for his treatment, or by a very favorable relationship to the personal physician. Realistic awareness of the complexity of large organizations or simply the fact that among many competent and interested doctors and nurses there may always be a "few who are not competent" may at least put the patient on the alert. In the words of a male patient with gastro—intestinal illness this fear is expressed as follows:

When you are really sick, you are at the mercy of the hospital staff. In my opinion, you've got to have luck on your side. You've got to be lucky enough to get key people in the hospital who are really alert and who wish to do a job; and have someone on the shift at the time you need them who want to give the service or you are just out of luck. I think you could die in one of these hospitals of a heart attack before anybody came in to help you.

Perceptions of the patient role make it unlikely that such fears will be openly expressed by many patients. It is one of the obligations of a patient to have "trust and confidence" in those who care for him. The expression of these concerns could thus be interpreted as a failure to conform to these obligations. Also a free expression of concerns is inhibited by the belief that the courageous, sick persons rather than "sissies" are valued and rewarded.

Apprehensions of certain "dangers" may be directly derived from previous experiences which were, to the patient, indicative of lack of competence, neglect, or lack of interest. They also may be derived indirectly from certain widely held conceptions about the nature of "some" doctors and nurses and the conditions under which they work. Thus, the belief that some nurses do not like "demanding patients" leads to the concern of many patients that asking for too much may result in a slow response to a call or in reduced attention to their needs. The belief that some nurses and some physicians may be prone to oversights because they are inevitably overworked and rushed may further contribute to insecurity. Some patients observed with concern that physicians occasionally are "too busy" to spend enough time to listen to their patients or that a nurse "under the pressure of work" may overlook a physician's order or fail to carry it out in time.

There is evidence in the data that both physicians and nurses, in effect, continuously have to prove themselves. Beliefs such as "some doctors are only interested in money," "some doctors are not interested in their patients," "some doctors are hard-hearted," appear as conceptions about "possibilities" which the patient is ready to have dispelled or confirmed upon first contact with a nurse or a physician in the hospital. Negative conceptions about physicians and nurses, therefore, are typically limited to specific individuals. Without this "specificity" in orientation, patients would find it difficult to sustain the trust and confidence which they consider so important.

The patient's search for safety and security in the hospital may also be indirectly expressed in expectations of good physicians and good nurses. Their behavior or attitudes are seen by the patient as being instrumental in recovery and recuperation. The attitudes of others in the hospital function as clues which are symbolic of good care. From the patient's point of view, the "dedicated nurse" or the nurse who gives "spontaneous and willing services" is a reliable nurse; the "kind" physician who visits the patient regularly is "trustworthy" and "thorough."

Mistakes and neglect are more obviously avoided if the nurse responds promptly, if the physician "knows what is going on" and if the nurse is informed about the doctor's intent. A "prompt response" from a nurse appears as one of the most significant indices for establishing trust and confidence in nursing care.

Patient's perspectives are also shaped by the nature of the social process into which they have entered and by the nature of the interactions to which they are exposed. Those patients who were very responsive to the more impersonal phases of patient-care also tended to be among the more apprehensive. Such patients often felt that they were functioning in a situation in which they could not establish effective and meaningful relationships with others. Feelings of "unrelatedness" were expressed directly in the observation that other patients are often "lonely" and "fearful" or that one sometimes feels like "just a case":

> You're no more . . . no more a patient but just a number . . . you dare not ask a question; you know, they're too busy. And they come around, fine, that's it, "we'll see you next time" and that's it. . . .

The very isolation he fears may be aggravated by the patient himself. In his efforts to be "considerate" and "not demanding" he may intensify the consequences of the anonymity and segmentalization he observes in the modern hospital. Efforts to be a "good patient" may, therefore, trigger disappointments and criticisms of those who do not provide services "spontaneously." The demand for "spontaneous services" appears also to stem from the desire to obtain all necessary services and attentions without having to initiate action. Spontaneous services curtail those interactions in which the patient may be viewed as "too demanding" or "difficult."

The interviews suggest that conformity to the patient role may lead to discrepancies between the behavior and the emotional condition of a patient. The calm appearance of the "good patient" may often hide anxieties and tensions which may not come to the attention of physicians or nurses unless relationships develop which do not trigger fear of criticism or sanction. When patients fail to exercise the restraints on behavior which they think appropriate, guilt or fear may be the consequence. Deviation from the good patient model can be threatening to a patient, unless he is convinced that his behavior was, in the eyes of others, legitimate and/or justified by the condition of his illness:

> I know myself that I talked very rudely to my doctor on one occasion. Afterwards I was ashamed of myself. I was sick or I would never act that way. He is kind and understanding. When I apologized, he acted as if nothing happened. He didn't walk out of the room or tell me off or any of the things that I might do after someone talked to me that way. But I know they have to have a lot of patience with us.

Patients practice an economy of demands, based on their own "principles of exchange." They will indeed curtail their less urgent demands to assure for themselves a prompt response during times when they "really need it." Some patients appear to consider themselves entitled to a certain finite quantity of services which they use sparingly to draw upon during periods of crisis, and many patients seem to feel that their entitlement to service is more severely cut by a demand which does not meet the approval of doctors and nurses:

> I says, "I'm saving that button," I says, "When I push that thing you'll know I need help." She smiled . . . they kind of appreciate that. And from that day, all the times I've been in the hospital I have never pushed the button unless it was something that I actually needed . . . not like some people that drive these nurses crazy; pushing it to raise the bed up; five minutes later push it again. "Oh, that's a little too high." To me it paid dividends, because every time I pushed that button I got service, every dog-gone time.

Discussion

The hospitalized patient is a "captive" who cannot leave the hospital without serious consequence to himself. These consequences do not only apply to the patient's physical condition. Our society expects efforts of the sick to do everything in their power to get well as soon as possible. Open rebellion against the care by competent professional personnel is, therefore, subject to severe criticism. The obligation to be a "co-operative patient" is learned early in life and, as has been indicated, apparently taken very seriously by most patients. More aggressive interpretations of the patient role are not easily verbalized and, apparently, not often realistic alternatives for the patient. Prevalent images of the hospital as a crisis institution, the conception that rights and demands should be governed by the seriousness of the illness and consideration for other, possibly sicker patients, makes it extremely difficult to play the "consumer role" openly and without fear of criticism. Thus, self-assertion as a "client" is controlled by moral commitments to the hospital community as well as by considerations of practical and necessary self-interest.

The norms of our society permit the sick person conditionally passive withdrawal and dependence but, at the same time, emphasize the sick person's responsibility to co-operate in efforts to regain his health.[5] The prevailing image of the hospital increases the pressure to get well fast by enhancing the patient's awareness of the relative degree of the seriousness of his case. Many patients do not have to look far to find and hear about patients who seem more seriously ill. This pressure to get well also is intensified by the observation of "over-worked" and "rushed" nurses and physicians. The pattern of hospital relationships which, for the most part, prevents the development of those relationships which would reduce fears of being rejected or criticized, further discourage patients from exploiting the leniency to which illness *per se* may entitle them. A moral commitment to physicians and nurses is also strengthened by the gratitude and admiration of the sick for those who are "trying to help."

[5] Parsons, T., and R. Fox, "Illness, Therapy and the Modern Urban American Family," in E. G. Jaco (ed.), *Patients, Physicians and Illness*, New York: Free Press, 1st ed., 1958, p. 236.

Patterns of interaction are also affected by the controls which the participants can exert over each other and the understanding which they can have of the function of others. For a variety of reasons, the patient sees few areas in which he has control.

A prerequisite for controlling the actions of others is the capacity to feel competent to judge their achievements. Most patients feel quite helpless in evaluating the knowledge, skill and competence of nurses and physicians. This may be one reason for their intense emphasis on "personality." "Personality" is felt to be associated with, and an indicator of, those more technical qualities which patients do not feel qualified to judge.

Control does not only depend on the capacity to judge the competence or efficiency of others. It also involves the freedom to convey and impose judgments. Even if patients feel quite certain about their judgments, they may feel reluctant to express them if such action may portend a reduction in good patient care.

The institutional context affects the way the patients balance their perceived claims and obligations. They manage to communicate the conditional nature of their claims, the undesirability of their state and, therefore, the importance of their obligations. Their persistent verbal assertions that they should co-operate, that they must not be demanding, underscore their motivation to get well. The problem of patients does not stem from a rejection of major social values but rather from the dissonance created between the desire to broaden the boundaries of what seems a legitimate sphere of control and the tendency to adhere compulsively to behavior which reflects conformity to obligations.[6] The data confirm Parsons'

[6] At times the patient and his significant others among hospital functionaries may be less in disagreement over proper role relationships than significant others involved in their social network. Thus, in some cases patients were found to define their obligations in terms of all the previously discussed considerations. Their relatives, however, emphasized the rights of the paying consumer and expressed their opinion

contention that dependence is, in our society, a primary threat to the valued achievement capacity and that the sick, to this extent, are called upon to work for their own recovery.[7]

Efforts to adhere to obligations are accompanied by the complementary hope that others will meet their obligations in turn and thus will satisfy the patient's expectations. Recognition of the limitations under which hospital functionaries work does not prevent patients from forming "ideal" expectations which call for a model of care which the on-going work processes of the hospital do not readily approximate.[8] The restraint which is exercised by the hospitalized patient is partly an expression of his fears that he may be deprived of important service if he should deviate from acceptable behavior. However, while patients have some notions of the sanctions which can be applied should they violate standards for appropriate behavior, they appear much less certain what they could do if nurses or physicians do not meet their obligations. The feeling of helplessness of patients is partly derived from an incapacity to judge adequately the competence of those who take care of them—in part, from the fact that their experiences do not provide easily defendable criteria for asserting their rights; and partly from their reluctance to use the controls which are available to them.

The interviews showed that patients always knew what they should not be like or what qualities or behavior would make them acceptable to others. Even much more difficult for them was to define what specific tasks they had a right to expect and what expectations could be transformed into active demands without deviating from general

that the patient was "not asking for enough." For a discussion of the role of the third party see W. J. Goode, "A Theory of Role Strain," *American Sociological Review*, 25:483–496, August, 1960.

[7] Parsons, "Definitions of Health and Illness. . . .," *op. cit.*, p. 185.

[8] Reactions to experiences in the hospital assume, therefore, meaning not only in relation to "realistic" anticipations but also in relation to more subtly held "ideal" expectations. The relative discrepancy between "realistic" and "ideal" experiences is a significant variable in the patients' responses to actual experiences.

norms for behavior. A lack of familiarity with what constitutes proper care and cure procedures as well as the fact that a slight change in their condition could alter the legitimacy of demands appears to contribute to this difficulty. Rigid adherence to general rules of conduct appeared to be one way out of this dilemma.

Patients were also limited in the expression of their feelings by the fact that personalized and supportive care was not considered to lie within the sphere of the essential. They clearly felt that they had to subordinate such demands to their own or other patients' needs for physical care. The point of view of patients parallels the common distinction between the legitimacy of somatic and mental illness—a distinction which is accompanied by the notion that somatic illness legitimately entitles the ill to accept dependence as a result of manifestly impaired *physical* capacity for task performance. This dependence is narrowly defined in terms of permitting hospital functionaries to do things for the patient only as long as it is really *physically* necessary. Emotional dependence or other deviations from adult role performance are considered legitimate by most patients only in cases of extreme illness.[9]

The opportunities to obtain personalized care are limited and they are further restricted by patients who as "good patients" withdraw from those on whom they depend and with whom they wish to communicate but whom they do not wish "to bother." The control of the desire to obtain and demand more personal care tends to intensify alienation.[10] The expression of such emotional needs is checked not only by the various pressures to conform to the patient role, but also by the fact that those patient-care activities which direct themselves to the emotional needs of the patient are not institutionalized as role obligations of personnel in the general hospital. Personal concern, support or other emotionally therapeutic efforts tend to be from the patient's point of view pleasant (often unexpected) attributes of otherwise task-oriented personnel. Such activities are quickly praised and even "ideally" seen as the major attributes of the "good" nurse and of the "good" physician. But, since these do not really belong to the manifestly legitimate obligations, they are only reluctantly criticized when missing and rarely directly demanded.

Efforts to adhere to rules of conduct involve also the desire to project a specific image of self.[11] Being accepted is of more than passing importance to the hospitalized patient.[12] Self-consciousness about the norms

---

[9] Patients were not interviewed during the critical phases of their illness when, indeed, their claims may have been different. However, only a few patients in the sample considered themselves recovered. The majority of patients in the cardio–vascular category were recuperating from severe illness and were under orders for bedrest. The majority of the patients in the gastro–intestinal category were under treatment for ulcers or hospitalized for other chronic or acute gastro–intestinal conditions. In all of these cases the conditional nature of rights was bound to create some difficulties—either because of the absence of visible symptoms of illness or because the illness was not considered very serious. Case studies of the more seriously ill patients indicate that anxiety may cause them to "break through" the limits set by their role but that such a breakthrough often demands added efforts since claims, demands or irritations have to be justified. To reestablish an acceptable view of themselves seems to often constitute a major effort for these patients.

[10] Parsons, "Definitions of Health and Illness . . .," *op. cit.*, p. 186. The author points out that the supportive treatment of the sick person "undercuts the alienative component of the motivational structure of his illness."

[11] Goffman, E., "The Nature of Deference and Demeanor," *Amer. Anthropologist*, 58: 473–502, June, 1956; E. Goffman, *Encounters: Two Studies in the Sociology of Interaction*, Indianapolis, Ind.: Bobbs-Merrill, 1961, pp. 99–105.

[12] Efforts to give verbal evidence of conformity may aim at protection from criticism. Deviations tend to be viewed as forgiveable as long as a person gives evidence of "good will." Goode emphasized that failure in role behavior tends to arouse less criticism than failure in emotional commitment to general norms. This principle may be particularly applicable to situations where it is also an obligation of alters to tolerate failures in role behavior. See W. J. Goode, "Norm Commitment and Conformity to Role Status Obligations," *Amer. J. Soc.*, 66: 246–258, November, 1960.

to which one tries to conform may also suggest that the role is in certain respects alien to the performers and that they are not secure in essential social relationships. Efforts to reiterate conformity to general rules of conduct may thus, at least in part, stem from the patient's limited knowledge of the reality of the institutional setting and from fears that he may not be able to measure up to institutionalized expectations. Thus, uncertain about how far he can go before violating prescribed rules for behavior, patients may find their security in efforts to live up to the "letter of the law."[13]

The frequently expressed obligation to co-operate and the persistent attempt to seek approval is, within this frame of reference, not only a diplomatic effort to manipulate relationships to one's own advantage, but also an expression of the patient's perception of the degree of dependency associated with his status. The associated attitudes are thus not merely psychological consequences of the sick role but also reflect the patient's common sense assessments of the abrogation of independence and decision-making associated with his status in the hospital.[14] These deprivations are communicated to the patient beginning with the possessive gesture of the identification bracelet affixed during admission to the hospital, and they are continuously reinforced in daily experiences. The hospital preempts control and jurisdiction, ranging from the assumption of accountability of body

13 See Merton's discussion of ritualism. Anxiety over the ability to live up to institutional expectations may contribute to compulsive adherence to institutional norms. R. K. Merton, *Social Theory and Social Structure*, New York: Free Press, Rev. Ed., 1957, pp. 184–187.

14 Parsons and Fox stressed the need for a "well-timed, well-chosen, well-balanced exercise of supportive and the disciplinary components of the therapeutic process." Institutional factors as well as widely held social values may tend to shift the emphasis too much to the disciplinary components particularly in the setting of the general hospital which incorporate structurally as well as in terms of explicitly or implicitly held attitudes the distinction between the emotionally sick and the physically sick (Parsons and Fox, *op. cit.*, p. 244).

functions to the withholding of information about medical procedures.[15]

The interviews reflect a degree of uncertainty whether physicians and nurses operate as effective teams in close communication or whether the patient ought to function as interpreter and intermediary between these two all important functionaries. Sometimes patients wonder whether they are sources of conflict and competition between medicine and nursing. The physician is seen as supreme authority and patients repeatedly stress that "if something is really seriously wrong," they would turn to the physician. The physician, however, is for the most part not present to observe, respond or intervene. The nurse is continually present, or at least within reach of the call system. She is the physician's representative and interpreter, but she also is the one who has to bear the brunt of work resulting from the physician's orders. She represents hospital rules, and yet she is not infrequently seen by the patient as a potential spokesman for his needs and interests. These perceptions reflect remarkably well the organization of the hospital and the ambiguous position of the nurse at the crossroads of the care and cure structures.[16]

This study suggests that the patient role, like other comparable behavior syndromes organized around a status, are not adequately described by isolating attitudinal and normative responses to the role theme itself, i.e., illness. The full repertory of role behavior must be placed into the context of organizational processes if it is to encompass realistic orientations and behavior display.

The patient role described in this paper is specific to the hospital. The data support and amplify the implication of Merton's use of the role-set as an analytic concept.[17] The patient gropes for appropriate criteria and distinctions in defining his role with

15 Mauksch, H. O., "Patients View Their Roles," *Hospital Progress*, 43: 136–138, October, 1962.

16 Mauksch, H. O., "The Organizational Context of Nursing Practice," in F. Davis (ed.), *The Nursing Profession*, New York: Wiley, 1966, pp. 109–137.

17 Merton, R. K., "The Role Set," *British J. Sociology*, 8:106–120, June, 1957.

reference to a variety of significant relationships. The concept points to the importance of the difference in the power of the members of the role-set *vis-à-vis* the status occupant who has to manipulate between correspondents and to the significance of the support which the status occupant receives from others in like circumstances. However, the relatively isolated patient in the modern single or double hospital room is frequently left to his own devices in coping with differences in real or perceived expectations. This adds to the conditions favoring manifestations of withdrawal or dependence on the approval of others as realistic responses to institutionalized impotence.

The data also suggest a further elaboration of certain aspects of the theoretical model of role behavior. The concept of the role-set refines the differential system of expectations attached to a status from the point of view of the range of counter roles. The data reported in this paper suggest that an additional dimension of role expectation would be a useful addition to theory. Expectations which define a role are normally attributed to the social system surrounding a status.[18] It is suggested that a distinguishable difference exists between the pattern of expectations arising from the structural aspects of the status and those expectations which are attached to the function ascribed to the role. Thus, the role concomitants of being ill can be defined as the functional role segment of the patient role while the consequences of hospitalization, be they perceived or real, could be termed positional role segments.

Concern with the functional segment of the patient role has been evidenced in most previous treatments of the sick role in the

[18] *Ibid.*, p. 113f.

literature.[19] The positional role segment in this study is specific to the hospital. Yet in other settings for patient behavior—be it the home, the clinic or the physician's office —these structural components of the patient role would also bear fruitful sociological investigation. This conceptual scheme aids in structuring the observations of potential strain and conflict between different aspects of the patient role.

This study suggests that a prevailing theme of successful role behavior is the ability of the status occupant to integrate into his own behavior and responses different components from the system of expectations surrounding him. In the case of the patient his efforts to be "a good patient," to meet the obligations as he perceives them and to strive to cooperate in recovery are handicapped by the inadequacy of the communications system within which he functions.[20] Were it more effective, it may permit the patient to cope with his role with greater certainty about rights and obligations, the controls at his disposal and the risks inherent in behavioral experimentation.

[19] Parsons, *The Social System, loc. cit.* Other writers, notably R. Coser, *Life in the Ward*, Lansing, Mich.: Michigan State Univ. Press, 1962, include positional considerations to a greater extent.

[20] Skipper, Jr., J. K., D. L. Tagliacozzo and H. O. Mauksch, "Some Possible Consequences of Limited Communication Between Patients and Hospital Functionaries," *J. Health and Human Behavior*, 5:34–39, Spring, 1964; J. K. Skipper, Jr., "Communication and the Hospitalized Patient", in J. K. Skipper and R. C. Leonard (eds.), *Social Interaction and Patient Care*, Philadelphia: Lippincott, 1965, pp. 61–82.

12

Physical Rehabilitation: A Social-Psychological Approach

Theodor J. Litman

THE IMPACT of a rather sudden, often unexpected, physical disability such as a stroke, polio or a paralytic injury may necessitate considerable personal adjustment on the part of the individual involved. Acts, formerly performed in an unthinking, almost automatic fashion soon represent new challenges to functionless nerve patterns and unresponsive joints and muscles. A rather robust mechanic and avid sportsman, for instance, may suddenly find himself unable to use his legs or grasp even the simplest eating utensils. Such common daily activities as washing, dressing and going to the bathroom become arduous chores. In addition to coming face to face with the realistic limitations and adaptations imposed on him by his condition, however, he may also be forced to modify his conception of self as well. In a society such as ours in which the so-called body-whole and body-beautiful have attained high social value, the disabled is often regarded by himself and others as inferior.

In general, physical rehabilitation envisions the maximum physical, mental, social, vocational and economic recovery possible for any given condition.[1] Cognizant that

the physician alone has neither the time nor skill essential to provide all the necessary services required by the severely involved patient during his course of treatment, the efforts of a highly trained team of medical and para-medical personnel are systematically mobilized to assist the patient achieve maximum independence within the limits of his condition. Although the goals attained may vary with each individual case, the ultimate success of the program lies in a remarkable interplay between the biogenic, sociogenic and psychogenic components of human behavior.

Since the end of the Second World War, the significant role that social and psychological factors may play in the rehabilitation of the physically disabled has been increasingly recognized by physicians and social scientists alike. Although of relatively recent origin, behavioral research in physical rehabilitation has essentially been multidisciplinary in scope. On the whole, three major approaches: psychological, psychotherapeutic and sociological may be delineated.

The Social Psychology of Rehabilitation: A Theoretical Overview

A PSYCHOLOGICAL APPROACH

Perhaps the most outstanding contribution to the development of a social psychology of physical injury has been the classic work of the Lewinean psychologists Barker, Wright, Dembo, *et al.*[2] Drawing

---

[1] The emphasis in this paper will be on physical rather than mental or vocational rehabilitation. The philosophy of most state and federal programs, however, tend to be essentially vocationally oriented. Although traditionally couched in humanitarian terms, such programs

have consistently been tied to a dependency–productivity model dominated by a utilitarian goal of employability. As a result, the so-called unemployed segment of our disabled population (housewives, the aged and children) have been systematically excluded from consideration. For a more penetrating historical analysis of the evolution of our governmental involvement in rehabilitation services, see R. Straus, "Social Change and the Rehabilitation Concept," in M. B. Sussman (ed.), *Sociology and Rehabilitation*, Washington, D.C.: American Sociological Association, 1966, pp. 1–34.

[2] Barker, R. G., *Adjustment to Physical Handicap and Illness*, Social Science Research Council, Social Science Research Bulletin no. 55, 1953.

upon a field theoretical approach, adjustment to physical disability has been conceived in terms of marginal group membership. The position of the disabled, they have suggested, is similar to that of an underprivileged ethnic or religious group. It is thus not only a consequence of the illness per se, but it is derived, in part, from the negative attitudes of the "normal" majority with whom the afflicted individual must live.[2] As an individual with a minority position which usually is not shared with others, he may be looked upon as either "unfortunate" or as a "person who has difficulties." Consequently he may feel a loss of status as a "normal" human being in the devaluative attitude of the "fortunate" to the "unfortunate."[3]

In a series of brilliant publications which have spanned the past two decades, Barker, Wright, Dembo, *et al.*, have dwelt extensively with such problems as acceptance of loss, "coping" with and "over-coming mourning," and adjustment to misfortune associated with physical disability.[4] The

disabled's feelings of shame and inferiority due to a loss in value, they maintain, may be overcome by: (1) an enlargement of his scope of values, (2) containment of the effects of disability, (3) subordination of physique and (4) transformation of comparative values to asset values.

The differential response of the disabled to the total treatment process has attracted the attention of a number of other investigators.[5] Zane and Lowenthal, for instance, proposed that rehabilitation therapy could be used to strengthen and develop positive motivation for treatment by re-channeling the patient's goals and activities so as to reduce stress and increase the likelihood of achievement.[6]

Seidenfeld, on the other hand, concluded that the behavior of the disabled was in large part directly related to the attitude of the patient toward his condition. This in turn, he noted, depended upon: (1) the amount of fear the individual experienced concerning his illness, (2) his pre-illness attitudes toward disability in general, (3) the amount of clear and accurate information available to him about the possible effect of the disease on his future, (4) the kind of experiences the patient had had

For a more detailed review of the psychology of physical rehabilitation see G. L. Leviton (ed.), *The Relationship Between Rehabilitation and Psychology*, Conference held at the Institute of Human Development, Clark University, June 11–13, 1959; L. H. Lofquist (ed.), *Psychological Research and Rehabilitation*, American Psychological Association, 1960; J. F. Garrett and E. Levine (eds.), *Psychological Practices with the Physically Disabled*, New York: Columbia Univ. Press, 1962.

[3] Barker, R. G., "The Social Psychology of Physical Disability," *J. Social Issues*, 4:32, 1948; T. Dembo, G. Ladieu and B. Wright, "Acceptance of Loss-amputations," in J. F. Garrett (ed.), *Psychological Aspects of Physical Disability*, Office of Vocational Rehabilitation, Rehabilitation Service Series no. 210, 1953, p. 80; P. H. Mussen and R. G. Barker, "Attitudes Toward Cripples," *J. Abnormal and Social Psychology*, 39:351–355, 1944.

[4] Dembo, T., G. Ladieu and B. Wright, "Adjustment to Misfortune—A Study on Social Emotional Relationships Between Injured and Non-injured People," Final Report: Army Medical Research and Development Board, Office of the Surgeon General, United States War Department, April 1, 1948; T. Dembo, G. Ladieu and B. Wright, "Adjustment to Misfortune—A Problem of Social Psychological Rehabilitation," *Artificial Limbs*, 3:4–62, Autumn, 1956; R. Barker and B. A. Wright, "The Social Psychology of Adjustment to Physical Disa-

bility," in J. F. Garrett, (ed.), *Psychological Aspects of Physical Disability*. Rehabilitation Services Series no. 210, Office of Vocational Rehabilitation, 1953, pp. 18–32; R. K. White, B. A. Wright and T. Dembo, "Studies in Adjustment to Visible Injuries: Evaluation of Curiosity by the Injured," *J. Abnormal and Social Psychology*, 43:13–28, 1948. An especially penetrating discussion of the concepts "Coping" with a disability and "Overcoming mourning" has been presented in B. A. Wright, *Physical Disability—A Psychological Approach*, New York: Harper, 1960.

[5] For perhaps one of the most comprehensive reviews of the influence of motivation on rehabilitation, see J. R. Barry and M. R. Malinovsky, *Client Motivation for Rehabilitation: A Review*, Univ. Florida Rehabilitation Research Monograph Series no. 1, February, 1965.

[6] Zane, M. D., and M. Lowenthal, "Motivation and Rehabilitation of the Physically Handicapped," *Arch. Physical Med. and Rehab.*, 41:400–407, January, 1960.

with his loved ones and his community as far as his disability was concerned and (5) his belief in his own capacity to be trained to attain independent activity, self-reliance and security.[7]

Shontz, on the other hand, has taken issue with those who have considered motivation as a unitary force. Although he acknowledges that some empirically valid predictive measures of success in specific aspects of rehabilitation might be developed, he has questioned whether any global or general motivational factor, as such, would be uncovered. Instead, he has concluded that client motivation might best be described in terms of a complex interaction of five factors or dimensions: (1) the client's degree of orientation, (2) cooperation, and (3) energy level as well as (4) his breadth of motivation and (5) his ultimate social placement.[8]

[7] Seidenfeld, M. A., "Psychological Problems of Poliomyelitis," in Garrett, *op. cit.*, p. 38; M. A. Seidenfeld and C. L. Lowman, "A Preliminary Report of the Psycho–Social Effects of Poliomyelitis," *J. Consulting Psych.*, 11:30–37, 1947.

[8] Shontz, F., "Concept of Motivation in Physical Medicine," *Arch. Physical Med. and Rehab.*, 38:635–639, October, 1957; F. C. Shontz, "Severe Chronic Illness," in J. F. Garrett and E. Levine, *Psychological Practices with the Physically Disabled*, New York: Columbia Univ. Press, 1962, pp. 410–446; F. C. Shontz and S. L. Fink, "A Method for Evaluating Psycho–Social Adjustment of the Chronically Ill," *Amer. J. Physical Med.*, 40: 63–69, April, 1961; and F. C. Shontz, S. L. Fink and C. E. Hallenbeck, "Chronic Physical Illness As Threat," *Arch. Physical Med. and Rehab.*, 41:143–148, April, 1960. Fink, *et. al.*, While recognizing the value of Shontz's notions, I feel that such a schema has neglected the importance of forces within the individual from which external motivation may be generated. Of particular note they specified two general levels of motivation: Deficiency needs, which arise from some deficit within the client and gross needs, which arise from the natural tendency of a person to strive for mastery of his environment. S. L. Fink, R. Fantz and J. Zinker, "The Growth Beyond Adjustment: Another Look at Motivation," unpublished paper presented at the annual meetings American Psychological Association, St. Louis, September, 1962; S. L. Fink, R. Fantz and F. Zinker, "Relevance of Maslow's Hierarchy to Rehabilitation," *Rehabilitation Counseling Bulletin*, 7: 41–48, December, 1963.

There has also been some attempt to apply reinforcement theory in developing techniques to assist rehabilitation.[9] Lofquist, *et al.*, for instance, have theorized that as the patient matures, he experiences differential reinforcement from the potential reinforcers in his environment and through this process specific needs and abilities become differentiated.[10] Tincher, as well as Maslow and Patterson, on the other hand, using a Rogerian framework, have emphasized the role of self-realization as a primary motivating force in the rehabilitation of the physically handicapped.[11]

In a somewhat different vein, Mueller, Mosak, Thom and Berger have emphasized the role of pre-traumatic personality factors in the motivational activity of the spinal cord injured. According to their reports, extroversion, high feeling tone and little intellectualization seem to be associated with a favorable reaction to disability. Patients whose pre-traumatic personalities have been marked by intense personal effort and ambition, however, often exhibited depression over their slow progress. Nevertheless, the most difficult patients seemed to be the so-called psychopathic deviates, who were inclined to be over-demanding and uncooperative, and demonstrated excessive temper tantrums, profanity and abuse toward the nurses and hospital staff.[12]

[9] Meyerson, L., J. L. Michael, O. H. Mowrer, C. E. Osgood and A. W. Staats, "Learning, Behavior, and Rehabilitation" in L. H. Lofquist, *Psychological Research and Rehabilitation*, American Psychological Association, 1963, pp. 68–111.

[10] Dawis, R. B., G. W. England and L. H. Lofquist, "A Theory of Vocational Adjustment," Minnesota Studies in Vocational Rehabilitation, Bulletin 38, Univ. of Minnesota Press, 1964; R. B. Dawis, G. W. England, L. H. Lofquist, J. R. Barry and W. M. McPhee, "Regional Rehabilitation Institutes," *J. Counseling Psychology*, 11:184–189, 1964.

[11] Tincher, D. H., "Self-Realization of the Handicapped," *J. Rehab.*, 27:24–25, 1961; A. Maslow, *Toward A Psychology of Being*, D. VanNostrand Co., 1962; C. H. Patterson, "A Unitary Theory of Motivation and Its Counseling Implications," *J. Individual Psychology*, 20:17–31, May, 1964.

[12] Mueller, A. D., "Personality Problems of the Spinal Cord Injured," *J. Consulting Psychology*, vol. 14, June, 1950; A. D. Mueller and C. E. Thompson, "Psychological Aspects of the

Siller, on the other hand, has advanced the theory that reaction to a handicap either in oneself or in others is a function of ego strength and the stability of interpersonal relationships.[13]

Finally, in view of their studies of patients undergoing treatment for muscular disabilities, Ripley and associates have concluded that such factors as: (1) biogenic and psychogenic influences; (2) the type of disability; (3) the muscles involved and the physiologic, economic and cosmetic significance of those muscles; (4) the age of onset; (5) the nature of the onset, i.e., acute or insidious; (6) the length of time the symptoms had been present; and (7) the course of the disability (whether constant, slowly progressive, rapid or variable) appeared to be more important in determining adjustment than the physical ailment itself.[14]

THE PSYCHO-THERAPEUTIC APPROACH

Since Adler first suggested that physical defects, whether congenital or acquired, may raise feelings of inferiority or inadequacy within a person which may subsequently create various compensatory mechanisms in behavior, there have been a number of psychiatric reports directed to the emotional aspects of paralytic illness.[15]

Among the more significant contributions have been those of Grayson, Cruickshank, Menninger, Robinson, Finesinger and Bierman.[16] Although rich in clinical insight, such studies, for the most part, have tended to be more impressionistic than empirical in nature. Nevertheless, Fishman, using projective techniques, found that self-image constituted one of the major factors underlying adjustment to leg prosthesis among 48 above-the-knee amputees. The substitution of more realistic life goals, however, seemed to lessen their frustration.[17]

Other investigators have dwelt at length with the mechanism of denial in physical disability. Not all patients are able to face the consequences of their condition. Fisher and Ashenhurst, Hurwitz and Gruen have suggested that anxiety over negative feelings in status or role relationships due to disability may prevent the patient from facing the need for help or effectively benefit from

Problems in Spinal Cord Injuries," *Occupational Therapy and Rehabilitation*, vol. 29, 1950; A. D. Mueller, "Psychological Factors in Rehabilitation of Paraplegic Patients," *Arch. Physical Med. and Rehab.*, 43:151–159, 1962; H. H. Mosak, *Personality Adjustment of Paraplegic Veterans*, Hines Paraplegic Center, 1948; D. Thom, C. F. VonSalzen and A. F. Frommer, "Psychological Aspects of Paraplegic Patients," *Med. Clinics N. Amer.*, 30:473–480, 1946; S. Berger, "Paraplegia," in Garrett, *op. cit.*, pp. 46–59; S. Berger and J. F. Garrett, "Psychological Problems of the Paraplegic Patient," *J. Rehab.*, 18:15–17, September–October, 1952.

13 Siller, J., "Reactions to Physical Disability by the Disabled and the Non-disabled," *Amer. Psychologist*, 14:351, 1959.

14 Ripley, H. S., C. Bohengel and A. T. Milhorat, "Personality Factors in Patients with Muscular Disability," *Amer. J. Psychiatry*, 99: 781–787, 1943.

15 Adler, A., "Study of Organ Inferiority and Its Physical Compensation," *Nerv. and Ment. Dis. Monograph*, no. 24, 1917; A. Adler *The Practice and Theory of Individual Psychology*,

New York: Harcourt-Brace, 1924; R. Dreikurs, "The Socio–Psychological Dynamics of Physical Disability; A Review of the Adlerian Concept," *J. Social Issues*, 4:44, 1948.

16 Grayson, M., A. Powers and J. Levi, *Psychiatric Aspects of Rehabilitation*, Rehabilitation Monograph no. II, Institute of Physical Medicine and Rehabilitation, New York: Bellevue Medical Center, 1952; "The Concept of Acceptance in Physical Rehabilitation," *Military Surgeon*, 107:221–226, September, 1950; W. M. Cruickshank, "The Impact of Physical Disability on Social Adjustment," *J. Social Issues*, 4:79, 1948; K. Menninger, "Psychiatric Aspects of Physical Disability," in Garrett, *op. cit.*, pp. 8–17; H. A. Robinson and J. E. Finesinger, "A Framework for the Psychology of Poliomyelitis," *Nervous Child*, 11:10–17, January, 1956; H. A. Robinson and J. E. Finesinger, "The Significance of Work Inhibition for Rehabilitation," *Social Work*, 2:22–31, October, 1957; H. A. Robinson, J. E. Finesinger and J. S. Bierman, "Psychiatric Considerations in the Adjustment of Patients with Poliomyelitis," *New England J. Med.*, 254:975–980, April–June, 1956.

17 Fishman, S., "Self-concept and Adjustment to Leg Prosthesis," unpublished doctoral dissertation, Columbia Univ., 1949; "Amputee Needs, Frustrations, and Behavior," *Rehabilitation Literature*, 20:322–329, November, 1959.

the services offered.[18] Barry and Malinovsky, however, feel that such a view greatly oversimplifies the case since it fails to take into account the rather complex network or extrapersonal determinants and personally valid reasons that may underlie the vacillations and conflict that accompany movement through the rehabilitation commitment.[19]

[18] Fisher, S., "Mechanisms of Denial in Physical Disabilities," *Arch. in Neurol. and Psychiatry*, 80:784, 1958; E. Ashenhurst, L. Hurwitz and A. Gruen, "Motivational and Structural Factors in the Denial of Hemiplegia," *Arch. in Neurology*, 3:315–317, 1960; J. R. Barry and M. R. Malinovsky, *op. cit.*, pp. 18–19.

[19] Davis, F., "Polio in the Family—A Study of Crisis in Family Process," unpublished doctoral dissertation, Univ. of Chicago, June, 1958; F. Davis, *Passage Through Crisis, Polio Victims and Their Families*, New York: Bobbs-Merrill Co., 1963; "Definition of Time and Recovery in Paralytic Polio Convalescence," *Amer. J. Soc.*, 61:582–588, May, 1956; H. R. Kelman, "Experiment in the Rehabilitation of Nursing Home Patients," *Public Health Reports*, 77:356–366, April, 1962; H. R. Kelman and J. N. Muller, "Rehabilitation in Nursing Home Residents," *Geriatrics*, 17:402–411, June, 1962; H. R. Kelman, "Evaluation of Rehabilitation for the Long Term Ill and Disabled Patient: Some Persistent Research Problems," *J. Chronic Dis.*, 17:631–639, 1964; J. N. Muller, "Rehabilitation Evaluation—Some Social and Clinical Problems," *Amer. J. Public Health*, 51:403–409, March, 1961; J. N. Muller, J. S. Tobis and H. R. Kelman, "The Rehabilitation of Nursing Home Residents," *Am. J. Public Health*, 53:243–247, February, 1963; H. R. Kelman, M. Lowenthal and J. N. Muller, "Community Status of Discharged Rehabilitation Patients: Results of a Longitudinal Study," *Arch. Physical Med. and Rehab.*, 47:670–675, October, 1966; H. R. Kelman, J. N. Muller and M. Lowenthal, "Post-hospital Adaptation of a Chronically Ill and Disabled Rehabilitation Population," *J. Health and Human Behavior*, 5:108–113, Summer–Fall, 1964; H. R. Kelman and J. N. Muller, "The Role of the Hospital and the Care of the Ambulatory Chronically Ill and Disabled Patient After Discharge," *Amer. J. Public Health*, 57:107–117, January, 1967; M. B. Sussman, *Family Unit Critique of Selected Scales and Indexes Available for Measuring the Relationship of Family Behavior to the Etiology in the Course of Chronic Illness and Disability*, unpublished paper, working draft, part I, Project 94U44, Association for the Aid of Crippled Children, 1960; "Social Psychological Factors to Individual Patient Needs," part of a larger study entitled: "Individual Patient's Needs," un-

THE SOCIOLOGICAL APPROACH

With such notable exceptions as Davis' pioneering work on family adjustment to poliomyelitis, Kelman's studies of after-care and Sussman's investigations into the relationships of social–psychological factors in rehabilitation, sociologists for the most part have been relatively slow in coming to grips with the theoretical and empirical implications of rehabilitation and disability. The classic conceptualization of the sick role by Parsons,[20] for instance, completely fails to take into consideration the consequences of long-term chronic illness. Moreover, as Freidson has pointed out, as formulated, such a concept is severely limited in its capacity to facilitate analysis of stigmatized roles imputed from what may be essentially incurable, though possibly improvable, deviance.[21]

But if sociological inquiry into the field of physical rehabilitation has generally paled before that of the other approaches, its contributions have none the less been significant. The theoretical orientation has essentially been one of social behaviorism. Litman, for instance, using an interactionist approach, found rather strong evidence that self-conception and rehabilitation response were directly associated. Orthopedically disabled patients who were able to maintain a favorable conception of self appeared to consistently respond well to treatment while those with negative self-conceptions tended to perform below expectations. This was true whether performance was measured by a composite physician–therapist evaluation or rating of his performance in each phase of therapeutic endeavor separately. Moreover, the relationship continued to remain

published paper, 1960; M. B. Sussman, *et al.*, "Rehabilitation in Tuberculosis: Predicting the Vocational Economic Status of Tuberculosis Patients," Western Reserve Univ., 1964.

[20] Kassebaum, G. G., and B. O. Baumann, "Dimensions of the Sick Role in Chronic Illness," *J. Health and Human Behavior*, 6:16–27, Spring, 1965.

[21] Freidson, E., "Disability As Social Deviance," in M. B. Sussman (ed.), *Sociology and Rehabilitation*, American Sociological Association, 1967, p. 81.

strong even when the patient's rehabilitation potential was held constant.

Interestingly enough, there was also a good deal of evidence that the nature of the self-conception, i.e., whether bitterness or resignation, may play an important part in determining the patient's rehabilitation response. A number of cases were reported of patients who, despite their negative conceptions of themselves and bitter feelings toward their physical condition, exhibited considerable motivation during their course of treatment and received excellent evaluative scores from the therapeutic staff. Apparently, such individuals possessed such a distasteful conception of themselves that they directed every effort toward the alteration of the physical state believed to be the cause of it. In Meadean terms, such patients were seemingly unwilling to give in to the depreciated perceived image of themselves as seen in the eyes of others, the "me," and consequently sought its modification through alteration of the physical state believed to be its source. The rehabilitation process, then, offered the "I" an opportunity to change the unfavorable "me."

Unfortunately, in such cases, once the patient's maximum physical capacity has been reached and he is forced to face up to the limitations of his condition, i.e., he will never again be physically "normal," productive effort begins to decline and a desperate search for miracle cures, new and different treatment procedures and facilities ensues.[22]

In addition, there was some indication that although such remedial measures, as more extensive public education concerning the potential value of rehabilitation and the importance of providing a more positive atmosphere within which the disabled's conception of self may develop, might indeed

be beneficial, the apparent inability of the populous to either *take the role* of the disabled when well or *play the role* at onset would seem to mitigate against their success.[23] Almost 70 per cent of the patients studied, for instance, expressed the belief that people outside the hospital really did not understand the problems of the physically disabled. The single, most consistent, theme advanced to explain this observation was an apparent inability to adequately take the role of the other. As one patient so succinctly put it:

No, they're healthy and strong, busy doing things. They don't understand how hard it is for us to do things that they take for granted every day. If you haven't experienced it, you just can't know.

Another expressed it this way:

I have seen new patients when they came in. They don't realize what polio is and how long it takes to get well. They don't realize it is a long process. Physical medicine is quite new and many don't realize it—even the doctors don't.

Interestingly enough, several staff members expressed a similar point of view in personal conversation and sincerely wondered how they, themselves, would respond under similar circumstances. Moreover, many patients were quick to admit that they too were completely unaware of the ramifications of physical disability, its limitations, implications and possibilities of recovery before they were stricken:

---

[22] Litman, T. J., "The Influence of Concept of Self and Life Orientation Factors upon the Rehabilitation of Orthopedic Patients," unpublished doctoral dissertation, Univ. of Minnesota, 1961; "Self-conception and Physical Rehabilitation," in A. M. Rose (ed.), *Human Behavior and Social Processes*, chap. 29, pp. 537–574; "The Influence of Self-conception and Life Orientation Factors in the Rehabilitation of the Orthopedically Disabled," *J. Health and Human Behavior*, 3:249–257, Winter, 1962.

[23] See W. Coutu, "Role-playing Versus Role-taking: An Appeal for Clarification," *Amer. Sociological Rev.*, 16:180–187, April, 1951. Role-playing in this sense, refers to behavior, performance and the conduct of overt activity. Role-taking, on the other hand, is conceived as strictly a mental or cognitive, empathic, activity in which a person momentarily pretends to himself that he is another and imaginatively projects himself into the other's perceptual field. In so doing, he is able to apprehend the other's point of view to anticipate that person's behavior and then act accordingly.

No, I didn't, until I came here—a person doesn't really understand what a paralysis is unless they have experienced it. A majority don't . . . I know my own experience. I don't think I ever saw a person crippled till I saw myself, i.e., this bad—people don't really think about it much till it happens to them or someone close to them or working with them.

In view of the Rose–Cottrell thesis that one's degree of adjustment to a future role varies directly with the degree of clarity with which that future role is defined, it is not surprising that such patients may find a great deal of difficulty coming to grips with their illness and its consequences.[24]

Rabinowitz and Mitsos, on the other hand, offer a highly sophisticated conceptualization of the rehabilitation process in terms of social change. Motivation for recovery, they argued, constitutes the manifestation of a complex of values and relationships which are shared by the patient as well as those who work with him. The process of rehabilitation, then, may be viewed as a sequence of planned re-socializations which involve both the disabled and their environment.[25]

[24] See A. M. Rose, *Theory and Method in the Social Sciences*, Univ. of Minnesota Press, 1954, p. 24; L. S. Cottrell, Jr., "Some Problems in Social Psychology," *Amer. Sociological Rev.*, 15: 709–711, December, 1950. On the other hand, the accomplishments of other patients with similar disabilities may serve not only to exemplify what can be accomplished, but to provide an atmosphere of hope and friendly competition as well. Such patients provide a ready reference for identity. "Oh yes," one patient commented, "look at the guys in the wheel chairs—they can move. They tell you what they went through, their treatment, how they improved in time. There's no encouragement when someone tells you, when they have not had it." Moreover, many rehabilitation centers regularly employ disabled individuals as staff members, i.e., psychiatrists and therapists, which in turn serves as a beneficial stimulus to patient response.

[25] Rabinowitz, H. S., and Spiro B. Mitsos, "Rehabilitation As Planned Social Change: A Conceptual Framework," *J. Health and Human Behavior*, 5:2–14, Spring, 1964; H. S. Rabinowitz, "Motivation for Recovery; Four Social–Psychologic Aspects," *Arch. Physical Med. and Rehab.*, 42:799–807, December, 1961. Moreover, a similar notion has been advanced by B. E. Cogswell, "Rehabilitation of the Paraplegic: Process of Socialization," unpublished paper presented before the 6th World Congress of Sociology, Evian, France, September 4–11, 1966.

Meanwhile, Thomas has reported on an attempt to analyze the problems of disability from the perspective of role-theory. Five disability-related roles are described: the "disabled patient," "handicapped performer," "helped person," "disability comanager," and the "public-relations man." In addition, the problems of role discontinuity, role conflict, conflict of role definition, role strain and the difficulties of role synchronization are elaborated.[26]

The relationship between social class and reaction to disability, however, seems to be somewhat less clear. Dow, for example, found neither the reaction to disability nor the emphasis attached to physique were distinguished by social class.[27] Yet Kronick, in a study of patients undergoing rehabilitation for stroke, noted a marked social class effect on familial reaction to illness. Families of higher socio–economic status, she observed, tended to respond more deliberately to the illness than those from the lower class. Lower-class patients and those cared for by people who were more anomic seemed to fare better than their higher class, less anomic fellows. The failure of the lower-class families to make special arrangements for the patient or disrupt their normal activities for him, she suggests, may force the patient to look after himself and consequently make greater use of his unimpaired muscles and residual abilities.[28]

Finally Kutner and associates have reported rather promising application of the therapeutic community concept to the treatment of the chronically ill.[29] Yet, as

[26] Thomas, E. J., "Problems of Disability from the Perspective of Role Theory," *J. Health and Human Behavior*, 7:2–13, Spring, 1966.

[27] Dow, T. E., Jr., "Optimism, Physique, and Social Class in Reaction to Disability," *J. Health and Human Behavior*, 7:14–19, Spring, 1966.

[28] Kronick, J., "The Rehabilitation of Stroke Patients: An Experimental Analysis of the Effects of Physical and Social Factors in Determining Recovery," unpublished report, Department of Social Work and Social Research, Bryn Mawr College, 1962.

[29] Kutner, B., *et al.*, "A Therapeutic Community in a General Hospital: Adaptation to a Rehabilitation Service," *J. Chronic Dis.*, 16: 179–186, 1963; B. Kutner, "Modes of Treatment of the Chronically Ill," *Gerontologist*, 4: 44–48, June, 1964; B. Kutner, "Modes of Treating the Chronically Ill," *Proc. Symposium on*

Sussman warned, such efforts may require considerable re-conceptualization to account for the differences that exist between disability and illness, the social roles associated with these conditions as well as the involvement of multiple social systems in the definition, identification and treatment of the disabled.[30]

Despite the significant contributions cited above, the potential value of sociological analysis to the field of rehabilitation probably was not fully crystallized until the so-called Carmel Conference of 1965. This symposium, held under the joint auspices of the American Sociological Association and the Vocational Rehabilitation Administration, was entirely devoted to an exploration of the usefulness and applicability of current sociological theory and research to the field of rehabilitation. The proceedings, which were later compiled and published as a monograph under the editorship of Sussman, received wide-spread distribution to all members of the association.[31] Although most of the participants were much better known for their contributions to empirical research, sociological knowledge and social theory than for their experience or involvement in rehabilitation per se, a number of stimulating proposals were put forth. One of the most promising of these was Freidson's analysis of disability and rehabilitation in terms of a model of social deviance. Unfortunately, he noted, disability may pose an analytic problem for the sociologist because of the juxtaposition between the stigma and social legitimation attached to long-term chronic illness.[32] Nevertheless, Scott points out that

the actual form the deviancy will take may well be determined by the rehabilitation process itself. That is, the process of rehabilitation tends to serve a socialization function, preparing the disabled to play a type of deviant role. In contrast to illness which is often curable, he notes that disability normally is not. While a person who is ill may return to a socially accepted normal role, the role of the disabled remains a deviant one.[33] Myers, on the other hand, in a penetrating discussion of the consequences and prognoses of disability, calls for greater use of control groups in research and suggests the possible value of applying theories of the middle range to the field of rehabilitation.[34] Finally, Suchman proposed two models for evaluative research in rehabilitation. The first, a basic research model, facilitates analysis of rehabilitation as an intervening variable. The second, an applied evaluative model, may be used to determine the effectiveness of rehabilitation agencies and personnel in influencing the relationship between the occurrence of disability and its consequences. He concluded that the major contribution sociological theory can make in this area is through conceptual analysis of the conditions and events which predate the rehabilitation process itself.[35]

71–99. Also see F. Davis, "Deviance Disavowal: The Management of Strained Interaction by the Visibly Handicapped," in H. S. Becker (ed.), *The Other Side, Perspectives in Deviance*, New York: Free Press, 1964.

[33] Scott, R. A., "Comments about Interpersonal Processes of Rehabilitation," in M. B. Sussman, (ed.), *ibid.*, p. 135. In a somewhat similar vein, Schlesinger noted that as far as the disabled are concerned, the transition from "ill" to "well" is not a clear one and the social transitions are not well established. As a result, the patient may well experience considerable difficulty in evaluating his post-dramatic state. See L. E. Schlesinger, "Psychological and Social Losses Associated with Cerebral Vascular Accidents," *Rehab. Counseling Bulletin*, June, 1964, p. 126.

[34] Myers, J. K., "Consequences and Prognosis of Disability," *ibid.*, pp. 35–51.

[35] Suchman, E. A., "A Model for Research and Evaluation of Rehabilitation," *ibid.*, pp. 52–70.

Research and Long-term Care, Jewish Hospital of St. Louis, September 25–27, 1963, pp. 48–57; F. Racker, E. F. Delagi and A. F. Abramson, "The Therapeutic Community: An Approach to Rehabilitation," *Arch. Physical Med. and Rehab.*, 44:257–261, May, 1963.

[30] Sussman, M. B., "Outcomes and Outlooks," in *Sociology and Rehabilitation, op. cit.*, p. 232.

[31] Sussman, M. B. (ed.), *Sociology and Rehabilitation*, American Sociological Association, 1966. Also see C. Safilios–Rothschild, *The Sociology of Rehabilitation*, New York: Random House, 1968; and J. Roth and E. Eddy, *Rehabilitation of the Unwanted*, New York: Atherton Press, 1968.

[32] Freidson, E., "Disability As Social Deviance," in M. B. Sussman (ed.), *ibid*, pp.

In summarizing the social–psychological approach, we find it to be an amalgamation of several theoretical approaches rather than a single, cohesive whole. While each of the disciplines has tended to conceive the field in terms of their own respective points of view, at least two things seem to be clear. First, there is considerable evidence that adjustment and reaction to physical disability is, to a large extent, dependent upon the attitudes of the patient himself and those of his non-injured fellows. Second, the individual's pre-traumatic personality, social experiences, family constellation patterns, etc., may also play an important part in determining his response to treatment.

Unfortunately, however, communication and interaction between the various disciplines involved has generally been somewhat less than desired. While most investigators have tended to confine publication of their results to their own specialty journals, few are either able or do take the time to keep abreast of the contributions made by others outside their own specific field. Thus, as Barry and Malinovsky note, concepts which have long been utilized in one field often are re-discovered and proposed by another as a tremendously new and important contribution when in fact they are hardly new at all. The consequence of such interdisciplinary parochialism has been an excessive degree of conceptual confusion, empirical fragmentation and theoretical eclecticism.[36]

The Social Psychology of Physical Rehabilitation: An Empirical Review

A PROBLEM OF MEASUREMENT

But if the social psychology of rehabilitation has been marked by a theoretical

[36] Barry and Malinovsky, *op. cit.*, p. 53. One attempt to breach this communication problem has been the publication: *Rehabilitation Literature*. For a more definitive discussion of the tautological relationship between theory and method and its consequences upon evaluative research, see A. M. Rose, "The Relation of Theory and Method," in L. Gross (ed.), *Colloquium on Sociological Theory*, New York: Harper & Row, 1966.

pluralism, attempts at more definitive empirical analysis have been no less plagued by the rudimentary nature of its system of measurement. Stinson, for instance, as well as Moskowitz and McCann have clearly demonstrated that medical diagnosis alone does not always accurately reflect the physical capacity of the ill or disabled.[37] The validity of using re-hospitalization as a criterion of rehabilitation success has been seriously questioned by Kelman, *et al.*[38] Finally Neff has suggested that any exploratory research must be preceded by better descriptive observation.[39]

In the past few years, however, the problem has attracted the attention of several investigators. Hoff and Mead, for instance, have sought to obtain a more objective evaluation of rehabilitation results through development of an ordinal scale.[40] Sokolow, Rusk and associates have developed a functional method of evaluating disability which takes into account the medical, social, psychological and vocational aspects of disability.[41] Along the same line, Ellwood,

[37] Stinson, M. B., "Medical Care and Rehabilitation for the Aged," *Geriatrics*, 8:226–229, April, 1963; E. Moskowitz and C. B. McCann, "Classification of Disability and Chronically Ill and Aging," *J. Chronic Dis.*, 5:342–346, March, 1957.

[38] Kelman, H. R., M. Lowenthal and J. N. Muller, "Community Status of Discharged Rehabilitation Patients: Results of a Longitudinal Study," *Arch. Physical Med. and Rehab.*, 47:670–675, October, 1966.

[39] Neff, W. S., "Research Needs and Perspectives," *Rehabilitation Record*, 5:17–20, March–April, 1964.

[40] Hoff, W. I., and M. Sedgwick, "Evaluation of Rehabilitation Outcome: An Objective Assessment of the Physically Disabled," *Amer. J. Physical Med.*, 44:113–121, 1965.

[41] Rusk, H. A., and J. Sokolow, *Developing and Standardizing a Method of Classifying the Physical, Social, Emotional, and Vocational Capacities of the Disabled Individual Functionally*, O. V. R. Project S. P. 154, New York Univ.–Bellevue Medical Center, Department of Physical Medicine and Rehabilitation; J. Sokolow, J. E. Silson, E. J. Taylor, E. T. Anderson and H. A. Rusk, "Functional Approach to Disability Evaluation," *J. Amer. Med. Assoc.*, 167:1575–1584, July, 1958; J. Sokolow, J. E. Silson, J. E. Taylor, E. T. Anderson and H. A. Rusk, "A Method for the Functional Evaluation of Disability," *Arch. Physical Med. and Rehab.*, 40:421–428, October, 1959; J. Sokolow, J. E. Silson, E. J. Taylor, E. T. Anderson and H. A.

et al., have been experimenting with the use of a multiphasic screening program using computers at the American Rehabilitation Foundation's Kenny Rehabilitation Institute.[42] In addition, the work of Nagi, Wylie, Katz, Shontz and Fink should be mentioned.[43]

The possible sources of error involved in making disability evaluations have been discussed at length by Kessler and Manning.[44] According to McBride, the results of disability should be correlated with subsequent rehabilitation and restoration.[45] Mueller, however, has suggested that all rehabilitation services should ultimately be judged qualitatively in terms of their success or failure in restoring a client's functioning to the limit of his potentialities. Therefore, a reliable measure of disability requires separation of the measurement of current

performance from estimates of prognosis.[46]

In perhaps one of the most discursive examinations of the problem of measurement in rehabilitation research to date, Kelman and Willner have cited the need for more objective, verifiable techniques. The development of more rigorous measuring instruments, they propose, would require greater precision in the specification of the goals of rehabilitation. Yet, clarification of the problem of criteria must precede measurement construction. The development of more precise measures, they concluded, thus depends upon improved differentiation and delineation of the physiological and structural components of the rehabilitation process from the mediating psychological and social influences.[47]

Behavioral Research in Physical Rehabilitation: A Status Report

In spite of its multi-disciplinary character and methodological imprecision, a rather impressive body of knowledge has evolved concerning the attitudes of the disabled and the influence of various social and psychological factors upon the rehabilitation of the physically disabled. Some of the more significant findings will be briefly examined below. As indicated earlier, there appears to be a good deal of evidence that adjustment and reaction to physical disability is to a large extent dependent upon not only the attitudes of the disabled themselves but those of their non-injured fellows as well.

ATTITUDES OF THE DISABLED

In 1953, Barker, *et al.*, noted that relatively little research had been done on assessing the attitudes of the disabled toward

Rusk, "A New Approach to the Objective Evaluation of Physical Disability," *J. Chronic Dis.*, 15:105–112, 1962.

[42] Schoening, H. A., L. Anderegg, D. Bergstrom, M. Fonda, N. Steinke and P. Ulrich, "Numerical Scoring of Self-care Status of Patients," *Arch. Physical Med. and Rehab.*, 46: 689–697, October, 1965.

[43] Nagi, S. Z., "A Study in the Evaluation of Disability and Rehabilitation Potential: Concepts, Methods, and Procedures," *Amer. J. Public Health*, 54:1568–1579, September, 1964; C. M. Wylie, "Measurement in Medicine and Public Health," *J. Chronic Dis.*, 15:381–387, 1962; C. M. Wylie and B. K. White, "A Measure of Disability," *Arch. Environ. Health*, 8:834–839, June, 1964; S. Katz, "Definitions of Terms for Index of Independence in Activities of Daily Living," *J. Chronic Dis.*, 9:55–63, 1959; S. Katz, A. B. Ford, R. W. Moskowitz, B. A. Jackson and M. W. Jaffe, "Studies of Illness in the Aged: The Index of ADL, A Standardized Measure of Biological and Psycho-Social Function," *J. Amer. Med. Assoc.*, 185:914–919, September, 1963; F. C. Shontz and S. L. Fink, "A Method for Evaluating Psycho–Social Adjustment of the Chronically Ill," *Amer. J. Physical Med.*, 40:63–69, April, 1961. For a more comprehensive discussion of the problems of measurement, see Barry and Malinovsky, *op. cit.*, pp. 40–51.

[44] Kessler, H., and G. C. Manning, "The Effect of Personal Opinion on Disability Evaluation," *J. Occupational Med.*, 5:411–417, September, 1963.

[45] McBride, E. D., *Disability Evaluation and Principles of Treatment of Compensable Injuries*, Philadelphia: J. B. Lippincott, 1963.

[46] Muller, J. N. "Rehabilitation Evaluation— Some Social and Clinical Problems," *Amer. J. Public Health*, 51:403–409, March, 1961.

[47] Kelman, H. R., and A. Willner, "Problems in Measurement and Evaluation of Rehabilitation," *Arch. Physical Med. and Rehab.*, 43:172–181, April, 1962.

their own disabilities. Yet, an extensive review of the pertinent literature, some 14 years later, led Yuker and associates to reach the same conclusion.[48] They found that most of the measures developed for use with the disabled were directed toward specific disabilities, i.e., the deaf, the blind, the orthopedically handicapped. Only a few had been designed for persons with various non-specialized disabilities and none could be considered appropriate for use with both the disabled and non-disabled. On the whole, three types of techniques had been used: self-inventories, attitude scales and projective sentence completion.

The attitudes of the disabled, either toward themselves or toward other disabled persons, tend to be rather difficult to measure, since they presumably deal with ego-involved attitudes with strong emotional components. Although most of the instruments available have been designed for specific disability groups, a significant number such as Christopherson and Swartz's Perceptual Modification Scale, Wright and Remmers' Purdue Handicapped Problems Inventory Scale, Berger's Sentence Completion Test, Braen and Weiner's Fielding Story Completion Test and our own (Litman) Disability Self-conception Scale can be used with a broader group of disabilities. In addition, Richardson, *et al.*, have devised a self-description technique that can be used by children with any type of disability.[49]

The use of Likert-type scales in the measurement of attitudes toward the disabled has been a relatively recent development. Only one other scale (Roeher's, 1959) in addition to Yuker and associates' own Attitudes Toward Disabled Persons Scale (ATDP) has been designed for disabled persons in general.[50] A number of other

[48] Yuker, H. E., J. R. Block and J. H. Younng, "The Measurement of Attitudes Toward Disabled Persons," Human Resources Study no. 7, Albertson, N.Y.: Human Resources Center, 1967. We are especially indebted to Dr. Yuker and his staff for compiling this extremely comprehensive compendium. Much of the discussion that follows concerning studies on the attitudes of the disabled and non-disabled has been drawn from it.

[49] *Ibid.*, pp. 14–16.   [50] *Ibid.*, p. 16.

investigators, however, have attempted to adapt the Osgood, Suci and Tannenbaum Semantic Differential technique to assess self-attitudes toward disability.[51]

ATTITUDES OF THE NON-DISABLED

In contrast to the paucity of activity noted above, there has been considerable effort devoted to the development of measures of the attitudes of the non-disabled toward disability. Perhaps the first to study comparative attitudes toward different disabilities and other groups was the psychologist E. K. Strong in 1931,[52] while the first person to investigate attitudes toward a specific disability group was Schaefer in 1930.[53] Probably the most extensive work in this area, however, has been that of Yuker and associates.[54] Experiments with the

[51] *Ibid*, p. 15.
[52] Strong, E. K., *Change of Interests with Age*, Stanford: Stanford Univ. Press, 1931.
[53] Schaefer, F. M., "The Social Traits of the Blind," unpublished Master's thesis, Loyola University, 1930; Yuker, *et al., op. cit.*, p. 6.
[54] Yuker, H. E., J. R. Block and W. P. Campbell, *A Scale to Measure Attitudes Toward Disabled Persons*, Human Resources Study no. 5, Albertson, N.Y.: Human Resources Center, 1960; H. E. Yuker, J. R. Block and W. P. Campbell, *Disability Types and Behavior*, Human Resources Study no. 6, Albertson, N.Y.: Human Resources Center, 1962; J. R. Block and H. E. Yuker, "A Scale to Measure Job Satisfiers and Dissatisfiers," paper presented before the annual meetings of the American Psychological Association, Los Angeles, Calif., September, 1964; J. R. Block, H. E. Yuker, W. J. Campbell and K. B. Melvin, "Some Correlates of Job Satisfaction Among Disabled Workers," *Personnel and Guidance J.*, 42:803–810, 1964; H. E. Yuker, "Attitudes As Determinants of Behavior," *J. Rehab.*, 31:15–16, November–December, 1965; H. E. Yuker, J. R. Block and J. H. Younng, *The Measurement of Attitudes Toward Disabled Persons*, Human Resources Study no. 7, Albertson, N.Y.: Human Resources Center, 1967. In light of extensive field study, Yuker, *et al.*, feel that the ATDP is an extremely valid measuring instrument. Although there is some question concerning its predictive value for any one individual, it appears to be an excellent summary measure for groups of individuals. Moreover, to the extent that the instrument correlates with other measures of behavior such as those involving prejudice toward other groups, they contend that it provides a general measure of prejudice toward disability groups as well. For a more extensive discussion of the ATDP, see *ibid*, pp. 75–81.

Attitude Toward Disabled Persons Scale indicate that attitudes toward the disabled seem to be correlated with attitudes toward specific disability group and "disabled people in general." Thus Bates notes that the term "disability" may have several connotations, although it usually refers to obvious physical impairments and sensory defects.[55]

While Bates appears to be the only investigator to examine differences between attitudes towards persons with a specific disability and attitudes toward persons who have been labeled "disabled" and "handicapped," Siller has experimented with a multi-dimensional attitude scale to assess factors analytically and various components underlying such attitudes. Attitudes toward the disabled, he concluded, are not only multi-dimensional and measurable, but they apparently are a function of the type and severity of the disability, specific experiences with handicapped persons and possibly certain other individual personality determinants as well.[56]

SOCIAL DISTANCE

A number of other investigators have been struck by the variations in social distance that accrue due to the differential perception of various disability categories. Although such studies have seldom been subjected to statistical test, their findings have generally tended to be consistent. When rated in terms of occupational capacity or professional relationship, the physically disabled seem to be more generally preferred over those afflicted with sensory impairments, i.e., deafness or blindness. The latter, in turn, tend to be more generally preferred over those with brain damage, i.e., cerebral palsy, epilepsy or aphasic hemiplegia.[57]

Such preferences, however, seem to be less clear cut when the rating is made in terms of personal qualities and social acceptance. Whiteman and Lukoff, for instance, found that blindness was considered to be more unpleasant than a physical handicap. Richardson, Hastorf, Goodman and Dornbusch reported that the more disfiguring disabilities were rated the least socially acceptable by both disabled and non-disabled children alike. Gowman, on the other hand, noted in a study of 104 high school students that there was a decided tendency to fear sensory loss (blindness, deafness) more than disfiguring losses, e.g., loss of an arm or a burn, when the self was the point of reference. Yet when the object of acceptance was a possible mate, the reverse was true. Apparently, as Yuker suggests, a disfiguring disability may seem less acceptable in others, while the functionally limiting handicaps are considered less acceptable for self and others when the relationship is merely one of education, training or employment.[58]

[55] Yuker, Block and Younng, op. cit., pp. 74–75; R. E. Bates, "The Meaning of 'Disabled' and 'Handicapped': Their Relationship to Each Other and Specific Defects,' unpublished doctoral dissertation, Univ. of Houston, 1965; R. E. Bates, P. Rothaus and S. E. Vineberg, "Limitation of the Term 'Disabled' in Attitude Measurement," paper presented before the annual meetings of the American Psychological Association, Chicago, September, 1965.

[56] Siller, J. and A. Chipman, "Factorial Structure and Correlates of the Attitudes Toward Disabled Persons Scale," Educ. and Psychol. Measurement, 24:831–840, 1964; J. Siller, "Reactions to Physical Disability," Rehab. Counseling Bull., 7:12–16, 1963; J. Siller, "Personality Determinants of Reaction to the Physically Disabled," Amer. Found. for Blind Res. Bull., 7:37–52, 1964; J. Siller and A. Chipman, "Response Set Paralysis: Implications for Measurement and Control," J. Consulting Psychol., 27:432–438, 1963; J. Siller and A. Chipman, "Perceptions of Physical Disability By the Non-disabled," paper presented at the annual convention of the American Psychological Association, Los Angeles, September, 1964; J. Siller, "Components of Attitudes Toward the Disabled: Theory and Experimental Schema," paper presented at the annual meetings of the American Psychological Association, New York, September 2, 1966.

[57] Yuker, Block and Younng, op. cit., pp. 75–77.

[58] Whiteman, M., and I. F. Lukoff, "Attitudes Toward Blindness and Other Physical Handicaps," J. Social Psychol., 66:135–145, 1965; S. A. Richardson, A. H. Hastorf, N. Goodman and S. M. Dornbusch, "Cultural Uniformity

Finally, Siller's analysis of the reaction to physical disability suggests the following underlying themes: (1) Exclusion from a high degree of personal intimacy may be accounted for more in terms of inferred dependency than in terms of personal feelings of aversion; (2) emotional attitudes toward the disabled do not seem to be unitary— there is a striking tendency for feelings to be sharply differentiated in terms of the type and severity of the illness; (3) specific experiences with the disabled seem to be highly influential in conditioning attitudes toward not only specific disabilities but disabilities in general; (4) efforts designed to minimize aversion should be directed toward their emotional base; (5) although initial reaction may well serve as a major stumbling block to successful interaction between disabled and non-disabled persons, once the initial deterrent has been broached, the possibility of a more satisfactory relationship improves. Moreover, as far as the majority of the non-disabled are concerned, the best chance to promote receptivity would seem to lie in stressing the disabled's legitimate vocational capability and the ability of the disabled themselves to very clearly face-up to their own responsibility in helping define the situation for those with whom they interact.[59]

Empirical analysis of organizations responsible for dispensing rehabilitation services, Wessen has observed, have been relatively limited. This may be attributed in part to the fact that rehabilitation services have not as yet become crystallized into a typical organizational format.[60] Nevertheless, there seems to be considerable evidence that the organization of services and the attitudes of the staff does play an important part in the rehabilitation process itself. Schlesinger, for instance, has described as a participant–observer the debilitating impact of poor staff morale on the attitudes of patients with cerebral vascular accidents. Specific management problems, he observed, often arose from the social interaction of those involved in the rehabilitation process itself. Ultimately, the patient's course of treatment seemed to rest upon the balance between the patient's feelings of rejection and doubt, on the one hand, and their trust and acceptance, on the other. The nature of the relationship appeared to stem from not only the structure of established procedures, but the attitudes and kinds of

and Reaction to Physical Disabilities," *Amer. Sociological Rev.*, 26:241–247, April, 1961; "Varient Reactions to Physical Disabilities," *Amer. Sociological Rev.*, 28:429–435, June, 1963; S. A. Richardson, A. H. Hastorf and S. A. Dornbusch, "Effects of Physical Disability on the Child's Description of Himself," *Child Development*, 35:893–907, 1964; N. Goodman, *et al.*, "Variant Reactions to Physical Disabilities," *Amer. Sociological Rev.*, 28: 429–435, June, 1963; A. G. Gowman, "Attitudes Toward Blindness," in A. G. Gowman (ed.), *The War Blind in American Social Structure*, Amer. Found. for Blind, 1957. In addition, see Yuker, *et al.*, *op. cit.*, pp. 75–76.

[59] Siller, J., "Reactions to Physical Disability," *Rehab. Counseling Bull.*, September, 1963, pp. 12–16; "Reactions to Physical Disability by the Disabled and the Non-disabled," *Amer. Psychologist*, 14:351, 1959; "Personality Determinants of Reaction to the Physically Handicapped," *Amer. Psychologist*, 17:338, 1962.

[60] Wessen, A. F., "The Apparatus of Rehabilitation: An Organizational Analysis," in Sussman, *Sociology and Rehabilitation, op. cit.*, pp. 148–178. A classic hospital care model is compared with one consonant with the goals of rehabilitation services. The definition of health in terms of optimal, physical, psychological and social well-being, he notes, has never been accepted as an *operant* goal by the great majority of medical care institutions and practitioneers. Whereas the classical model emphasizes acute, short-term and emergency situations, the rehabilitation model deals with chronic handicaps which if they respond to treatment at all, do so only over a relatively long period of care. In contrast to the classical emphasis on disease, diagnosis and therapeutic procedure, the rehabilitation model stresses restoration and normal function, prognosis and adjustment and re-training. Thus the patients are defined not as passive recipients but as persons whose motivation to master their handicap is vital to the joint endeavor between patient and staff. See *ibid.*, pp. 170–176. M. Grayson, A. Powers and J. Levi, *Psychiatric Aspects of Rehabilitation*, Monograph II, Institute of Physical Medicine and Rehabilitation, New York Univ.–Bellevue Med. Center, 1952.

relations fostered in the rehabilitation center as well.[61]

In a somewhat similar vein, Shatin, *et al.*, in a study of chronically ill physical medicine patients undergoing treatment at a veteran's hospital, found that successful remotivation was often related to the staff's acceptance of the patient and the enthusiasm they demonstrated over the latter's improvement. Kelman has reported that patient apathy and reluctance to participate in therapeutic activities appeared to be markedly less when such activities were embedded in a social framework.[62]

[61] Schlesinger, L. E., "Patient Motivation for Rehabilitation: Integrating Staff Forces," *Amer. J. of Occupational Therapy*, 17:5–8, January–February, 1963; "Staff Authority in Patient Participation and Rehabilitation," *Rehab. Literature*, 24: 247–249, August, 1963; "Staff Tensions and Needed Skill in Staff–Patient Interactions," *Rehab. Literature*, 24:362–365, December, 1963; "Psychological and Social Losses Associated with the Cerebral Vascular Accident," *Rehab. Counseling Bull.*, 1964.

[62] Shatin, L., P. Brown and M. Loizeaux, "Psychological Re-motivation of the Chronically Ill Medical Patient: A Quantitative Study in Rehabilitation Methodology," *J. Chronic Dis.*, 14:452–468, October, 1961; H. R. Kelman, "An Experiment in the Rehabilitation Nursing Home Patients," *Public Health Reports*, 77: 356–366, April, 1962. But not all health professionals are related to in the same way. Our own work has revealed rather striking differences in the patients' perception of the medical therapeutic staff as compared with the nursing service. To some extent, this may be explained by the different functions served by each. Whereas therapy may be perceived in terms of the hopes and desires for return to normality, the hospital ward stands as a constant reminder of the patient's complete helplessness and dependency on others. Moreover, his feelings of hopelessness and insignificance may be further heightened when the communication channels are restricted and/or he is treated indifferently by aids and orderlies. In addition, it should be remembered that as a custodial and housekeeping facility, the nursing service is constantly exposed to the patient's daily irritations and frustrations. Consequently it is not surprising that they should be the recipient, justifiably or not, of the bulk of the criticism. See T. J. Litman, "The Influence of Concept of Self and Life Orientation Factors upon the Rehabilitation of Orthopedic Patients," unpublished doctoral dissertation, Univ. of Minnesota, 1961, pp. 128–131.

GOAL HIATUS

The patient's response to treatment may also be greatly affected if there is a disparity between his goals and those of the staff. This differential perception of therapeutic needs and goals may reflect a major goal hiatus between patient and staff. As Pilisuk has noted, a patient may give the appearance that he is unmotivated when in fact his performance merely reflects a disparity between his own conception of his needs and those of the therapist. Moreover, in many cases, as Barry and Malinovsky suggest, staff complaints about a patient's motivation may be traced to the former's dismay over the latter's failure to do what the staff feels he ought to do. The tendency for the staff to label some patients as "unmotivated," Phillips warns, may belie an incomplete understanding of the dynamics of the patient's behavior and goals.[63]

But while the treatment center can and does play a major role in promoting physical recovery, it often has little or no control over the social and psychological milieu outside its walls. Thus emerging from the relatively sheltered cloisters of the therapeutic setting, the patient is often ill-prepared to face the lack of understanding and rejection of the outside world exhibited by his family, friends and employer.

[63] Pilisuk, M., "Motivation for Therapy: The Gap Between Ego Skills and the Self-image," *Amer. J. Occupational Therapy*, 17:111–115, May–June, 1963; Barry and Malinovsky, *op. cit.*, p. 20; E. L. Phillips, "The Problem of Motivation: Some Neglected Aspects," *J. Rehab.*, 23:10–12, 1957. In a somewhat different vein, Roth has raised a significant question concerning the ethical legitimacy of institutional established goals for the rehabilitation of older patients. Although perhaps somewhat unjustly hard in his criticism of public facilities, the point he raises is an extremely important one which offers many important ramifications for successful rehabilitation treatment. See J. A. Roth, "The Public Hospital: Refuge for Damaged Humans," *Trans-Action*, July–August, 1966. For a more extensive statement of this position, see Roth and Eddy.

New, *et al.*,[64] for instance, have noted that the problem of predicting the patient's progress or performance after discharge may be confounded by the conveyance of his self-image (and attendant goal expectations) to *his* public. While the patient may view himself as either still sick or well, at the same time his support system or "significant others" also must determine whether to view him as being sick-dependent/well-dependent or independent. The patient then must convince his public, or at least those to whom he refers, of his new status and related expectations through his "presentation of self." Similarly, his significant others must decide whether to grant him the status he desires. If there is mutual agreement between patient and those to whom he refers, New, *et al.*, argue, the support system may aid the rehabilitation process. On the other hand, in the absence of such agreement or accommodation, the ultimate consequence may be quite dysfunctional.

THE FAMILY

The notion that the family may play an important part in determining the patient's response to treatment was first given prominence in Richardson's classic treatise *Patients Have Families*.[65] Since then there has been considerable interest on the part of both physicians and social scientists alike in the role of the family in adjustment to and response to illness.

In the field of rehabilitation, Sussman, *et al.*, several years ago undertook an extensive critical literature review to determine the applicability of various measures of family solidarity and integration to the study of chronic illness and disability. They concluded that not only could the family be studied as a social system undergoing change due to the impact of chronic illness but there were a number of sufficiently developed instruments available to measure this relationship as well. Davis, on the other hand, examined the impact of poliomyelitis upon family processes. Deutsch and Goldston found in a study of disabled polio patients at the New York Respirator Center that re-establishment of the home situation for the disabled seemed to rest upon the degree of role reversal involved. Mueller has reported that the patient's attitude toward his family may be instrumental in over-coming dependency induced by extensive, long-term hospitalization.[66]

Nevertheless, our own investigations among orthopedically disabled patients undergoing rehabilitation at two Midwestern therapeutic centers revealed little significant relationship between one's degree of family solidarity and his response to treatment. We would suggest, however, that the apparent failure of the family solidarity concept to account for variation in patient response to treatment may actually lie in the very nature of the therapeutic program itself. That is, during the particular phase of rehabilitation

[64] New, P., A. Ruscio, R. Priest and D. Petritsi, "The Support Structure of Heart and Stroke Patients: A Study of the Role of Significant Others in Patient Rehabilitation," paper presented at the National Rehabilitation Association annual meeting, Denver, October, 1966, and to be published in *Social Science in Medicine*, forthcoming. Similar findings have also been reported by J. Kronick *et al.*, "The Rehabilitation of 'Stroke' Patients: An Experimental Analysis of the Effects of Physical and Social Factors in Determining Recovery," unpublished paper, Bryn Mawr College, 1962.

[65] Richardson, H. B., *Patients Have Families*, New York: Commonwealth Fund, 1945.

[66] Sussman, M. B., *Family Unit Critique of Selected Scales and Indexes Available for Measuring the Relationship of Family Behavior to the Etiology and Course of Chronic Illness and Disability*, unpublished working draft, part I, Project 94U44, Association For the Aid of Crippled Children, 1959; F. Davis, "Polio in the Family—A Study of Crisis and Family Process," unpublished doctoral dissertation, Univ. of Chicago, June, 1958; *Passage Through Crisis, Polio Victims and Their Families*, Indianapolis, Bobbs–Merrill Co., 1963; C. P. Deutsch and J. A. Goldston, "Patient and Family Attitudes and Their Relationship to Home Placement of the Severely Disabled," paper presented before the annual meetings of the American Psychological Association, Cincinnati, September 4, 1959; P. Deutsch and J. A. Goldston, "Family Factors in Home Adjustment of the Severely Disabled," paper presented before the annual meetings of the American Orthopsychiatric Assoc. Convention, San Francisco, April 1, 1959; A. D. Mueller, "Psychologic Factors in Rehabilitation of Paraplegic Patients," *Arch. Physical Med. and Rehab.*, 43:151–159, 1962.

studied (the active therapeutic one), the family must more or less relinquish all responsibility for the care and treatment of their loved ones. To provide ample time for extensive therapy, visiting hours are severely restricted. Consequently, once the patient has been released from this somewhat sheltered setting, we would suspect to find family integration to prove a far more crucial variable in determining the patient's post-discharge adjustment, since from that point on, the family can no longer share with, or abrogate their responsibility to, the hospital. Accommodations and adjustments must be made with the family unit as an active participant. The very foundations of a happy marriage or family life may be put to the severest test. The implications are many, and additional research would certainly seem warranted.[67]

While there appeared to be little significant relationship between rehabilitation response and degree of family integration per se, there was considerable evidence that the family, as an interacting unit, may well play an important *supportive* role in the patient's convalescence. For the most part the patients studied tended to look to, and receive comfort and encouragement from, their immediate families. In the absence of such familial reinforcement, therapeutic performance declined. Finally, there was some indication that the patient's response seemed to be enhanced when therapy could

be conceived in terms of re-entry into an established family constellation, rather than as an individual or personal matter.[68]

More recently, New, *et al.*, have undertaken a project somewhat along the lines already mentioned. Sociologists from four major treatment centers began a joint exploratory study of the career of the patient and his family from time of the onset of his illness. The main emphasis of this examination will be on the impact of the family upon the eventual rehabilitation of the patient. According to their preliminary prospectus, data from approximately 400 patients (100 from each center) will be collected during the first year.[69]

AREAS OF NEGLECTED RESEARCH

Although rich in insight and theoretically rewarding, research to date on the behavioral aspects of physical rehabilitation has really only barely scratched the surface. Much remains to be done. Among the more promising areas of future inquiry, we would suggest the following:

First, we would propose a more intensive examination of the rehabilitation process

[67] Litman, T. J., "The Family and Physical Rehabilitation," *J. Chronic Dis.*, 19:211–217, 1966; "The Influence of Self-conception and Life Orientation Factors in the Rehabilitation of the Orthopedically Disabled," *J. Health and Human Behavior*, 3:252–254, Winter, 1962; "An Analysis of the Sociological Factors Affecting the Rehabilitation of Physically Handicapped Patients," *Arch. Physical Med. and Rehab.*, 45:12–13, January, 1964. Similarly, a study of discharged chronically ill disabled patients by Kelman, *et al.*, revealed that those who were living alone were subject to greater risk of being re-hospitalized sooner than those living with families or in boarding homes, while those who were hospitalized because of social changes, i.e., an unsatisfactory home arrangement, were at a greater risk to become permanent residents of a chronic care facility. See H. R. Kelman, J. N. Muller and M. Lowenthal, "Post-hospital Adaptation of a Chronically Ill and Disabled Rehabilitation Population," *J. Health and Human Behavior*, 5:4, Summer–Fall, 1964.

[68] Hoberman and Springer, for instance, have suggested that failure to provide an atmosphere of warmth, acceptance, encouragement, etc., may well deter rehabilitation when the client returns home (Hoberman, H., E. F. Cicenia and G. R. Stephenson, "Useful Measurement Tools and Physical Rehabilitation Programs of Preschool Orthopedically Handicapped Children," *Arch. Physical Med. and Rehab.*, 32:456–461, July, 1951).

[69] New, P. K., *et al.*, "Pathways to and from the Rehabilitation Institute: A Study of Heart and Stroke Patients," unpublished progress report, Vocational Rehabilitation Administration R–T7, Social Science Research Unit of Rehabilitation Institute: New England Medical Center Hospitals, July, 1967. The centers involved are: American Rehabilitation Foundation in Minneapolis, Univ. of Colorado Department of Physical Medicine and Rehabilitation, Emory University School of Medicine and Tufts University School of Medicine. The sample will include 100 patients from rehabilitation centers in Atlanta, Boston, Denver and Minneapolis, respectively.

itself, up to and beyond discharge in order to discern alterations in the patient's concept of himself, over time. The possibility of a longitudinal rather than a cross-sectional design is envisioned. In addition, more is needed to be known about the composition of the patient's reference group—who comprise the significant others—staff, family, friends? The process by which the disabled induce and perpetuate stigmatization of themselves and the role played by others in this labeling process also seem worthy of further analysis.[70]

Second, we would like to see more intensive social–psychological analysis of the patient's "career" following his release from the treatment setting. Despite the tremendous amount of time and effort invested by the therapeutic staff in preparing the patient for release to the outside world, once discharged, he and his family are often forced to fend for themselves. Such problems as: the acceptance of the disabled member within the family constellation, familial role reversal, family reaction to the stress and strains caused by curtailed family income and reliance upon public financial support, all pose interesting and stimulating questions for the behavioral scientist.[71]

Third, the morass of organizational, institutional and legal instrumentalities which constitute the so-called rehabilitation reference network would seem to lend themselves to systemic analysis.[72] Moreover, a comparative study of the levels of functioning of hospital-based versus independent therapeutic centers along the lines suggested by Wessen might also be explored.[73]

Fourth, the marginal position of physical medicine and its problems of emergence as an acceptable field of scientific medicine and the problem of male role conflict in a female-dominated profession such as physical therapy would seem to lend themselves to role analysis.[74]

Finally, the development of more refined measuring techniques to assess: rehabilitation response, disability self-conception, attitudes toward disability, as well as greater

[70] See Friedson, op. cit. More recently, Petroni has attempted to delineate the variations in the perception of the sick role between self and other, husband and wife and chronic and acute illness. F. Petroni, "Variations in Perception of Legitimacy in the Sick Role: The Influence of Significant Others, Chronicity, Sex and Generational Factors," unpublished doctoral dissertation, Univ. of Minnesota, 1968. Also see New, Ruscio, Priest and Petritsi, op. cit.

[71] Although highly desirable, Krause has presented a rather extensive methodological criticism of the use of follow-up studies. See E. A. Krause, "After the Rehabilitation Center," Research Report no. 7, New England Rehabilitation–For Work Center of Morgan Memorial, Inc., Boston. For some excellent examples of post-hospital follow-up studies, see: H. Freeman and O. Simmons, The Mental Patient Comes Home, New York: John Wiley, 1963; A. Donabedian and L. S. Rosenfeld, "Follow-up Study of Chronically Ill Patients Discharged from Hospitals," J. Chronic Dis., 17:847–862, September, 1964; E. Scull, et al., "A Follow-up Study of Patients Discharged from a Community Rehabilitation Center," J. Chronic Dis., 15:

207–213, February, 1962; J. Kronick, et al., "The Rehabilitation of 'Stroke' Patients: An Experimental Analysis of the Effects of Physical and Social Factors in Determining Recovery," unpublished paper, Bryn Mawr College, 1962; H. R. Kelman and J. Muller, "The Role of the Hospital and the Care of the Ambulatory Chronically Ill and Disabled Patient After Discharge," Amer. J. Public Health, 57:107–117, January, 1967; G. J. Vlasak and H. T. Phillips, "What Comes After Discharge: A Study of Post-hospital Experience of Patients Discharged From an Active-treatment Chronic Disease Treatment Hospital," unpublished preliminary report, Bureau of Chronic Disease Control, Massachusetts Department of Public Health, 1967.

[72] See S. Olshansky and R. J. Margolen, "Rehabilitation As a Dynamic Interaction of Systems," J. Rehab., 24:1–3, May–June, 1963; D. K. Rice, "Measuring Concepts in Long-term Care Research," Gerontologist, 4:34–37, June, 1964: "The Organization of Care for the Chronically Ill in General Hospitals—A Preliminary Discussion," unpublished paper presented at "Symposium on Research in Long-term Care," Jewish Hospital of St. Louis, September 25–27, 1963.

[73] Wessen, op. cit.

[74] See Sussman, "Occupational Sociology and Rehabilitation," op. cit.; B. E. Cogswell and B. D. Weir, "A Role in Process: The Development of Medical Professionals—Role in Long-term Care of Chronically Diseased Patients," J. Health and Human Behavior, 5:95–102, Summer–Fall, 1964; E. A. Krause, "Structured Strain in a Marginal Profession: Rehabilitation Counseling," J. Health and Human Behavior, 6:55–62, Spring, 1965.

use of experimental design in evaluative research and development of behavioral models and middle range theories to explain rehabilitation behavior deserve further exploration.

Summary and Conclusion

The problems of physical disability and rehabilitation thus involve a rather remarkable interplay between the biogenic, sociogenic and psychogenic components of human behavior. A theoretical pluralism reflects this multi-disciplinary focus. Yet despite the eclectic nature of its approach and the imprecision of its methodology, a fairly impressive body of knowledge has developed. The influence of such factors as conception of self, social distance, staff–patient interaction and the family have been explcred. Still, however, much remains to be done. For the behavioral scientist interested in an opportunity to test his theories and methods and develop new ones, the field of physical rehabilitation offers a stimulating challenge.

13

Disclosure of Terminal Illness

Barney G. Glaser

ONE OF THE MOST difficult of doctor's dilemmas is whether or not to tell a patient that he has a terminal illness. The ideal rule offered by doctors is that they should decide for each patient whether he really wants to know and can "take it." However, since, depending on the study, 69 to 90 per cent of doctors favor not telling their patients about terminal illness,[1] rather than making a separate decision for each patient, it appears that most doctors have a general standard from which the same decision flows for most patients—that he should not be told. This finding also indicates that the standard of "do not tell" receives very strong colleagueal support.

Many conditions reduce a doctor's inclination to make a separate decision for each case. Few doctors get to know each terminal patient well enough to judge his desire for

[1] Feifel, H., "Death," in N. L. Farberow (ed.), *Taboo Topics*, New York: Atherton Press, 1963, p. 17.

disclosure or his capacity to withstand the shock of disclosure. Getting to know a patient well enough takes more time than doctors typically have. Furthermore, with the current increase of patient loads, doctors will have less and less time for each patient, which creates the paradox: with more patients dying in hospitals, more will not be told they are dying. Even when a doctor has had many contacts with a particular patient, class or educational differences or personality clashes may prevent effective communication. Some doctors simply feel unable to handle themselves well enough during disclosure to make a complicated illness understandable. If a doctor makes a mistake, he may be liable for malpractice. Some doctors will announce an impending death only when a clear-cut pathologist's report is available. Others do not tell because they do not want the patient to "lean" on them for emotional support, or because they simply wish to preserve peace on the ward by preventing a scene.

Similarly, a number of conditions encourage disclosure of impending death regardless of the individual patient's capacity to withstand it. Some doctors disclose to avoid losing the patient's confidence should he find out indirectly through other sources, such as changes in his physical condition, accidentally overhearing the staff discuss his case or comparing himself with other patients. Telling also justifies radical treatment or a clinical research offer; it also reduces the doctor's need to keep up a cheerful but false front. Some tell so that the patient can put his affairs in order, plan for his family's future or reduce his pace of living; others, because family members

From Journal of Health & Human Behavior, *Vol. 7: 83–91, Summer, 1966; by permission of the author and publisher.*

This paper derives from an investigation of terminal care in hospitals supported by N.I.H. Grant NU 00047. I wish to thank Anselm Strauss for helpful comments and criticisms on an earlier draft. Other papers from this study are: A. Strauss, B. G. Glaser and J. Quint, "The Non-accountability of Terminal Care," *Hospitals*, 36:73–87, January 16, 1964; B. G. Glaser and A. Strauss, "The Social Loss of Dying Patients," *Amer. J. Nursing*, 64:119–121, June, 1964; B. G. Glaser and A. Strauss, "Awareness Contexts and Social Interaction," *Amer. Soc. Rev.*, 29:669–678, October, 1964; B. G. Glaser and A. L. Strauss, "Temporal Aspects of Dying as a Non-scheduled Status Passage," *Amer. J. Sociology*, July, 1965; B. G. Glaser and A. L. Strauss, "Discovery of Substantive Theory: A Basic Strategy Underlying Qualitative Research," *Amer. Behav. Scientist*, 8:5–12, February, 1965; J. C. Quint and A. Strauss, "Nursing Students, Assignments and Dying Patients," *Nursing Outlook*, Vol. 12, January, 1964; B. G. Glaser, "The Constant Comparative Method of Qualitative Analysis, *Social Problems* 12:436–445, Spring, 1965; two books, B. G. Glaser and A. Strauss, *Awareness of Dying*, Chicago: Aldine Press, 1966, and B. G. Glaser and A. L. Strauss, *Discovery of Grounded Theory*, Chicago: Aldine Press, 1970.

request it. Of course, if the chances for recovery or successful treatment are relatively good, a doctor is naturally more likely to disclose a possibly terminal illness; disclosing a skin cancer is easier than disclosing bone cancer.

The combined effect of these conditions—some of which may induce conflicting approaches to the same patient—is to make it much easier for doctors to apply to all patients a flat "no, he should not be told." For when people are in doubt about an action, especially when the doubt arises from inability to calculate the possible effects of many factors on which there is little information, it is almost always easier and safer to not act.[2]

Response to Disclosure

The intent of this paper is to formulate a descriptive, process model for under-

patient's initial response is almost invariably *depression*, but after a period of depression he either *accepts* or *denies* the disclosure, and his ensuing behavior may be regarded as an affirmation of his stand on whether he will, in fact, die. Acceptance may lead to active preparation, to passive preparation or to fighting the illness. A particular patient's response may stop at any stage of the process, take any direction, or change directions. The outcome depends on the manner in which he is told, and then managed by staff, as well as his own inclinations. The response process is diagrammed in Figure 13–1, and the characteristic forms of staff–patient interaction that occur at each stage, often precipitating advance to the next stage, are discussed in the remaining pages.

FIGURE 13-1 *The response process*

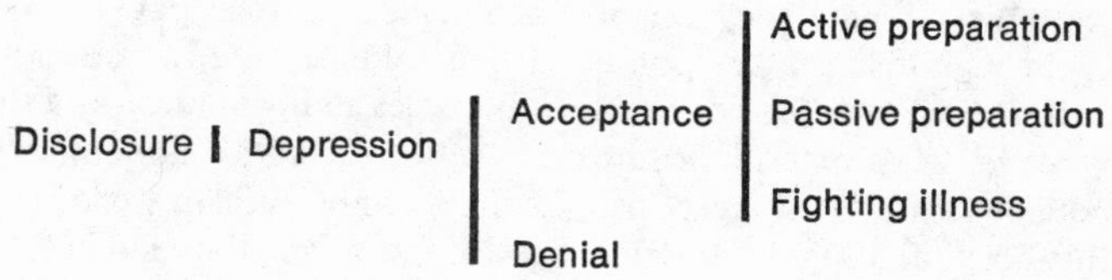

standing disclosure of terminal illness. This model combines *both* (1) the stages typically present in the response process stimulated by such disclosure *and* (2) the characteristic forms of interaction between the patient and staff attendant to each stage of the response process. Thus the focus in the following pages is just as much upon how hospital staff initiates, and attempts to guide and control the response process through interaction with the patient as upon the patient's responses per se.

First, the response process is stimulated by a doctor's *disclosure* to the patient. The

Method and Research Site

This conception of the characteristic stages of a patient's response to disclosure of terminal illness is based largely on field observations and interviews with patients, doctors, nurses and social workers on the cancer wards of a Veterans' Administration Hospital in the San Francisco Bay Area. In this hospital the normal procedure is to disclose the nature of his illness to every patient; as a result, many patients are told of a fatal illness.[3]

[2] For a conceptual analysis that applies to why there is less risk for doctors in not disclosing terminality, see T. J. Sheff, "Decision Rules, Types of Error, and Their Consequences in Medical Diagnosis," *Behavioral Science*, 8:97–107, April, 1963.

[3] This norm may be considered an aspect of "batch" treatment of captive inmates of a total institution. It is also the procedure on the medical ward of the state penitentiary in California. See E. Goffman, "Characteristics of Total Institutions," in A. Etzioni (ed.), *Complex Organizations*, New York: Holt, Rinehart and Winston, 1961, pp. 312–340.

By and large, the patients in these wards are in their middle or late years and in destitute circumstances. Since their care is free, they are captive patients—they have little or no control over their treatment, and if they do not cooperate, their care may be stopped. If a man goes "AWOL," the hospital is not obliged to re-admit him, or it can re-admit him but punish him by denying privileges. Because the patients lack financial resources, they typically have no alternative to their current "free" care, and their lower-class status accustoms them to accepting or to being intimidated into following orders from people of higher status. Since these captive lower-class patients are unable to threaten effectively the hospital or the doctors, disclosure of terminal illness occurs regardless of the patient's expected reaction.

These patients seemed to exhibit a full *range* of responses to disclosure of impending death, which it is our only purpose to set forth here. (How differently, if at all, from higher socio–economic patients they might be distributed throughout the response process is unascertainable with the collected data.) So many cases of direct disclosure and the consequent variety of response patterns made this hospital a highly strategic research site for studying the problem. In other hospitals we found only a few cases of direct disclosure of terminal illness and the general aspects were the same as those of the VA cases.

Disclosing Terminal Illness

Disclosure of terminal illness to patients in this hospital has two major characteristics. First, the patient is told that he is certain to die, but not when he will die. Expectations of death have two dimensions: *certainty* and *time* of demise, and the first is the more readily determined in advance.[4] As one doctor put it: "In my opinion, however, no doctor should take it upon himself to say to a patient, 'You have ten weeks to live'—

[4] See Glaser and Strauss, "Temporal Aspects . . .," *op. çit.*, for a full discussion of death expectations.

or three months, or two years or any time whatsoever." And another doctor said: "Doctors simply do not know when patients are going to die." Stopping short of full disclosure tends to soften the blow to the patient and reduces chances of error for the doctor.

Second, the doctors typically do not give details of the illness, particularly mode of dying, and the type of patient under consideration usually does not ask for them. Primarily, this is a problem of communication: a doctor finds it hard to explain the illness to a working-class patient, while lack of familiarity with the technical terms, as well as a more general deference to the doctor, inhibits the patient's impulse to question him. In addition, not giving details is a tactic doctors use to cut down on talk with the patient and to leave him quickly.

In combination, these two characteristics of disclosure often result in *short, blunt announcements* of terminal illness to the patient. Even the nurses are often shocked by the doctor's bluntness. Nevertheless, they often feel that the patient is better off for being told because, as one nurse put it, he "becomes philosophical in a day or two."

A short, blunt announcement may be softened, however, in various ways. One way is to add a religious flavor: "You've had a full life now, and God will be calling you soon." This manner is perhaps most appropriate for older patients. Another is to muffle the language. To the patient's question, "Is it cancer, Doc?" the doctor responds, "We don't call it that . . ." and then gives it a technical name that the patient can understand only vaguely. The "suspicion" announcement also dulls the blow: "There is a high clinical suspicion that the tumor removed was cancer. However, we won't have a pathological report on it for ten days." The announcement that there is "nothing more to do" (to cure the patient) can be muffled with a hopeful lie such as by adding "but then who knows, next week, next month or maybe next year there may be a drug that will save you," or by suggesting to the patient that he join an experimental program that may help him, as well as mankind.[5] Finally, there is the important

[5] If the patient takes the experimental drug, he

statement that softens any form of disclosure: "We can control the pain."

In some forms, the blunt announcement *sharpens* the blow of disclosure by forcing a *direct confrontation* of the truth with little or no preamble. The doctors are quite aware of, and favor the use of, this approach by colleagues. One doctor says, "With average patients, we tell them what they got." Another says, "I don't think the staff as a whole goes along with the hard-boiled approach, but me, I try to tell them the truth." The "hardboiled" announcement is often linked with a report to the patient of the results of his surgery. In this hospital, patients are customarily told, two or three days after surgery for cancer, whether they will die. For example, one doctor walks into the patient's room, faces him, says, "It's malignant" and walks out. To be sure, this tactic also eliminates having to answer the patient's questions. Another rather direct confrontation is, "We weren't able to get it (the malignant tumor) all out." Another form of sharp announcements is the *direct retort*: when a patient asks, "Doctor, do I have cancer?" the doctor replies, "Yes, you do." (One doctor commented, "If they ask directly, we answer as directly as possible.") Lastly, the *implied, but sharp, confrontation* of terminal illness is exemplified by the doctor who greeted a patient returning to the hospital with the order to sell her house and all her things, for she would not leave the hospital again.

In this group of doctors who favor the short, blunt disclosure there is one who does not. He refuses to disclose in this fashion because he has had previous experience with errors due to changing pathology reports, and because he tries, through surgery, to make the patient's last weeks more comfortable. Other doctors tend to disagree that his "comfort surgery" is useful, but he continues because sometimes he actually saves the patient for years. This doctor, continually

maintains a cheerful and optimistic manner, never directly disclosing to the patient that he will die. What actually occurs when he offers the patient comfort surgery or participation in a clinical experiment is *silent disclosure*: both doctor and patient know of the latter's fatal illness, and both know the other knows, but they do not talk to each other about it.[6] The doctor reveals the patient's fatal illness by oblique references to it in proposing comfort surgery or experimental participation, the meaning of which the patient clearly understands. The patient thus begins his process of response-to-disclosure without the customary stimulus of direct disclosure.

Depression

The initial response of the patient to disclosure is depression. The large majority of patients come to terms with their depression sufficiently to go on to the next stage of the response process. A few do not. Their depression precipitates a *withdrawal* from contact with everyone, and they remain in a state of hopelessness. In this limiting sense they become non-interacting, non-cooperative patients; the nurses can not "reach" them. Depression is usually handled by staff with sedation until the patient starts relating to them again. In one case a nurse observed that a patient visibly shortened his life because of his period of anxiety and withdrawal.

Acceptance or Denial?

After the initial period of acute depression, the patient responds to the announcement by choosing either to accept or to deny the imminence of his death. In effect, he takes a stand on whether and how he will die, and this stand profoundly affects his relations with the staff from that time on.

---

continually checks his condition by asking the doctor: "What next, Doc?" "What now?" "Am I better?" "Am I getting well?" When the experiment is over and the patient is still going to die, he must start through the response process again with a depressing "now what" feeling.

[6] See Glaser and Strauss, "Awareness Context . . .," *op. cit.*, for a discussion of the "mutual pretense awareness context" which silent disclosure institutes.

In general, sharp, abrupt disclosure tends to produce denial, and dulled disclosure, acceptance.[7] When the disclosure is sharp, the depression is more immediate and profound, and denial starts right in as a mechanism to cope with the shock.[8] To predict an individual's response, however, one needs the kind of intimate knowledge of the patient that doctors would prefer to have. Without it, it is very difficult to say which path to death a patient will take, or for how long. In some cases, the patient's response changes; he cannot hold out against accumulating physical, social and temporal cues. The usual change is from denial to acceptance, though when patients improve briefly before growing worse or a new drug helps for a few days, acceptance may change, for a time, to denial. The direction an individual takes depends not only on how he is told, but also on a variety of social and psychological considerations impinging on the passage from life to death.

Acceptance—Patients may demonstrate acceptance of impending death by actively preparing for death, passively preparing, or fighting against it. *Active preparation* may take the form of becoming *philosophical* about dying, death and one's previous life; patients review and discuss how full their life has been with family, nurses, social workers and chaplain. They may pose the destiny question: "Why me?" and try to work through it with the philosphical help of others. This approach leads the patients to draw the nurses into the discussion which can be very difficult for them. Nurses

[7] These hypotheses complement the discussion by Feifel on the importance of "how telling is done" (*op. cit.*).

[8] For another discussion of denial of illness upon disclosure, see H. D. Lederer, "How the Sick View Their World," in E. Gartly Jaco (ed.), *Patients, Physicians and Illness*, New York: Free Press, 1958, pp. 247–250. Denial of dying is characteristic of our society as shown by R. Fulton's data: see "Death and the Self," *Journal of Religion and Health*, 3:359–368, July, 1964. See the analysis of denial of death in American Society by T. Parsons, "Death in American Society," *Amer. Behav. Scientist*, May, 1963, pp. 61–65.

are still only trained by and large to help motivate patients to live, not to die! If a nurse is to help a patient prepare himself she too must accept his impending death and refrain from chastising him for not fighting to live. Otherwise she is likely to consider the patient "morbid" and tends to avoid his invitations to help him face death squarely. She will usually try to transfer the burden to the social worker, sister or chaplain when they are available.

Some patients start immediately to prepare themselves for death through religion. For others it is an easy transition to slip from philosophical to religious terms, a transition often aided by the chaplain, who then helps the patient prepare himself.

Another form of active preparation for death is to *settle social* and *financial affairs*, perhaps linking this effort with philosophical or religious preparation. The typical helpers in settling affairs are family members and social workers. For example, upon learning that he was going to die, the patient turned to his wife and said, "Well, we've got to get everything lined up; I promised (so and so) my . . ." This immediate getting down to the provisions of a will was considered abnormal by one nurse who said, "I've never seen a reaction like that, it was almost morbid." Another patient began discussing with the social worker the various veteran's benefits they could obtain for his wife, and another tried to marry his wife, who was emotionally very dependent on him, to a hospital corpsman. One patient gave up his pain medication long enough to put his financial affairs in order with the aid of a social worker, for he knew that as soon as he was too drugged to operate effectively, his family would try to take over his estate.

To give the patient a chance to settle his affairs, to plan for the future of his family, is, of course, an important consideration when a doctor decides whether to disclose terminal illness. He can seldom be sure, however, that the patient's response will take this direction or advance so far. Moreover, some affairs to be settled are less important than social or financial ones, though they do allow patients to pick up loose ends or accomplish unfinished business. For example, before entering the hospital for cancer surgery one woman said, "I am going to do three things before I enter the hospital —things I've been meaning to do for a long time. I'm going to make some grape jelly. I've always dreamed of having a shelf full of jelly jars with my own label on them. Then I'm going to get up enough nerve to saddle and bridle my daughter's horse and take a ride. Then I'm going to apologize to my mother-in-law for what I said to her in 1949." Another patient with leukemia quit work and bought a sail boat. He planned to explore the delta region of the Sacramento and San Joaquin rivers until his last trip to the hospital.

Another form of active preparation is to attempt a "*full life*" before death.[9] This pattern is characteristic of younger patients (in contrast to older patients who review the fullness of their life) like the 22-year-old who, when told he had three months to three years to live, married a nurse. "If we have only two months," she said, "it will be worth it." The patient lived two years and had a son. Faced by certain death, he had achieved the most he could from life.

Auto-euthanasia (*suicide*) is another way of actively preparing for death.[10] It eliminates the sometimes very distressing last weeks or days of dying. One patient, who had no friends to visit him, felt that he was very alone and that no one in the hospital cared, so he tried to hasten his death by suicide. Some patients try to end their lives while they are physically presentable, not wanting their families to see their degeneration. Other stresses that encourage auto-euthanasia are unbearable pain and the discipline imposed by a clinical experiment to which one may be irrevocably committed. Others decide to end their life when they can no longer work.[11] Still others prefer

auto-euthanasia as a way of controlling their dying as they controlled their living, thus wresting this control from the hands of the staff and the rigors imposed by hospital routine.[12]

Passive preparation for death, among patients who accept their terminal illness, also has some characteristic forms. One is to take the news in a *nonchalant* manner. Nurses sometimes find this response disturbing; one put it: "But some take it quite nonchalantly. We've had several very good patients—right to the end. One that upset me was here when I came. He was the hardest for me to see die—he was young and not only that—such a wonderful fellow. Even as sick as he was, he was always kind and courteous." Apart from the social loss factor —"young" and "wonderful"—which usually upsets nurses,[13] this nurse also found such a passive outlook on death rather disquieting.

Nurses, however, are grateful to patients who approach death with *calm resignation*. This response relieves them of the responsibility for cheering up the patient and improves their morale, too. Since it would not do for a nurse to be less calm or resigned than her patient, a patient who responds in this fashion raises and supports the nurse's morale. The *nonverbal* patient, who simply accepts his fate and does not talk about it, also relieves the nurse of possible stress in having to talk, as she often does with the more actively preparing patient. He makes few or no demands on nurses or social workers. A disquieting aspect of this response is the loss of contact with the patient: "It is very hard for us 'well people' to really grasp how they feel." One social worker bridges

---

[9] This form of active preparation is appropriate in American society which stresses the value that death is unacceptable until one has had a full life; see: Parsons, *op. cit*.

[10] Shneidman feels a question deserving of research is "why so many cancer patients *do not* commit suicide." E. S. Shneidman, "Suicide," in Farberow, *op. cit*.

[11] For an account of a cancer patient who planned to commit auto-euthanasia after he could no longer work, see L. Wertenbaker, *Death of a Man*, New York: Random House, 1957.

[12] A growing problem that medical staff and hospitals must face is that people wish to control their own way of dying; they do not want it programmed for them by medical staff and hospital organization. To achieve this end, many patients also wish to die at home. (Fulton, *op. cit*., pp. 363–364); see the analysis of this problem in J. Quint, "Some Organizational Barriers to Effective Patient Care in Hospitals," paper given at the American Medical Association convention, June 24, 1964.

[13] Glaser and Strauss, "The Social Loss . . .," *op. cit*.

this gap by sitting with the patient for a time each day. She reports, "Sometimes it's a matter of just touching their hand—whatever is natural—to make them feel that you understand and care." Another version of the passive response is expressed by the patient who emerges from his depression only to turn his face to the wall, "the spirit drained out of him," and "passively wait to die."

Some patients accept their terminal illness but decide to *fight* it. Unlike denial behavior, this fight indicates an initial acceptance of one's impending death together with a positive desire to somehow change it. Three forms of fighting behavior are *intensive living*, *going to marginal doctors or quacks*, and *participating in an experiment*. One patient, for example, started going out on passes, and living it up, asserting, "I'll beat it," as if he could hold death off by living life to the full. He kept getting thinner and eventually died. This mode of fighting off death can be readily transformed into active preparation for death if it increases the patient's fullness of life before death.

Taking an outside chance with quacks or marginal doctors[14] gives some patients a feeling that they are actively combatting the disease. A regular physician usually permits his patient to go to a marginal doctor, since the visits keep the patient hopeful and busy and his permission allows the physician to see that the marginal treatments do not injure his patient. Denied this permission, a patient who wants to fight his disease in some way may break off relations with his physician, so that the physician loses control over both the patient and the marginal doctor. A rupture like this makes it difficult for the patient to return to the original doctor when, as is typical, the marginal treatment fails.[15]

The search for a way to fight the fatal illness can also lead a patient into a clinical

experiment. If he does not win his own battle, he at least may help future patients with theirs. The chance to contribute to medical science does not, however, sustain the motivation of *all* research patients.[16] Some, when they see it is hopeless for themselves and find the experimental regime too rigorous to bear, try to extricate themselves from the experiment. If the doctors will not let them off, these patients sometimes interfere with the experiment by pulling tubes out, by not taking medicine or by taking an extra drink of water. Some attempt autoeuthanasia. Doctors may carry on the fight regardless of the patient's desire to give up. One nurse, at least, feeling that the lives of research patients are excessively prolonged, bitterly said: "They (doctors) keep them alive until the paper (the research report) is written."

Denial—Some patients deny they are approaching death and proceed to establish this stand in their interaction with staff members. Typical denying strategies are juggling time, testing for denial, comparing oneself to other patients, blocking communication, becoming intensely active, emphasizing a future orientation, and forcing reciprocal isolation. In the cancer ward, it is relatively easy to deny impending death by *juggling time*, for, as we have noted, disclosure implies certainty that death will occur, but no assurance as to *when* it will occur. Patients can therefore invent a time, and this becomes a way of denying that one is truly dying.[17] Some literally give themselves years. But even when a denying patient is given a time limit, he is still likely to start thinking, as one nurse said, "in terms of years, when it really is a matter of a month or two."

---

[14] In this connection see B. Cobb, "Why Do People Detour to Quacks?" in Jaco, *op. cit.*

[15] For an illustration of how the doctor allowed, hence could control, a dying patient's submission to the rigorous treatment of a marginal doctor, see J. Gunther, *Death Be Not Proud*, New York: Harper Bros., 1949.

[16] Cf, R. Fox, *Experiment Perilous*, New York: Free Press, 1959. One gets the feeling that the patients in Fox's sample were all highly motivated to go on with the experiments to the bitter end.

[17] That in the case of dying, patients will tend to give themselves *more* time than they actually have, contrasts with studies of recovery which show that patients are likely to give themselves *less* time than it takes to recover. See F. Davis, *Passage Through Crisis*, Indianapolis: Bobbs–Merrill, 1963, and J. Roth, *Timetables*, Indianapolis: Bobbs–Merrill, 1963.

A patient can *test* the staff in various ways *to establish* his *denial*. A negative way is not to test, by failing to ask the questions called for. For example, the doctor who tells the patient he has a tumor adopts a grave manner, indicating that the tumor is malignant, and expects the patient to try to verify it. The patient never asks the doctor or anyone else. Other patients test the nurses, indirectly, by asking, "Why aren't I feeling better?" "Why aren't I gaining weight?" Since these patients can be assumed to know why, the nurse understands that they want these physical cues interpreted in such a way as to deny that they indicate impending death. Patients often ask nurses to manage temporal cues in the same way, by interpreting extended stays in the hospital or slow recuperation in ways that point away from death.

Another form of testing for denial is the *polarity game*. By questioning a nurse or social worker about the most extreme living or dying implications of his illness, the patient forces her to give a normalizing answer, which usually locates him a safe distance from death. For example, focusing on the dying implications, the patient asks, "Am I getting worse? The medicine isn't helping." The forced answer is, "Give yourself a chance—medicine takes a long time." Or focusing on the living implications, to a social worker trying to figure out his VA benefits for his family a patient replies, "Well, all right—but it won't be for long, will it?" Since the social worker cannot confront the patient with coming death if he "really doesn't know," she in effect denies it for him by classifying him with the living but disabled. "This is what welfare is for—to help the families of men who are disabled and can't work." Here, the social worker understood the patient's words as a request "for assurance that he wasn't going to die," and she responded appropriately.

Patients may deny their fate by using other patients as *comparative references*. Two common types of comparison are the exception and the favorable comparison. A patient using the first approach becomes very talkative about other patients with the same disease. He adopts a manner, or style, like that of staff members, that is, people

who do not have the illness. In the end this borrowed objectivity and immunity leads him to conclude that he is an exceptional case, that somehow the illness that caused so many others to die will not kill him: he will be cured. The favorable comparison is a distorted effort to include one's illness in a non-fatal category: one patient said, "The doctor says I *only* have a (severe illness)." Another literally dying patient said, "Thank God, I am not as bad off as (another patient near death)."

Some patients try to prove they are not terminal by *engaging in strenuous activities*. One patient, having been told he had a bad heart, left the hospital and started spading up his garden to prove the doctor wrong, that is, his denial correct. Another patient wouldn't stick to his diet. The death impending in the present can also be denied through *future-oriented talk* with the nurses. One patient began making plans to buy a chicken farm when he left the hospital—as soon as he learned he was going to die. *Communication blocks* of various sorts aid denial. Some patients simply don't hear the doctor, others refuse to admit it, others cannot use the word "cancer" in any verbal context, and still others avoid any discussion of the nature of their illness or the inevitability of death.

A denying patient can start an accumulating process of *reciprocal isolation* between himself and nurses, doctors, family members and social workers. After disclosure, others expect him to acknowledge his impending death, so they attempt to relate to him on this basis. Doctors speak to him and nurses give treatment on the understanding that his impending demise can be mentioned, or at least signaled. Family members and social workers may refer to plans for his burial and his finances. A patient who avoids the subject when he is not expected to avoid it forces others to avoid it, too, and thus renders them unable to help and prepare the patient. One social worker said, hopelessly, about a denying patient, "There was nothing I could do for him." At this first stage of the isolation process, the patient has forced an implicit agreement between himself and others that the topic of his illness will not be discussed.[18] In the next stage, some of these people may avoid all contact with the patient because he has frustrated their efforts to help him. Nurses, doctors and social workers tend to spend their time with patients they can help, to prevent the feeling of helplessness that often overcomes them while engaged in terminal care. As a result, the patient finds himself alone, apart from receiving the necessary technical care to insure painless comfort, thus his isolation is complete.

Avoidance of the denying patient occurs because he refuses to act as a dying patient, although it has been clearly pointed out to him that this is exactly what he is. In contrast, an unaware patient, who is not expected to act like a dying patient, will not be avoided on these grounds. Rather, he is likely to attract others who will gather around him in silent sympathy, wishing they could tell him and help him. In the end, both the denying patient and the unaware patient may die without preparation for death. But a denying patient had the chance to accept his impending death and prepare himself with the help of others, while the unaware patient's chances for preparation are mostly dependent on his doctor's decision not to disclose his terminal illness.

Implications for Disclosure

Many of the standard arguments given by doctors for and against disclosure anticipate a single, permanent impact on the patient.[19] The patient is expected to "be brave," "go to pieces," "commit suicide," "lose all hope," or to "plan for the future" and such. But the impact is not so simple. Since disclosing the truth sets off a response process

18 Thus, instituting a "mutual pretense awareness context" is part of this process: see Glaser and Strauss, "Awareness Contexts . . .," op. cit.

19 For an illustration of this kind of argument, see the discussion between two doctors in "How Should Incurably Ill Patients Be Dealt with: Should They Be Told the Truth," *Parent's Magazine*, 71:196–206, January, 1963.

through which the patient passes, to base the decision as to whether to disclose on a single probable impact is to focus on only one stage in the response process, neglecting the other stages and how each stage may be controlled through appropriate forms of interaction by hospital staff. For example, to predict that the patient will become too despondent is to neglect the possibility that he will overcome this despondency and with the aid of a nurse, chaplain, social worker or family member prepare adequately for his death and for his family's future. Or, to expect a patient simply to settle his affairs is to fail to evaluate his capacity for overcoming an initial depression, as well as the capacity of the staff to help him at this stage.

A doctor deciding whether to tell the patient therefore should consider not a single impact as a desiderata, but how, in what direction and with what consequences the patient's response is likely to go, and what types of staff are available and how will they handle the patient at each stage. A doctor who says "no" to disclosure because the patient will "lose hope" need not be in conflict with one who says "yes," to give the patient a chance to plan for his family. Each is merely referring to a different stage of the same process. For both, the concern should be to judge whether the patient can achieve the acceptance–active preparation stage.

Once again, the benefits and liabilities of unawareness (non-disclosure) as opposed to disclosure and the possibilities for acceptance or denial, depend on the nature of the individual case. But on the whole, there is much to recommend giving more patients than are presently given an opportunity actively to manage their own dying and prepare for death. As a strong controlling factor, staff members in interaction with the patient could self-consciously soften the disclosure, handle the depression so as to encourage acceptance, and guide the patient into active preparations for death. They could also find interaction strategies that would convert a patient's denial to acceptance. Yet staff members may hesitate to tamper with a patient's choice of passage to death. For example, one social worker said of a denying patient, "I'm loathe to play

God on this. Unless it could serve a useful purpose—would it really be helpful. Where a man shies away from something—maybe you should let him—why make him face this most terrible reality?"

The understanding that the descriptive model presented here affords will, we trust, give doctors as well as other parties to the dying situation, such as family members, nurses, social workers and chaplains, a perspective that is of use in deciding the advisability of disclosing terminal illness to a patient, and if advisable, how best it might be done, and how to guide the patient through the response process. Thus perhaps this understanding will reduce some of the

current reluctance of medical staff to disclose and to tamper with patients' responses to disclosure. This model also provides sociologists with a beginning basis both for entering into, as consultants, the discussion on whether or not to disclose and for the needed social psychological research on the problem. For instance, further research could specify what types of terminal patients follow what kinds of patterns of movement through the response process under what conditions of patient–staff interaction—a problem only hinted at in this paper.

14

Client Control and Medical Practice

Eliot Freidson

THAT THE MEDICAL practitioner is typically a colleague in a structure of institutions and organizations, the patient being an essentially minor contingency, is the picture presented in the general discussions of Carr-Saunders and Wilson,[1] Parsons,[2] Merton,[3] and Goode,[4] as well as in studies of medical practice by Hall,[5] Solomon,[6] Hyde,[7] Peterson,[8] and Coleman, Menzel, and Katz.[9] The nature of medical practice is seen as determined largely by the practitioner's relation to his colleagues and their institutions and by the profession's relation to the state.

But practice cannot exist without clients and clients often have ideas about what they want that differ markedly from those supposedly held by the professionals they consult. As anthropologists have so copiously illustrated,[10] the client's choice is guided by norms that differ from culture to culture and even within a single complex culture.[11] And, after the client has exercised his choice to see a practitioner, normative or cultural differences between patient and physician qualify the relationship considerably.[12] These characteristics, in the client, obviously are a systematic source of pressure on the practitioner. To understand medical practice, therefore, one must learn the circumstances in which the pressure is initiated and sustained, and this requires regarding the client and the practitioner in a single analytical system in which one explores the sources of strength of each.

[1] Carr–Saunders, A.M., and P. A. Wilson, *The Professions*, Oxford: Clarendon Press, 1933.

[2] Parsons, T., "The Professions and Social Structure," in his *Essays in Sociological Theory Pure and Applied*, New York: Free Press, 1949, pp. 185–199.

[3] Merton, R. K., "Some Preliminaries to a Sociology of Medical Education," in R. K. Merton, G. G. Reader and P. L. Kendall (eds.), *The Student–Physician*, Cambridge, Mass.: Harvard Univ. Press, 1957, pp. 73–79.

[4] Goode, W. J., "Community Within a Community: The Professions," *Amer. Soc. Rev.*, 22:194–200, April, 1957.

[5] Hall, O., "The Informal Organization of the Medical Profession," *Canadian J. of Econ. and Pol. Science*, 12:30–41, February, 1946; "The Stages of the Medical Career," *Amer. J. Soc.*, 53:327–336, March, 1948; and "Types of Medical Careers," *ibid.*, 55:243–253, November, 1949.

[6] Solomon, D. N., "Career Contingencies of Chicago Physicians," unpublished Ph.D. dissertation, Chicago: Univ. of Chicago, 1952.

[7] Hyde, D. R., and P. Wolff, with A. Gross and E. L. Hoffman, "The American Medical Association: Power, Purpose and Politics in Organized Medicine," *Yale Law Journal*, 63: 938–1022, May, 1954.

[8] Peterson, O. L., *et al.*, "An Analytical Study of North Carolina General Practice, 1953–1954," *J. Med. Educ.*, 31:1–165, part II, December, 1956.

[9] Menzel, H., and E. Katz, "Social Relations and Innovation in the Medical Profession: The Epidemiology of a New Drug," *Public Opinion Quart.*, 19:337–352, Winter, 1955–1956; J. Coleman, E. Katz and H. Menzel, "The Diffusion of an Innovation Among Physicians," *Sociometry*, 20:253–270, December, 1957; H. Menzel, J. Coleman and E. Katz, "Dimensions of Being 'Modern' in Medical Practice," *J. Chronic Dis.*, 9:20–40, January, 1959.

[10] E.g., B. D. Paul (ed.), *Health, Culture and Community*, New York: Russell Sage Foundation, 1955, and the studies cited in G. K. Foster, *Problems in Intercultural Health Programs*, Social Science Research Council Pamphlet, no. 12, New York, 1958.

[11] E.g., E. L. Koos, *The Health of Regionville*, New York: Columbia Univ. Press, 1954, and the excellent summary and bibliography of O. G. Simmons, *Social Status and Public Health*, Social Science Research Council Pamphlet, no. 13, New York, 1958.

[12] E.g., L. W. Saunders, *Cultural Differences and Medical Care*, New York: Russell Sage Foundation, 1954.

From American Journal of Sociology, *Vol. 65: 374–382, January, 1960; by permission of the author and the University of Chicago Press.*

Revision of a paper read at the 1959 meetings of the American Sociological Association, Chicago.

To bring the two together, analysis must proceed on a model of society that is more common to anthropological than to sociological studies. Practice seems usefully analyzed not only as a set of practitioners interacting with each other[13] but as a concrete local situation in which two systems touch to form a larger whole in which there are characteristic norms, positions, and movements. To isolate the whole, the model is not that of a society within which there are practitioners and clients,[14] or of a consultation room in which there are a practitioner and a client,[15] but of a system in which representatives of the medical profession practice in consultation rooms located in local communities of prospective clients. In recognizing practitioners as members of a profession, reference may be made to their organization and culture. In recognizing clients as members of a specific local community, reference may be made to their own organization and culture. In joining the two within a community, instances studied by anthropologists in which professional practitioners find it difficult to get clients can find as much of a place in the analysis as instances in which professional practice is so thoroughly accepted by clients as to be almost (but never quite) routine.

It is the purpose of this paper to use such a model to organize analysis of aspects of client experience that may significantly affect medical practice and to outline a descriptive typology of such practice, the analysis being put in a sufficiently general fashion to allow application to other types of professional practice.

Characteristically, the professional practitioner claims that his skills are so esoteric that the client is in no position to evaluate them. From this stems his privilege to be somewhat removed from the market place

and to accept the evaluation of his colleagues rather than of his clients.[16] And this claim is one mark of his separation as a member of a professional "community."[17]

But, while his own "community" may be without physical locus, he must *practice* in a spatially located community among more or less organized potential clients. Thus, while he is a member of a professional "community," accepting its norms and formally dependent on its institutions, the practitioner is always a kind of stranger in the community of his practice, for his reference group is his colleagues, not his clients.

However, while the physician may share special knowledge, identity, and loyalty with his colleagues rather than with laymen, he is dependent upon laymen for his livelihood. Where he does not have the power to force them to use his services, he depends upon the free choice of prospective patients.[18] But, since these prospective clients are in no position to evaluate his services as would his colleagues, and insofar as they do exercise choice, it follows that they must evaluate him by non-professional criteria and that they will interact with him on the basis of non-professional norms. Hence practice generically consists in interaction between two different, sometimes conflicting, sets of norms.

Consequently, we have two systems, the professional and the lay. In any concrete

[13] Hall's stress on the "inner fraternity" implies this even though he has some important things to say about clients (see Hall, "Informal Organization," *op. cit.*, pp. 30–31). He is primarily concerned with how a physician obtains a clientele already organized into practices.

[14] Goode, *op. cit.*, exploits this perspective.

[15] Cf. T. Parsons, *The Social System*, New York: Free Press, 1954, pp. 428–473.

[16] See E. C. Hughes, "Licence and Mandate," in E. C. Hughes, *Men and Their Work*, New York: Free Press, 1958, pp. 78–87.

[17] Goode, *op. cit., passim*. Goode uses the term "community" in the sense of shared interests and identity. Thus all American physicians belong to the medical "community," just as all American Catholics belong to the Catholic "community." I use the term to mean locality.

[18] It is not predicated here that clients choose particular practitioners—that is, that practice is characteristically solo, fee-for-service in nature. Choice of physician is made to some degree by clients in the United States but hardly in other countries (cf., on Israel, J. Ben–David, "The Professional Role of the Physician in Bureaucratized Medicine: A Study in Role Conflict," *Hum. Relations*, 11:255–274, 1958). The choice the client must make everywhere is not which doctor to see but whether to see one at all.

situation the two touch: the local physician may be seen as the "hinge" between a local lay system and an "outside" professional system. Structurally, the practitioner's support theoretically lies outside the community in which he practices, in the hands of his colleagues, while his prospective clientele are organized by the community itself. Culturally, the professional's referent is by definition "the great tradition" of his supra-local profession, while his prospective clientele's referent is the "little tradition" of the local community or neighborhood.[19] The lay tradition of the local community may, in one place or another, absorb varying amounts of the professional tradition, but by the nature of the case, as Saunders and Hewes have so persuasively argued,[20] lay medical culture seems unlikely ever to become identical with professional medical culture.

How are the physician and his prospective clientele brought together? How is consultation initiated and sustained? Obviously, the prospective client must perceive some need for help and that it is a physician who can help him. And, if solo practice is the rule, he must determine who is a "good" practitioner. These perceptions seem to emerge from a process of interpersonal influence similar to that studied in other areas of life, a process organized by the culture and structure of the community or neighborhood through which "outside" knowledge and evaluation is strained.

In one locality,[21] conceiving the need for

19 The terms and image are those of R. Redfield. See his *Peasant Society and Culture*, Chicago: Univ. of Chicago Press, 1956, pp. 43–45, and his "A Community Within Communities," *The Little Community*, Chicago: Univ. of Chicago Press, 1955, pp. 113–151. In industrial society the "little tradition" seems less stable than in peasant society and more dependent upon the "great tradition" for its content.

20 Saunders, L. W., and G. H. Hewes, "Folk Medicine and Medical Practice," *J. Med. Educ.*, 28:43–46, September, 1953.

21 The following sketch stems from intensive interviews with 71 patients of a metropolitan medical group, in which they were asked to give detailed chronological accounts of the way in which they were led to seek medical care. It is not intended to describe the average experience

"outside" help for a physical disorder seems to be initiated by purely personal, tentative self-diagnoses that stress the temporary character of the symptoms and to end by the prescribing of delay to see what happens. If the symptoms persist, simple home remedies such as rest, aspirin, antacids, laxatives, and change of diet will be tried. At the point of trying some remedy, however, the potential patient attracts the attention of his household, if he has not asked for attention already. Diagnosis then is shared, and new remedies may be suggested, or a visit to a physician. If a practitioner is not seen, but the symptoms continue (and in most cases the symptoms do *not* continue), the diagnostic resources of friends, neighbors, relatives and fellow workers may be explored. This is rarely very deliberate; it takes place in daily intercourse, initiated first by inquiries about health and only afterward about the weather.

This casual exploring of diagnoses, when it is drawn out and not stopped early by the cessation of symptoms or by resort to a physician, typically takes the form of referrals through a hierarchy of authority. Discussion of symptoms and their remedies is referral as much as prescription—referral to some other layman who himself had and cured the same symptoms, to someone who was once a nurse and therefore knows about such things, to a druggist who once fixed someone up with a wonderful brown tonic, and, of course, to a marvelous doctor who treated the very same thing successfully.

Indeed, the whole process of seeking help involves a network of potential consultants, from the intimate and informal confines of the nuclear family through successively more select, distant, and authoritative laymen, until the "professional" is reached.[22] This

but is a synthetic construct designed to portray the full length to which the process may go before professional practice is reached. The data suggest that, the longer the process that intervenes between first perception of difficulty and contact with a practitioner, the greater the likelihood that the symptoms are ambiguous and not unbearable: a broken leg has different consequences from a "cold" of excessive duration.

22 For data on the referral process and the network of consultants see E. E. Evans–Pritchard,

network of consultants, which is part of the structure of the local lay community and which imposes form on the seeking of help, might be called the "lay referral structure." Taken together with the cultural understandings involved in the process, we may speak of it as the "lay referral system."

There are as many lay referral systems as there are communities, but it is possible to classify all systems by two critical variables —the degree of congruence between the culture of the clientele and that of the profession, and the relative number of lay consultants who are interposed between the first perception of symptoms and the decision to see a professional. Considerations of culture have relevance to the diagnoses and prescriptions that are meaningful to the client and to the kinds of consultants considered authoritative. Consideration of the extensiveness of the lay referral structure has relevance to the channeling and reinforcement of lay culture and to the flowing-in of "outside" communications.

These variables may be combined so as to yield four types of lay referral system, of which only two need be discussed here— first, a system in which the prospective clients participate primarily in an indigenous lay culture and in which there is a highly extended lay referral structure and, second, a system in which the prospective clients participate in a culture of maximum congruence with that of the profession and in which there is a severely truncated referral structure or none at all.

The indigenous, extended system is an extreme instance in which the clientele of a community may be expected to show a high degree of resistance to using medical services. Insofar as the idea of diagnostic authority is based on assumed hereditary or divine "gift" or intrinsically personal knowledge of one's

Witchcraft, Oracles and Magic Among the Azande, Oxford: Clarendon Press, 1937; M. R. Yarrow, C. G. Schwartz, H. S. Murphy and L. C. Deasy, "The Psychological Meaning of Mental Illness in the Family," *J. Social Issues*, 11:12–24, 1955; J. A. Clausen and M. R. Yarrow, "Paths to the Mental Hospital," *J. Social Issues*, 11:25–32, 1955; E. Goffman, "The Moral Career of the Mental Patient," *Psychiatry*, 22:123–142, May, 1959.

"own" health being necessary for effective treatment, professional authority is unlikely to be recognized at all. And, insofar as the cultural definitions of illness contradict those of professional culture, the referral process will not often lead to the professional practioner. In turn, with an extended lay referral structure, lay definitions are supported by a variety of lay consultants, when the sick man looks about for help. Obviously, here the folk practitioner will be used by most, the professional practitioner being called for minor illnesses only, or, in illness considered critical, called only by the socially isolated deviate, and by the sick man desperately snatching at straws.

The opposite extreme of the indigenous extended system is found when the lay culture and the professional culture are much alike and when the lay referral system is truncated or there is none at all. Here, the prospective client is pretty much on his own, guided more or less by cultural understandings and his own experience, with few lay consultants to support or discourage his search for help. Since his knowledge and understandings are much like the physician's, he may take a great deal of time trying to treat himself, but nonetheless will go directly from self-treatment to a physician.

Of these extreme cases, the former is exemplified by the behavior of primitive people and the latter by the behavior of physicians or nurses when taken ill. (Paradoxically, they are notoriously "uncooperative" patients, given to diagnosing and treating themselves.) Between these two extremes, in the United States at least, members of the lower class participate in lay referral systems resembling the indigenous case, and members of the professional class tending toward the other pole, with the remaining classes, taking their places in the middle ranges of the continuum.[23]

As Goode has noted, "Client choices are a form of social control. They determine the survival of a profession or a specialty, as well as the career success of particular pro-

[23] See the review of studies in Simmons, *op. cit.*

fessionals."[24] The concept of lay referral system, thus, provides a basis not only for organizing knowledge about the patient's behavior but also for understanding conditions under which he, a layman, to some extent controls professional practice. Indeed, the lay referral system illuminates the ways in which the client's choice is qualified and channeled and how the physician's sex, race and ethnic background affect his success— though it is often said that professions rest upon achieved status.[25] We can now see why a practitioner may never get any clients, and why, on the other hand, he may get clients but then lose them; for the lay referral system not only channels the client's choice but also sustains it or, later on, leads him to change his mind. Interviews with urban patients reveal that the first visit to a practitioner is often tentative, a tryout. Whether the physician's prescription will be followed or not, and whether the patient will come back, seems to rest at least partly on his retrospective assessment of the professional consultation. The client may form an opinion by himself, or, as is often the case, he may compare notes with others—indeed, he passes through the referral structure not only on his way to the physician but also on his way back, discussing the doctor's behavior, diagnosis, and prescription with his fellows, with the possible consequence that he may never go back.

One might assume that all but the most thick-skinned practitioner soon become aware of lay evaluations, whether through repeated requests of their patients for vitamins or wonder drugs or through repeated disappearances or protests following the employment of scientifically acceptable prescriptions such as calomel or bleeding. Whether their motive be to heal the patient or to survive, professionally, they will feel pressure to accept or manipulate lay expectations, whether by administering harmless placebos[26] or by giving up unpopular drugs.[27]

In a relatively organized community,

channels of influence and authority that exist independently of the profession may guide the patient toward or away from the physician and may more or less control not only the latter's success but, to some extent, also his professional technique and manner,[28] in short, the lay referral system is a major contingency of medical practice. Practice in an indigenous extended system must adjust itself to the system in order to exist: when involving patients who are themselves professionals, it may make fewer adjustments.

The above discussion of the lay referral system should be taken to show that, in being *relatively* free, the medical profession should not be mistaken for being *absolutely* free from control by patients. Indeed, we may classify various kinds of professional practice on the basis of relative freedom from client control. But, to do so, we must examine sources of professional freedom that lie not in a complaisant clientele but in the nature of professional organization itself.

Enough has been written about the privileged position that the organized power of the state grants the practitioner. (Indeed, this support by power located outside the community is often crucial to practice in

---

24 *Op. cit.*, p. 198.
25 E.g., T. Parsons, "The Professions," *op. cit.*, pp. 189 and 193; note the qualification on p. 197.

26 The placebo might be used as an index of control by the client of the terms of practice. On rationalizing sleight-of-hand as the placebo see Evans–Pritchard, *op. cit.*, pp. 235–236.
27 "This helplessness of regular physicians, coupled with popular distaste for bleeding and vile medicines, goes far to explain the success enjoyed by large groups of irregular practitioners. . . . A not uncommon shingle advertisement in those early years was: Dr. John Doe; No Calomel" (T. N. Bonner, *Medicine in Chicago, 1850–1950*, Madison, Wis.: American History Research Center, 1957, p. 12). When doctors began to do less dosing in the late eighteenth and early nineteenth centuries, the public went out and bought its own medicine. Cf. R. H. Shryock, *The Development of Modern Medicine*, New York: A. A. Knopf, 1947, pp. 248 ff.
28 Cf. the devices used in China and in Europe to avoid offending the patient's sense of modesty —H. Dittrick, "Chinese Medical Dolls," *Bulletin of the History of Medicine*, 26:422–429, September–October, 1952; J. Friedenwald and S. Morrison, "The History of the Enema with Some Notes on Related Proceedings," *Bull. History of Med.*, 8:68–114, January, 1940, and *ibid.*, February, 1940, pp. 239–276. On modern practice, articles in *Medical Economics* provide evidence.

"underdeveloped" countries where the prospective patients do not have a high opinion of modern physicians.) At the same time, political support sets severe limitations on competition,[29] both by prosecuting irregular "folk" or "quack" practice and by allowing restriction of the number of professional practitioners, two measures which greatly contribute to the stability and independence of the professional role.

Beyond these measures, however, we must note an additional important source of strength: Insofar as there are two "traditions" and two structures in a community, the lay referral system is one, and what we might call the "professional referral system" is the other. The professional referral system is a structure or network of relationships with colleagues that often extends beyond the local community and tends to converge upon professionally controlled organizations such as hospitals and medical schools. Professional prestige and power radiate out from the latter and diminish with distance from them. The authoritative source of professional culture—that is, medical knowledge—also lies in these organizations, partly created by them and partly flowing to them from the outside.

The farther this professional referral system is penetrated, the more free it is of any particular local community of patients. A layman seeking help finds that, the farther within it he goes, the fewer choices can he make and the less can he control what is done to him. Indeed, it is not unknown for the "client" to be a petitioner, asking to be chosen: the organizations and practitioners who stand well within the professional referral system may or may not "take the case,"

according to their judgment of its interest.

This fundamental symmetry, in which the client chooses his professional services when they are in the lay referral system and in which the physician chooses the patient to whom to give his services when he is in the professional referral system, demonstrates additional circumstances of the seeking of help. When he first feels ill, the patient thinks he is competent to judge whether he is actually ill and what general class of illness it is. On this basis he treats himself. Failure of his initial prescriptions leads him into the lay referral structure, and the failure of other lay prescriptions leads him to the physician. Upon this preliminary career of failures the practical authority of the physician rests, though it must be remembered that the client may still think he knows what is wrong with him.

This movement through the lay referral system is predicated upon the client's conception of what he needs. The practitioner standing at the apex of the lay referral system is the last consultant chosen on the basis of those lay conceptions.[30] When that chosen practitioner cannot himself handle the problem, it becomes *his* function, not that of the patient or his lay consultants, to refer to another practitioner. At this point the professional referral system is entered. Choice, and therefore positive control, is now taken out of the hands of the client and comes to rest in the hands of the practitioner, and the use of professional services is no longer predicated on the client's lay understandings—indeed, the client may be given services for which he did not ask, whose rationale is beyond him. Obviously, the patient by now is relatively helpless, divorced from his lay supports.

From the point of view of the physician,

29 To cite a dramatic instance of earlier competition: two tenth-century physicians who were competing for the favor of a king ended by poisoning each other at the king's dinner table. The one who knew the antidotes obtained the king's patronage (L. C. MacKinney, "Tenth Century Medicine As Seen in the *Historia* of Richer of Rheims," *Bull. History of Med.*, 2: 367–368, August, 1934. The veracity of this is questioned in P. O. Kristeller, "The School of Salerno," *Bull. History of Med.*, 17:143–144, February, 1945, but as the historian L. Gottschalk once said, "Se non è vero è ben trovato." For modern times Hall's observations on the "individualistic career" are relevant.

30 The actual specialty of the practitioner's standing in the lay referral system varies; certainly the general practitioner is almost always within it. Often pediatricians, gynecologists, internists, and ophthalmologists are to be found within it, particularly in communities of the professional classes; pathologists, anesthesiologists, and radiologists are unlikely ever to be within it.

position in the process of referrals is also of importance. If he is the first practitioner seen in the lay referral structure, and if he sends no cases further on, he is subjected only to the lay evaluation of his patients as they pass back through the hands of their lay consultants after they leave him. If he refers a case to another practitioner, however, his professional behavior becomes subject to the evaluation of the consultant. In turn, when the patient leaves the consultant, he often passes back to the referring practitioner, so in this sense the professional consultant is subjected to the evaluation of the referring physician. Thus the physician who subsists on patients referred by colleagues is almost always subject to evaluation and control by his colleagues, while the practitioner who attracts patients himself and need not refer them to others is subject primarily to evaluation and control at the hands of his patients.

These observations suggest two extreme types of practice, differing in the relation of practice to the lay and to the professional referral systems. At one extreme is a practice that can operate independently of colleagues, its existence predicated on attracting its own lay clientele.[31] In order to do so, this "independent practice" must offer services for which those in a lay referral system themselves feel the need. In reality, of course, it will be conditioned both by the existence of competitors and by the particular lay system in which it finds itself, but on the whole, one should expect it to be incapable of succeeding unless conducted in close accord with lay expectations. To survive without colleagues, it must be located within a lay referral system and, as such, is *least* able to resist control by clients, and *most* able to resist control by colleagues.

At the other extreme is postulated a "dependent practice" that does not in and by itself attract its own clientele but, instead, serves the needs of other practices, individual or organizational. The lay clientele with whom the practice must sometimes deal

does not choose the service involved: a professional colleague or organization decides that a client needs the services of a professional in a dependent practice and transmits the client to him: the colleague or organization, alone, in many cases are told the results of the consultation. Obviously, by definition, dependent practice could not exist in a lay referral system. To survive without self-selected clients, it must be in a professional referral system where clients are so helpless that they may be merely transmitted. As such, dependent practice is *most* able to resist control by clients and *least* able to resist control by colleagues.

The logical extreme of independent practice does not seem fully applicable to any professional practice, if only because a professional practitioner is trained outside the lay community before he enters it to practice and because his license to practice ultimately depends upon his colleagues "outside" and may be revoked. The "quack" seems to fit this logical extreme, for not only does he not require outside certification but, as Hughes defined him, he is one "who continues through time to please his customers but not his colleagues."[32] He, like the folk practitioner, is a consultant relatively high in the structure of lay referrals, with no connection with an outside professional referral system.

Close to this extreme in the United States is the independent neighborhood or village practice (usually general in nature) that Hall calls "individualistic,"[33] with, at best, loose co-operative ties to colleagues and to loosely organized points in the professional referral system. All else being equal in this situation of minimal observability by colleagues and maximum dependence on the lay referral system, we should expect to find the least sensitivity to formal professional standards[34] and the greatest sensitivity to the local lay standards.[35] This differential sensitivity

[31] See my paper, "Specialties Without Roots: The Utilization of New Services," *Human Organization*, vol. 18, Fall, 1959.

[32] Hughes, *op. cit.*, p. 98.

[33] See Hall, "Types of Medical Career," *op. cit.*, pp. 249–252, and Solomon, *op. cit.*, chaps. vi and vii on physicians connected with Group II hospitals.

[34] This, rather than medical education, might be an important determinant of the findings in Peterson, *et al.*; *op. cit.*

[35] As examples of the effect of clients' prejudices of success and location, see J. J. Williams,

should show up best where the lay referral system is indigenous and extended.

Moving toward the position of dependent practice is what Hall called the "colleague practice," in close connection with a well-organized "inner fraternity" of colleagues and rigidly organized service institutions.[36] This practice tends to revolve around specialties, which in itself makes for location outside particular neighborhoods or villages, and therefore reduces the possibility of organized control by the clients.

Finally, the closest to the extreme of dependent practice is a type that overlaps somewhat with the "colleague practice" but that seems sufficiently significant to consider separately. It might be called "organizational practice." Found in hospitals, clinics, and other professional bureaucracies,[37] it involves maximal restriction on the client's choice of individuals or services: clients are referred by other practitioners to the organization, or, if they are seeking help on their own, they exercise choice only in selecting the organization itself, functionaries of which then screen them and refer them to a practitioner. Here, practice is dependent upon organizational auspices and equipment.

"Patients and Prejudice: Attitudes Toward Women Physicians," *Amer. J. Soc.*, 51:283–287, January, 1946; and S. Lieberson, "Ethnic Groups and the Practice of Medicine," *Amer. Soc. Rev.*, 23:542–549, October, 1958. For the effect of the type of legal practice on participation in community affairs see W. I. Wardwell and A. L. Wood, "The Extra-professional Role of the Lawyer," *Amer. J. Sociology*, 61:304–307, January, 1956; A. L. Wood, "Informal Relations in the Practice of Criminal Law," *Amer. J. Soc.*, 62:48–55, July, 1956.

[36] See Hall, "Types of Medical Careers," *op. cit.*, pp. 246–249; see also Solomon, *op. cit.*, chaps. vi and vii, on physicians connected with Group I hospitals. In "colleague practice" it seems that the colleagues' racial or ethnic prejudice determines success, not the clients'.

[37] This term is defined in D. C. McElrath, "Prepaid Group Medical Practice: A Comparative Analysis of Organizations and Perspectives" unpublished Ph.D. dissertation, New Haven, Conn.: Yale Univ., 1958; its problems are analyzed in M. E. W. Goss, "Physicians in Bureaucracy: A Case Study of Professional Pressures on Organizational Roles" unpublished Ph.D. dissertation, New York: Columbia Univ., 1959). See also Ben–David, *op. cit.* Unfortunately for our present purposes, none of these studies paid much attention to the role of the client.

The client's efforts at control are most likely to take the form of evasion. The events of the referral process being systematically recorded and scrutinized, and ordered by hierarchical supervision, the practitioner is highly vulnerable to his colleagues' evaluations: we should expect him to be most sensitive to professional standards and controls and least sensitive to the expectations of his patient.

This paper has stressed two notions—that variation in the culture and organization of patients and in the location of medical practice in the community is decisive in the introducing and sustaining of practice and in the technical and interpersonal modes of procedure in established practice. These closely interrelated notions were derived by conceiving of practice in relation to organized lay communities as well as to organized professional systems and by following the prospective patient through the two referral systems. The outcome emphasized was the relative extent to which control lay in the client's or in the practitioner's hands.

Like any analysis in which one must hold much of reality in abeyance, this has produced a certain amount of exaggeration. Where practice is already established, as opposed to where it is struggling to establish itself, much of what goes on is routine and conflict between the patient and the physician is rarely open but is masked by evasion and depends upon the practitioner's justified assumption that incompatible clientele will stay away or can be discouraged easily. Within this routine, such breaks and irritations as do exist are, of course, strategic areas to study, but the very routine, with the stable set of selected patients it implies, when compared from place to place, practice to practice, should reveal the compromises necessary to establish and maintain practice in the face of varying lay systems and varying positions in the lay and professional systems. Thus, the abstractly conceived professional role as described by such writers as Parsons may be qualified—indeed, sometimes, compromised—by the cultural and structural conditions in which it must be played.

15

The Doctor-Patient Relationship in the Perspective of "Fee-for-Service" and "Third-Party" Medicine

Mark G. Field

As MEDICINE BECOMES more complex and costly, the problem posed by the organization and particularly the financing of professional medical services on an equitable and socially adequate basis has become one of perhaps the thorniest social and political issues of mid-century America. Rare indeed is today's layman or physician who, publicly at least, would echo the statement made some twenty-five years ago by a professor of medicine in a grade A medical school that he did "not believe a patient was entitled to free medical care any more than he was entitled to free housing, free clothing and free feeding."[1]

And yet, with the growing realization that the health of a nation is a societal problem and not, as some thought and still think, the exclusive concern of the individual and his private physician, there has arisen substantial and understandable controversy on the modes of organizing and financing medical services. And it is significant to note that arguments about one or another such mode rarely fail to bring forth a discussion of its impact (real, alleged, or fancied) upon the doctor–patient relationship and, indirectly, on the quality of the professional services offered by the physician.

Purpose of the Study

The aim, in this exploratory study, is limited to an examination of certain aspects of the doctor–patient relationship as they might be affected by the institutional structure in which this relationship takes place. By institutional structure is meant here the complex of arrangements, predictable patterns, and social relationships whereby an activity of some importance to the society is supported and carried out.

The starting point is that the increasing complexity of modern medicine (a technological factor) and the growing functional significance of health (a social factor) have led both to an increase in the costs of medical services and to the rise of "organizational" as against the more traditional "solo" type of practice. This, in turn, has led to important changes in the mode of employing and

[1] Sigerist, H. E., "Socialized Medicine," in M. E. Roemer (ed.), *On the Sociology of Medicine*, New York: M.D. Publications, 1960, p. 39. It may be noted, however, that the same basic argument (upgraded as a result of prosperity to include luxury transportation) was recently taken up by a spokesman of the Health Insurance Association. "Why," he asked, "should we use tax money to buy everybody health insurance? We might as reasonably buy everybody a Cadillac. It's the same argument." Quoted in R. W. Tucker, *The Case for Socialized Medicine*, New York: The Call Association, 1961, p. 6.

From Journal of Health & Human Behavior, *Vol. 2: 252–262, Winter, 1961; by permission of the author and publisher.*

A revised version of a paper originally presented to the Alpha Omega Alpha Society at the Harvard Medical School, February, 1959. I am grateful to the discussants, particularly Drs. H. K. Beecher, A. M. Butler and D. D. Rutstein for their critical and insightful comments. Drs. J. Aronson and W. R. Burack read subsequent drafts and gave valuable suggestions. Eliot Freidson's book, *Patients' Views of Medical Practice*, New York: Russell Sage Foundation, 1961, was also very useful in clarifying certain issues. Finally Drs. E. Freidson and G. A. Silver made very valuable comments, most of which I was unfortunately unable to use because of publication deadlines. I alone, of course, bear the responsibility for the contents and interpretations expressed here.

This work was supported, in part, by research grants (RG 6318 and RG 9644) from the National Institutes of Health, Division of General Medical Sciences, U. S. Public Health Service.

remunerating the physician for his work. The emphasis in this paper is on the relevance of this mode for the doctor–patient relationship. It is also assumed that this relationship has some emotional connotation or meaning for the patient and is, in most cases, an element of the therapeutic process (though this element is not always recognized as such either by the patient or the physician). It is also assumed that the mode of employing and particularly, remunerating the physician is analytically distinct from the mode of organizing medical services though empirically the two often cannot be separated (physicians working in a hospital, for example, may either be salaried or paid by their private patients and yet be bound by the same hospital rules).

These above considerations grew out of a study conducted some years ago on certain aspects of medicine in the Soviet Union, and particularly on the performance of professional functions in a highly mobilized and directed society.[2] In one sense, every Soviet physician is a "company" physician, the company being the state. In the course of that study, the writer administered a written questionnaire to 1,650 former Soviet citizens then residing in Western Germany and in the Eastern United States.[3] The purpose of the questionnaire was to gain an insight into what it meant to be a patient under Soviet conditions. Of particular interest was the fact that the émigrés had experienced, in the course of their lifetime, at least two basic types of medical systems: "third-party" medicine in the Soviet Union and in Germany, and "fee-for-service" medicine in the United States. They were, therefore, in a fairly good position to make comparative judgments and evaluations qua patients. In the German sample, for example, about three-quarters of the respondents preferred the German system of medical care (i.e., insurance medicine) over the Soviet type, primarily because the former delivered, in actuality and in quality, what the latter often

[2] Field, M. G., Doctor and Patient in Soviet Russia, Cambridge: Harvard Univ. Press, 1957.
[3] Field, M. G., "Former Soviet Citizens' Attitudes Toward the Soviet, the German and the American Medical Systems," Amer. Soc. Rev., 20: 674–679, 1955.

only promised. The picture was the reverse in the United States, where 73 per cent of the respondents, when specifically asked which system of medical care they preferred, opted in favor of the Soviet system over the American. The reason they adduced was that in the Soviet Union, however inadequate medical care had been, they at least had a legitimate claim to it, not as charity, but as a right spelled out in the Constitution. Most émigrés also thought it was the duty of the state to provide free medical care to the people. In the United States, on the other hand, they had to pay what they felt were exorbitant fees to physicians in private practice, or suffer the indignities of charitable medical care. One of the anonymous respondents who, at the time, was living in New York, after answering the many questions put to him, epitomized what he, as a patient, felt was the difference between private medical care as practiced in the United States and Soviet socialized medicine: "In the Soviet Union," he commented in the margin of the questionnaire, "the physician is a slave of the state . . . in America he is the slave of the dollar."

Whatever the personal experiences behind this statement, and however excessively critical and over-dramatic the respondent may have been, his subjective assessment of the physician's position reflects some insight into certain structured tensions in "third-party" and "fee-for-service" medicine. It meant that the physician, either by being beholden to the state or dependent on the fee, was not exclusively devoted to the patient's interests, at least not to the degree wished by the patient. Stripped of its emotional connotation it signified, there were, in the two systems, certain "built-in" flaws that were, actually or potentially, detrimental to the clinical relationship. Before considering, in some detail, what these flaws might be, it may be necessary briefly to place medical services within a sociological framework.

From the viewpoint of society as an on-going and functioning social system, the provision of medical care to the members of that body must be seen as part of its "maintenance" mechanisms. Insofar as human beings can be viewed (from a narrow perspective, of course) as specific social investments (gestation, support, education, and training) before they become self-sufficient and self-supporting and insofar as they have specific adult roles to perform (occupational, kinship, political, religious, *et cetera*) the inability to perform such roles (either because of premature death or disability of any kind) poses for society a severe functional problem. The role of medicine, taken in its broadest sense, is to deal with that problem, and the physician's to eliminate, mitigate, minimize, neutralize (and sometimes prevent) the disruptive effects of illness, injuries, mental disorders, and premature death.

Within this context, two further elements seem of particular import: one is that of control over the professional actions of the physician. There must be some mechanism that will assure both society and the patient that the physician will perform his functions according to certain established and accepted standards, that the patient's helplessness will not be exploited by the physician, and that the interests of the patient will be safeguarded.

The other element derives from the fact that medicine is a specialized occupation and is part of the general division of labor; as such it *must* depend on the exchange processes and the market mechanisms for its economic maintenance and ongoing operations. In other words, the *outflow* of specialized professional services must be matched by a corresponding *inflow* of resources (usually expressed in money terms, but sometimes in services such as room and board during internship); the physician, in order to perform his medical functions has to be compensated, in one way or another, for his time and services. There are, of course, a variety of ways in which these costs can be met, but basically let us assume the two polar types mentioned earlier of "fee-for-service" and "third-party" medicine, and let us examine certain issues relevant to the doctor–patient relationship in each.

In this arrangement, usually associated with solo practice, the norm is that the patient directly compensates the physician in the form of an honorarium or fee. The physician renders a specific service to the patient, and in exchange the patient transfers to the physician an agreed-upon amount of money (or as the case may be, goods or services). The exchange transaction arising from the division of labor and specialization of functions is a private matter that need concern only the physician and the patient (or his representatives). The "sale" of professional services, therefore, is a direct one involving no middle-man. But, in this context, the transaction involves the physician in the traditional role of the small serviceman or businessman: He charges a fee for services rendered, accepts money, sends bills and reminders, and occasionally sues or may use the services of a collection agency. And yet, it is only necessary to point to certain commercial practices which the medical profession rejects to realize that the medical relationship is qualitatively different from the commercial relationship. The ideology of the profession, for example, places great stress on the obligations of the physician toward the patient's welfare and the exclusion of the profit motive in professional decisions. Nor is the physician expected to advertise, to give bargain fees, to promise "double your money back," to guarantee a cure, to refuse a patient because he is a poor credit risk, to split fees with referring colleagues, or to refrain to send his bill if the patient dies. The assumption is that the physician does his best in the interest of the patient's welfare under all circumstances. There is thus, in theory and in practice, *a complete segregation between the exchange aspect on the one hand, and the performance of services on the other.*

The foregoing, as Parsons has pointed out, should not be construed, however, as meaning that the physician is by nature *altruistic* and the businessman *egotistic*. This dichotomy is not only too simple, it is basically inaccurate. We can assume that both physician and businessman are concerned with occupational success in their respective field of endeavor. Success in the business world is measured by profits and failure by losses, all expressed in monetary terms; it is therefore expected of a businessman that he will strive to maximize profits. To do otherwise, would be contrary to the accepted definition of the businessman's role. Occupational success in the professional, and particularly the medical, role is only indirectly measured by monetary criteria. The criteria used to determine success in this field are different: training, knowledge, professional performance, intelligence, publications, contributions to science and medicine, new clinical procedures, respect on the part of professional colleagues and of the lay community. These conditions, furthermore, are the functional prerequisites for the establishment of a physician–patient relationship based on confidence; this confidence, which is of undeniable therapeutic value, could hardly exist in a typical buyer–seller relationship governed by the rules of the market.[4]

Control over the professional actions of the physician appears to be vested primarily in an internalized and self-enforced code of professional behavior of the type mentioned above and in the lay community (what Freidson calls the "lay referral system"). In such a system the physician is under some pressure to please his patients in order to acquire clientele. Word-of-mouth recommendations become an important element in building a practice, and inability to please the clientele will be reflected (in a competitive situation, at least) in mediocre success and a correspondingly poor income. In a noncompetitive situation there is, of course, less of a pressure to please patients.

Third-Party Medicine

If it is part of the ethos of the medical profession to provide services independently of the likelihood of being paid for them and, if we assume that the physician cannot live

on air, prestige, and good works alone, some mechanism must exist to compensate the physician for services rendered to those who cannot pay on a fee-for-service basis either from past savings, current income or a mortgaging of the future. The device of the sliding-scale is such a mechanism. Fundamentally it is an expression of the rough social justice dispensed by Robin Hood[5] in which the rich patient is robbed to help the poor one.[6] The sliding-scale as a device for financing medical care typically is an informal mechanism controlled and operated by the physician who determines, although he has no special training or competence to do so,[7] how much a patient can afford to pay. The sliding-scale as applied by the physician belongs primarily to solo practice. With the increased costs of medical care (including medical education which is part of these costs), with the increased proportion of individuals who depend on a salary for their livelihood, and with the development of organizational medicine (medical groups, clinics, health centers, hospitals), as the major setting for medical practice in the community, it becomes clear that the medical profession is not in the position any more to close, in one way or another, the financial gap caused by medical indigency. Furthermore, the rise of medical insurance has led to the progressive standardization of fees so that the sliding-scale tends to be progressively discarded. Some other way has to be devised

[5] I am indebted to R. W. Tucker, *op. cit.*, for pointing to the analogy.

[6] In a personal communication based on his work in Wellesley, Mass., Dr. W. T. Vaughan, Jr., pointed out to me that wealthy patients and clients expect to be overcharged by their physicians and lawyers, and develop a feeling of being unfairly exploited. Under these circumstances, the one-price situation of the store and supermarket is a much more comfortable one. It might be pointed out that the sliding scale also obtains in education in the form of scholarships and aids for deserving, but poor, students, and in the expectation that wealthy persons and alumni will make substantial gifts to the school, college, or university.

[7] This function has tended to pass to the social worker.

[4] Parsons, T., "The Professions and the Social Structure," in *Essays in Sociological Theory*, New York: Free Press, 1949, pp. 185–199, and in *The Social System*, New York: Free Press, 1951, pp. 428–479.

to compensate the physician for his work on other than a fee-for-service basis paid by the recipient of the service. Typically a fund is created, either through voluntary, regular contributions or through involuntary contributions (salary deductions) or through other methods such as taxation. (In this last case, it is understood that some persons who benefit from this fund do not make any contributions to it, this to the distress of some who are forced to make contributions but do not benefit from it.) The physician may draw his remuneration from this fund either on a fee-for-service basis, a flat fee, or a regular salary. For the purpose of this discussion it matters little *how* this fund was created and in what form payment is made available to the doctor. The critical point is that now the physician draws his compensation not directly from the patient but from a third-party (insurance, cooperative group, closed panel, company, school, army, state and so on). Schematically the outflow of services (—————→) to the patient and the inflow of compensation to the physician (— — — →) and the contributions to the third party (– – – – – →) can be represented as shown in Figure 15–1.

FIGURE 15-1

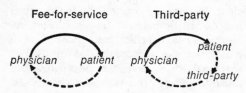

Fee-for-service   Third-party

The "third-party," whatever its nature or organizational form, is always under some obligation to see to it that the funds, for which it is responsible, are expended in what it believes to be the wisest, most economical, most effective, and most honest way possible. In order to carry out this mandate, some kind of review often is exercised over the recipient of funds, in this case, the physician. Institutional safeguards may be built that will reduce such review to the minimum and will allow the physician absolute professional freedom and discretion; on the other hand, certain restrictions may be

imposed for purposes of economy, as, for example, in prescribing. Further pressure may be imposed in the choice of modalities of treatment and in the assignment of certain standards that must be fulfilled if the physician is to remain in good standing with the third-party. Finally, there may be direct interference in, and dictation over, professional matters, coupled with professional or lay disciplinary power over medical personnel, e.g., under certain military, industrial or political conditions. Admittedly, the latter is an extreme situation but it does represent certain implications that can flow from third-party medicine, as will be seen below.

A Comparative Summary

It may be useful, before proceeding any further, to recapitulate, in summary form, the major dimensions of the two arrangements just described. It may be noted that, in the tabular presentations in Table 15–1, those aspects of the doctor–patient relationship that are not directly related to the mode of payment have been placed into square brackets. As pointed out earlier, empirically they often cannot be so clearly distinguished.

It will readily be seen that the two types of arrangement outlined above are polar types, models so to speak, each one doing violence to reality, and yet useful as tools of analysis. It is only through picturing the theoretical extremes that one can distinguish the nuances of the intermediate types. Thus, for instance, in the United States while the general picture traditionally has been that of fee-for-service medicine, there is an ever increasing amount of third-party medicine (insurance-financed medical care, closed panels, industrial, military, institutional medicine, Veterans' Administration, and so on). In the Soviet Union, on the other hand, while the official norm is that of third-party medicine, there is still, according to most reports, a fair amount of fee-for-service practice, and even privately operated medical installations.[8] England might well represent a midway point with strong elements or

[8] Snegireff, L. S., "Review of Doctor and Patient in Soviet Russia," *Amer. Slavic and East European Rev.*, 17:548–549, 1958.

Table 15–1

	Fee-for-Service Medicine Also Known As "Private" or "Entrepreneurial" Medicine	Third-party Medicine "Socialized" or "Organizational" Medicine
Physician's Working Conditions:	["Solo," "independent," "individualistic" practice; physician typically works in relative isolation from his colleagues, responsible primarily to his patient; control of his professional acts rests in code of professional behavior and the lay clientele.]	["Group," "dependent," "closed-panel" practice; physician typically works within context of a professional collectivity, to whose members he is oriented and primarily responsible; what physician does, in one sense, commits or involves his colleagues in the collectivity; control of his professional acts rests in code of professional behavior, his colleagues and the collectivity more than in the lay clientele.]
Physician's Source of Income:	Typically the patient directly or his representatives.	Typically a group or organization but not the patient (except *indirectly* through contributions to group).
Settlement of Terms of Exchange:	Physician typically must settle terms with his "employer," the patient or his representative. Basis for settlement is service performed (regardless of outcome); fee theoretically tailored to ability to pay, while service is not. Physician must keep accounts, send bills, reminders, sometimes sue for his fee.	Physician typically relieved of necessity to settle terms with patient, but must settle terms of employment with collectivity (in the form of a salary, flat-fee or fee-for-service); collectivity responsible to settle terms both with physician and with patient (premium) or other source of income (company, state).
Potential Advantages to Physician:	[Independence from group or colleague pressures, supervision and control;] possibility to maximize income through hard work, successful practice and good reputation in lay and professional community.	[Assistance, cooperation, support, advice from colleagues; availability of "stand-ins" to relieve physician of professional responsibilities (weekends, nights, holidays)]; no need to attract clientele from lay community since patients are available as "captive audience"; regularity and predictability of [work load and] income.
Potential Disadvantages to Physician:	[No regular assistance from readily available colleagues and assistants; no provision for "stand-ins" to cover for physician; need to always be available to patient, long hours and unpredictability of work load and income;] income dependent on physician's health and ability to work, and no provisions are made for maintenance of income if he is disabled; need to attract lay clientele; potential incompatibility between professional ethics and demands of patients.	More patients come to physician than would if they had to pay a fee; there usually is limitation of income by comparison with equivalent fee-for-service practice; "paper work"; physician more or less dependent on collectivity that employs him and subject to its demands, pressures and control; potential incompatibility between professional ethics and bureaucratic norms.
Potential Advantages for Patient:	Physician in competition with other physicians interested in doing good job because his reputation and income depend on it; client can therefore "manipulate" physician; this is client-centered practice; patient typically deals with only one physician, "his" own physician; this permits a personal relationship to exist between patient and physician.	Physician can help patient independently of patient's financial resources; no tendency to give unneeded treatment to increase own income; [physician usually has ready access to consultants; colleague-oriented medicine likely to be better than independent, isolated practice.]
Potential Disadvantages for Patient:	Tendency to please patient may be detrimental to patient's best interests (requests for popular but contraindicated treatment) (lack of supervision by colleagues and isolation of physician may affect quality of care); commercialism, exploitation of patient, selection of patient on financial grounds, unneeded treatment, over-treatment, quackery, charlatanism, fee-splitting, "slavery to the dollar."	Tendency to please or obey organization on part of physician may be detrimental to patient's best interests (requests of the organization for standardization of treatment or prescription); "politics," bureaucratism, under-treatment, indifference because of lack of competition, availability of patients and regular income; [patient typically deals with multiplicity of essentially interchangeable physicians leading to a depersonalization of physician–patient relationship; patient becomes organization's patient rather than physician's patient;] control, pressures, demands by organization may lead to "slavery to the state."

combinations of elements of the two basic types outlined above.[9]

Pitfalls and Temptations in the Two Systems

The contention is that these two types of institutional arrangements may give rise, under certain social conditions and pressures, to pitfalls and temptations and to the "dependencies" mentioned earlier and which are detrimental to the patient. In a system of private medical care coexisting with widely accepted commercial practices in the larger society, as in the United States, physicians would be less than human if they did not feel that their training, qualifications, working conditions, and the importance of their functions did not entitle them to the same status, financial rewards and creature comforts gleaned by those in the commercial world with equivalent (and sometimes more limited) education, work-load and responsibilities. It may well seem unfair to the physician that some people begrudge him his Cadillac and other visible signs of status[10] that are commonplace in the business world, particularly when he can point to statistics showing that the public may spend more on cigarettes and entertainment than on medical care. As Parsons has pointed out:

Actual achievements may fail to bring recognition in due proportion and vice versa achievements either of low quality or in unapproved lines may bring disproportionate recognition. Such lack of integration inevitably

[9] Eckstein H., *The English Health Service*, Cambridge: Harvard Univ. Press, 1958.

[10] There is, indeed, increased evidence of general resentment against the physicians and the fees they charge. In a poll conducted only a few years ago, Elmo Roper and his organization found out that doctors' bills were the ones most resented by the American public. Among the well-to-do, doctors placed a close second after plumbers. And yet, as Tucker points out, computed on an average work-week of slightly over 60 hours a week in terms of hourly rates with overtime, and doubletime for Sunday, the average base pay of doctors comes to $4.13 as against $4.25 for union bricklayers in New York City. *op. cit.*, pp. 10 and 13.

places great strain on the individual placed in such a situation and behavior deviant from the institutional pattern results on a large scale. It would seem that, seen in this perspective, so-called "commercialism" in medicine and "dishonest" and "shady" practices in business have much in common as reactions to these strains.[11]

In a society where status must be conspicuously displayed to count, the temptation may be to slip into commercialism, and even for the patient with the slightest persecution complex, the feeling of being exploited may sometimes intrude itself uncomfortably between himself and the physician. The fact that the overwhelming majority of physicians do not succumb to this temptation is a tribute both to their integrity and to the effectiveness of the system of institutional controls mentioned earlier. There are, of course, other stresses inherent in medical practice everywhere (the strain of uncertainty, the inability to help in many conditions, the unrealistic expectations of the public) but these are unrelated to the institutional arrangements of medicine and are not relevant to the argument at hand. While the advantages and the pitfalls of private medicine are well known to most American physicians, much less is really known of the strains inherent in socialized or public medicine, particularly as practiced under Soviet conditions. It is to these that the writer would like now to turn his attention.

Soviet society may be characterized as a large-scale social system of the national type in a state of forced-draft industrialization and urbanization. Furthermore, it may be described as a politically monolithic society in which all the power, including control over the means of mass communications, has been concentrated into a single party, and eventually into the hands of a few persons or even one person. This party considers itself the embodiment, the corporate expression so to speak, of a body of doctrine or an ideology in the name of which it governs and rules the country. It has defined a series of goals and subgoals toward which it harnesses most social processes in the society, a process

[11] Parsons, "Professions and the Social Structure," *op. cit.*, p. 195.

facilitated by the political monopoly of the party. One of these goals is industrialization at a rapid pace without importation of capital from abroad. Capital formation is the result of enforced savings at the expense of the working population, and is facilitated by the absolute political control over all national means of production. Thus, the twin factors of industrialization and monolithic political control must be kept in mind when one examines all aspects of that society, including the medical system. As a mobilized society in which maximum performance is expected from the population, the medical profession is also mobilized to help contribute to the goals of the regime by keeping the population healthy and fit to produce. The quantitative achievements of the Soviet regime in medicine over the last forty years are impressive, to say the least. A medical contingent that has increased about 18 times since the revolution, a complement of hospital beds that increased 6 to 7 times, a 75 per cent drop in the death rate, a doubling of the life expectancy at birth are just some crude indices of accomplishments.[12] And yet this progress has been accompanied by far-reaching changes in the status and working conditions of the physician, such as the elimination of the medical profession as an independent corporate body,[13] the bureaucratization and centralization of most medical services under the administration of the Health Ministry, the subordination of that Ministry to the needs of the state, and the transformation of the physician into a salaried state employee. In the study the writer conducted of the Soviet medical profession, it soon became apparent that these working conditions carried certain implications for the physician, especially with respect to the doctor–patient relationship. It should be added, parenthetically, that the conditions examined were those of the late thirties and early forties, the years

12 *Zdravookhranenie v SSSR Health Protection in the USSR*, Moscow: Gostatizdat, 1960; also, see M. G. Field, "Soviet Health Services," *Soviet Survey*, No. 35, January–March, 1961, pp. 100–105.
13 Field, M. G., "Medical Organization and the Medical Profession," in C. E. Black (ed.), *The Transformation of Russian Society*, Cambridge: Harvard Univ. Press, 1960, pp. 541–552.

of massive purges, terror, war preparations, and other stressful events in the Soviet Union. These must have been years in which pressures upon physicians were maximal, and there is little doubt that, at the present time, they have considerably abated.[14] Yet, it is perhaps under extreme conditions that the potential fault-lines are most clearly visible for analytical examination.

Stress in the Soviet System

Testimony from former Soviet physicians indicated many areas of stress in the practice of medicine under Soviet conditions, in addition to the usual problems of medical practice everywhere. But it soon became clear that interference into strictly medical problems on the part of the state, and the intrusion of considerations extraneous to the clinical situation, made it difficult for the physician to perform his functions exclusively in terms of the best interests of the patient. One problem, in particular, loomed large as a source of difficulty both for the physicians and for patients: this was the question of the certification of health and illness.[15] Peterson, in his study of the British Health Service, has pointed to the importance of this medical function:

> Medical certification is necessary and correct in a society in which the individual is insured against illness and disability. There is no other obvious way to do justice to the individual. ... The situation is further complicated by the fact that the practitioner is often busy and probably does not have the time to perform a more extensive investigation which might occasionally satisfy the doctor that no certificate of disability should be given.[16]

It is probable that the physician's certification function constitutes one of the import-

14 Personal observations in the course of two trips in 1956 and 1961.
15 See Field, *Doctor and Patient in Soviet Russia, op. cit.*, pp. 146–180.
16 Peterson, O. L., *A Study of the National Health Service of Great Britain*, New York: Rockefeller Foundation, 1951, mimeo.

ant *hinges* between the social and the medical systems. As the one person qualified to do so, the physician testifies as to the fitness or the unfitness, physical and mental, of the individuals he is asked to examine, from the chief of state to the new draftee, from the applicant for a life insurance policy to the aircraft pilot. In the Soviet Union, in the period immediately preceding the Second World War, medical work was complicated by the existence of rigid and extremely harsh disciplinary measures in industry and agriculture, brought about by the regime's frantic efforts to industrialize as the war was approaching and its inability to provide the necessary incentives in consumer goods to the population.[17] Relief from some of these measures could sometimes be obtained from a physician through a medical certificate. As might have been expected, this resulted in malingering and the exaggeration or exacerbation of symptoms and signs in order to obtain the necessary dispensation. As one physician recalled:

There were workers who burned their hands. They would put a piece of ice on the skin to anesthetize it, and would burn it either with a piece of hot metal or a cigarette. Then they would put salt on it and they would do all they could to retard healing.[18]

Or as another one put it, in a slightly different context:

Let us say a patient comes to your office and says: "Look here, doctor, I am healthy, but I have four children and a wife to support, and we are starving; if you write a certificate stating I have gastritis, I will then be entitled to a better kind of ration. If you can do this, then I can feed my children a little better; I ask this, not for myself but for my family. . . ." You witnessed the terrible situation of a person and by empathy you decided, no, I must help this person, I cannot follow the laws of the government.[19]

[17] See, among others, R. A. Bauer, A. Inkeles and C. Kluckhohn, *How the Soviet System Works*, Cambridge: Harvard Univ. Press, 1956; and A. Inkeles and R. A. Bauer, *The Soviet Citizen*, Cambridge: Harvard Univ. Press, 1959.
[18] Protocols of the *Harvard Refugee Interview Project*, Bulletin no. 1379, pp. 31–32.
[19] *Protocols*, Schedule B11 no. 1758, pp. 41–42.

What the physician meant, by the "laws of the government" was the complex of regulations and pressures to which he himself was subject, as a medical employee, to prevent him from being too lenient, too softhearted in his medical role, and thereby from undermining or short-circuiting the elaborate system of controls devised by the regime. Both physicians and former patients indicated the imposition on them of standardized devices to restrict the latitude and the discretion of physicians in their medical functions. One of these devices was simply the setting of a body-temperature level below which a patient should not be excused from work; another consisted in providing physicians with only a limited number of certificate blanks to give out in a given period. Any supplementary blanks had to be formally requested from the clinic chief. The physician who consistently showed more "liberalism" than his colleagues would then be called to account for his actions. He might be accused of either disloyalty to the regime, or suspected of having accepted money for the certificate, charges that might lead to severe penalties.[20] Altogether, the physician's position as a state employee and civil servant placed him at the mercy of the medical organization that employed him. This organization could, if it felt the conditions warranted it, place powerful pressures upon him; these, in turn, might affect the clinical relationship and the performance of strictly professional functions. Such conditions of work naturally have an impact on the doctor–patient relationship.

Generally speaking, most Soviet émigrés who were queried on the subject held a favorable opinion of the Soviet physician. They believed that, basically, he was a good human being, ready and willing to help them, in medical as well as in non-medical situations; but that the political system and the organization of the medical services often transformed him into a willing or unwilling tool of the regime, who, as such, placed (or had to place) the interests of the state and of production ahead of those of individual patients. State or organizational pressure upon the physician to discover who was and

[20] Field, *Doctor and Patient, op. cit.*, pp. 165–167.

who was not faking illness, or aggravating an injury, negatively affected mutual trust between patient and physician. As one physician recalled: "Every person who was sick and knew about fakers tried to aggravate his case in order to receive the medical treatment to which he was entitled."[21] Inability on the physician's part to play what the émigrés believed to be his proper medical role and his over-dependence on organizational or "third-party" dictates undoubtedly constituted the "slavery to the state" mentioned earlier. Abundant comments in the questionnaires make this explicit:

[I do not like] Soviet medicine's subordination to the government, i.e., if there is a possibility of non-fulfillment of the plan, the doctor receives orders to cut down the number of [excused] sick workers.[22]

The [Soviet] doctor was not independent. Very often he had to act against his own conscience.[23]

Soviet doctors feared to give sick leave lest they be accused of sabotage or bribe-taking.[24]

English Medicine

It is in the light of this, and other similar evidence, that one can understand the initial reluctance of medical practitioners to work under systems of third-party medicine.[25] As Eckstein has pointed out, with reference to English medicine, "those doctors who claimed before the Appointed Day that under a comprehensive public medical service the doctor's loyalty would be torn between his patient and the State were not just talking reactionary nonsense."

What the doctors meant was that the State, whatever the nature of its intervention, would inevitably subject the practitioner to demands

irrelevant to the clinical situation and potentially destructive of it: demands for economy, for fitting patients into generalized classifications, for treatment along standardized lines, for an annoying amount of paper work. . . . The chief threat to medical practice in this respect was stereotyping—the gradual replacement of the spontaneous clinical relation by bureaucratic rules and standards.[26]

In many respects it appears that the fears of the British doctors were unjustified, or that these doctors were powerful enough to shape the National Health Services so as to minimize the potential pitfalls of socialized medicine. An important factor in this was the existence and the influence of the medical profession as an organized corporation that was free to state its position and make its demands known to the state, the Health Ministry and the public. There is, as far as the writer knows, no similar countervailing force under the Soviet political system. It may therefore be suggested that the "third-party" does not have uniform significance but that the professional association (or the lack of it) is an analytically as well as empirically important intervening variable.[27]

Conclusion

In conclusion, it may be stated that the Soviet version of third-party medicine may well exacerbate, rather than mitigate, certain structural defects of this type of medical organization and that this must be seen as the result of certain features of Soviet society, as defined earlier. Moreover, the data on which this study was based came, as pointed out earlier, from some of the worst periods in Soviet history, and naturally the medical scene has reflected these tensions and social upheavals. With the gradual improvement that has taken place in the life situation of the population since Stalin died, some of these extreme distortions in the medical field have, doubtless, disappeared. Nonethe-

[21] *Protocols*, Schedule B11 no. 607, p. 23.
[22] *Respondent* no. 531, Paper and Pencil Questionnaire.
[23] *Respondent* no. 1116, *ibid.*
[24] *Respondent* no. 1210, *ibid.*
[25] Apart, of course, from ideological considerations and possible income losses, at least in the American situation. In England, apparently, most physicians earn more money under the British Health Service than they did formerly. D. Cook, "Socialized Medicine, Ten Years Old," *Harpers*, May, 1959, p. 34.

[26] Eckstein, *op. cit.*, p. 174.
[27] Freidson, E., personal communication.

less, these defects are inherent in this type of medical organization as other defects are inherent in fee-for-service medicine.

As an ever increasing proportion of our population and of the medical profession will receive and give care within a "third-party" framework it becomes important that the basic problems and structural defects of such a framework be recognized by the parties concerned, and that they neither be swept under the rug by enthusiastic reformers nor magnified out of all proportion by equally adamant opponents. It would seem to be a major task of the organized medical profession to recognize the existence of changes in the nature of contemporary medical practice, i.e., both its complexity and its cost, and to devise the same types of safeguards and codes of professional behavior that have been so successful in insulating the clinical relationship from the temptations inherent in "the business ethic" or "commercialism." Indeed it might be said that the temptations of the "bureaucratic ethic" or of the "organization mentality" are no less potent nor less destructive of the doctor–patient relationship than those arising from the "acquisitive" society.

16

TEN YEARS AGO the writer terminated his article on "basic functional roles in nursing" with the statement that "nursing, with which the role of mother surrogate is so completely associated, will still be nursing [in the future], but it will be carried on by persons of other occupational affiliations, not the professional nurse."[1] Responses and comments to this statement came from many sources, chiefly from practicing nurses, nurse–educators and students in schools and colleges of nursing. Some were overtly hostile, others incredulous, others in agreement. Now a decade has passed and there is no longer any doubt that professional nursing has left the patient's bedside and that a majority of professional nurses have resolved the mother surrogate–healer role conflict by abandoning, circumventing or sublimating the mothering functions of the nurse's role. Although such a resolution is lamented by leaders in professional nursing,[2] it is difficult, if not impossible, to deny. The sociologist Rushing states that ". . . the conditions of social reality that sustain an image of the nurse as mother surrogate no longer exist."[3]

The obvious question which must then be raised is "Why?" What has happened to nursing and in nursing that has forced this resolution? This writer proposes that pressures from without as well as from within the discipline have molded, and are molding, the "new nurse," and that they have forced mother surrogate functions into the background if not into antiquity. There is no single factor which will explain the change: it is multi-causal with some factors immediate and apparent, others diffuse and evasive.

Mother Surrogate—After a Decade

Sam Schulman

External Factors

Perhaps the most evasive factor which has affected the nurse's predominantly non-affective performance today is rooted in the American family. The mother surrogate role may be said to develop out of the multi-faceted functions of the traditional mother–parent. Long before the decade of change we are considering, the American mother–parent role had begun to change. As if in a geometric progression, the initial changes in this role were few, slow to reach fruition and episodic; latter changes have been many, rapid and virtually constant. The American family and its constituent norms have come quickly to modernity. Familial affect has not been lost; in fact, as Parsons and Fox have noted, it has been intensified and has become strain-producing.[4] It does not depend, however, on the constant and multiform emotional and physical presense of a mothering figure. The mothering figure, for an ever-growing number of middle-class American families, is a spasmodic one. Part-time or full-time jobs, community participation, Leagues of Women Voters, as well as the many time-saving devices which have "liberated" women from "children, kitchen, and church"—all have served to reduce

[1] Schulman, S., "Basic Functional Roles in Nursing: Mother Surrogate and Healer," in E. G. Jaco (ed.), *Patients, Physicians and Illness*, New York: Free Press, 1958, chap. 54, p. 537.

[2] Reiter, F., "The Nurse–Clinician," *Amer. J. Nursing*, 66:278, February, 1966; F. Flores, "Role of the Graduate Nurse Today," *New England J. Med.*, 267:488, September 6, 1962; B. G. Schutt, "Conflicts in Medicine Raise Questions for Nursing," *Amer. J. Nursing*, 66:2419, November, 1966.

[3] Rushing, W. A., "The Hospital Nurse As Mother Surrogate and Bedside Psychologist: A Sociological Approach," *Mental Hygiene*, 50:74, January, 1966.

[4] Parsons, T., and R. Fox, "Illness, Therapy, and the Modern Urban American Family," *J. Social Issues*, 8:2–3, 31–44, 1952; reprinted in E. G. Jaco (ed.), *Patients, Physicians, and Illness*, New York: Free Press, 1958, chap. 25.

home contacts of children with mother once infancy has been conquered. Both boys and girls are affected by this lack of contact with a traditional mothering figure. Girls, who later become young women and, hence, constitute the "manpower" pool available to professional nursing, are of primary interest to us.

In essence, a great many—if not most—of the young women who are recruited into the ranks of professional nursing have lacked an adequate model of a mother–parent. However highly motivated they may be (as the writer's earlier presentation had indicated) to enact the role of mother surrogate, they have seldom been sufficiently exposed to an immediate and intimate example to whom they may refer. To many young women the mother surrogate role, however commendable and desired it may be, is an alien role.

Dean Dorothy Smith of the College of Nursing of the University of Florida has specifically blended into the four-year curriculum of her students self-perceptive psychological group work at each stage of their nursing education. All her teaching staff, in addition, are prompted to allow their students the fullest possible expression of "self" even as they are subjected to the demanding discipline of their clinical experiences. Although there are, indeed, psychotherapeutic benefits garnered from such an approach in the preparation of professional nurses, a basic goal is that of permitting young women the opportunity of voicing their inabilities as "mother surrogates." Bringing these inadequacies into the open and examining them under sympathetic and competent guidance helps these young women achieve an affective potential which otherwise they might not have.

But Dean Smith's educational philosophy is not yet found in many schools and colleges of nursing. It is assumed, where such assumption is made at all, that nursing students will absorb the mother surrogate functions somehow—and most do not. In the analyses of nurses' roles where the lack of these functions is indicated there is a failure to comprehend that large numbers of professional nurses began their careers without them and do not possess them now.

Two-thirds of all professional nurses work in hospitals.[5] Prior to and during the past decade the hospital as a working environment has changed. It would be extraordinary, as Florence Flores states, that with momentous changes in the hospital that nursing would emerge today "unscathed and undisturbed."[6] The modern hospital must share in the responsibility of changes in nursing: it, too, is a causative agent in the move away from the mother surrogate role. Hospitals today are "big business" and, with the extension of hospital care through growing public and private medical programs, can only grow "bigger." The pragmatic necessities of business force the hospital to utilize its personnel, professional and non-professional, to its most economical. With the relative scarcity of nurses, the major professional group in the therapeutic process over which the hospital exercises immediate control, and with the increasing utilization of non-professional nursing help, hospital administration has been forced to remove the nurse from the bedside. As seen by hospital administrators, nurses are more economically used in managerial and supervisory positions than in bedside nursing. Tasks involved in patient care run from the simple to the sophisticated, and hospital administration prefers, where it can, to use less-skilled and less expensive, but competent, personnel in simple tasks. Many of the jobs which relate directly to the immediate "custodial care" of hospitalized patients are classified as simple and, hence, are assigned to auxiliary nursing personnel. In 1963 the Surgeon General's office reported that 70 per cent of all bedside contacts with patients by all nursing personnel were made by auxiliaries. "I would suggest," states Rushing, "that the persons most suited for the mother surrogate role are nursing auxiliaries."[7]

It must be borne in mind that a great many hospital administrators are not ignorant of the fact that professional nurses, in large part, are better equipped to give bedside nursing care than are ancillary nursing

[5] Rushing, *op. cit.*, p. 74.
[6] Flores, *op. cit.*, p. 489.
[7] Rushing, *op. cit.*, p. 76.

personnel and that some—certainly not all —professional nurses regret their paucity of patient contacts. The director of a large southern medical center remarked to the writer, "It is a sorry affair, I know, to run a hospital like a machine tool plant. But when we can get our books to balance, and this isn't easy, we have to try to do so. And part of this is pushing the graduate nurse off the floor and behind a desk." The hospital, then, finds it necessary to optimize the services of professional nurses by substituting much of their patient-centered functions by managerial functions and by reducing their few actual patient contacts to those which demand greater skill and responsibility.[8] The professional nurse today is prevented from personally giving total care to her patients. States Rushing:

There are certain constraints placed on the nurse's hospital role that deter her from giving comprehensive nursing care. Furthermore, the types of nurse–patient interaction that are becoming increasingly frequent deter the development and reinforcement of the sentiments and attitudes that are at the heart of programs designed to encourage interaction with patients as "whole" persons [i.e., as persons with psychologic, interpersonal and social, as well as medical, needs].[9]

In the therapeutic process there are three essential role complexes which are systematically interrelated: those of patients, physicians and nurses. These constitute a fairly classic triadic relationship.[10] It is inevitable that any change in role performance of a member of the triad will affect the role performance of the other members. In this light, it might be said that changes in the behavior and attitudes of patients and physicians will produce change in the behavior and attitudes of nurses. This writer thus feels that it is justified to find some of the causal factors for changes in nursing in the medical profession and in the patient population.

Within the context of the hospital milieu

[8] See M. Jahoda, "A Social Psychologist Views Nursing As a Profession," *Amer. J. Nursing*, 61:54–55, July, 1961.

[9] Rushing, *op. cit.*, p. 71.

[10] Johnson, M. M., and H. W. Martin, "A Sociological Analysis of the Nursing Role," *Amer. J. Nursing*, 58:373–374, March, 1958.

the physician typically cannot be present to perform personally nursing functions for his patients. He must depend on the hospital's nursing service to see that his patients are afforded the correct care associated with a therapeutic regimen which he designs. The physician sees professional nursing as the keystone of effective hospital care. It is quite probable that he would prefer that all care tasks performed for his patients were done by a professional nurse, for he respects her preparation, knowledge and abilities. In this regard, Flores relates the following anecdote:

Some years ago I was a member of a group of doctors, hospital administrators and nurses (all appointed by their respective professional organizations) who were attempting to define the unique functions of the nurse. There was general agreement regarding matters of personal hygiene, nutrition and the like. When it was suggested that the nurse must meet some of the patient's emotional and psychologic needs, the physicians not only disagreed with the rest of the group but also disagreed with each other. Strangely enough, there was agreement that if the doctor didn't meet these needs, the nurse must.[11]

Physicians, however, recognize that total patient care given by professional nurses is not within the realm of possibility in modern hospitals. They, too, must abide the extension of care tasks to non-professional personnel. It is a "necessary evil." If, however, the care regimen is entrusted to a host of variously titled nursing personnel, the physician wants the leader of the team to be a professional nurse. If this means that the "leader" sits at a desk and manipulates others who are "hands and feet," then he directly supports the diminution of face-to-face nursing–patient contacts.

Medicine itself has for years been many medicines and is exaggeratedly so today. The family doctor of yore in medicine has gone the way of the mother surrogate in nursing. Medical specialties have grown in both number and diversity. The needs of medical specialists have demanded complementary professional nursing specialists.

[11] Flores, *op. cit.*, p. 490.

The cardiac surgeon, as an example, cannot accept whatever help may be assigned to him: he must have a nurse co-worker who has special interest, abilities and experience in working with cardiac patients and a highly profound knowledge of the intricate machines, techniques and medications involved in the treatment of heart conditions. When a medical specialist states that a particular nurse "is worth her weight in gold," he indicates that she can be trusted to execute the intricacies of the procedures within "their" specialty with ability and dispatch. There are probably few things as disturbing to a medical specialist than to find an unfamiliar and untried replacement for a nurse in whom he has confidence. With the possible exceptions of psychiatrists[12] and pediatricians, medical specialists are more "procedure-oriented" than "patient-oriented," and they prefer to work with professional nurses who have developed expertness in procedures. The pressure applied by the medical profession has not only supported the elevation of professional nurses to administrative and supervisory positions, but has also forced these nurses more-and-more into patient contacts mediated by gauges, tubes and electronic devices.

Patients, too, have been instrumental in helping nurses dissociate themselves from mother surrogate functions. Like physicians, patients would undoubtedly prefer to have the most capable of nursing personnel, i.e., professional nurses, minister to their needs. Distinct from physicians, however, they do not usually distinguish "one kind of nurse from another" among the squadrons of women in white who enter and leave their hospital rooms. Their needs are many and it is their right to call upon nursing service to satisfy these needs. Researchers have shown that patients have difficulty in communicating the depth of their needs, especially those who ask for emotional support.[13] Those patients who

do vocalize their requirements ask for such things as bedpans, a more comfortable body position, the alleviation of pain, medications to induce sleep—simple things to ease their discomfiture. They do not overtly request emotional comfort. The simple things are supplied, in general, by non-professional personnel. Except in rare cases, since patients do not well express their insecurities and fears, their worries over their jobs or their homes, few members of nursing personnel, professional and non-professional alike, attempt to alleviate them. Hospitals are not warm nests where patients are coddled; they are efficient centers for the purpose of curing or ameliorating ailments, or they try to be so. Nurses of all rank and description fall prey to this ethos and help to maintain it. "Mother-surrogateness" is seldom encountered: in large measure, it is not asked for by patients nor is it given by nurses.

Patients, who are the clients of the big business of hospitals, want to achieve maximum benefit and return for their payments. Even though they cannot easily distinguish among the many women in white, their emphasis on optimal service for their money does so distinguish. The best possible service to patients parallels the physician's desire for the best possible internal organization for this service: physicians directly, and patients indirectly, demand the professional nurse head the team of non-professionals. In this sense, patients are supportive of the removal of professional nurses from patients' —their own—bedsides.

It bears mention that patients are parts of a greater collective, the lay public; they are that part of the lay public who are temporarily out of the usual run-of-things and in the hospital. Whereas inside hospital walls few patients would easily recognize the professional nurse, there is little doubt that the lay public, as a whole, has an altered image of the professional nurse today than yesterday. Professional nurses are no longer seen as "just anyone" who assumes the white uniform. The neighbor's daughter who is a university graduate must be a higher order of nurse. At one time most nurses were recruited from among lower- and lower-middle-class rural and small-town families who "worked" their way through three

[12] Olson, B. J., and J. E. Lubach, "Innovations in the Nursing Role in a Psychiatric Research Program," *Amer. J. Nursing*, 66:317–318, February, 1966.

[13] Elder, R. G., "What Is the Patient Saying?," *Nursing Forum*, 2:25–37, 1963.

arduous years of hospital "training". Today, ever increasing numbers of young women from well-situated middle-class families of large urban centers earn their caps and pins after four or five years of "education" at highly respected and accredited universities. It is inevitable that the changes in origin and background of newer recruits into professional nursing as well as the changes in nursing education programs will have had some impact on the public image of the professional nurse. This new nurse should be a leader, an authority, and well removed from menial tasks—these same simple tasks which have for many decades been associated with mother surrogate functions.

Internal Factors

Since the termination of World War II there has been a movement of great consequence to all nursing that can be best described as a "drive towards professionalization." The National League for Nursing, a younger organization dominated by the leading figures in nursing education, and the American Nurses Association, an older organization more dedicated to the rights and duties of nurses, have been prime movers in this direction. The League, specifically, has been able to challenge old ideas and sponsor new ideas in the professional preparation of nurses. The basic premises involved in the professionalization movement might be said to be: (1) in the past, the potential for nurses to do more responsible, involved and demanding tasks had not been realized; (2) decisions regarding the manner, magnitude and intensity of patient care could best be made by competent well-educated nurses; and (3) competent, well-educated nurses were not, in general, the products of weak and sometimes haphazard programs in schools of nursing in many hospitals where, at best, "training" was a three-year apprenticeship in simply hard work. Professionalization, then, has been approached from two major avenues: the upgrading of nursing education and, hence, of hospital nursing service; and a striving for more appropriate recognition and higher status within the health-asso-

ciated disciplines in the hospital community.

Even prior to this drive towards professionalization a few universities (beginning with the University of Minnesota as early as 1909) recognized the need to offer more than hospital training as the proper preparation for better nurses. The program at these universities combined both hospital training and a baccalaureate program without sacrificing the specific merits of either. Their students "worked" alongside diploma students for a complete hospital experience and "studied" at the university. It was the exceptional early university nursing student who completed her dual curriculum in less than five or six years.

In the late 1940s and early 1950s many other universities, most of these with medical schools or colleges, joined the effort. They cut back on the work experience and magnified the study program, usually limiting the total curriculum to four years. The stress was, and still is, on a full and enriching university-level education. Following the pattern of medical colleges, nursing colleges may be associated primarily with a single medical center (such as that of the University of Texas) or may eclectically choose clinical affiliations from several cooperating institutions (such as that of Boston University).

Although there is no complete unanimity in educational philosophy or practice in university programs, the National League for Nursing, the national accrediting agency, demands a rigid minimum in clinical facilities, well-prepared teaching staffs and true university instruction. All university nursing programs, however, share an emphasis on the fact that their graduates are, indeed, well-prepared and capable professionals.

The elevation of nursing into the realm of a higher educational discipline has had its effects elsewhere in the education of nurses. Many of the once-proliferating weak hospital schools have disappeared, and those that remain have been upgraded and modernized. Sub-baccalaureate programs at junior colleges, usually of two-year duration, have emerged as an intermediary type, producing "graduate" nurses (those who may be licensed within a state and who may affix the "R.N." to their names, as do hospital and university graduates) who are not afforded the same status within the discipline as are their better-educated associates. Even the programs for "practical" nurses have been made "courses of study" rather than short and over-simplified periods of on-the-job training. On the other hand, the move upward has prompted university graduates of special talent or ambition to pursue even higher academic recognition through achieving graduate degrees.

Professionalization has brought a greater dignity to nursing, it is true. Even in the decade under consideration one senses the the change that 10 graduate classes of modern professional nurses (and the subsequent retirement of 10-years-worth of nurses of the older tradition) have wrought. Esther Brown has described situations where professionally responsible nurses have challenged, and even admonished and corrected, medical authority when physicians have made incongruous or erroneous decisions.[14] At the University of Colorado Medical Center there has been initiated an experimental program of specialized education for a limited number of nurses where, under medical supervision and with medical approval, nurses are assuming certain physicians' functions in public health. A few years ago the writer proposed a program for the preparation of nurse–obstetricians (not nurse–midwives) who would replace and assist obstetrical specialists in hospitals, and the proposition was well-received by both physicians and nurses. Frances Reiter speaks of a "master practitioner" in nursing of great experience, special abilities and advanced education (the "nurse–clinician") who, in the not-too-distant future, would provide even more outstanding guidelines for patient care and who would be members of an Academy of Nursing.[15] The professional nurse is far from being a "hand-maiden," and her days as a drudge are in the remote past. She insists that she cannot be taken for granted as just a "professional employee" in the hospital. She has achieved, and is still achieving, a new status-role of greater authority and respect than she has ever had. And, even when the admission of this new status-role is only grudgingly made, she strives for this recognition.

Professional nurses have fought for, and received, acknowledgment in some difficult battles with other groups. The Fairview "incident," where a well-integrated sub-professional group set up barriers against them and where nurses tore them down, is a case in point.[16] In 1966, the status striving of nurses overcame their "ethical convictions" when they "struck" against the hospitals of a major American city—San Francisco—demanding greater monetary compensation in keeping with their professional status. Ten years earlier the San Francisco "strike" would have been unthinkable.

The drive towards professionalization has, almost inadvertently, assisted in diminishing mother surrogate functions of professional nurses. Many of these functions seem to be "dirty work" and beyond the pale of professionals. As a nurse mentioned to the writer, "A girl doesn't go through four years of college to do *scut* work. There are other people who can do that." Rushing states that "professionals" must have exclusivity of functions, and, hence, professional nurses cannot "adopt the mother surrogate core of skills, for it is clearly an ability that requires no special expertise."[17]

An interesting study using the technique of factor analysis by Raskin and his associates has illustrated the intense concern of professional nurses with their person-to-person interactions. It is striking, however, that their desires for interaction are not primarily with patients, but are oriented towards acting as leaders, interacting with others by ordering them about.[18] A British

[14] Brown, E. L., *Newer Dimensions of Patient Care*, New York: Russell Sage Foundation, 1962, part 2, pp. 61–64.

[15] Reiter, *op. cit.*, p. 280.

[16] Lewis, E. P., "The Fairview Story," *Amer. J. Nursing*, 66:64–70, January, 1966.

[17] Rushing, *op. cit.*, p. 77.

[18] Raskin, A., J. K. Boruchow and R. Golob, "Concept of Task Versus Person Orientation in Nursing," *J. Applied Psychol.*, 49:182–187, June, 1965. It is also of interest to note that another

physician involved in a one-year period of special study in the United States found American nurses to be rigid and disciplined, fond of their desks at nurses' stations and of the paraphernalia and norms of these stations. The visitor, W. Bryan Jennett, notes that American nurses do not "waste time" on patients: nor, for that matter, do they "waste time" on physicians.[19] He rather cynically notes:

> The convention of escorting doctors round the wards has long since lapsed. . . . Indeed, I was there for a long time before I ever saw a doctor and a nurse speaking to each other. A large notice reminded all comers that verbal orders were on no account to be accepted. The doctors wrote orders for the nurses, who in turn wrote reports for the doctors, and each stood around reading each other's writing with never a word exchanged.[20]

It is evident that nurses themselves have contributed to the diminishing, if not the disappearance, of the mother surrogate role: it no longer fits the profession's own image of itself. It is either archaic or inoperable.

Conclusion

Ten years ago this writer noted that there was a conflict in nursing, and within nurses, between two sets of role expectations, those of the mother surrogate and of the healer. He further suggested that mother surrogate functions were rapidly decreasing among professional nurses and were becoming the proper functions of nursing non-professionals. However lamentable this may be— and it is, indeed, a moot question that it *is* lamentable—the past 10 years have strengthened and corroborated this opinion. It is his further opinion that this change was impossible to avoid, for there have been pressures from without nursing and from within nursing that could neither be abated nor negated. It might well be said that mother surrogate functions in professional nursing are dying or, to be stringent, that they are dead. It has been the purpose of these paragraphs to explain their demise.

It may very well be that as a *functional* role the mother surrogate has withered away within the realm of professional nursing. This does not imply that it does not have importance in another sense: that the *novice* nurse—even the pre-novitiate—does not have the ministering mothering image in mind as an ideal when she imagines what she shall be like when she wears white.[21] Like the novice lawyer who dreams of rescuing the defenseless from injustice, the novice clergyman who dreams of lifting hardened hearts to salvation, the novice physician who dreams of conquering all affliction, the novice sociologist who dreams of using the scientific method to make societies sound, the novice nurse still has her dream of tenderly ministering to those who are ill and in pain. In this sense, there shall always be a mother surrogate shadow that falls upon the nurse-to-be.

---

major configuration in the factor analysis showed that there was a definite inclination for the nurses tested to exhibit a profile of characteristics attributed to the very rigid, politically conservative, "authoritarian personality"!

[19] Jennett, W. B., "Taking the Nursing out of Nursing: Trans-Atlantic Trends," *Lancet*, 2:95, July 8, 1961.

[20] Jennett, W. B., *Ibid.*

[21] Mauksch, H. O., "Becoming a Nurse: A Selective View," *Annals Amer. Acad. Pol. and Soc. Sciences*, 346:88–98, March, 1963, as reprinted in J. K. Skipper, Jr., and R. C. Leonard, *Social Interaction and Patient Care*, Philadelphia: J. B. Lippincott, 1965, pp. 335–336.

17

Poverty, Illness, and the Use of Health Services in the United States

William C. Richardson

IN THE PAST DECADE, increasing attention has been focused on the relationships among poverty, health levels, and use of health services. The conclusion drawn by most of those who have studied the problem, stated in its simplest form, is that the poor are sicker than the nonpoor, and yet they use fewer health services. Put another way, the conclusion is that as a group, those who need health services the most actually use them the least. The intent of this article is to review some of the data underlying this general conclusion and to discuss briefly the usefulness of the conclusion as a guide to action.

Poverty has several dimensions, and there are a great variety of ways to distinguish between the poor and nonpoor. Every measure of poverty, however, is based on some concept of "basic need." And even elaborate and sophisticated attempts at measuring and quantifying need are, in the final analysis, based on a series of assumptions about what Americans consider decent living.

When need is translated into an income requirement, perhaps adjusted for family size, region, changes in the consumer price index, and so forth, one can then clearly distinguish between those whose family incomes put them above the particular poverty line being used and those who fall below it.

However, it can not be assumed that there would be general consensus that all those falling below a given line are "really" poor and all those above are not. The poverty income level most often used is the one developed by the Social Security Administration, which for an urban family of four is currently about $3,300.

It is not only impossible to arrive at a particular poverty line on which there would be universal agreement, but the standards of decency and need on which a poverty line might be based tend to increase over time. As a result, it makes more sense to compare high and low income persons with respect to characteristics such as use of health services than to attempt a judgment of the adequacy of services received by a group designated as "the poor" at a given point in time. Because of our changing standard of decency, our concern with respect to medical care is likely to be more with narrowing the gap between the poor and nonpoor in terms of health status and both quantity and quality of services than with simply raising everyone's use to some minimum level.

The questions concerning health status and use of health services, then, become ones involving differences between higher and lower income persons, without much regard for the absolute levels of income involved. Rather than asking the question "Is the average number of physician visits per year for persons with family incomes below $3,000 at a satisfactory level?" what we generally ask is "Is the average lower than the corresponding averages for persons in families with incomes over $10,000?"

Health Levels

Measures that have been used to examine the relationship between illness and poverty have ranged from clinical examination to lay reporting of general level of health. Measurements of illness for large populations have typically been accomplished through health surveys using one or more of several types of measures such as reporting of specific medical conditions, reporting of symptoms, or reporting of disability days. Illness con-

From Hospitals, Vol. 43: 34–40, July, 1969; by permission of the author and publisher.

ditions tend to be underreported with the use of household interview surveys; however, when one is interested in looking at differences between classes of individuals with respect to illness, the assumption is made that the tendency to underreport is evenly distributed throughout the population. Studies done to date suggest that this is a plausible assumption.

One of the prime sources of health survey data is the National Center for Health Statistics. The Center conducts intensive interviews with a sample of 42,000 households each year, obtaining health status and utilization information on about 135,000 persons. The National Health Survey data presented below in all cases represent estimates for the noninstitutional civilian population of the United States. The annual periods during which data on the various measures were collected vary as indicated in the tables. The relationships over a four- or five-year period are stable enough, however, that these differences in data collection periods should make little or no difference.

With respect to medical conditions, the Center provides data on both acute and chronic conditions. Income differentials for acute conditions are very small taken as a whole. The incidence of all acute conditions per hundred persons per year for the period July 1962–June, 1963, age adjusted, for the income categories under $2,000, $2,000 to $3,999, $4,000 to $6,999, and $7,000 or over, were 216, 204, 216, and 232 respectively. By definition, all acute conditions included in these rates were either medically attended or caused at least one day of restricted activity. Thus, these rates combine the effects of an underlying illness and the individual's

Poverty, Illness, and the   231
Use of Health Services
in the United States

response to that illness. The fact that the incidence rate is somewhat higher for the highest income group may reflect a greater inclination on the part of higher income persons to consult a doctor for relatively minor acute conditions rather than a greater incidence of underlying illness.

Chronic Conditions

Turning to chronic conditions, a clearer picture emerges with respect to the relationship between this type of illness and income than was the case for acute conditions. Chronic conditions may be divided into two types: those that result in limitation of activity and those that do not. As may be seen in Table 17–1, for every age category the proportion of the lowest income group with one or more activity limiting chronic conditions is greater than any of the higher income groups. In fact, with the exception of children under the age of 17 years, there is a steady decline in the proportion with limiting chronic illness as one moves from the lowest to the highest income categories.

The prevalence of chronic illness with activity limitation increases dramatically with age, with slightly less than 2 per cent of the United States population under age 17 reporting such illness in contrast to 45 per cent of those over 65. It is also the case that up to age 65, the difference in prevalence between the lowest and highest income categories becomes relatively larger as age increases.

Table 17–1—Per cent of population with chronic conditions causing, activity limitation by age and family income, United States July 1965–June 1966

Age	All Incomes	Under $3,000	$3,000– $4,999	$5,000– $6,999	$7,000– $9,999	$10,000+
			FAMILY INCOME			
All Ages	11.2	25.4	12.1	7.9	6.9	6.8
Under 17 Years	1.9	2.6	1.6	1.5	1.6	1.7
17–44	7.3	13.1	8.6	6.4	5.8	5.4
45–64	18.9	38.5	22.5	15.9	13.8	10.4
65 and Over	45.1	50.6	42.4	42.1	38.8	38.6

Source: Limitation of Activity and Mobility Due to Chronic Conditions, United States, July 1965–June 1966, National Center for Health Statistics, series 10, no. 45.

Children in poor families are about half again as likely as those in families with incomes of $10,000 or more to report an activity-limiting chronic condition; persons age 17 to 44 with family incomes below $3,000 are almost three times as likely to report one or more conditions when compared to the highest income category, and finally, the low-income group from ages 45 to 64 had a rate almost four times higher than the rate for persons with incomes of $10,000 or more.

Prevalence rates have been computed for several specific condition categories causing limitation of activity, namely: heart conditions, arthritis and rheumatism, mental and nervous conditions, high blood pressure, visual impairments and orthopedic impairments. Using the same four age categories—under 15 years, 15 to 44, 45 to 64, and 65 or older—the difference between low- and high-income persons reflects an inverse relationship between prevalence and income for every age group. Comparing all those persons with family incomes below $2,000 to those with family incomes of $7,000 or more, the lower income group reported four times the number of heart conditions, six times as many cases of arthritis and rheumatism, mental and nervous problems, and high blood pressure, eight times the number of visual impairments, and more than three times as many orthopedic impairments (Table 17–2).

It was mentioned above that chronic conditions may be divided into those causing activity limitation and those causing no limitation. We have seen that the former are clearly related to level of family income, with the poor reporting more limiting illness. The prevalence of chronic illness conditions that do not cause any activity limitation has a much weaker association with income, and the relationship goes in the opposite direction. That is, higher income persons are somewhat more likely to report nonlimiting chronic conditions, as may be seen in Table 17–3.

Question of Causality

In an analysis of the relationship between illness and poverty, the question of causality

Table 17–2—Number of conditions causing activity limitation per 1,000 population by condition category and family income, United States, July 1962–June 1963

Selected Conditions	FAMILY INCOME			
	Under $2,000	$2,000–$3,999	$4,000–$6,999	$7,000+
Heart Conditions	53.8	26.6	12.6	11.9
Mental and Nervous Conditions	26.4	13.3	6.6	4.2
High Blood Pressure	23.8	9.2	4.1	3.9
Visual Impairments	23.4	9.0	3.4	2.7
Orthopedic Impairments (Excluding Paralysis and Absence of Extremities)	54.4	28.1	18.1	14.9

Source: White, E. L, "A Graphic Presentation on Age and Income Differentials in Selected Aspects of Morbidity, Disability, and Utilization of Health Services," *Inquiry*, Blue Cross Association, vol. 5, no. 1, March 1968.

Table 17–3—Per cent of population with nonlimiting chronic conditions by age and family income, United States, July 1965–June 1966

Age		FAMILY INCOME				
	All Incomes	Under $3,000	$3,000–$4,999	$5,000–$6,999	$7,000–$9,999	$10,000+
All Ages	37.9	34.5	35.4	36.9	39.4	42.4
Under 17 Years	20.5	18.9	17.6	19.6	21.8	23.8
17–44	46.6	42.6	43.4	46.7	49.3	49.5
46–64	51.7	40.8	50.6	52.5	54.8	57.6
65 and Over	40.1	37.6	43.2	40.1	41.1	46.2

Source: *Limitation of Activity and Mobility Due to Chronic Conditions, United States, July 1965–June 1966*, National Center for Health Statistics, series 10, no. 45.

may arise. One of the outcomes of poverty may be greater illness due to inadequate diet, unhealthy living conditions, or lack of access to health services. On the other hand, the onset of serious chronic illness may substantially reduce family income. A classic study of the relationship between chronic illness and socioeconomic status by Lawrence,[1] reported in 1948, found relationships similar to the findings presented above. Lawrence, however, was able to go further and explore causality by having resurveyed 20 years later the same families as were in the original study. His conclusions were that socioeconomic status in and of itself does not materially influence the chances of developing chronic disease. On the other hand, chronic illness did appear to be a factor in changing socioeconomic status.

Although in general the causality may be in the direction of illness causing low income, it is hardly a simple relationship. Further, there are certain chronic diseases for which the susceptibility of the poor is greater than that of the nonpoor. Suggestive of this is the fact that in New York City in 1961 the incidence of tuberculosis (rate of new cases per 100,000 persons) for Negroes, Puerto Ricans, and whites was 158, 99, and 33 respectively. In terms of the general conclusion that has been reached regarding illness and use of health services—namely, that the poor have more illness and yet use fewer services—it matters little what the direction or nature of causality is. If we observed the poor using fewer health services

not be a serious issue. It is the fact that lower use seemingly can not be accounted for by less illness, which makes it a matter of concern. Whether the environment of poverty results in higher morbidity or whether morbidity results in poverty, or both, there remains the fact that a commensurately greater level of use of health services does not accompany the illness differential.

Disability Days

So far we have looked at the reporting of acute and chronic illness conditions. A summary measure of illness often used to compare the health status of the poor and nonpoor is the number of disability days incurred per year due to illness or accident. There are three types of disability days: restricted activity day (one on which a person substantially reduces the amount of activity normal for that day because of a specific illness or injury), bed disability day (one on which a person stays in bed for more than half the daylight hours because of a specific illness or injury), and work loss day (one on which a person over 17 who is currently employed did not work because of a specific illness or injury). For persons aged 6 to 16 the equivalent measure is school loss day.

Table 17–4, shows the relationship be-

Table 17–4—Age–sex adjusted rates per person per year of selected disability days by family income, United States, July 1965–June 1966

	FAMILY INCOME				
	Under $3,000	$3,000–$4,999	$5,000–$6,999	$7,000–$9,999	$10,000+
Restricted Activity Days	22.8	15.9	14.9	13.4	13.8
Bed Disability Days	9.2	6.2	6.2	5.3	5.8
Work Loss Days	7.9	7.2	6.5	5.1	4.8

Source: Disability Days, United States July 1965–June 1966, National Center for Health Statistics, series 10, no. 47.

and at the same time noted less illness among the poor, the differential in use would

[1] Lawrence, P. S., "Chronic Illness and Socio-Economic Status" in E. G. Jaco (ed.), *Patients, Physicians and Illness*, 1st Ed., New York: Free Press, 1958, Chap. 5.

tween these types of disability days and family income. The age–sex adjusted rates per person per year for the United States for the period July 1965, through June 1966, for those with family incomes below $3,000 compared to those with family incomes above

$10,000 are 22.8 vs. 13.8 restricted activity days; 9.2 vs. 5.8 bed disability days; and 7.9 vs. 4.8 work loss days. The difference in average number of days lost from school comparing the lowest and the highest income groups was 6.1 days compared to 5.3 days. For every type of disability day, we see that the poor have a rate that is at least 50 per cent higher than the equivalent rate for the nonpoor.

Use of Health Services

The evidence that the poor use fewer health services generally includes income differentials with respect to number of physician visits, interval since last physician visit, dental visits, hospital admissions, and lengths of stay. These indicators are crude at best, ignoring as they must systematic differences between the types of visits or admissions reported by the poor and those of the nonpoor. As will be seen below, there are only moderate differences on a national basis for these overall measures of volume. On the other hand, differences along other dimensions such as race are substantial, as are income differentials on certain qualitative factors, such as use of medical specialists.

Looking first at physician visits, it may be seen in Table 17–5, that the proportion of each income group having had a physician visit within the year preceding the interview increases steadily, moving from the lowest income category of under $3,000 up to the highest of $10,000 or more. Sixty-four per cent of the poor compared to 73 per cent of

the highest income group had a physician visit within the year. At the other extreme of the distribution, those with low incomes were three times as likely as those with high incomes not to have seen a physician within the previous five years (9 per cent compared to 3 per cent).

For the 1966–67 period, there were an average of 4.3 physician visits per person in the United States. Children under age five and persons over 65 have the highest number of visits per year, while children between the ages of 5 and 14 have the lowest number. The disproportionately large number of the aged found in the under $3,000 category contribute to the average number of visits for this income category being as high (4.6) as the number found in the $10,000 and over category. Of greatest interest in Table 17–6, however, are the differences by income within certain age categories. It will be recalled that the differences in the prevalence of activity-limiting chronic illness as well as the absolute levels become larger with increasing age, while the prevalence of serious illness was lowest among children. However, it is among children that we find the greatest difference in use of physician services. The average number of visits per year for children under five in the lowest income group is 4.4 in contrast to 7.2 for children under five in families with incomes over $10,000. For children ages 5 to 14 the comparable averages are 1.5 and 3.5. The physician utilization differences by income that are so pronounced among children do not obtain in the older age groups. It may be that increased illness, particularly activity-limiting chronic illness among wage earners in the older age groups, results in an equalized use of services when

Table 17–5—Per cent distribution of persons by time interval since last physician visit and family income, United States, July 1966–June 1967

| | INTERVAL SINCE LAST PHYSICIAN VISIT | | | | |
	Less than 1 Year	1–4 Years	5+ * Years	Interval Unknown	Total**
All Incomes	68	25	5	1	99
Under $3,000	64	26	9	1	100
$3,000–$4,999	65	27	6	1	99
$5,000–$6,999	67	27	5	1	100
$7,000–$9,999	70	25	4	1	100
$10,000+	73	23	3	1	100

* Includes "Never"
** Percentages may not add to 100 due to rounding.
Source: Unpublished Data, National Center for Health Statistics.

higher and lower income persons are compared. One might expect to see greater utilization by the poor if serious chronic illness were the only determinant of use. But clearly these illness conditions, on which we have data, are not the only reason to see the doctor. To the degree that there is a more or less discretionary component of physicians visits, including certain preventive services, we would expect to see differences between the poor and nonpoor. It appears that the greatest differences in use occur in the age range when a large component of physician visits are in fact preventive.

Race-Related Differences

In areas of concentrations of the poor and particularly the black poor, the disturbing

Poverty, Illness, and the 235
Use of Health Services
in the United States

picture emerging from national data becomes a matter of great concern.

If *income* differentials with respect to the use of physician services are not too startling for the nation as a whole, the same cannot be said for racial differences. Although two-thirds of the poor (with family incomes below $3,000) are white, the most severe problems of poverty and a great deal of the national concern is focused on the nonwhite third of the poor. Table 17–7, shows the average number of physician visits by income, age, and color for the United States in the period 1966–67. White children under the age of 15 in families with incomes under $5,000 had an average of 3.3 visits. This was well below

Table 17–6—Number of physician visits per year by family income and age, United States, July 1966–June 1967

Age	All Incomes	Under $3,000	$3,000–$4,999	$5,000–$6,999	$7,000–$9,999	$10,000 or More
			FAMILY INCOME			
All Ages	4.3	4.6	4.1	4.2	4.3	4.6
Under 5 Years	5.7	4.4	4.7	5.4	6.4	7.2
5–14	2.7	1.5	1.9	2.7	2.9	3.5
15–24	4.0	4.3	3.7	4.1	4.2	3.8
25–34	4.4	4.2	4.3	4.3	4.5	4.6
35–44	4.3	3.8	4.7	4.2	4.0	4.7
45–54	4.3	5.2	4.6	3.9	4.0	4.7
55–64	5.1	5.1	5.4	4.9	5.1	5.4
65–74	6.0	6.2	5.3	6.8	6.3	6.8
75+	6.0	5.6	6.1	7.7	6.1	5.9

Source: *Volume of Physician Visits, United States July 1966–June 1967*, National Center for Health Statistics, series 10, no. 49.

Table 17–7—Number of physician visits per person per year by family income, age, and color

Family Income and Age	Average Number of Visits	White	Nonwhite
		AVERAGE NO. OF VISITS BY COLOR	
Under $5,000			
Under 15 Years	2.8	3.3	1.9
15–44	4.2	4.4	3.5
45–64	5.1	5.2	4.4
65 and Over	5.8	6.0	4.7
$5,000 and Over			
Under 15 Years	4.1	4.2	2.2
15–44	4.3	4.3	3.6
45–64	4.6	4.7	3.3
65 and Over	6.6	6.7	5.5

Source: *Volume of Physician Visits, United States July 1966–June 1967*, National Center for Health Statistics, series 10, no. 49.

the 4.2 average of higher income white children, but the equivalent number for lower income nonwhites was only 1.9. Indeed, for every age and income category the average number of visits per year for nonwhites was well below the number for whites.

In a large-scale health interview survey conducted by the author in a low-income black area of Atlanta, Ga., in 1968, the findings on both illness and use of health services suggested that income made relatively little difference *within* the area. However, the poor and nonpoor in this area had a uniformly higher level of illness and lower level of use of physicians' and hospital services than would have been expected on the basis of national figures. For example, the proportion of the population reporting chronic illness with activity limitation was 18 per cent, 50 per cent higher than for the nation as a whole despite the fact that it was a younger population. The average number

of physician visits in the year preceding the interview was about three.

Qualitative Indicators

There are, in addition to the volume measures, some qualitative indicators that document the common observation that a doctor contact for the poor is not likely to be the same type of visit as received by the nonpoor person. There are differences, for example, in the place of contact. Those in families with incomes under $3,000 are more than twice as likely as those in the highest income group to see the physician in a hospital clinic or emergency room and only half as likely to make contact over the telephone (see Table 17–8). The proportion of visits in a clinic or emergency room for the lowest income group is 14 per cent of all visits, compared to 6 per cent for those with family incomes over $10,000. One quarter (25.8 per cent) of all visits made by non-

Table 17–8—Per cent distribution of physician visits by place of visit according to income and according to color

Family Income	Office (Including Pre-paid group)	Hospital Clinic or Emergency Room	Telephone	Other	Total
Under $3,000	68.9	13.6	6.2	11.3	100
$ 3,000–$4,999	70.6	12.3	8.9	8.2	100
$ 5,000–$6,999	70.8	10.3	12.0	6.9	100
$ 7,000–$9,999	72.8	7.5	13.8	5.9	100
$10,000+	73.9	6.1	13.2	6.8	100
Color					
White	72.9	7.7	12.0	7.4	100
Nonwhite	60.3	25.8	4.0	9.9	100

Source: Volume of Physician Visits, United States July 1966–June 1967, National Center for Health Statistics, series 10, no. 49.

Table 17–9—Selected physician utilization characteristics by income, United States, July 1963–June 1964

	Per Cent of Visits* for Preventive Services	Per Cent of Persons* Under 17 Having Routine Physical	Per Cent of Persons** Under 17 with Visit to a Pediatrician	Per Cent of Women **with Visit to Obstetrician–Gynecologist
Under $2,000	10.8	15.7	7.5	2.8
$ 2,000–$3,999	11.6	25.1	11.3	5.5
$ 4,000–$6,999	12.3	35.0	18.3	8.7
$ 7,000–$9,999	14.4	43.1	23.8	11.0
$10,000+	17.5	53.9	33.0	12.5

* Source: White, E. L., "A Graphic Presentation on Age and Income Differentials in Selected Aspects of Morbidity, Disability, and Utilization of Health Services," Inquiry, Blue Cross Association, vol. 5, no. 1, March, 1968.
** Source: Characteristics of Patients of Selected Types of Medical Specialists and Practitioners, United States July 1963–June 1964, National Center for Health Statistics, series 10, no. 28.

whites, compared to 7.7 per cent of visits by whites, were to a hospital clinic or emergency room.

Of all visits occurring in the 1963–64 period, 10.8 per cent of those made by families with incomes below $2,000 were for preventive services (general check-up or immunization), in contrast to 17.5 per cent for those with family incomes above $10,000 (Table 17–9). Comparing the same two income groups, the per cent of low income children under age 17 having had a routine physical examination within the year was 15.7, while 53.9 per cent of the children in the highest income group reported a routine physical.

Another indicator of differences in the nature of the care received is obtained by comparing income groups on the proportion having seen various specialists. In general, the proportion of the higher income categories seeing specialists is larger than the proportion for the lower income categories. This is true for every specialty. It is most pronounced in the cases of obstetrics–gynecology and pediatrics. As may be seen in Table 17–9, 2.8 per cent of all low-income women, compared to 12.5 per cent of high income women, had seen an obstetrician or gynecologist in the 1963–64 period. Similarly, one third of all children under age 17 in families with incomes of $10,000 or more had seen a pediatrician, while only 7.5 per cent of children in families with incomes under $2,000 had seen one.

Dental Service Patterns

Income and racial differences with respect to dental services are considerably larger

Poverty, Illness, and the 237
**Use of Health Services
in the United States**

than those found for physicians' services. As shown in Table 17–10, the proportion of high-income persons having seen a dentist within a year is almost three times higher than the proportion for those in families with incomes under $2,000. Sixty-four per cent of the highest income group, compared to 23 per cent of the lowest income group, had seen a dentist. At the other end of the distribution, 22 per cent of the low-income persons versus only 7 per cent of high-income persons reported that they had never seen a dentist.

The average number of dental visits per person per year for the 12 months ending June 1964 for the United States was 1.6. The average for persons in families with incomes below $4,000 was 0.9, whereas it was 1.7 for persons with family incomes of $4,000 and above. It is also worth noting that the non-white average was close to half that of whites (0.9 vs. 1.7). Considering only persons in families with incomes below $4,000, the white average is one visit per year, while the nonwhite average is 0.6 visit per year.

As with physician visits, the nature of the service differs between high-income and low-income users. Particularly for dental services, differences in the type of service rendered are of interest. If we consider the proportion of all visits in a year that are for extractions or other surgery (Table 17–11), we see that for all ages there is a strong relationship between income and proportion of visits for extraction. The higher the income, the less likely is a visit to be for extraction. Twenty-six per cent of all visits for persons with family

Table 17–10—Per cent distribution of persons by time interval since last dental visit and family income, United States, July 1963–June 1964

| Income | INTERVAL SINCE LAST DENTAL VISIT | | | | |
	Less Than 1 Year	1 Year and Over	Never	Unknown	Total
Under $2,000	22.7	53.4	21.7	2.2	100
$ 2,000–$3,999	28.3	47.2	22.5	2.0	100
$ 4,000–$6,999	39.8	40.0	19.1	1.1	100
$ 7,000–$9,999	51.3	35.0	12.8	0.9	100
$10,000–Over	64.3	27.7	7.2	0.8	100

Source: *Dental Visits: Time Interval Since Last Visit, United States July 1963–June 1964*, National Center for Health Statistics, series 10, no. 29.

incomes under $4,000 were for extractions, compared to 8.5 per cent of the visits for persons in families with incomes of $10,000 or more. Comparing whites and nonwhites, 14 per cent of all visits made by whites, compared to 30 per cent of all visits made by nonwhites, were for extractions.

As is the case with other types of health services utilization, the national data give some idea of the disadvantaged state of those who are poor, but a more relevant picture is obtained by looking at indicators for smaller geographic concentrations of the poor. For example, in the study of a low-income area of Atlanta referred to earlier, we found that for those persons who had had a dental visit within the preceding 12 months, fully half

of the most recent visits had been for extraction only. As was the case for other indicators, it mattered little whether the family was very poor or was in the middle income group. The extraction proportion was uniformly high in this neighborhood of 25,000 persons.

Turning finally to hospital discharges and lengths of stay, we find that in general, lower income persons tend to be admitted to the hospital at a higher rate and have longer lengths of stay than higher income persons. For the 12 months ending June 1967, for the United States the discharge rate per hundred population for persons with family incomes under $3,000 was 15.7. Each income category has a rate that is lower than the category preceding it, with the highest income group, $10,000 or more, having an annual discharge

Table 17–11—Per cent of distribution of dental visits by family income and age, United States, July 1963–June 1964

Income and Age	Fillings	TYPE OF SERVICE			
		Extractions and Other Surgery	Examination and Cleaning	Other	Total
Under $4,000					
Under 5 Years	*	*	62.1	*	100.0**
5–14	41.4	22.5	30.8	16.0	100.0
15–24	31.6	29.2	20.2	18.2	100.0
25–44	34.3	28.4	26.7	23.7	100.0
45–64	28.9	24.6	24.1	33.2	100.0
65+	21.3	24.7	19.3	39.2	100.0
$4,000–$6,999					
Under 5 Years	49.2	*	33.8	*	100.0**
5–14	46.5	13.3	35.5	12.7	100.0
15–24	46.1	21.7	24.9	15.2	100.0
25–44	40.2	22.2	27.5	18.1	100.0
45–64	28.8	18.7	29.2	29.9	100.0
65+	21.1	9.1	12.4	50.8	100.0
$7,000–$9,999					
Under 5 Years	41.4	*	73.6	*	100.0**
5–14	44.0	10.6	37.5	18.2	100.0
15–24	51.5	7.4	30.8	18.7	100.0
25–44	38.2	14.0	39.5	22.8	100.0
45–64	30.8	16.2	33.3	29.2	100.0
65+	27.1	*	16.5	42.7	100.0
$10,000+					
Under 5 Years	18.9	*	88.8	*	100.0**
5–14	34.4	6.5	45.0	24.7	100.0
15–24	48.1	5.7	36.0	20.7	100.0
25–44	39.6	8.2	43.4	20.2	100.0
45–64	29.8	11.9	36.6	20.1	100.0
65+	15.7	16.0	49.9	31.0	100.0

* Figure does not meet NHS standards of reliability or precision.
** Includes unknown types of services. More than one type of service may be performed during a single visit, therefore, per cent may actually add to more than 100.0.
Source: Volume of Dental Visits, United States July 1963–June 1964, National Center for Health Statistics, series 10, no. 23.

rate of 10.7 per 100 (Table 17–12). The higher rates for the poor generally have been interpreted as evidence of either a tendency for the poor to avoid seeking care until illness has reached a serious stage and therefore more often requiring admission to the hospital or simply a use of hospital inpatient services as a substitute for ambulatory care by the physician because of the inadequacies of the ambulatory care system for the poor.

Concluding Observations

The data presented here support the conclusion that the poor in the United States are sicker than the nonpoor and use fewer ambulatory health services. If anything, however, these crude volume measures of utilization applied to a national sample tend to understate both the severity and complexity of the problem.

The matter for concern is not simply that the low-income segment of the population has fewer visits than the rest despite more illness. Rather, it is that for sub-groups of the poor, in part defined by race and place of residence, services are not economically or

**Poverty, Illness, and the 239
Use of Health Services
in the United States**

geographically available despite very high levels of illness relative to the nonpoor. In addition, the nature of services provided for the poor generally do not compare favorably with those provided to the rest of the population.

Neither the day-to-day frustrations of the poor as they come in contact with health services providers, nor the frustrations of many providers as they struggle to deliver health services to low-income persons in a more adequate way can be seen in the data presented in this paper. The outcome of those frustrations, however, are in large part the income differentials with respect to health status and health services documented here. With the increasing concentration of poor persons in urban areas, and their rising dissatisfaction with the health services available to them, the unmet needs and unfulfilled demand of the disadvantaged will plague the nation's health care system until an adequate response is evidenced.

Table 17–12—Discharge per 100 population from short-stay hospitals by family income and age, United States, July 1966–June 1967

Age	All Incomes	Under $3,000	FAMILY INCOME $3,000–$4,999	$5,000–$6,999	$7,000–$9,999	$10,000 or More
All Ages	12.6	15.7	14.3	12.7	11.7	10.7
Under 17 Years	6.9	7.4	7.1	7.4	7.2	5.8
17–44	14.9	17.9	19.2	16.5	14.1	12.5
45–64	14.2	17.0	15.9	13.5	14.4	14.1
65+	19.7	19.5	19.9	20.4	21.2	18.6

Source: Unpublished data, National Center for Health Statistics.

18

Social Class, Social Integration, and the Use of Preventive Health Services

Philip M. Moody
and
Robert M. Gray

IT IS NO EXAGGERATION to observe that one of the major problems in the field of medicine in the United States concerns the delivery of medical care to the people and their acceptance and utilization of health services. For example, a number of studies have pointed out that a sizable portion of the population, even when they have physical disorders, fails to utilize health services.[1] Even

greater difficulties have been encountered by medical and public health officials in securing participation in preventive health programs, especially among persons from lower social classes who are frequently the main target of public health and preventive care programs.[2] The purpose of this paper is to present further information on why persons in the lower socio–economic class utilize available preventive health services less frequently than do persons in higher social classes.

A review of the literature indicates a wide range of factors which have been studied in attempts to identify why people in all social classes do or do not utilize available health services.[3] On the one hand, researchers have attempted to explain the under-utilization of preventive health services in terms of personal beliefs and motives.[4] For example,

[1] See B. Blackwell, "The Literature of Delay in Seeking Medical Care for Chronic Illnesses," *Health Education Monographs*, 16:3–31, 1963; E. L. Koos, *The Health of Regionville*, New York: Columbia Univ. Press, 1954; J. D. Stoeckle, I. K. Zola and G. E. Davidson, "On Going to See the Doctor, the Contributions of the Patient to the Decision to Seek Medical Aid, A Selected Review," *J. Chronic Disease*, 16:975–989, September, 1963; I. K. Zola, "Illness Behavior of the Working Class: Implications and Recommendations," in A. Shostak and W. Gomberg (eds.), *Blue Collar World*, Englewood Cliffs, N.J.: Prentice-Hall, 1964, pp. 351–361; E. Freidson, *Patients' Views of Medical Practice*, New York: Russell Sage Foundation, 1961; I. K. Zola, "Culture and Symptoms–An Analysis of Patients' Presenting Complaints," *Amer. Socio-*

logical Review, 31:615–630, October, 1966; and D. Mechanic, *Medical Sociology*, New York: Free Press, 1968.

[2] See, for example, O. W. Anderson, "The Utilization of Health Services," in H. Freeman, *et al.* (eds.), *Handbook of Medical Sociology*, Englewood Cliffs, N.J.: Prentice-Hall, 1963, pp. 349–367; I. M. Rosenstock, "Why People Use Health Services," *Milbank Memorial Fund Quarterly*, 44:94–127, July, 1966; B. S. Hulka, "Motivation Technics in a Cancer Detection Program: Utilization of Community Resources," *Amer. J. Public Health*, 57:229–241, February, 1967; and E. A. Suchman, "Preventive Health Behavior: A Model for Research on Community Health Campaigns," *J. Health and Social Behavior*, 8:197–209, September, 1967.

[3] See, for example, Koos, *op. cit.*; A. L. Knutson, *The Individual, Society, and Health Behavior*, New York: Russell Sage Foundation, 1965; Suchman, *op. cit.*; Rosenstock, *op. cit.*; S. V. Kasl and S. Cobb, "Health Behavior, Illness Behavior and Sick Role Behavior, I. Health and Illness Behavior," *Archives of Environmental Health*, 12:246–266, February, 1966; and S. V. Kasl and S. Cobb, "Health Behavior, Illness Behavior, and Sick-Role Behavior, II. Sick-Role Behavior," *Archives of Environmental Health*, 12:531–541, April, 1966.

[4] Rosenstock, *op. cit.*; I. M. Rosenstock, M. Derryberry and B. K. Carriger, "Why People Fail to Seek Poliomyelitis Vaccination," *Public Health Reports*, 74:98–103, February, 1959; and

Abridged and revised from part of a larger report by Philip M. Moody entitled "The Inter-related Effects of Socio–Economic Status, Social Participation, and Alienation on Oral Polio Immunization Participation," unpublished Ph.D. dissertation, University of Utah, 1967. This paper is also a revised version of an address presented at the Annual Meeting of the American Sociological Association, August, 1968. The authors are indebted to Joseph Kesler, Elton Newman, John R. Ward and Jane Van Wey for their assistance in the presentation of these data. This study was supported in part by a Vaccination Assistance Project Grant from the U.S. Public Health Service.

Rosenstock, Derryberry and Carriger, after a critical review of studies on why people fail to seek poliomyelitis vaccination, postulated that polio vaccine acceptance was dependent on a person's perceived susceptibility to the disease, his conception of the safeness of the vaccine and the perceived seriousness of the disease.[5] They suggested, however, that the extent to which social class influence on taking polio vaccine operated independently of the factors described above would have to await further research. Two studies on preventive health behavior utilizing the psychological model suggested by Rosenstock, et al., are relevant in this connection.[6] First, Hochbaum in studying factors underlying the decision to seek chest x-ray for the detection of tuberculosis found that perceived susceptibility to the disease and perceived benefits from this diagnosis played a major role regardless of socio-economic status.[7] Similarly, socio-economic status was found to be independently associated with having taken voluntary chest x-rays. Kegeles, et al., in investigating relationships among the use of Papanicolaou tests, socio-economic status and beliefs in the benefits of early detection of cancer, found that beliefs and socio-economic status made independent contributions to the understanding of preventive health behavior.[8]

Kasl and Cobb in their review articles suggested that health behavior was a function of two factors: the perceived threat of disease and the attractiveness of value of the health behavior.[9] Furthermore, Kasl and Cobb noted that "both of these perceptions seem to be influenced by education, occupa-

tion, and income," which helps to account for the significant relationships between social class and use of preventive health services.[10] In sum, those studies which have examined the relationships among personal beliefs and motives, socio-economic status and the utilization of preventive health services have concluded that each of these factors has an independent influence on the use of these services.

On the other hand, research within a sociological framework has stressed the influence of group memberships, group pressures and role definitions of the individual as determining factors in preventive health behavior.[11] For example, Suchman in his survey [12] of approximately 1,800 respondents in an ethnically heterogeneous section of New York City found that:

1. Those subjects from a "cosmopolitan" group orientation or from those groups who tend to be "progressive, individualistic, instrumental or open," more frequently utilize "scientific," e.g., "formal, complex, impersonal, objective, disease- rather than patient-oriented and specialized, types of medical care."

2. Those respondents from a "parochial" type of group orientation, or from groups who tend to be "traditional, dependent, closed, and local," utilize more frequently a "non-scientific approach" to illness and medical care.

3. Persons from lower classes as compared with subjects from upper socio-economic status were more likely to be "parochial" and less "cosmopolitan."

G. M. Hochbaum, *Public Participation in Medical Screening Programs*, Washington: U.S. Government Printing Office, U.S. Public Health Service, Publication no. 572, 1958.

[5] Rosenstock, *et. al., op. cit.*

[6] Rosenstock, *et. al., op. cit.*, and Rosenstock, *op. cit.*

[7] Hochbaum, *op. cit.*

[8] Kegeles, S. S., J. P. Kirscht, D. P. Haefner and I. M. Rosenstock, "Survey of Beliefs About Cancer Detection and Taking Papanicolaou Tests," *Public Health Reports*, 80:815-824, September, 1965.

[9] Kasl and Cobb, "Health Behavior, Illness Behavior and Sick Role Behavior," Parts I and II, *op. cit.*

[10] *Ibid.*, Part II, p. 540.

[11] Suchman, *op. cit.*, p. 198; J. Cassel, "Social and Cultural Considerations in Health Innovation," *Annals of New York Academy of Science*, 57:739-747, 1963; and A. L. Johnson, C. D. Jenkins, R. Patrick and T. J. Northcutt, Jr., *Epidemiology of Polio Vaccine Acceptance*, Jacksonville, Fl.: Florida State Board of Health Monograph no. 3, Miami, Fla., 1962, pp. 1-100.

[12] Suchman, E. A., "Social Patterns of Illness and Medical Care," *J. Health and Human Behavior*, 6:2-16, Spring, 1965 (see Chap. 20 herein).

Furthermore, Suchman indicated that the utilization of preventive health services is more a function of socio–economic status than of group structure or health attitudes.

Numerous other studies have shown that socio–economic status affects an individual's propensity to utilize preventive health services, particularly immunization services.[13] Whether the specific measure is occupation, income, education or some combination of any or all of these indicators into an index of "social class," the results are most uniform: the higher the social status of those involved, the greater the participation in preventive health programs.

It is a basic assumption of the present study that social integration, defined by a low level of alienation and a high degree of social participation, may account in part for the differential utilization of preventive health services among the various social classes, and may help explain why persons in the lower socio–economic class utilize these health services less frequently than do persons in higher social classes. This supposition is based upon several research findings.

For example, studies have indicated that individuals who are involved in voluntary organizations tend to utilize preventive health services and receive vaccines at a higher rate than those who do not become so involved in voluntary organizations.[14]

Among the measures used to describe organizational involvement are membership in organizations, frequency of attendance at meetings including church meetings, committee appointments, financial contributions to organizations and offices held.

Other researchers have shown that organizational involvement or social participation is positively associated with socio–economic status.[15] Regardless of the

mons, "Family Culture and Participation in a Rheumatic Fever Clinic," paper presented at Skytop Conference, Social Science Research Council Committee on Preventive Medicine and Social Science Research, June, 1958 (mimeographed); R. W. Jessee and H. S. Bacon, "Resistance to Immunization in Southwestern Virginia," *Virginia Medical Monthly*, 88:649–652, November, 1961; T. J. Northcutt, Jr., C. D. Jenkins and A. L. Johnson, "Factors Influencing Vaccine Acceptance," in J. S. Neill and J. O. Bond (eds.), *Hillsborough County Oral Polio Vaccine Programs*, Jacksonville, Fla.: Florida State Board of Health, Monograph Series no. 6, 1964, pp. 31–55.

[15] See, for example, W. L. Warner and P. S. Lunt, *The Social Life of a Modern Community*, New Haven: Yale Univ. Press, 1941, pp. 329–338; M. Axelrod, "Urban Structure and Social Participation," *Amer. Sociological Review*, 21: 13–18, February, 1956; L. Reissman, "Class, Leisure and Social Participation," *Amer. Sociological Review*, 19:76–84, February, 1954; H. E. Freeman, E. Novak and L. G. Reeder, "Correlates of Membership in Voluntary Association," *Amer. Sociological Review*, 22:528–533, October, 1957; M. Komarovsky, "The Voluntary Associations of Urban Dwellers," *Amer. Sociological Review*, 11:686–698, December, 1946; P. F. Lazarsfeld, B. Berelson, and H. Gaudet, *The People's Choice*, New York: Columbia Univ. Press, 1948, p. 145; J. C. Scott, Jr., Membership and Participation in Voluntary Associations," *Amer. Sociological Review*, 22:315–326, June, 1957; C. R. Wright and H. H. Hyman, "Voluntary Association Memberships of American Adults: Evidence from National Sample Surveys," *Amer. Sociological Review*, 23:284–294, June, 1958; B. G. Zimmer and A. Hawley, "The Significance of Membership in Associations," *Amer. J. Sociology*, 65:196–201, September, 1959; G. Knupfer, "Portrait of the Underdog," *Public Opinion Quarterly*, 11:103–114, Spring, 1947; B. G. Zimmer, "Participation in Urban Structures," *Amer. Sociological Review*, 20:219, April, 1955; J. M. Foskett, "Social Structure and Social Participation," *Amer. Sociological Review*, 21: 433–436, February, 1956; D. L. Phillips, *op. cit.*; and W. Erbe, "Social Involvement and Political Activity: A Replication and Elaboration," *Amer. Sociological Review*, 29:198–215, April, 1964.

[13] Glasser, M. A., "A Study of the Public's Acceptance of the Salk Vaccine Program," *Amer. J. Public Health*, 48:141–146, February, 1958; J. S. Clausen, M. A. Seidenfeld and L. C. Deasy, "Parents' Attitudes Toward Participation of Their Children in Polio Vaccine Trials," *Amer. J. Public Health*, 44:1526–1536, December, 1954; L. C. Deasy, "Socio–Economic Status and Participation in the Poliomyelitis Vaccine Trials," *Amer. Sociological Review*, 21:185–191, April, 1956; R. S. Weiss, "Factors Affecting Participation in the Polio Vaccine Evaluation Experiment," presented at the annual meeting of the American Sociological Society, 1955; R. M. Gray, J. P. Kesler and P. M. Moody, "The Effects of Social Class and Friends' Expectations on Oral Polio Vaccination Participation," *Amer. J. Public Health*, 56:2028–2032, December, 1966.

[14] Johnson, *et al.*, *op. cit.*; Koos, *op. cit.*; P. B. Cornely and S. K. Bigman, "Some Considerations in Changing Health Attitudes," *Children*, 10:23–28, January–February, 1963; L. W. Sim-

measures of social participation and status, these studies indicate that the higher the socio–economic status, the higher tends to be the rate of participation in organizations.

Only one of these many studies has ever attempted to meet the problems of possible misinterpretation implied by these findings.[16] For example, people in upper socio–economic groups might participate more in preventive health programs than lower-status people because they tend to become more involved in organizations. Or one might assume that persons highly involved in organizations are more likely to participate in preventive health programs because they tend to have high status and would be seeking these services whether they were highly involved in organizations or not.

These considerations raise the question: To what degree are socio–economic status and formal social participation independently related to preventive health behavior? Johnson and his colleagues, in attempting to answer this question with respect to oral polio vaccine acceptance, wrote:

Is social participation associated with vaccine acceptance patterns by virtue of its association with social class, with other facets of social class actually being the process leading to the taking of vaccine? Or is social participation the factor more intimately tied in with vaccine taking with social class being the variable with the gratuitous association?[17]

Their conclusions were that "social class and social participation have independent influences on preventive health behavior" and that "there is something about group membership that encourages cooperation with health programs, irrespective of social class." This supposition will be further investigated in this study.

Alienation, which may also account for the differential rates of utilization of preventive health programs among the various social classes, has been found to be associated with health behavior in that those persons who are alienated from society participate less frequently in health programs than do non-alienated persons.[18] Alienation in this

context referred to feelings of powerlessness, normlessness, social isolation, meaninglessness, self-estrangement and other feelings of uneasiness or discomfort which reflect an individual's exclusion or self-exclusion from social and cultural participation.

The association of alienation with preventive health behavior raises two additional problems. A number of studies have shown that such factors as alienation and anomia are highly associated with socio–economic status[19] and social participation.[20] The relationship is in each case negative; that is, the higher the rate of organizational participation and the higher the socio–economic status, the lower the level of alienation.

These findings raise a provocative question: Are persons from lower social classes as compared with persons from higher socio–economic groups participating less frequently in preventive health programs because a

Rocky Mountain Social Science J., 4:161–168, April, 1967; Johnson, *et al.*, *op. cit.*; C. N. D'Onofrio, *Reaching Our "Hard to Reach"—The Unvaccinated*, Berkeley: California Office of State Printing, n.d.; J. Spencer, "The Multi-problem Family," in B. Schlesinger (ed.). The *Multi-problem Family*, Toronto: Univ. of Toronto Press, 1963, pp. 3–55; and D. Rosenblatt and E. A. Suchman, "The Underutilization of Medical-care Services by Blue-collarites," in A. B. Shostak and W. Gomberg (eds.), *Blue Collar World*, Englewood Cliffs, N.J.: Prentice-Hall, 1964, pp. 341–349.

[19] Dean, D. G., "Alienation: Its Meaning and Measurement," *Amer. Sociological Review*, 26: 753–758, October, 1961; W. E. Thompson and J. E. Horton, "Political Alienation As a Force in Political Action," *Social Forces*, 38:190–195, March, 1960; W. Bell, "Anomie, Social Isolation and the Class Structure," *Sociometry*, 20:105–116, June, 1957; and E. L. McDill, "Anomie, Authoritarianism, Prejudice and Socio–Economic Status: An Attempt at Clarification," *Social Forces*, 39:239–245, March, 1961.

[20] Rose, A. M., "Alienation and Participation: A Comparison of Group Leaders and the 'Mass,'" *Amer. Sociological Review*, 27:834–839, December, 1962; D. L. Meier and W. Bell, "Anomia and Differential Access to Life Goals," *Amer. Sociological Review*, 24:189–202, April, 1959; E. Mizruchi, "Social Structure and Anomia in a Small City," *Amer. Sociological Review*, 25:645–654, October, 1960.

[16] Johnson, *et al.*, *op. cit.*
[17] *Ibid.*
[18] Gray, R. M., J. P. Kesler and P. M. Moody, "Alienation and Immunization Participation,"

larger portion of them are alienated from society? It might well be that the crucial factor accounting for the lower utilization rates among persons from lower socio–economic groups is their comparatively lower level of integration into the main stream of societal life.[21] As such, they simply do not respond to activities organized within the context of a social structure of which they are not or do not feel a part. In short, it might be that social integration may be more of a determining factor of the under-utilization of preventive health services than is socio–economic status.

The present study was undertaken to investigate the independent associations that socio–economic status and social integration have upon persons' participation in a state-wide oral polio immunization program. The independent associations of socio–economic status and social integration, as measured by indices of alienation and social participa-tion, are to be investigated, taking into account either or both of the other factors. The following hypotheses are to be tested in the present investigation:

1. Persons from high socio–economic groups will receive oral polio immunizations at a greater rate than will subjects from lower socio–economic groups.

2. The greater the subjects' social par-ticipation in voluntary associations, the higher will be their participation in an oral polio vaccination program.

3. The higher the subjects' alienation scores, the lower will be their rate of oral polio immunization participation.

4. Each of the relationships predicted in hypotheses 1, 2 and 3 will persist when either or both of the other variables are controlled.

In order to adequately test hypothesis 4, the following subhypotheses are tested:

5. The higher the subjects' socio–economic status, the greater will be their oral polio vaccination rate when controlling for their social participation scores.

[21] Suchman, "Preventive Health Behavior," *op. cit.*

6. The higher the subjects' socio–economic status, the greater will be their rate of oral polio immunization participation when con-trolling for their alienation scores.

7. The higher the subjects' socio–economic status, the greater will be their oral polio vaccination rate when controlling for both their social participation and alienation scores.

8. The higher the subjects' social partici-pation scores, the greater will be their rate of oral polio immunization participation when controlling for socio–economic status.

9. The higher the subjects' social partici-pation scores, the greater will be their oral polio vaccination rate when controlling for their alienation scores.

10. The higher the subjects' social partici-pation scores, the greater will be their rate of oral polio immunization participation when controlling for their alienation scores and socio–economic status.

11. The higher the subjects' alienation scores, the lower will be their oral polio vaccination rate when controlling for socio–economic status.

12. The higher the subjects' alienation scores, the lower will be their rate of oral polio immunization participation when con-trolling for their social participation scores.

13. The higher the subjects' alienation scores, the lower will be their oral polio vaccination rate when controlling for both their social participation scores and socio–economic status.

Methods

The study population was restricted to mothers with children under five years of age.[22] Ninety-five per cent of the sample by

[22] Reasons for subjects being mothers with children under five are:
1. Sample had to meet public health as well as sociological considerations in that two surveys were conducted simultaneously.
2. Considerations of time and money had to be taken into account.

For further discussion see R. E. Serfling and I. L. Sherman, *Attribute Sampling Methods for Local Health Departments with Special Reference to Immunization Surveys*, Washington, D.C.: U.S. Government Printing Office, PHS Pub. no. 1230, 1965.

observations were categorized white. The remaining 5 per cent of the sample was comprised of Indian, Negro, Oriental and Spanish–American. The subjects (N = 959) were selected from eight communities in a Western state by the use of a two-stage area probability sampling technique.[23] These eight communities can be grouped into three categories on the basis of population. There were two urban areas of intermediate size (6,000 to 9,000). The remaining five were rural communities of 2,500 or less. The primary source of data in this study was an interview with the mother at home which was conducted approximately two months following a state-wide oral polio immunization program.

The immunization data was obtained from the subjects by a public health nurse who was well acquainted with oral polio immunization practices. The subjects' self-reports on vaccine participation were assumed to be valid indicator of their taking of the oral polio vaccine since a correlation coefficient of 0.80 was found between self-reports and actual behavior of selected subjects residing within two of the eight communities.[24]

The standardized questionnaires containing Dean's Alienation Scale,[25] Chapin's Social Participation Scale[26] and Hollingshead's Two Factor Index of Social Position[27] were administered to subjects by a trained interviewer following the immunization level surveys.[28]

Dean's Alienation Scale consists of a combination of three subscales measuring the elements of powerlessness, normlessness and social isolation.[29] This 24-item scale is of the Likert type on which subjects had five alternatives to rate the strength of her agreement or disagreement with each statement. The responses to each item were then converted into a five-point scale and tabulated to give a total alienation score. For purposes of χ^2 analysis, the total scores were categorized into groups ("high" and "low") using the median of a sample of subjects as the cutting point.

Chapin's Social Participation Scale is a Guttman-type scale designed to measure the degree of a person's or family's participation in community groups and organizations.[30] The five components of this scale are (1) membership, (2) attendance, (3) financial contributions, (4) member of committees

surveys and an attempt was made to have sociological interviews with all of these subjects. Of the total number of 1,076 possible interviews, 959 were completed which represents an 89 per cent completion rate. In the 117 cases in which a sociological interview was not completed the following reasons for not doing so were:

51—Out-of-town or not at home (on vacation during the time interviews were in community)
29—Refused
20—Moved
17—Miscellaneous (language difficulty, etc.)

A comparison was made between the total study group and variables obtained from the immunization level questionnaires. It was concluded from this analysis that there were no significant differences between completed cases and the total study group who participated in the immunization level surveys. See P. M. Moody, "The Interrelated Effects of Socio–Economic Status, Social Participation, and Alienation on Oral Polio Immunization Participation," unpublished Ph.D. dissertation, University of Utah, 1967, for further discussion of methods used in this study.

[23] Serfling, R., R. G. Cornell and I. Sherman, "The CDC Quota Sampling Technic with Results of 1959 Poliomyelitis Vaccination Surveys," *Amer. J. Public Health*, 50:1847, December, 1960.

[24] When obtaining oral polio vaccine during the statewide program, participants were asked to record their name on a slip of paper. The names of those participants in two of the eight selected communities were recorded by the public health nurse after each polio vaccine type was given. This record provided the data for correlating subjects' self-reports and behavior.

[25] Dean, *op. cit.*

[26] Chapin, F. S., *Experimental Designs in Sociological Research*, New York: Harper, rev. ed., 1955.

[27] Hollingshead, A. B., *Two Factor Index of Social Position*, New Haven, Conn.: privately mimeographed, 1957.

[28] A total number of 1,076 cases were selected in the sample during the immunization level

[29] Dean, *op. cit.* The total-scale score is reported to have a split-half reliability of 0.78. The subscales, which Dean considers to be independent enough to treat as independent variables, have reported split-half reliability coefficients ranging from 0.73 to 0.84.

[30] Chapin, *op. cit.*

and (5) offices held. The reported reliability ranges from $r = 0.89$ to 0.95.[31] Correlations with other measures have been reported to range from 0.52 (with income class) to 0.76 (between husband and wife). Each individual in the sample was given a total social participation score. For purposes of χ^2 analysis, the total scores were categorized into two groups as described above.

Hollingshead's Two Factor Index of Social Position utilized occupation and education level of heads of households to determine social position.[32] The subjects were then divided into one of four social classes, into one of three occupational groupings and into one of four educational categories.[33] They were further placed in one of three groups depending on whether they had received none, one or two, or three oral polio vaccinations.

Results

As expected, the associations between oral polio immunization participation and two more commonly used measures of socio–

[31] See D. C. Miller, *Handbook of Research Design and Social Measurement*, New York: David McKay, 1964, p. 209.

[32] Hollingshead, *op. cit.*

[33] To further investigate the notion that socio-economic status has an independent influence on oral polio immunization participation, three measures of this construct are utilized: subjects' education level, occupation of household head and social class as measured by the Hollingshead *Two Factor Index of Social Position*. It is felt that by using three measures the results of the study may be generalized more readily. Classes I and II were combined into one group due to the few number of subjects in Class I. The categories of subjects' education and husband's occupation were divided into the following categories according to Hollingshead's classification:

Occupation
1. Professional and Semi-professionals; Proprietors of Large Businesses.
2. Clerks and Skilled Workers.
3. Semi-skilled and Unskilled Workers; Proprietors of Small Businesses.

Education
1. College Graduate
2. Some College
3. High School and Some High School
4. Grade School or less

economic status, education and occupation, as well as the relationship of oral polio vaccination with the Hollingshead's Two Factor Index of Social Position were found to be statistically significant. (See Table 18–1.) These data supported the first hypothesis in that persons from the higher socio–economic groups were immunized for polio more frequently than were those from the lower socio–economic groups.

The association between subjects' oral polio vaccination and social participation was also significant. The greater the mothers' social participation score the higher were their level of oral polio immunization participation (Table 18–2). These data supported the second study hypothesis.

Subjects' alienation scores were found to be significantly related to oral polio immunization participation in that the higher the subjects' alienation scores the lower their oral polio vaccine acceptance (Table 18–3). Upon the basis of these data the third hypothesis was supported.

The study data thus far have shown that the present sample of mothers from high socio–economic groups were immunized against polio more frequently than were subjects from low socio–economic groups. The data also revealed that mothers who had high participation in voluntary organizations received oral polio vaccine more frequently than did subjects who had low social participation. Finally, the study data have indicated that mothers with high alienation scores were not immunized as frequently as those with low alienation scores. Inasmuch as these data, including the intercorrelations among socio–economic status, social participation and alienation (see Table 18–4) supported previous findings, the following problem must be examined: Are these three predictor variables independently associated with oral polio immunization participation? Tables 18–5 through 18–8 present data examining the association of each of the independent variables with oral polio immunization participation while holding one or both of the others constant. The statistical procedure used was partial correlation with F ratios.

When holding subjects' social participation scores constant, the relationships between

Table 18–1—Subjects' oral polio immunization participation by measures of socio–economic status—(in percentages)

| | NUMBER OF ORAL POLIO IMMUNIZATIONS RECEIVED | | | | | | |
	0	1–2	3	Total	N	df	χ^2
A. Education							
College Graduate	7%	2	91	100	(57)		
Some College	2%	7	91	100	(168)	6	34.58*
High School	10%	12	78	100	(628)		
Grade School	25%	20	55	100	(40)		
B. Occupation							
Professionals and Semi-professionals; Proprietors of Large Businesses	4%	7	89	100	(171)		
Clerks and Skilled Workers	5%	9	86	100	(323)	4	23.86*
Semi-skilled and Unskilled Workers; Proprietors of Small Businesses	13%	12	75	100	(352)		
C. Socio–Economic Class							
I–II	3%	7	90	100	(143)		
III	6%	9	85	100	(216)	6	18.07*
IV	10%	10	80	100	(362)		
V	15%	12	73	100	(129)		

* p < 0.01

Table 18–2—Mothers' oral polio immunization participation by social participation score—(in percentages)

| Social Participation | NUMBER OF ORAL POLIO IMMUNIZATIONS RECEIVED | | | | | | |
	0	1–2	3	Total	N	df	χ^2
High	4%	9	87	100	(388)	2	18.65*
Low	12%	11	77	100	(499)		

*p < 0.01

Table 18–3—Subjects' oral polio immunization participation, by alienation score—(in percentages)

| Alienation | NUMBER OF ORAL POLIO IMMUNIZATIONS RECEIVED | | | | | | |
	0	1–2	3	Total	N	df	χ^2
High	12%	11	77	100	(519)	2	17.54*
Low	5%	9	86	100	(368)		

* p < 0.01

Table 18–4—Inter-correlations among measures of socio–economic status, social participation and alienation (Pearson r)

Components	Occupation	Socio–Economic Status	Social Participation	Alienation
Education	0.179*	0.170*	0.307*	−0.006
Occupation	—	0.654*	0.268	−0.307*
Socio–Economic Status	—	—	0.216*	−0.250*
Social Participation	—	—	—	−0.153*

* p < 0.01   N = 959

mothers' oral polio vaccination participation and each of the variables of socio–economic status, education and occupation are not significant (Table 18–5). On the basis of these data, hypothesis 5—which stated that the higher the subjects' socio–economic status, the greater will be their oral polio vaccination rate when controlling for their social participation scores—was rejected.

In addition, although holding mothers' alienation scores constant, only the subjects' education maintained a significant relationship with their oral polio vaccination rate (Table 18–5). This finding indicated that the higher the subjects' education the greater was their rate of oral polio immunization participation. There were no significant associations of subjects' immunization participation and occupation and socio–economic status while controlling for their alienation scores. On the basis of these findings, hypothesis 6 is rejected.

Subjects' social participation scores maintained a significant relationship with their oral polio immunization participation, even when controlling for subjects' measures of socio–economic status and alienation, in that the greater the social participation, the higher the oral polio immunization rate (Table 18–6). These findings supported hypotheses 8 and 9.

When controlling for measures of socio–economic status and social participation, the relationship between alienation and rate of oral polio vaccination was maintained (Table 18–7). On the basis of these data hypotheses 11 and 12 are supported.

In summary, the independent relationships between subjects' measures of socio–economic status and oral polio immunization participation, when controlled for their social participation scores, were not significant. The same was found to be the case when controlling for mothers' alienation scores with the exception of the significant relationship between subjects' education and oral polio immunization participation. Furthermore, the relationship between subjects' social participation scores and rate of oral polio vaccination remained significant when controlling either for measures of socio–economic status or for measures of alienation. Finally, the independent relationship of alienation and oral polio immunization participation remained significant when controlling either for measures of socio–economic status or for social participation.

On the basis of these findings, when controlled for either of the other variables, hypothesis 4 was supported for social participation and alienation, but was rejected for socio–economic status. In addition, the findings reported above indicate that more correlational analysis is desirable. For example, the first-order relationship of subjects' education and oral polio immunization participation while controlling for alienation might be an artifact of the relationship between social participation and education. To determine whether or not the first-order significant relationships are spurious, or instead might be explained through some pattern of association between the other two independent variables, a second-order partialling operation was performed again utilizing the partial correlation method.

The data in Table 18–8 indicated that subjects' socio–economic status, education

Table 18–5—First-order partial correlation coefficients between mothers' oral polio immunization participation and measures of socio–economic status, holding social participation and alienation scores constant

Independent Variable Held Constant	Independent Variable Correlated with Oral Polio Immunization Participation	N	r_p	F Ratio*	P
Social Participation	Education	(893)	0.057	3.09	NS
Alienation	Education	(893)	0.083	6.49	0.05
Social Participation	Occupation	(846)	0.050	2.39	NS
Alienation	Occupation	(846)	0.038	1.35	NS
Social Participation	Socio–Economic Status	(850)	0.006	0.03	NS
Alienation	Socio–Economic Status	(850)	0.005	0.02	NS

* Degrees of freedom to test significance of F ratio are unity for the numerator and N-k-1 for the denominator where k represents the number of independent variables.

Table 18–6—First-order partial correlation coefficients between subjects' oral polio immunization participation and social participation scores, holding measures of socio–economic status and alienation scores constant

Independent Variable Held Constant	Independent Variable Correlated with Oral Polio Immunization Participation	N	r_p	F Ratio*	P
Education	Social Participation	(887)	0.067	4.28	0.05
Occupation	Social Participation	(887)	0.072	4.95	0.05
Socio–Economic Status	Social Participation	(887)	0.085	6.93	0.01
Alienation	Social Participation	(887)	0.077	5.63	0.05

* Degrees of freedom to test significance of F ratio are unity for the numerator and N-k-1 for the denominator where k represents the number of independent variables.

Table 18–7—First-order partial correlation coefficients between subjects' oral polio immunization participation and alienation, holding measures of socio–economic status and social participation scores constant

Independent Variable Held Constant	Independent Variable Correlated with Oral Polio Immunization Participation	N	r_p	F Ratio*	P
Education	Alienation	(887)	−0.119	13.51	0.01
Occupation	Alienation	(887)	−0.101	9.72	0.01
Socio–Economic Status	Alienation	(887)	−0.115	12.75	0.01
Social Participation	Alienation	(887)	−0.106	10.74	0.01

* Degrees of freedom to test significance of F ratio are unity for the numerator and N-k-1 for the denominator where k represents the number of independent variables.

Table 18–8—Second-order partial correlation coefficients between subjects' oral polio immunization participation and measures of socio–economic status, social participation and alienation, holding two independent variables constant

Independent Variable Held Constant	Independent Variable Correlated with Oral Polio Immunization Participation	N	r_p	F Ratio*	P
Alienation and Social Participation	Education	(893)	0.063	3.82	NS
Alienation and Social Participation	Occupation	(846)	0.022	0.44	NS
Alienation and Social Participation	Socio–Economic Status	(850)	−0.019	0.33	NS
Alienation and Education	Social Participation	(887)	0.049	2.26	NS
Alienation and Occupation	Social Participation	(887)	0.065	4.01	0.05
Alienation and Socio–Economic Status	Social Participation	(887)	0.074	5.23	0.05
Social Participation and Education	Alienation	(887)	−0.109	11.47	0.01
Social Participation and Occupation	Alienation	(887)	−0.096	8.76	0.01
Social Participation and Socio–Economic Status	Alienation	(887)	−0.107	11.03	0.01

* Degrees of freedom to test significance of F ratio are unity for the numerator and N-k-1 for the denominator where k represents the number of independent variables.

and occupation are not significantly related to their oral polio immunization participation, when controlling for both social participation and alienation scores. On the basis of these findings hypothesis 7 was rejected.

Furthermore, the second-order relationships between subjects' social participation scores and their oral polio immunization participation are significant when controlling for socio–economic status and alienation and when controlling for occupation and alienation (Table 18–8). When controlling for subjects' education and alienation, the relationship between mothers' social participation scores and their rate of oral polio vaccination was not significant. These findings partially substantiated hypothesis 10 in that the higher the subjects' social participation scores, the greater their level of oral polio immunization participation when their alienation scores and socio–economic status were held constant.

The relationships of mothers' alienation scores to rate of oral polio vaccination indicated that the higher the subjects' alienation scores, the lower their oral polio immunization participation rate when controlling for both measures of socio–economic status and social participation (Table 18–8). On the basis of these findings hypothesis 13 was supported.

In summary, the second-order partial correlation coefficients indicated that subjects' socio–economic status does not have an independent relationship with their oral polio immunization participation rate, when controlling for both social participation and alienation scores. However, the coefficients indicated that subjects' social participation scores maintained their independent relationship in the predicted direction with rate of oral polio vaccination when controlling for socio–economic status and alienation scores. This was not found to be the case when controlling for subjects' education and alienation scores. The data also supported the hypothesis that the higher the mothers' alienation scores, the lower their oral polio vaccination rate when controlling for both their social participation scores and socio–economic status.

On the basis of these findings, when controlled for both of the other variables, hypothesis 4 was supported in that the independent relationships between subjects' oral polio immunization and their alienation and social participation—with the exception of the combined control of subjects' education and alienation scores—were maintained. Hypothesis 4 was rejected as it pertained to subjects' socio–economic status and their oral polio immunization participation.

Discussion

In this report an attempt has been made to analyze the interrelationships of social integration and social class as they affect the utilization of a state-wide oral polio program. In summary, the results of this research indicated that social integration, as measured by social participation and alienation, was an important antecedent of the willingness of subjects to receive oral polio vaccine. This was true regardless of the higher-order partialling operations. It was also found that although socio–economic status might be of some importance in leading to oral polio immunization participation, statistical analyses raise doubts as to whether this influence is independent of the level of social integration. Most of its association with the rate of oral polio vaccination seems to be due to the fact that subjects of high socio–economic status (and the highest oral polio immunization participation) are also the highest in their level of social integration (i.e., high social participation scores and low alienation scores).

The data of this study suggest that the independent associations between socio–economic status and oral polio immunization participation may be considered to a degree to be either spurious or explained by the fact that socio–economic status is antecedent to either alienation or social participation. Furthermore, on the basis of these findings, the notion that there is something about participation in voluntary organizations that encourages cooperation with health programs irrespective of social class is further substantiated. However, the supposition that "social class has an independent influence on preventive health behavior,"[34] regardless of level of social participation, is not supported in this study.

The discrepancy of results between the present study and the study reported by Johnson, et al., may be due to the characteristics of the samples surveyed.[35] In Dade County, Florida, the subjects were urban, both male and female, ages ranged from 20–39, and comprised of 15 per cent "Negro," 9 per cent "Latin," or recent immigrants to Florida from Cuba and Puerto Rico, and 76 per cent "Anglo." In the present study, the subjects were urban and rural, all females with children under five years of age, and comprised of 95 per cent "White" and 5 per cent "Non-white." Both studies, however, had a similar research design in that field interviewing began after oral polio vaccine distribution was terminated. Furthermore, in Dade County 74 per cent of the target population were immunized during the oral vaccine program compared with 79 per cent of the subjects and their families in the present study who were immunized against poliomyelitis.

The question which remains unanswered in this report is whether social class would maintain independent relationships with other kinds of preventive health behavior, as reported in earlier studies by Hochbaum, Kegeles, Rosenstock and Suchman, had level of social integration been taken into account. Further studies into the relationship of social class and other demographic variables, social integration as measured by indices other than Dean's Alienation Scale and Chapin's Social Participation Scale and preventive health behavior might provide an answer to this question.

Implications

The problem of persuading people to use health services is an ultimate aim of physicians and public health officials.[36] Rosenstock, in reviewing factors which induce change in health behavior, wrote:

A decision to take a health action is influenced by the individual's state of readiness to behave, by his socially and individually determined beliefs about the efficacy of alternative actions, by psychological barriers to action, by interpersonal influences and by one or more cues or critical incidents which serve to trigger a response. No a priori reason may be found to indicate that action directed toward any one of these will in the long run prove more effective than action directed toward the others. Therefore, action programs to modify behavior could legitimately focus on any one or more of the determinants.[37]

Although changing the health beliefs and motives of individuals might secure more public participation in preventive health programs, the results of the present study suggest that additional activities would be warranted. For unless something is done to alter the prevailing conditions of alienation and anomie, in addition to merely providing health services, "one may safely predict the continued under-utilization of health services for this type of individual and community."[38] Such an activity, which might increase the utilization of health services, would consist of educating health personnel concerning the effects of bureaucracy in medicine upon some lower-class clients and other persons who are alienated and not integrated into community life. Because of the changes now occurring in medicine and the concomitant increase of bureaucracy in the delivering of medical care, the health worker needs to be made aware that this condition will tend to alienate some persons even more and further decrease their likelihood of utilizing health services. Such an education program might be directed toward educating health personnel about the needs and cultural patterns of lower-class groups in the community. In sum, it might be more effective to alter the perceptions and behavior of health personnel and the system of the delivery of health care than altering those of the clientele.[39]

[34] Johnson, et al., op. cit.
[35] Ibid. Also see Moody, op. cit.
[36] Rosenstock, op. cit., p. 113.

[37] Ibid.
[38] Rosenblatt and Suchman, op. cit.
[39] Rosenstock, op. cit., p. 127.

19

Social Patterns of Illness and Medical Care

Edward A. Suchman

PEOPLE SEEKING medical care and the practitioners of medical care may be viewed as two components of an interacting social system.[1] To some extent these two components have divergent and, at times, conflicting interests. People, as patients, are more likely to be concerned with their painful and incapacitating symptoms rather than the underlying organic disease and to be oriented toward a return to normal social functioning rather than to a healthy physiological state. Doctors, on the other hand, as professionals, are more likely to be interested in the clinical illness *per se* rather than in its physical discomforts or its social consequences. Moreover, patients and physicians may differ not only in their perceptions and interpretations of symptoms and illness but

also in the relative reliance they place upon the scientific or formal approach to medical care as compared with the more personal, popular or folk means of treating illness.[2] These varying definitions, objectives, and methods may generate conflict, or at least a lack of congruence, between professionals in the health field and their patients. These potential sources of disagreement underlie many of the problems in medical care today.[3]

The present research attempts to study this conflict in terms of the influence of social group forces upon individual illness behavior. We propose that certain socio-cultural background factors will predispose the individual toward accepting or rejecting the approach of professional medicine and, hence, increase or decrease the possibility of conflict between patient and physician.[4] Our fundamental postulate is a familiar one; that is, behavior is constrained by the expectations and directives of the social groups which bear significance for the individual. Medically relevant behavior, rather than being an exception, is, for many important reasons, a type of behavior on which the constraining mould of society rests

[1] Parsons, T., *The Social System*, New York: Free Press, 1951, chap. 10; I. T. Sanders, "Public Health in the Community," in H. Freeman, *et al.*, (eds.), *Handbook of Medical Sociology*, Englewood Cliffs, N.J.: Prentice-Hall, 1963, pp. 369–396; E. Freidson, *Patients' Views of Medical Practice*, New York: Russell Sage Foundation, 1961.

[2] For a discussion of some of the problems in patient–physician relationships, see R. N. Wilson, "Patient–Practitioners Relationships," in H. Freeman, *et al.*, (eds.), *op. cit.*, pp. 273–295. Also S. W. Bloom, *The Doctor and His Patient*, New York: Russell Sage Foundation, 1963.

[3] Good reviews of current problems in medical care may be found in H. H. Somers and A. R. Somers, *Doctors, Patients, and Health Insurance*, Washington: The Brookings Institution, 1961; and M. M. Davis, *Medical Care for Tomorrow*, New York: Harper and Brothers, 1955.

[4] This analysis will be limited to the patient side of the physician–patient equation. King offers the relevant suggestion that the health professional's own perceptions and beliefs about illness influence his behavior as a medical practitioner. See S. H. King, *Perceptions of Illness and Medical Practice*, New York: Russell Sage Foundation, 1962.

From Journal of Health & Human Behavior, Vol. 6: 2–16, Spring, 1965; by permission of the author and publisher.

Revision of a paper read at the annual meeting of the American Sociological Association, August, 1963. This investigation was supported in whole by U.S. Public Health Service Grant no. CH 0001005 from the Division of Community Health Services, Dr. George James, principal investigator. Field work was aided by the Health Research Council of the City of New York, Grant no. U-1053, Dr. Jack Elinson, principal investigator. Margaret C. Klem and Sylvia Gilliam (deceased) played a major role in the planning of this project, while field work and analysis were aided by Marvin Belkin, Martin Goldman, Martin Smolin, Raymond Maurice and Daniel Rosenblatt. John Colombotos and Annette Perrin O'Hare were in charge of interviewing, with Regina Loewenstein responsible for sampling and data-processing.

heavily. Illness is a frequently recurring phenomenon which generates fundamental concerns and anxieties and which intimately involves many other people besides the sick individual. As a consequence, significant group norms and mores have evolved which strongly influence individual attitudes and behavior in the health area.

In this study, we plan to investigate these constraints through an analysis of certain aspects of the social relationships which the individual has to other members of his community, friendship, and family groups. Our hypothesis is that those individuals who belong to relatively more homogeneous and cohesive groups will be more likely to react to illness and medical care in terms of the social group's definition and interpretation of appropriate medical behavior rather than the more formal and impersonalized prescriptions of the official medical care system.

Definition and Measurement of Concepts

We propose to test our hypothesis by determining the interrelationships between the following sets of indices of social group organization and individual medical orientation:

Social Group Organization
1. Ethnic Exclusivity
   (Community level)
2. Friendship Solidarity
   (Social group level)
3. Family Tradition and Authority
   (Family level)

Individual Medical Orientation
1. Knowledge about Disease
   (Cognitive)
2. Skepticism of Medical Care
   (Affective)
3. Dependency in Illness
   (Behavioral)

Each of the indices listed above was constructed by means of Guttman scaling procedures. Social group organization was determined by a series of questions indicative of the degree of social cohesion or homo-

geneity on three levels of interaction. On the community level, we employed a scale of *ethnic exclusivity* which referred to the tendency of the individual to interact with individuals from the same ethnic or social background as himself; on the social group level, we measured *friendship solidarity* which referred to the degree to which the individual belonged to a close friendship group of long duration; on the family level, we used a scale of *orientation to family tradition and authority* which referred to the importance placed by the individual's family upon customs and traditions and the degree of authority possessed by the head of the household.[5]

To study individual variations in response to illness and medical care, we employed a series of operational measures indicative of the cognitive, affective, and behavioral aspects of illness and medical care. These indices referred to, first, *knowledge about disease* (cognitive) as measured by the correctness of responses to thirteen questions

[5] The specific questions asked were: "I am going to read some statements. Just tell me whether you agree or disagree with each of these statements." (Agreement is indicative of a higher degree of cohesion.)

1) *Ethnic Exclusivity* (*Community level*)
The parents of most of my friends come from the same country as my parents come from.
I prefer to deal in stores where clerks are the same kind of people as we are.

2) *Friendship Solidarity* (*Social group level*)
Almost all my friends are people I grew up with.
Most of my close friends are also friends with each other.
Most of my friends have the same religion as I do.
Most of my friends come from families who know each other well.

3) *Family Tradition and Authority Orientation* (*Family level*)
Everybody in my family usually does what the head of the house says without question.
My family usually waits until the head of the house is present before we have dinner.
In my family we think the old-time customs and traditions are important.

dealing with etiology, symptoms, and prognosis of various diseases; second, *skepticism of medical care* (affective) which dealt with the doubts the individual had about the claims of professional medicine and his desire to check on who the doctor was and what he was doing; and third, *dependency in illness* (behavioral) which measured the need of the sick individual to rely upon other lay individuals for help and support during illness.[6]

Our working hypotheses, based on the above operational indices, is that those individuals who belong to community groups which are highly exclusive ethnically, to friendship groups which are highly cohesive, and to family groups which are highly oriented to tradition and authority will be found to have a lower level of knowledge about disease, higher skepticism of medical care, and greater dependency in illness.

The above formulation of the problem, thus, seeks to relate social group factors to the individual medical orientation. We recognize the inherent complexity of each of the individual concepts proposed and the usual problems of reliability and validity associated with our present operational indices. They are offered at the present time only as first approximations to a more fully developed and defined conceptual model for linking social factors to illness responses.

[6] The specific questions asked were:

1) *Knowledge about Disease* (*Cognitive dimension*)
   Thirteen questions dealing with causes, symptoms and prognoses of various diseases.
2) *Skepticism of Medical Care* (*Affective dimension*) (Agreement is indicative of skepticism)
   I have my doubts about some things doctors say they can do for you.
   When I am ill, I demand to know all the details of what is being done to me.
   I believe in trying out different doctors to find which one I think will give me the best care.
3) *Dependency in Illness* (*Behavioral dimension*) (Agreement is indicative of dependency)
   When I think I am getting sick, I find it comforting to talk to someone about it.
   When a person starts getting well, it is hard to give up having people do things for him.

Space limitations prevent us from developing the definition and theoretical rationale for each of these six major indices in more detail.

We would like, however, to offer the following more theoretical statement of the problem before proceeding to a presentation of our data. On a broad scale of generalization, we might speak of variations in social group background in terms of cosmopolitanism–parochialism.[7] On the parochial side we would characterize social groups as traditional, shared, affectual, and closed, while on the cosmopolitan side, they would tend to be more progressive, individualistic, instrumental, and open. In relation to medical care, we would hypothesize that cosmopolitan social structures would be more congruent with the highly impersonal, complex organization of modern medicine and that the more the individual's social group memberships could be characterized as cosmopolitan, the easier would be his acceptance and adaptation to modern medical practices.

Similarly, on the same broad scale of generalization, we might speak of variations in medical orientation in terms of scientific vs. popular health approaches.[8] We would

[7] Freidson employs a similar cosmopolitan–parochial distinction in characterizing lay referral structures in medical care (E. Freidson, *op. cit.*). Gouldner develops a cosmopolitan–local differentiation in his analysis of bureaucratic structures (A. W. Gouldner, "Cosmopolitans and Locals: Toward an Analysis of Latent Social Roles—I," *Admin. Science Quart.*, 2:281–306, December, 1957). R. K. Merton utilizes a similar framework in his paper, "Patterns of Influence: A Study of Interpersonal Influence and of Communications Behavior in a Local Community," in P. Lazarsfeld and F. Stanton (eds.), *Communications Research, 1948–1949*, New York: Harper and Bros., 1949, pp. 180–219.

[8] We are not here proposing a strict scientific–popular dichotomy regarding medical care. The two approaches are too closely interwoven to permit this separation. However, we do feel that this distinction is valid as a general measure of one's overall view of medical care. See, e.g., S. Polgar, "Health and Human Behavior," *Current Anthropology*, 3:159–205, April, 1962; and S. H. King, *op. cit.*, pp. 91–120. Saunders and Hewes propose an operational scheme for the analysis of folk or popular medicine in terms of places one can visit, things one can buy, or individuals one can visit (L. W. Saunders and G. W. Hewes, "Folk Medicine and Medical Practice," *J. Med. Educ.*, 28:43–46, September, 1953).

characterize as scientific, an objective, formal, professional, independent approach to illness and medical care, and as popular, a subjective, informal, lay, dependent health orientation. Modern medicine is highly oriented toward the scientific approach and we would hypothesize that conflict is less likely to occur among those individuals sharing this scientific commitment to health and medical care.

Our most general hypothesis linking social group influences to individual medical responses is that a cosmopolitan type of social background will be more highly related to a scientific approach to health and medical care than a parochial type of background which will be more highly related to a popular health orientation. In terms of conflict between the public and the professional medical care system, the greatest degree of congruence would exist among the scientific-oriented individuals belonging to cosmopolitan groups while the greatest degree of conflict would occur among the popular-oriented individuals belonging to parochial groups.

Method of Procedure

This study is based upon information obtained by a trained staff of interviewers from a representative cross section of adults, 21 years of age or older, living in the Washington Heights community of New York City. According to the U.S. Census of 1960, the Washington Heights Health District has 100,000 dwelling units and 270,000 people. The area contains a great deal of ethnic variation with about a quarter of the population being non-white and another quarter being foreign-born whites. There is also a wide range of socio–economic statuses from slum areas to luxury apartment houses. The area contains a large number of public and private medical facilities including the Columbia University-Presbyterian Medical Center.[9]

[9] Lendt, L. A., *A Social History of Washington Heights, New York City*, Columbia–Washington Heights Community Mental Health Project, Columbia University, Faculty of Medicine, February, 1960 (mimeo.).

Sampling—The sampling design utilized a stratified, two-stage, cluster plan. Eleven substrata were used as defined by geographical location, average rent, and racial composition of blocks according to the 1950 census. Data were obtained for a probability sample of 5,340 persons comprising some 2,215 families by means of personal household interviews conducted from November 1960 through April 1961. The initial interview in each household was conducted with an adult member of the family, usually the female head of the household. This interview obtained the basic demographic data for all members of the household, an inventory of all chronic conditions and impairments, and a record of all medically attended illnesses experienced by any family member during the past year, together with an account of all medical care and the sequence in which such care was received. All adult members of this initial sample were then listed and a random sample of 1,883 respondents over 21 years of age selected for a more detailed follow-up interview on social group memberships, symptoms of illness, and related medical knowledge, attitudes and behavior. This is the sample upon which the current report is based. A weighted completion rate of over 90 per cent was obtained from all eligible respondents.[10]

Findings

First, let us examine briefly the interrelationships of the operational indices used to define our dependent (individual medical

[10] This weighted completion rate is based upon a 76.3 per cent return on first interviews combined with returns, from a one-third random sampling of non-respondents (weighted 3X). A comparison of the obtained sample with the 1960 census on a large number of variables showed no major demographic category differing by more than 3 per cent. For a description of sampling procedures and results see J. Elinson and R. Loewenstein, *Community Fact Book for Washington Heights*, New York: Columbia University School of Public Health and Administrative Medicine, 1963.

orientation) and our independent (social group memberships) variables.[11] As can be seen from Table 19–1, low knowledge about disease, high skepticism of medical care, and high dependency in illness go together. For example, individuals who report high dependency in illness are almost twice as likely to score low on knowledge about disease and almost three times as likely to register high skepticism of medical care compared to those with low dependency in illness. These differences are all statistically significant at or beyond the 0.01 level of probability.[12]

Similarly, from Table 19–2, we find that high ethnic exclusivity, high friendship

[11] The individual questions used in each of the six indices of socio–medical orientation and socio–cultural background were tested for inter-item reliability and, in each case, the items combined in a single index were found to have highly significant coefficients of correlation. The reader is cautioned, however, against the error of "operationalism" and is urged to keep the content meaning of specific questions clearly in mind. Until these hypothetical constructs have been tested further by means of additional indices, it is wise to accord them only tentative acceptance.

[12] In the tables to be presented, chi square (upper-tail test) has been used as an indication of the level of statistical significance. These values were obtained using the 7090 computer. They should be viewed as approximate since the tables presented do not always coincide exactly with the tables as run, although only minor changes have been made.

solidarity, and high family orientation to tradition and authority are also associated with each other. These relationships are even more pronounced than those for medical orientation. Individuals who belong to community groups characterized by high ethnic exclusivity are three times as likely as those coming from groups with lower ethnic identification to belong also to friendship groups which are highly cohesive and to come from families with a high orientation toward tradition and authority.

From these results, there appears to be sufficient empirical justification for treating the three indices of socio–medical orientation and social group structure in combination. Each index, and, in fact, each separate question, of course, taps a somewhat different area of health orientation or social organization, but a detailed discussion of each of the separate indices or questions would be of limited value. Our major concern in this report is with general patterns only. This restriction also applies to other medical and social indices studied, the results of which will be discussed in further reports.[13]

[13] These included such social group measures as a sociometric index of degree and intensity of cohesion among specifically listed members of the individual's friendship group and an index of degree of reliance on one's friends. These indices were found highly related ($p < 0.001$) with the index of friendship solidarity and showed the same relationships to medical orientation as friendship solidarity. Religiosity, as measured by extent of religious attendance, also is related

Table 19–1—Interrelationships of individual medical orientation factors

	DEPENDENCY IN ILLNESS		
	High	Medium	Low
% Low Knowledge about Disease **	38.0	28.8	20.6
% High Skepticism of Medical Care **	31.4	21.1	12.4
Total Cases	(493)	(840)	(550)

	SKEPTICISM OF MEDICAL CARE			
	High	Med. High	Med. Low	Low
% Low Knowledge about Disease *	32.8	29.9	25.8	24.7
Total Cases	(399)	(728)	(569)	(174)

* p < 0.01.
** p < 0.001.
(X² = based upon the total number of categories)

Relating these independent and dependent variables to each other in Table 19–3, we find that in all instances, our hypotheses are strongly confirmed. Thus, ethnic exclusivity, friendship solidarity, and family orientation to tradition and authority are all individually related in the predicted direction to knowledge about disease, skepticism of medical care, and dependency in illness.[14]

Table 19–4 shows the relationship between the combined score for the three indices of social group structure and the combined score for three indices of medical orientation. As we move from scores indicative of membership in social groups tending toward "cosmopolitanism" to those tending toward "parochialism," we have a dramatic decrease in the proportions adhering to a "scientific" health orientation and an increase in the proportions with a "popular" health orientation. In general terms, membership in closely-knit, ethnocentric, traditionalistic community, friendship, and family groups appears to symbolize a parochial way of life which finds expression in the health area as a popular or non-scientific orientation characterized by low factual knowledge about disease, suspicion of outside professional medical care, and reliance upon members of one's own group for help and support during illness.[15]

DEMOGRAPHIC CHARACTERISTICS AND
MEDICAL STATUS

The remainder of this report will examine this relationship between social group structure and individual medical orientation in terms of three other sets of major variables: demographic characteristics, health status, and medical care. On the sociological side, we will look at the demographic variables of social class, including sex and age differences. On the medical side, we will look at health status in terms of medically attended conditions, chronic conditions, and mental illness, and at medical care in terms of the source of medical services for attended illnesses.

We hypothesize the following relationships of these social and medical variables to social group structure and individual medical orientation:

1) Socio–economic classes will differ in social group structure, with the lower social class tending toward a "parochial" social structure. Therefore, this lower

---

positively to the three indices of social group structure with high religious attendance being associated with high community, friendship, and family integration. In regard to medical orientation, we find that an index of preventive medical behavior is related to knowledge of disease (low knowledge = low use of preventive measures), that agreement with statements indicative of low physician interest in the welfare of his patients is associated with high skepticism of medical care, and that resistance to going to bed and staying in bed when ill is related to high dependency in illness (p < 0.001). Only the latter relationship did not coincide with our hypothesis. It seems that acceptance of the sick role as measured by ease of going to bed and staying in bed is indicative of a scientific health orientation while high dependency on others in illness indicates a popular health orientation. In retrospect, this seems to make sense in terms of a "rational" acceptance of illness and medical care.

[14] It has been suggested that an "acquiescent response set" might account for some of the observed interrelationships. However, it must be remembered that the possibility of this kind of artifact being introduced is greatly reduced by the use of scale scores instead of individual item relationships. Furthermore, the thirteen knowledge items obviously must be free of such possible spuriousness and this score gives us some of our highest correlations. Other indices to be reported elsewhere did not contain the possibility of this bias and still showed the same relationships, i.e., a friendship group cohesiveness score based upon the closeness of specifically named members of the individual's social group to each other; a religious attendance score; a preventive medical behavior score based on such behavioral items as polio immunizations and periodic doctor visits.

[15] This characterization of social structure as "cosmopolitan" or "parochial" and medical orientation as "scientific" or "popular" requires a great deal of further careful and rigorous conceptualization and measurement, far beyond what was attempted in the present study. We are aware of the many theoretical arguments which surround the use of both typologies, especially in anthropology as applied to folk-urban cultures, and to scientific–popular ideologies. We offer them here only as promising guidelines for future research.

Table 19-2—Interrelationships of social group structure factors

	ETHNIC EXCLUSIVITY		
	High	Medium	Low
% High Friendship Solidarity*	61.7	45.8	20.7
% High Family Authority*	51.5	33.1	16.5
Total Cases	(282)	(771)	(830)

	FRIENDSHIP SOLIDARITY		
	High	Medium	Low
% High Family Authority*	45.5	23.4	14.4
Total Cases	(699)	(513)	(671)

* p < 0.001.

Table 19-3—Relationship between social group structure factors and medical orientation

	ETHNIC EXCLUSIVITY		
	High	Medium	Low
% Low Knowledge about Disease*	48.0	32.3	19.0
% High Skepticism of Medical Care*	36.5	22.3	15.1
% High Dependency in Illness*	44.3	27.9	18.4
Total Cases	(282)	(771)	(830)

	FRIENDSHIP SOLIDARITY		
	High	Medium	Low
% Low Knowledge about Disease*	37.8	29.6	18.8
% High Skepticism of Medical Care*	27.5	18.9	16.5
% High Dependency in Illness*	36.1	23.2	18.2
Total Cases	(699)	(513)	(671)

	FAMILY ORIENTATION TO TRADITION AND AUTHORITY		
	High	Medium	Low
% Low Knowledge about Disease*	40.5	28.1	18.0
% High Skepticism of Medical Care**	27.3	21.0	19.7
% High Dependency in Illness*	37.0	25.3	19.2
Total Cases	(432)	(499)	(595)

* p < 0.001.
** p < 0.01.

Table 19-4—Relationship between social group structure and medical orientation*

		(COSMOPOLITAN)		SOCIAL GROUP STRUCTURE			(PAROCHIAL)	
		1	2	3	4	5	6	7
Socio-Medical Orientation								
1. (Scientific)	(%)	40	36	32	21	14	7	1
2. ↓	(%)	28	29	29	28	28	15	12
3. ↓	(%)	21	21	21	28	28	28	24
4. (Popular)	(%)	11	14	18	23	30	50	63
Total Per Cent		100	100	100	100	100	100	100
Total Cases		206	353	364	348	310	211	91

* p < 0.001.

socio–economic group will also show a more "popular" orientation toward health and medical care, while the upper social class will tend toward a "scientific" health orientation.

2) Health status, per se, will be little affected by social group structure or medical orientation, but will reflect the underlying social class, sex, and age differences. Source of medical care, on the other hand, will vary with social group structure and medical orientation with the "cosmopolitan-scientific" individuals making greater use of modern medical services.

Thus, our analytical framework might be diagrammed as follows in terms of the hypothesized sequence of independent, dependent, and intervening variables.

Social Status → Social Group Structure → Individual Medical Orientation → Source of Medical Care

In the tables that follow, we shall present the data on the relationships between these four sets of variables and attempt to test the hypothesized causal sequence.

Social Characteristics — Socio – economic status constitutes one of the most important sources of social and medical differentiation in the United States. Almost all studies have shown that upper and lower social classes, however defined, have different values and norms and vary in both their health status and utilization of health facilities.[16] Our study is no exception. Using a classification of social class based upon an individual's income, education, and occupation,[17] we find in Table 19–5 that lower class

[16] Anderson, O. W., "The Utilization of Health Services," in H. Freeman, *et al.* (eds.), *op. cit.*, pp. 349–367; and O. G. Simmons, *Social Status and Public Health*, New York: Social Science Research Council, pamphlet 13, 1958.

[17] The Social Class index was formed from the person's education, occupation, and total family income as follows: Education was divided into five categories: some college, high school graduate, some high school, grammar school graduate, and some grammar school. Occupation was divided into four categories: professional and managerial, clerical and sales, craftsmen and operators, and household, service workers, etc. Total family income was divided into four categories: $7,500 plus, $5,000 to $7,500, $3,000 to $5,000, and less than $3,000. These were scored

status as compared to upper class status is much more likely to be associated with "parochialism" and a "popular" health orientation. Each of the specific subdivisions of lower income, less education, and blue collar occupation are significantly related to the individual measures of greater ethnic exclusivity, friendship solidarity, and family authority, on the one hand, and to lower knowledge about disease, higher skepticism toward medical care, and greater dependency in illness, on the other hand.[18]

When we look at the relationship of social group structure to medical orientation for the different socio–economic levels, we find that, within each social class, higher "parochialism" continues to be significantly related to a less "scientific" health orientation. Thus, it would seem that the relationship between "parochialism" and a "popular" health orientation cannot be explained solely by the lower social class status of the "parochial" group. However, neither can we account for social class differences in health orientation solely in terms of social group factors.

On the basis of this evidence, our hypothesis that socio–economic status reflects varying forms of social group organization which in turn produce different medical orientations needs to be revised to show separate and independent "causal" relationships between socio–economic status, social

and distributed on an index which ranged from a score of 13 for highest SES to 3 for lowest SES. Where information was not ascertained for one of the 3 index components, the score was based upon a linear interpolation of the remaining 2 components.

[18] This is consistently the case for each of the individual social status measures of income, education, and occupation related to each of the separate indices of community, friendship, and family group integration, and to knowledge about disease, skepticism of medical care, and illness dependence ($p < 0.01$ or < 0.001).

group structure, and individual medical orientation—diagrammed as follows:

Socio–Economic Status → Individual
↓ Medical
Social Group Structure → Orientation

Sex and Age—Unlike social class, sex and age do not represent group statuses so much as role variations within social groups. When we look at sex and age variations in social group structure and medical orientation (Table 19–6), we find a puzzling reversal. While women tend to be somewhat more "parochial" than men, they actually show a lower commitment to a "popular" health orientation, especially the older women. Analyzing the indices separately, we see that women are likely to be better informed about disease than men and to be less skeptical of medical care, but to be about equally high in illness dependency. It may be that health and medical care are areas of greater salience for women, as mothers responsible for the health of their families, and that, for this reason, they learn more about disease and place more faith in doctors.

The relationship of social group structure to individual medical orientation holds within each separate age, sex, and social class grouping. Socio–economic differences appear even more sharply when controlled on sex and age. Of all three variables, social class is by far the most highly related to both social group structure and medical orientation. The cumulative effect of all three factors, as given in Table 19–7, is worth noting; older, lower class, males in "parochial" groups are *twelve* times as likely to hold a "popular" health orientation (61.2 per cent) as compared to older, upper class, females in "cosmopolitan" groups (5.1 per cent).

Each of these comparisons of different demographic groups supports our previous interpretation of demographic characteristics and social group structure as contributing independently to medical orientation. On a descriptive level of analysis, we find that "cosmopolitanism" is related to a "scientific" approach to health and medical care among all social class, sex, and age

groups, even when these are analyzed simultaneously. On an explanatory level, we find that the observed demographic group differences in health knowledge, attitudes towards medical care, and responses to illness cannot be accounted for in terms of the social group structural differences in ethnic exclusivity, friendship group solidarity, or family orientation to tradition and authority. We therefore conclude that *both* demographic characteristics and social group structure independently contribute to medical orientation.

Health Status and Medical Care

We now turn our attention to the final set of variables—health status and source of medical care. The relationship of social factors to health status is, of course, an area of primary concern to social epidemiology. This study was not intended to investigate health status in any detail and our data are limited to subjective reports on symptoms, attended illness, and chronic conditions without any objective medical verification.[19] While these subjective reports may constitute doubtful indices of actual disease conditions, they do represent a valid picture of health status of the individual *as he perceives it*, and may, in fact, be more predictive of how he behaves in the face of illness that the correct medical diagnosis itself.[20] For purposes of sociological analysis, we

[19] Several studies have shown the relatively low validity of household interviews as a source of morbidity data. J. J. Feldman, "The Household Interview Survey As a Technique for the Collection of Morbidity Data," *J. of Chronic Dis.* 11: 535–557, May, 1960. However, data on utilization of medical services appears to have higher validity, J. A. Solon, C. G. Sheps, S. S. Lee and J. P. Barbano, "Patterns of Medical Care: Validity of Interview Information on Use of Hospital Clinics," *J. of Health and Human Behavior*, 3:21–29, Spring, 1962.

[20] Suchman, E. A., B. S. Phillips and G. F. Streib, "An Analysis of the Validity of Health Questionnaires," *Social Forces*, 36:223–232, March, 1958.

Table 19–5—Relationship between socio–economic status, social group structure and medical orientation*

Social Class		% "Parochial" Social Structure	% "Popular" Health Orientation
Upper	(246)	20.3	12.0
Middle Upper	(652)	22.9	36.2
Middle Lower	(623)	38.4	43.1
Lower	(277)	53.1	57.1

| | | SOCIAL GROUP STRUCTURE** | | | | |
Social Class	Cosmopolitan		Mixed (% "Popular" Health Orientation)		Parochial	
Upper	10.4	(106)	10.0	(90)	12.0	(50)
Middle Upper	11.2	(251)	15.5	(252)	36.2	(149)
Middle Lower	14.4	(153)	26.5	(230)	43.1	(239)
Lower	29.6	(27)	33.0	(103)	57.1	(147)

* p < 0.001.
** p < 0.001 for all comparisons except upper class.

Table 19–6—Social group structure and medical orientation according to sex, age, and social class*

		% "Parochial" Social Structure	% "Popular" Health Orientation
Male			
21 to 44 Years			
Upper Social Classes	(203)	19.2	21.7
Lower Social Classes	(143)	32.9	37.8
Over 44 Years			
Upper Social Classes	(185)	23.2	22.6
Lower Social Classes	(230)	33.5	41.3
Female			
21 to 44 Years			
Upper Social Classes	(288)	26.0	14.9
Lower Social Classes	(195)	31.3	34.4
Over 44 Years			
Upper Social Classes	(221)	26.7	8.1
Lower Social Classes	(332)	36.7	29.0

* p < 0.01 for entire table. Individual sub-group comparisons vary as discussed in text.

Table 19–7—Relationship between social group structure and medical orientation according to social class, sex, and age*

| | | | SOCIAL GROUP STRUCTURE | | | |
	Cosmopolitan		Mixed (% "Popular" Health Orientation)		Parochial	
Male						
21 to 44 Years						
Upper Social Classes	12.5	(96)	18.1	(72)	54.3	(35)
Lower Social Classes	26.7	(30)	28.1	(57)	53.6	(56)
Over 44 Years						
Upper Social Classes	10.8	(65)	22.9	(70)	37.3	(51)
Lower Social Classes	14.0	(50)	32.5	(77)	61.2	(103)
Female						
21 to 44 Years						
Upper Social Classes	13.6	(118)	9.2	(109)	27.9	(61)
Lower Social Classes	20.0	(45)	27.5	(69)	48.1	(81)
Over 44 Years						
Upper Social Classes	5.1	(78)	9.9	(91)	9.6	(52)
Lower Social Classes	10.9	(55)	26.9	(130)	37.7	(146)

* p < 0.01 for entire table.

may usefully distinguish between the *disease* entity, as diagnosed by the physician, and the *illness*, as experienced by the individual.[21] The following data on health status are based on individual reports of illness during the study year.

First, in relation to demographic factors, Table 19–8 confirms the expected higher occurrence of illness among the old as compared to the young. This holds true for each separate sex and socio–economic status group in relation to chronic conditions, medically attended conditions, and mental disability, with the single exception of upper class males for whom we find more mental disability among the young than the old.[22] Women report significantly more chronic conditions, medically attended conditions, and mental disability than men within each age and social class group. In regard to social class, differences are smaller than for sex and age, with the lower socio–economic groups reporting somewhat more chronic conditions (except among the young males, where there are no differences), fewer medically attended conditions (except among the old males, where the lower groups report more conditions), and much higher mental disability, especially among the old males.

Of more direct concern to our present analysis is the relationship of health status to social group structure and medical orientation. As can be seen from Table 19–9, the relationship of social group structure and medical orientation to health status is slight and variable. There is a tendency for groups with "parochial" characteristics to

report somewhat more illness than the groups with "cosmopolitan" characteristics, but these differences are not entirely consistent for the different health orientation groups. Controlling on demographic characteristics fails to change this picture materially. Thus we would conclude that social group structure, as we have measured it, has little relationship to health status, as reported by the respondent.

There is a significant and consistent relationship, however, between mental health status and individual medical orientation. The "popular"-health oriented individuals are more likely than the "scientific"-oriented individuals to score high on mental disability. This is the case regardless of social group structure and the relationship continues to exist when controlled on demographic characteristics. Since our medical orientation score to some extent indirectly reflects degree of adjustment to illness and medical care, it is not surprising that this should also relate to psychological adjustment and ability to meet one's daily problems as indexed by our mental health score. This relationship is particularly high for the specific medical orientation index of "dependency in illness" with high mental disability being associated with high illness dependency [32 per cent of the high mental disability cases showing high dependency during illness compared to 19 per cent of the low disability cases ($p < 0.01$)].

If we reverse the question and now ask what effect does experience with illness and medical care have upon one's socio–medical orientation, we see from Table 19–10 that the more one is exposed to illness and medical care, the more likely is one to have a "scientific" health orientation. This holds true regardless of socio–economic class or social group structure. The cumulative effect of all three variables may be seen in the comparison between lower class "parochials" with no chronic conditions, 50 per cent of whom have a "popular" health orientation, and the upper class "cosmopolites" with two or more chronic conditions, only 5.8 per cent of whom maintain a "popular" health orientation.

In regard to utilization of medical services, our main comparison deals with the use

---

21 Elinson, J., "Methods of Sociomedical Research," in H. Freeman, *et al.*, *op. cit.*, pp. 449–472.

22 *Chronic conditions* were determined by asking, "Have you had any of these conditions during the past 12 months?" with the interviewer reading a list of 29 chronic conditions taken from the National Health Survey. *Attended conditions* were determined by asking, "Were you sick at any time in the past 12 months and talked to a doctor about it?" Mental disability was determined from a score based on 22 indices of mental disability developed by Srole and his associates, L. Srole, *et al.*, *Mental Health in the Metropolis: The Midtown Manhattan Study*, New York: McGraw-Hill, 1962.

Table 19–8—Relationship between social class, sex, age and health status

		% with Chronic Conditions	% with Attended Conditions	% High Mental Disability
Male				
21 to 44 Years				
Upper Social Classes	(203)	24.8	42.4	25.6
Lower Social Classes	(143)	24.6	39.9	29.3
Over 44 Years				
Upper Social Classes	(185)	40.5	47.6	18.3
Lower Social Classes	(230)	55.2	55.7	31.3
Female				
21 to 44 Years				
Upper Social Classes	(288)	32.3	56.3	25.0
Lower Social Classes	(195)	39.4	52.3	37.9
Over 44 Years				
Upper Social Classes	(221)	47.5	64.3	30.8
Lower Social Classes	(332)	58.7	57.5	44.3

Table 19–9—Relationship between social group structure, medical orientation and health status

Medical Orientation	SOCIAL GROUP STRUCTURE		
	Cosmopolitan	Mixed	Parochial
	(% with Chronic Conditions)		
Scientific	40.8	40.0	49.3
Mixed	40.5	46.1	45.5
Popular	31.9	49.0	37.0
	(% with Attended Conditions)		
Scientific	55.0	52.4	50.0
Mixed	57.0	54.6	54.2
Popular	44.3	47.7	52.1
	(% with High Mental Disability)		
Scientific	24.2	19.4	27.6
Mixed	33.9	34.1	32.0
Popular	31.4	37.7	38.9
Number of Cases upon which Percentages Are Based			
Scientific	211	191	58
Mixed	277	370	297
Popular	70	151	257

Table 19–10—Relationship between health status and medical orientation according to social group structure and socio–economic status

	UPPER SOCIAL CLASSES			LOWER SOCIAL CLASSES		
*Number of Chronic Conditions**	Cosmopolitan	Mixed	Parochial	Cosmopolitan	Mixed	Parochial
	(% "Popular" Medical Orientation)					
None	12.3 (228)	15.0 (213)	37.9 (132)	19.4 (93)	27.2 (162)	50.0 (208)
One	10.4 (77)	14.7 (75)	17.9 (39)	10.3 (39)	30.8 (78)	45.7 (94)
Two or More	5.8 (52)	9.4 (53)	10.7 (28)	15.9 (44)	29.3 (92)	47.0 (83)
*Number of Attended Conditions**						
None	15.8 (152)	16.9 (172)	34.7 (95)	16.3 (92)	31.3 (150)	48.0 (179)
One	7.6 (131)	14.0 (107)	30.0 (60)	20.0 (50)	22.7 (97)	51.8 (139)
Two or More	6.8 (74)	6.3 (63)	20.5 (44)	13.2 (38)	30.2 (86)	42.6 (68)

* $p < 0.05$ for entire table.

of a private physician as the primary source of medical care.[23] As can be seen from Table 19–11, recourse to the private sector of medical care is closely related to age and social class, and only slightly related to sex. The upper social classes and the older people are much more likely than the lower classes and younger people to make use of private physicians. Thus, social status and age markedly affect where an individual turns for medical help when ill.[24]

Looking at the relationship of social group structure and medical orientation to source of medical care, we find in Table 19–12 that "parochial" groups, regardless of socio–economic status, are more likely than "cosmopolitan" groups to make use of private physicians. This preference for personalized care, as hypothesized, probably reflects the stronger need of the "parochial" group member for more informal patient–physician relationships and the greater willingness of the "cosmopolite" to utilize the more impersonal sources of medical care.

There are no strong or consistent relationships between socio–medical orientation and source of medical care. Among the upper socio–economic groups, there is a slight tendency for the scientifically oriented individual to make greater use of private physicians but this difference does not occur among the lower socio–economic groups.

Table 19–11—Relationship between social class, sex, age, and source of medical care

| | MALE | | | | FEMALE | | | |
| | 21–44 Years | | Over 44 Years | | 21–44 Years | | Over 44 Years | |
	Upper	Lower	Upper	Lower	Upper	Lower	Upper	Lower
Source of Medical Care								
Family and Private Physician	41.8	26.3	63.6	45.3	51.2	25.4	63.5	59.2
Outpatient Clinic and Private Physician	24.4	21.1	22.7	21.9	29.6	36.3	17.6	18.1
Outpatient Clinic Only	15.1	29.8	8.0	16.4	9.3	26.5	5.6	15.4
HIP* and Private Physician	4.7	7.0	—	6.2	6.8	2.0	7.7	1.6
Other	14.0	15.8	5.7	10.2	3.1	9.8	5.6	5.7
Total Per Cent	100.0	100.0	100.0	100.0	100.0	100.0	100.0	100.0
Total Cases**	86	57	88	128	162	102	142	191

* Health Insurance Plan.
** For respondents reporting medically attended conditions only.

Table 19–12—Relationship between source of medical care, social group structure, and medical orientation according to socio–economic status

	Upper	Middle Upper	Middle Lower	Lower
	(% Family and Private Physician)			
*Social Group Structure**				
Cosmopolitan	59.3 (59)	54.1 (146)	32.1 (78)	—**
Mixed	46.5 (43)	52.8 (127)	48.1 (129)	40.7 (54)
Parochial	72.4 (29)	57.3 (75)	50.0 (124)	42.2 (83)
*Medical Orientation****				
Scientific	66.7 (51)	55.4 (112)	44.6 (56)	33.3 (15)
Mixed	52.2 (69)	57.0 (186)	45.1 (175)	50.0 (68)
Popular	54.5 (11)	42.0 (50)	45.0 (100)	37.5 (64)

* $p < 0.01$.
** Less than 10 cases.
*** $p < 0.05$.

[23] Types of facilities used for all attended conditions were ascertained from the following question: "(Let's start with the first doctor you talked to in the past 12 months) where did you see him? Was it at a clinic or health center, at a doctor's office or at home?"

[24] In general, very little research has been done on the sociological aspects of the use of health services. See O. W. Anderson, *op. cit.*, pp. 349–368.

For each type of social group structure and medical orientation, choice of a private physician for medical care increases steadily with a rise in socio–economic status. It would appear that the choice of a medical care facility is largely a reflection of socio-economic factors rather than social group structure or health orientation.

Several other indices of medical behavior support this finding concerning the relatively greater influence of socio–economic status as compared to social group structure or health orientation upon the individual's medical behavior. Buying health insurance, getting a periodical medical check-up, receiving polio immunizations, eating a balanced diet, and seeking dental care or an examination for eye glasses occur less frequently among the lower socio–economic classes than among the upper classes. When controlled on socio–economic status, we do not find any consistent relationship between either group structure or medical orientation and any of the above items. While in each case the upper socio–economic groups continue to be more likely to engage in these activities, within each socio–economic group these activities do not appear to be affected by social group structure or medical orientation. This would indicate that, to a large extent, the utilization of preventive services and health insurance is also more a function of socio–economic status than group structure or health attitudes.

type of social group structure was not found to be related to either health status or source of medical care. The chart below summarizes the presence or absence of significant relationships, on the whole, for our five sets of variables.

It now remains for us to reconstruct our framework for the hypothesized "causal" sequence among the five sets of variables studied. We fully recognize the limitations of the present exploratory study for this purpose, both theoretically in terms of the broad and superficially defined concepts employed, and methodologically in terms of the relatively non-rigorous and imprecise measures of the operational indices used. However, we share the conviction of others that the field of medical sociology is badly in need of attempts to build conceptual frameworks based upon empirical data[25] and tentatively offer the following model (Figure 19–1):

	Demographic Factors	Social Group Structure	Medical Orientation	Health Status	Source of Medical Care
Demographic Factors	—	yes	yes	yes	yes
Social Group Structure	yes	—	yes	no	no
Medical Orientation	yes	yes	—	no	yes
Health Status	yes	no	no	—	yes
Source of Medical Care	yes	no	yes	yes	—

Summary and Discussion

In this report we have attempted to analyze the relationship between social and medical factors in terms of a framework which linked demographic factors to social group structure and both of these to health status and medical care by means of an intervening set of medical orientation factors generally indicative of a "scientific" or "popular" approach to health and medical care. In summary, we found that demographic factors and social group structure were independently related to medical orientation and that demographic factors and medical orientation were independently related to source of medical care. By and large, the

FIGURE 19-1

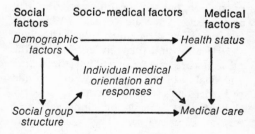

25 The need for the development of such theoretical frameworks in the field of medical sociology has been stressed by many writers. See comments by E. Freidson and J. Cassel in S. Polgar, *op. cit.*, pp. 159–205; and E. A. Suchman, *Sociology and the Field of Public Health*, New York: Russell Sage Foundation, 1963.

The arrows indicating the direction of causality are, of course, largely arbitrary, but, as Freeman, Levine and Reeder have pointed out:

"Often, of course, the ordering of variables is purely arbitrary and 'causal sequence' is not a relevant issue. Nevertheless, from the standpoint of the field of medicine, knowledge becomes relatively useless unless some ordering can be identified or at least assumed. Given the present status of knowledge, it is essential that careful explication of the actual or assumed ordering of variables be undertaken in all but solely descriptive studies. If it is not done, the practitioner does it anyway, and the medical sociologist finds himself in the position of contending with false inferences for which, through omission, he is at least in part responsible. The problem of 'as if it were causal' has always plagued sociology but takes on particular importance in a field where findings may potentially, no matter how tentatively they are noted, be put to immediate use."[26]

Cause and effect are reciprocal to some degree and the mutual interaction of two variables often creates a reversible equation. We might briefly note four such "actions and reactions" in the above model.

1. Social factors predispose toward illness, but illness may also affect social factors as when medical costs reduce economic status.

2. Health status influences one's medical orientation, but such health orientation may also affect one's state of health especially in the area of preventive medical behavior.

3. Health status largely determines the medical care one receives, but the nature and quality of such care may, in turn, aid or hinder one's return to health.

4. Medical orientation influences the medical care one seeks, but good or bad experiences with medical care may affect subsequent health orientation.

Socio–medical research, to date, has been almost entirely limited to the relationships

[26] Freeman, H. E., S. Levine and L. G. Reeder, "Present Status of Medical Sociology," in H. E. Freeman, et al., op. cit., pp. 484–485.

between social factors, health status and medical care. As far as we know, this study represents the first major empirical attempt to collect systematic data on the two sets of social factors which constitute the focal points of the present analysis—social structure and medical orientation. The highly significant relationship of these two factors to each other and to health and medical care, it would seem to us, has been sufficiently indicated to warrant further research along these lines in the future.

Implications for Medicine and Public Health

These findings have many implications for the provision and utilization of medical care which can be mentioned only briefly. To the extent that modern medicine is becoming increasingly "scientific," e.g., formal, complex, impersonal, objective, disease rather than patient oriented, and specialized, it will come into increasing conflict with the "parochial" types of social groupings in our society, e.g., traditional, dependent, closed, and local, which feel more at home with a "popular" or non-scientific approach to illness and medical care. In fact, it may be argued that many of the current physician–patient conflicts stem from the former's emphasis on scientific medicine, while the latter still clings to popular or folk medicine. King has characterized this incongruence as a form of "cultural lag" between scientific medicine and popular beliefs and attitudes about disease.[27]

This problem is most apparent where the medical or public health practitioner attempts to introduce new and more "scientific" medical practices or public health programs into highly traditional or parochial settings. Thus various studies have shown that the underdeveloped areas of the world resist many modern medical programs,[28]

[27] King, S. H., op. cit., pp. 156–157. The continued strong appeal of folk medicine in the United States today is evidenced by the best seller popularity of such books as D. C. Jarvis, Folk Medicine, New York: Henry Holt, 1958.

[28] Paul, B. D. (ed.), Health, Culture and Community, New York: Russell Sage Foundation, 1955.

public health programs for the American Indians in the Southwest have to be adapted to local customs,[29] lower class minority groups in our large cities constitute centers of non-cooperation and malutilization of medical care services,[30] and farmers in rural areas resent urbanized medical care.[31]

In a similar way, on the level of individual patient behavior, diverse findings from numerous studies have indicated that the more an individual tends towards a "parochial–popular" approach to illness and medical care, the more likely he is to seek lay diagnosis and help,[32] to delay treatment,[33] to stress folk remedies and self-medication,[34] to react more strongly to pain symptoms,[35] to be more concerned with immediate symptom relief than long-term cure of disease,[36] to use marginal or quasi-practitioners,[37] to find it difficult to adjust to hospital routines,[38] to be less favorable toward group health practice,[39] and, in general, to be poorly informed about health or medical services.[40] Thus, in terms of

[29] Adair, J., "The Indian Health Worker in the Cornell–Navajo Project," *Human Organization*, 19:59–63, 1960.

[30] Cornely, P. B., and S. K. Bigman, "Acquaintance with Municipal Government Health Services in a Low-income Urban Population, *Amer. J. Public Health* 1877–1886, November, 1962.

[31] Hassinger, E. W., and R. L. McNamara, *Relationship of the Public to Physicians in a Rural Setting*, Columbia, Mo., University of Missouri Research Bulletin 653, January, 1958.

[32] Freidson, E., "Client Control and Medical Practice," *Amer. J. Sociology*, 65:374–382, January, 1960 (see Chap. 15 herein).

[33] Kutner, B., and G. Gordon, "Seeking Care for Cancer," *J. Health and Human Behavior*, 2:171–178, Fall, 1961.

[34] Berle, B., *Eighty Puerto Rican Families in New York City: Health and Disease Studied in Context*, New York: Columbia University Press, 1958.

[35] Zborowski, M., "Cultural Components in Responses to Pain,"*J. Social Issues*, 8:16–30, 1952.

[36] Jeffreys, M., "Social Class and Health Promotion: Some Obstacles in Britain," *Health Education J.* 15:109–118, May, 1957.

[37] Steiner, L. R., *Where Do People Take Their Troubles*, Boston: Houghton Mifflin, 1945.

[38] Coser, R. L., "A Home Away from Home," *Social Problems*, 4:3–17, 1956.

[39] Freidson, *Patients' Views of Medical Practice, op. cit.*

[40] Koos, E. L., *The Health of Regionville*, New York: Columbia University Press, 1954.

modern medical care and public health programs, "parochialism" and an "antiscientific" health orientation are major sources of resistance and malutilization.

The obvious, but difficult, answer to this problem lies in the development of a greater congruence between modern, scientific medical and public health practice and the needs of a still largely popular or folk-oriented public. On the one hand, medical care must become more rather than less personalized with a greater accent on the patient and his family as whole units, as currently advocated by the practice of comprehensive medicine,[41] and public health programs must "reach out" into the community adapting their services to local customs and bringing them to the people rather than waiting for the people to show up at public clinics.[42]

On the other side, the public must become more sophisticated and knowledgeable about health and medical care. This may require a new form of health education which stresses "rationality" in the seeking and finding of medical care rather than traditional factual information about the disease etiology and symptoms. What is needed is a more intelligent medical consumer who is better able to decide when and how to purchase, and to evaluate, medical care. To some extent such increased public sophistication may conflict with private medicine's traditional authoritative control, but if scientific medicine is to become acceptable to the people it must be more willing to take an informed public into its confidence.

[41] Matarazzo, J., "Comprehensive Medicine: A New Era in Medical Education," *Human Organization*, 14:4–9, Spring, 1955.

[42] A movement in this direction has been made by the New York City Health Department with demonstration–research projects designed to offer comprehensive medical care on an integrated interagency basis such as the Cornell Medical Center Welfare Demonstration Project headed by Dr. Goodrich and the Queensbridge Housing Project Center for the Aged, headed by Dr. Kuo. See G. James, "The Present Status and Future Development of Community Health Research—A Critique from the Viewpoint of Community Health Agencies," *Annals of N. Y. Acad. of Sciences*, 107:760–770, May 22, 1963.

Implications for Social Action

On the broadest level of generality, we feel that an analysis of congruence between social group structures characterized according to relative cosmopolitan or parochial organization and professional sub-systems characterized according to relative emphasis upon a scientific or popular orientation provides a useful framework for research on many current social problems. This framework postulates social conflict as the result of a discrepancy between the basic values and approaches of the professional sub-system and the customary modes of thought and behavior of the public. We may envision the following four general situations (Figure 19–2):

FIGURE 19-2

Professional
subsystem
orientation   Scientific
                     popular

Social group structure

Cosmopolitan   Parochial
    A   C
    B   D

To the degree that a scientific-oriented professional sub-system operates within a cosmopolitan social group structure or a popular-oriented system within a parochial structure, as in cells A and D, there will be congruence of profession and public with a minimum of conflict. On the other hand, to the extent that a cosmopolitan group is exposed to a popular-oriented system, or a parochial group to one that is scientifically oriented, as in cells B and C, there will be an incongruence of social structure and professional sub-system values with a maximizing of potential conflict.

We may cite a few examples. In the case of our present concern—the medical sub-system—congruence is more likely to occur between a complex, highly organized medical service in an urban, cosmopolitan community or a small, personal medical practice in a parochial, rural area. Incongruence and conflict, on the other hand, are more likely to result from trying to impose a complex medical organization upon a non-cosmopolitan area, as can be seen today in the difficulties encountered by efforts to introduce modern medicine into underdeveloped areas, or from attempting to continue a personalized medical service in a highly urban area, as evidenced by the rapidly disappearing general practitioner.

Other examples besides the medical may be mentioned briefly dealing with the religious and educational sub-systems. Unlike medicine, religion is largely characterized by a popular or non-scientific orientation. This would make it more congruent with parochial social groups and less congruent with cosmopolitan groups and thus help to explain the greater strength of the church in rural areas and among parochial groups. It would also help to account for current attempts to make religious beliefs and practices more "rational" in order to increase their acceptability to a cosmopolitan people. In education, the conflict stems from the use of "progressive" methods and forms of organization representative of a scientific approach and hence more in congruence with a cosmopolitan people as opposed to the more "traditional" or popular approach favored by some parochial groups.

To the extent that the major direction of social change today is from parochial to cosmopolitan forms of social organization and from popular to scientific sub-system value orientations, the existence of such conflict may be viewed as a consequence of cultural lag. Professional sub-systems, such as medicine and education, respond more readily to the need for reorganization in line with modern scientific and technical advances than do the values and behavior of the people. A major problem of modern times is to reduce the gap between a rapidly advancing scientific technology looking forward and a hesitant, parochial public looking backward. This can probably be done more successfully by seeking new organizational forms and modes of operation which, while taking advantage of scientific advances, still are translated into terms acceptable to the parochial segments of the public. These parochial groups in modern society, often those most in need of the services being offered, constitute the core of resistance to and non-participation in many of the more advanced medical and educational programs. It makes no sense to talk about "calling a halt" to scientific progress, but much can be done to frame such progress so that it appears less foreign to traditional forms and methods. Similarly, while insofar as possible people need to be "educated" to this new scientific approach, they cannot be threatened or exhorted to change. The major share of responsibility must remain with the changing social institutions to seek ways of reaching out to the people with new ideas and techniques fitted as closely as possible into old and traditional clothing.

Society and Health Care Administration

AS ORGANIZATIONS and institutions become established to detect, comprehend, care for, and cope with disease and disability, the need to maintain these varying, complex, and often uncoordinated health and medical care services and facilities becomes a demanding and significant effort for the community and total society. The often unrelated, independent, and divergently developed health care programs, services, and facilities, as they have survived and expanded through time, have tended to develop cooperative and interdependent relationships that eventuate into "health care systems." These health care systems are organized and coordinated efforts to stabilize and maintain existing facilities, services, and related enterprises, and they attempt to legitimize previously established ways and means of producing, distributing, and consuming health services into a socially sanctioned health care "Establishment." Different societies, particularly in the western world, have therefore evolved divergent health care systems in the delivery of health and medical care to their constituents.

In most western societies, especially in the United States, many voluntary associations, groups, organizations, and religious sects have developed, organized, and maintained a wide array of health care services and facilities (such as hospitals, clinics, sanitaria, medical and nursing schools, medical research organizations and units) to augment similar services and facilities provided by governmental and public agencies, such as federal hospitals (including the military hospitals), state, county and city hospitals, and clinics for curative services, not to mention public health agencies and programs aimed at prevention and control of disease in the community.

Hospitals and other kinds of health care facilities, for example, evolve and establish their own kinds of social organizations and systems of roles and statuses defining the various skills and functions that come to be regarded as needed to maintain their institution in the community and in the health care industry. Administrators become needed to recruit personnel, collect and pay the bills, prepare and supervise operating budgets, maintain the physical plant, arbitrate personnel conflicts, and manage the facility within the framework of the system of health care. In time, any deficiencies and weak spots inherent in the earlier evolutional phases of the various components of the total establishment may become problems in maintaining that system, both from internal and external sources involved in the total health industry of a society.

These problems may, in turn, accumulate to the stage where they become public issues. Arenas develop in which antagonists and protagonists form lines of disputation, debate, and controversy in attempts to resolve such conflicts and restore the system on their own terms or as a compromise between opposing forces.

Thus, social and behavioral scientists have studied total health care systems in different societies and specific aspects of the organization and management of health care systems and facilities. Their studies often lead them into areas of conflict between opposing vested interests, and they often venture into areas where the existing health care system fails to cope adequately with the health and medical needs of certain groups and segments of society. The results of such inquiries may often contribute toward implementing public policy for health care.

Organizing and Managing Health Care Services and Facilities

The health service systems of the United States and other nations are critically compared in the chapter by Odin Anderson, who has conducted first-hand many studies of health systems in various societies.

A major feature of the voluntary health care system in American society is the board of trustees responsible for operating hospitals and related facilities. The relationship of trustees to their community and to the health care system is analyzed in the article by Ray Elling and Ollie Lee.

A cogent description of the social organization of the general hospital for acute illness is presented in the article by Basil Georgopoulos and Floyd Mann.

The analysis of decision-making behavior by hospital boards of trustees and their organizational structure is presented in the chapter by Robert Holloway, Jay Artis and Walter Freeman.

The general hospital with its divergent categories of personnel may become a "house divided within itself" as administrative, medical, nursing, and paramedical, ancillary, and technical personnel evolve divergent ideologies and impair channels of communication related to patient care. Albert Wessen's original article depicting these elements of hospital ideology and communication between various types of personnel in the hospital ward is repeated from the first edition.

General hospitals are continually confronted with high rates of turnover of personnel. A study of this problem by Llewellyn Gross, Elliott Grosof and Constantine Yeracaris has culminated in a theory to account for such turnover in hospitals.

A significant conceptual framework in terms of an exchange system is presented by Sol Levine and Paul White to account for relationships prevailing among health and welfare agencies in the contemporary community.

Toward a Public Policy for Health Care: Some Current Issues

That the present health and medical care system in American society, perhaps also the western world, is in ferment and that many changes and innovations are forecast have been reported in many media of mass communication and in health, medical, scientific, and professional publications. There have been significant changes in the health and medical care systems of many European societies and Canada in the past few decades, and there has been the recent introduction of new health programs in American society. Medicare and Medicaid, federal and state governmental programs, prepaid group medical practice, health maintenance organizations, an increasing concern for better health care for the poor, and increasing alarm over rapidly rising financial costs for health services are symptomatic of growing public concern and dissatisfaction with many facets of the American health care system. Such concerns are stimulating efforts to develop a public policy for health care and to provide means whereby the role of government and lay consumers of medical services will likely expand considerably in the provision of health care services in the future.

The remaining articles of this volume represent only a few of the current health care issues emerging in contemporary American society. Such issues will very likely be an area of increasing interest and study by social scientists and an area toward which they can make sound contributions.

Speculation as to what physicians in the United States would do to oppose the initiation of the governmental Medicare program stimulated the interesting study by John Colombotos, which includes an analysis of the effects of legislation on attitudes related to health care.

A critical analysis of the failure of the American health system to provide adequate and appropriate medical care for the poor segments of American society is presented in the provocative article by Anselm Strauss.

The need to clarify such concepts and issues as "good" medical care, "quality" of care, "best" care, and to develop a philosophy of medicine and medical care are discussed in the concluding chapter by John Stoeckle and Irving Zola, another contribution to some current issues involving the development of public policy for health care in contemporary western and American society.

20

Health-Services Systems in the United States and Other Countries: Critical Comparisons

Odin W. Anderson

THE HEALTH SERVICES that have developed in Europe, Great Britain and the Commonwealth countries and the United States share basic similarities. They are products of advances in medical science that occurred from the late nineteenth century to World War I, when these countries were being transformed from agricultural to industrial economies. The discovery that bacteria caused a number of widespread diseases and the discovery and application of anesthesia in surgery provided the specific stimuli that led to the development of the modern hospital, the nursing profession and the hospital-based medical services. The medical profession was in existence in large numbers by the time the bacteriologic revolution swept through it. The infusion of new medical knowledge took a generation or more to accomplish, and the impact of the general hospital on medical practice was not fully felt until the turn of the century and later.

In Western countries the medical profession was engaged primarily in private practice on a fee-for-each-service basis. Physicians were individual entrepreneurs licensed by the government. General hospitals now emerged as indispensable places to provide certain types of medical services. At this time they were financed by tax funds in Europe, partly tax and partly private philanthropic funds in Great Britain and largely private philanthropic funds in the United States and Canada.

In Europe and Great Britain, the hospitals were built primarily for charity and low-income patients—even hospitals financed by philanthropic sources. In the United States and Canada, with a larger middle class, the hospitals built by philanthropic funds were immediately open to private-pay patients as well as charity patients. Physicians practicing in hospitals generally provided free care to charity patients in all countries, but in the United States and Canada, they were able to admit private patients, who paid for the hospital service directly, as well as the fees charged by physicians. In other countries there was a tendency for private hospitals to develop parallel to the tax-supported hospitals. These private hospitals were for the benefit of a small segment of the population who could pay for their own care. In all countries mentioned, then, the private practice of medicine was well established by the time the general hospitals became indispensable for modern medical care. The chief differences between the United States and Canada on this side of the Atlantic and the countries on the other side were the type of control, source of funds and pay status of patients admitted. The dentists and pharmacists were private practitioners like the physicians. Fundamentally, the structures of the personal health services were much the same.

In Europe and Great Britain the chief impact that the development of general hospitals made on the medical practitioners was the creation of a class of hospital-based specialists, who also had the option to treat private patients for a fee, and the exclusion of all other physicians from hospital practice. For the growing but small middle and upper classes private hospitals, usually called nursing homes or cottage hospitals, where hospital-based specialists could send their private patients, were established. Physicians without hospital appointments were assumed to refer patients to specialists in the hospitals when indicated. In the United States and Canada the hospitals had no less an impact

From New England Journal of Medicine, *Vol. 269: October 17 & 24, 1963; by permission of the author and publisher.*

on medical practitioners than in other countries. Physicians, instead of becoming a class of hospital-based specialists, sought hospital appointments to permit the admission of their patients while retaining their private offices outside the hospital.

The usual public-health programs that developed in the latter part of the nineteenth century and the early part of the twentieth were tax supported, such as sanitary environmental control, control of epidemic and communicable diseases and well-baby and maternity care.

The curative health services—that is, health services for individuals—evolved with various degrees of support and control from public funds during the latter quarter of the nineteenth century. The North American continent had primarily a privately supported health-services establishment, with tax-supported hospitals for the indigent. In Europe the hospitals were wholly tax supported; in Great Britain they were supported by both private and public funds.

In all countries the hospital and the clinics attached for outpatient services became the main site for the care of the low-income patients and the indigent. Physicians normally provided their services free because the hospital was the only place where the latest medical technics and knowledge were being introduced systematically; it was a place where such technics and knowledge could be applied to relatively large numbers of patients.

The valuable experience gained in hospitals by hospital-based specialists enhanced their ability to attract patients from the growing middle classes. Finally, the provision of free care by the medical profession was a natural continuation of the traditional expectation of the profession as providing a service "clothed with the public interest."

For physicians with hospital connections it was a usual way of discharging their social responsibility at the same time that they had the privilege of earning a living as private entrepreneurs from the steadily growing middle class. Private practice without middle-class patients is inconceivable. The values of free choice of physician and confidentiality of the physician–patient relationship took on increasing importance as the middle-classes began to use health services. These are middle class values associated with basic human rights as well as a highly regarded condition of good medical practice.

In all countries free choice and confidentiality were accepted as integral values in the health-services establishment for private patients. Countries shared this development in various degrees, depending on the relative size of the population that could afford private-practice medicine either in or out of the hospital. For the indigent the government was able to enlist the services of physicians at little or no cost to the public treasury. The very grouping of indigent patients in the large charity hospitals permitted rather large-scale empirical medical experimentation, which accelerated the development of the medical sciences. Hospital-based physicians were able to use knowledge thus gained in their private practices, an interesting example of the intertwining of the public and private sectors.

It should be evident from the foregoing that the health services did not develop according to any preconceived plan. The resources and social values existing at the time the modern basis for health services was laid seem to have been drawn on quite ingeniously. The latter nineteenth century was a period of fundamental social, political and economic changes, stimulated by industrialization and urbanization. There were then too many imponderables for intelligent planning. An important by-product was the changing role of women, which enabled the rapidly growing hospitals to expand and improve their nursing forces. The nurses' training schools in hospitals became a place where families could send their daughters at no cost to them. The girls were supervised, fed, sheltered and trained for a skill useful in both the hospital and marriage.

Not until the health-services establishment was already taking the essential form that it has today in all Western countries, the facilities constructed, particularly in cities, and the increasing effectiveness of medical care demonstrated, was there much public concern for making these services available to large segments of the population through health insurance. The poverty-class orientation of the health services was pervasive, and it is only within living memory that public policy began to include the middle and upper-middle classes as well.

It was assumed that those who were not poor could afford to buy hospital and physicians' services in the open market without health insurance. In time it was realized that not even the middle classes could be reasonably expected to pay for all services, because medical-care episodes were becoming increasingly more costly as the hospital and surgery grew in medical importance. The early governmental programs in Germany (1883) and Great Britain (1911), for example, were for the working class, and in Great Britain for the wage earner only. Since the general hospitals of these times were designed for low-income patients, who comprised a relatively large proportion of the population, these early health-insurance plans were then limited to out-of-hospital physicians' services. Physicians' services in the hospital were given free, as I have already mentioned.

The early pattern of development of paying for services was some form of government-sponsored health insurance for the lower-income sectors of the population. For the skilled workman, the white-collar worker and other middle-class groups governmental provisions were supplemented or paralleled by a proliferation of benefit associations, mutual-aid societies, provident associations and similar agencies. Eventually, government-sponsored health insurance was expanded to cover large segments of the population above the low-income group. Many existing private health-insurance associations became the administrative organizations for governmental payment for hospital and physicians' services.

Exceptions to this usual development are found in the United States, and until recently, and then only in part, in Canada. The shift in many countries from privately sponsored health insurance to government-sponsored health insurance has been regarded as an inevitable historical process by both those who favor and those who oppose government-sponsored health insurance. Some regard privately sponsored health insurance as inherently inadequate, and

others as the beginning of the trend toward governmental intervention. In this country many believe that a vigorous voluntary health-insurance establishment would indeed assure the perpetuation of an essentially non-governmental health-services establishment.

It should be noted that health insurance in some form and with either non-governmental or governmental sponsorship, or more commonly both, has emerged in all industrialized countries. An orderly method for the public to pay for health services is associated with the economic risks inherent in an industrial society, and the costs of health services are recognized as a contingency—that is, a risk that can jeopardize family solvency.

In this connection two concepts of facilitating access to health services exist side by side and are frequently confused. In the first place, it should be observed that in Western countries the government is partly a provider of services and partly a buyer of services— important distinctions. Generally in other countries, through government-sponsored health insurance, governments provide hospital care, including in-hospital physicians' services. However, governments buy physicians' and other services outside the hospital by some kind of mutual agreement. In effect, even specialists on salaried hospital staffs are contracting agents, particularly the department heads, analogous to professors in universities, and enjoy a similar type of autonomy.

Secondly, as mentioned earlier, the governments in other countries, through some form of health insurance, became largely buyers of health services without changing the prevailing organization of the existing health-services system. There is a tendency to perpetuate the organization of services in existence when government-sponsored health insurance becomes the chief source of funds.

Range of Health-Services Systems

The literature on health services and health insurance in different countries gives the impression that all countries are different. There is a basic core of similarities in how services are organized, but a wide range of differences in the proportion of funds coming from private and public sources. In organization the chief difference between the North American Continent and other areas is the method of staffing general hospitals: in North America the physicians are not salaried members of the hospital staff, but have access to hospitals as private practitioners. Elsewhere, the usual pattern is salaried posts for specialists, and all other physicians are excluded from hospital practice.[1-5]

The health-services systems in various countries can be classified according to several criteria that give some indication of the public policies underlying them. They can be arranged according to the proportion of funds that comes from the government and from private sources. They can be arranged according to the extent to which insurance is provided by government-sponsored health insurance or by some kind of private plans. They can be arranged by the extent to which health insurance covers all types of health services, hospital, physician, drugs and medications, and others, and among services that are insured whether all or only part of the charges are paid by insurance. The countries can be arranged by the extent to which the entire population is covered by insurance. Finally, they can be arranged according to the extent to which

[1] Abel–Smith, B., *Paying for Health Services: A Study of the Costs and Sources of Finance in Six Countries*, Geneva: World Health Organization, WHO Public Health Papers no. 17, 1963.

[2] Follmann, J. F., *Medical Care and Health Insurance: A Study in Social Progress*, Homewood, Ill.: R. D. Irwin, 1963, chap. 2, 3.

[3] Francis, C. L., J. E. Sparks and J. E. Osborne, "Health Care Programmes: Financial Aspects in Seven Countries," *Canadian Tax J.*, 2:12–19, January–February, 1954.

[4] Moutin, J. W., and G. St. J. Perrot, "Health Insurance Programs and Plans of Western Europe: Summary of Observations," *Pub. Health Reports*, 62:369–399, 1947.

[5] Roemer, M. I., "General Hospitals in Europe," in J. K. Owen (ed.), *Modern Concepts of Hospital Administration*, Philadelphia: Saunders, 1962, pp. 17–37.

the government is a provider of services, actually controlling and using the facilities, or simply a buyer of services, contracting with the hospitals, physicians and so on.

It might be assumed that health services and health insurance in all countries are evolving in a certain direction—that is, past evolution will continue to its logical conclusion unless it is deflected, arrested or modified. In all countries certain adjustments and accommodations were made because of the amount of money available and allocated, the perceptions of the population, the desires of the providers of service and the prerogatives that they valued, the difficulties of covering certain groups of people, or of including certain types of services and so on.

It seems that past trends indicate the polar type or ultimate form that a health-services system and methods of paying for it would take if there were no countervailing forces. I do not imply that the ultimate form is good or bad, but simply the result of forces pushing it in a certain direction. The chief characteristics would be as follows: all health services would be completely tax-supported according to a graduated income tax so that the higher-income families would pay more than the lower-income families; all health services would be provided at no direct charge to anyone; all facilities would be owned by the government; all health personnel would be salaried; and all curative and preventive services, including immunization, periodic physician examinations and so on, would be available.

The other polar type is completely supported by private funds in the open market. Although a purely private health-services system has in fact never existed, it may be useful to conceptualize the opposite of a polar-type governmental system. All the facilities, services and personnel are established on a profit basis for those who wish to invest in them. There are no gifts or subsidies. Service is "sold" only to those who can and wish to pay for it at the going rates. There is no free care. The government could conceivably purchase care for its wards on an open-bid system. The hospitals need not be open all night or on weekends unless they consider it of competitive advantage to have a stand-by service like an all-night filling station. Physicians can tailor their services to the market regardless of need or even type of disease that may be unprofitable to treat.

The first polar type exists almost in its pure form in the U.S.S.R. In the Western countries the National Health Service in Great Britain comes closest to this ultimate in development. The opposite polar type of system has not existed even approximately. Health services have always been "clothed with the public interest."

Among Western countries three might be selected to represent a range of types of health-service systems that have in substance the same health-services organization, but vary considerably in how these services are paid for and by what sources; they vary in the extent to which the government pays for services and facilities, and the extent to which health insurance pays for all types of personal health services. These countries are the United States, Sweden and Great Britain in order of increasing governmental support, degree of comprehensiveness of services paid by insurance and the extent to which the government controls the services or contracts for them from independent providers of service.

Briefly, the dominant characteristics of the health-services systems in the three countries are as follows:

THE UNITED STATES[6]

The dominant characteristics of the organization and financing of personal health services in the United States are general hospitals owned largely by nonprofit corporations sponsored by private citizens and sectarian groups. The physicians are predominantly in private practice, own their equipment and own or rent their offices. Dentists are in the same situation. Pharmacists are largely in their own retail stores, with a small proportion in hospitals.

For direct services 80 per cent of the cost is paid by the private sector and 20 per cent by all levels of the Government. Within the private sector most of the expenditures for general hospital care and less than half the

[6] "Government and Medicine in the United States," *Current History*, 45:1–114, August, 1963.

physicians' services are paid by voluntary health insurance. Other goods and services are not covered by insurance, with some exceptions.

Over 70 per cent of the population is covered by some type of insurance, and by a great variety of insurance agencies. To an increasing extent employers are contributing to the costs of health insurance. Consequently, there are now many sources of funds.

Government on various levels provides care for special groups such as veterans, the elderly and certain types of indigency, maternal and child health and special diseases, such as mental illness and tuberculosis.

The federal Government has assisted since 1946 in grants to the states for the construction, expansion and renovation of general hospitals, but not in payment for services, except for special purposes and groups as mentioned.

The health-services establishment is, then, relatively loosely organized, and policy decisions regarding expenditures and other matters are diffused.

SWEDEN[7]

Enrollment in government-sponsored health insurance is mandatory for the total population. The dominant characteristic of the health services in Sweden is government ownership of the general hospitals, but exclusively by the county and municipal governments. They are responsible for the total cost of building, maintaining and providing services, including specialists who are salaried members of the hospital staffs. The central Government pays the general hospitals a very nominal sum per diem for each patient from the health-insurance fund, and the counties are responsible for the rest.

General practitioners provide care outside

[7] Persson, K., *Social Welfare in Sweden: A Summary Account*, Stockholm: Föreningen för Främjande av Pensionsstyelsens Verksamhet, 1959.

the hospitals exclusively and make referrals to specialists on the hospital staffs. General practitioners do not have hospital appointments. Even so, patients can go directly to specialists without first being referred by general practitioners. General practitioners own or rent their offices and are paid a fee for each service, and the health-insurance fund refunds the patient approximately 75 per cent of the physicians' charges. The general practitioners do not negotiate a fee schedule with the Government, but are supposed to charge according to norms established in the professional associations.

Drugs are included in the health-insurance benefits, but the patient pays half the costs for prescriptions of more than 60 cents except for lifesaving drugs. Pharmacists in their own retail outlets contract with the Government for prescription drugs. With a few exceptions, dental care is not included.

The health-services system is financed from a variety of sources: payments from employers and employees; direct charges to patients; funds from county and municipal governments for general hospital care; and funds from the federal Government for mental and tuberculosis hospitals. It is reasonable to assume that approximately 65 per cent of the funds come from governmental sources.

GREAT BRITAIN[8]

The entire population has virtually free access to private health services by signing up with a general practitioner. About 95 per cent have done so. The main characteristics of the British National Health Service can be easily described, because the central Government owns and operates the entire hospital system. All services and goods are provided by the system, and almost the entire cost is paid from general tax funds collected by the central Government. Only a small portion is paid by payroll deductions.

[8] Lindsey, A., *Socialized Medicine in England and Wales: The National Health Service, 1948–1961*, Chapel Hill, N.C.: Univ. of North Carolina Press, 1962.

As in Sweden, the specialists are salaried members of the hospital medical staffs, but, unlike those in Sweden, their services may not be sought directly by patients within the health-insurance system. They must be referred by the general practitioners, who do not have hospital appointments. The general practitioners own or rent their own offices, but they are paid on a capitation basis arrived at by negotiations between the practitioner representatives and the Government. Dental care is provided at a small initial charge to patients, and dentists are paid a fee for each service, arrived at by negotiations with the Government. Prescription drugs are provided at a small charge for prescriptions, and pharmacists are paid according to a schedule arrived at by negotiation with the Government.

It is seen that, in contrast to the United States and Sweden, the British National Health Service is highly structured and almost entirely financed by the central Government. Hence, the costs of the services are in direct competition with other obligations of the Treasury. The size of the private sector is not known but is very probably small. There are estimates that 10 to 25 per cent of the population carry some limited type of private health insurance, mainly to supplement the National Health Service. It is reasonable, then, to assume that over 85 per cent of the funds come from governmental sources.

It is seen that the health-services system and methods of paying for services are "loosest" in the United States, and "tightest" in Great Britain, with Sweden occupying a position between the two countries. It can be said that the situation is more dynamic and in greater ferment in the United States than in Sweden and Great Britain, because the latter two countries already have a rather well-defined public policy regarding the proper sharing of governmental and private responsibilities and methods of organizing and providing services. It cannot be said that the United States has yet arrived at a definite policy in this regard because the issue of medical care for the aged regardless of income is still unresolved and a variety of existing methods of organizing and paying for services are vying for attention.

If there were agreed-on measures of efficiency and effectiveness of various health-service systems there would be little difficulty in deciding which one would provide the best service at the least cost to the most people and satisfy three important parties: the recipients of service; the providers of service; and those who must raise and allocate the money. Because hard-and-fast criteria are lacking, debates on public policy then become very opinionated. Differences of opinion are based on philosophic differences regarding the proper role of the government, nebulous concepts of adequate care, unmet need and many others.

It seems, however, that regardless of sponsorship there is confusion regarding the primary purpose of health insurance. Is this purpose to provide comprehensive health services for the population, or is it to spread the high magnitude of costs from individuals to groups? The one approach tends to "provide" services, and the other approach to "buy" services. Those who support the first approach believe that services should be provided with no direct charge to the patient, to encourage prevention and early diagnosis. But, more basic, this approach enables direct control over the providers of service in terms of cost, quantity and quality. Those who support the second approach believe that costs of large magnitudes, rather than the first dollar, are the ones that need to be covered. The proponents of this point of view do not, of course, deny the value of early diagnosis and prevention, but believe that a risk approach does not preclude adequate use of services. And, indeed, it is believed that some charges for services will encourage wiser use of services and help to contain costs. The controls over the providers of service are minimal.

Although there are variations between countries in methods of organizing and paying for health services, it is very doubtful if differences in various health indexes can be attributed to the type of health service prevailing. The usual indexes of infant mortality, the age-specific mortality, leading causes of death and so on are much too similar among Western countries. Various

mortality rates are a product of so many factors, health services among them, and they are such crude measurements anyway, that I take no stock in comparing mortality rates between the United States, Sweden and Great Britain and attributing the differences to the different health-service systems described.

The most easily demonstrable criterion for comparing countries is the extent to which the costs of services incurred by families is spread. Since expenditures vary, the extent to which a method of payment spreads cost can then be easily demonstrated. With this criterion, Great Britain easily leads both Sweden and the United Sates, although other objectives may have higher priority in the British system.

If one wishes to use the criterion of public satisfaction, the British public has shown a very high degree of satisfaction. This is also true in general for the American public, but there is dissatisfaction with the present level of health-insurance benefits. The Swedish population has not been polled. The level of satisfaction of the providers of service can also be used as a criterion, particularly the physicians. Here, the evidence is fragmentary and inconclusive, because no systematic studies have been done in any country. Chronic problems in all countries, however, appear to be method and amount of payment to physicians rather than direct interference with medical practice itself.

Another criterion is the volume of use of services. Although there are no standards for a proper level of services there is a consensus that the increase in use during the last thirty years is a good thing. The general level of use in all countries, however, is causing concern because of fear of "overuse" precipitated by increasing costs. There are interesting and currently unexplainable variations in levels of use between countries and areas. The three countries, the United States, Sweden and Great Britain, are illustrative. In the United States people are admitted to hospitals at the rate of 130 per 1000 population per year, stay an average of eight days and see physicians approximately five times a year. In Sweden patients are admitted to hospitals at the same rate, 130 per 1000, stay an average of fifteen days and see a physician three times a year. In Great Britain the respective figures are rate of 88 per 1000, fifteen days and five times a year, the latter rate being the same as that in the United States.[9-12]

The different methods of providing and paying for services in the three countries do not explain these gross differences. In the United States, where physicians' calls are rarely free, people see physicians as often as they do in Great Britain, where they are free, and a third more often than in Sweden, where they are almost free.[13]

Some believe that illness rates and patterns vary sufficiently among the three countries to account for the variations in rates of use of services. I do not believe this to be tenable because the patterns of causes of death are similar for the three countries, and morbidity surveys in the United States and Great Britain do not reveal differences gross enough to account for the variations in use of services (Sweden has not had a morbidity survey of the general population). I am, then, left with the assumption that variations in use are to be accounted for by a combination of social custom in the use of the health services by the general population, the practice habits of physicians and the organizational patterns channeling patients in and out of the health-services system. In other words, it is not known why these variations exist.

[9] Health Information Foundation, *The Changing Pattern of Hospital Use*, New York: The Foundation, 1958.

[10] Health Information Foundation, *The Increased Use of Medical Care*, New York: The Foundation, 1958.

[11] Great Britain, Ministry of Health and General Register Office, *Report on Hospital In-patient Enquiry for Two Years, 1956–1957*, London: Her Majesty's Stationery Office, 1961.

[12] Great Britain, General Register Office, W. P. D. Logan and A. A. Cushion, *Morbidity Statistics from General Practice*, London: Her Majesty's Stationery Office, Studies on Medical and Populational Subjects no. 14, 1958.

[13] Sverige, *Inrikesdepartmentet: Statens Offentliga Utredningar 1963. 21. Sjukhus och Öppen Vard*, Stockholm, 1963.

Another criterion is the cost to the economy for value received. Although it seems that public policy should be related to what health services are worth in productivity, health and happiness, it is not possible to measure worth but only cost. So one is left with the subjective criterion of how great a cost, in relation to other goods and services, an economy will bear. It appears that the United States spends relatively more for health services per capita and per cent of gross national product than either Sweden or Great Britain. Sweden spends more than Great Britain. At best, however, international cost comparisons are extremely slippery, and the foregoing observations are made with the utmost caution.

A final criterion, although there may be others, is the quality of the services. This is the most nebulous criterion of all, particularly among Western countries with very similar scientific and medical traditions. Presumably, the range from excellent to bad practice exists in all countries, but one does not know how to determine the distribution within this range. Adequate methods of measuring quality are still in a primitive stage of development.

Composites of Possibilities

In the polar types of health-services systems and their variations described in the first section of this article it is a truism that each type has inherent advantages and disadvantages depending on the balance of objectives. One of the banes of the health field is that objectives are stated in Utopian terms rather than in terms of long-range possibilities. Because of the inability to test the effectiveness of health services and to set up scientifically verifiable criteria for determining who should receive what, in what volume, and at what level of quality, it is difficult to ascertain how much a health-service system should cost and to see if such cost can be borne by the economy. Cost, then, is related to the ability and willingness of the economy—whether the public treasury, voluntary health insurance or direct payments by patients—to pay for a certain level of services rather than related to "need," "effectiveness" or similar nebulous criteria.

Accordingly, an "open" system like the one in the United States, with its many sources of funds for health services and high proportion of discretionary income, is more likely to be generous in financing than a country like Great Britain, where the source of funds is centralized and there is a lower average of discretionary income. Likewise, Sweden, with a variety of funds and a high standard of living, is spending more than Great Britain and apparently less than the United States. This is not to say that a governmental system cannot be generous, but it seems that several sources—different levels of government, charges to patients, payroll deductions from employees and employer contributions—provide higher net expenditures than a single source. The private sector, a quasi-market mechanism, seems to provide the economic leeway necessary for continuing and rapid change. Furthermore, a single source of finance applied to the entire health-services system would tend to perpetuate the organization of that system as it was at the time when the payment method went into effect. Experimentation is inhibited, because changes in the system are difficult to accomplish.

In the United States, undoubtedly in part because sources of finance have not been centralized, a range of different methods of organizing and paying for services has developed, from solo practice to group practice, and limited health-insurance benefits to comprehensive benefits. Some of the arrangements are as comprehensive as those in Great Britain. The prevailing arrangement is an attempt to accommodate to the existing structure of practice. At the same time, some attempts are being made to reorganize the structure fundamentally. All of them represent varying balances between the patient, the providers of service and the paying agencies. No one system has proved universally acceptable.

Both Sweden and Great Britain have solved the problem of covering all the people, an inherent advantage in governmental systems. Great Britain has "provided" hospital basic services and guaranteed payments for virtually all other health goods and services. Sweden has "provided" hospital basic services and a selection of other services but not dental care.

A "loose" system is inherently untidy,—that is, some people are left out, and some services are inadequately covered—but there is room to maneuver in a service where new technology is being improved constantly and cost patterns are changing. It is more difficult to keep the lid on, as it were, because there is no central control on sources of funds, the lifeblood of a good health-services system.

Countries vary in their histories and the levels of their economies. In the United States private capital, mainly philanthropy, built the hospitals, resulting in a strong hospital association. The medical profession had time to become a cohesive body, to become the vehicle of modern medicine and, therefore, to gain great bargaining power, before government-sponsored health insurance became an issue. Furthermore, the medical market provided a large enough mass of buyers to sustain the essentially non-governmental character of the health services in the United States and the private control of methods of payment. None of these conditions have been present in other countries to the same degree.

In the United States public policy has developed on a broad base of consensus that is relatively conservative about the place of government. Other countries have developed public policy as a struggle between private ownership and control and public ownership and control, or between rival political ideologies of left and right. Eventually, a consensus has emerged accepting a degree of public ownership and control that is not seriously considered politically viable in this country. Each country works with what it has in the crucible of possibilities, aspirations and accommodations.

Mutual Lessons

It seems that all countries can learn from each other, but it is difficult to select one element in a health-service system from one country and introduce it into a system in another unless the traditions and experiences in each country are taken into account. However, several experiences stand out.

In this review of various systems it is seen that it is possible to pay for any and all goods and services on some sort of insurance basis, given certain controls. Differences in charges, financial controls and other "barrier" payments to services emerge, but the "catastrophic" nature of health services can be mitigated. The concept of "uninsurability" is not tenable.

It is not possible in a non-governmental system to have universal health insurance coverage although it can be approximated. Consequently, some means must be devised to help those who are not in the system. In itself, compulsory enrollment is a far less consequential problem than the usual concomitant of governmental control over funds. The one is basically a philosophic issue; the latter is an administrative issue. My framework of thinking is the primary practical one of determining what is necessary to maintain an adjustable and dynamic health-services system responsive to patients, providers of service and financing agencies. In Great Britain, for example, the patients are asked to assume extremely little responsibility. The providers of service are made part of a total system without much control over methods and amounts of payment. And the central Government has the stupendous task of raising and allocating virtually the total budget.

In Sweden the patients are asked to assume a fair amount of responsibility for some services, but nothing for hospital-based services. As for providers of services, the hospitals are owned and maintained by the counties and municipalities; general practitioners so far do not even negotiate fees, and the Government pays a certain proportion up to a maximum. Finally, the central Government is not responsible for the total cost of the health services, but it shares it with the counties and municipalities, employers and employees.

In the United States, with primarily a privately supported system, the providers of service have been very free to organize services as they deemed best, patients and insurance are paying the going "costs," with little examination of those costs until recently —countervailing forces of large private buyers and Government are now emerging. Furthermore, health-insurance benefits are inadequate but improving gradually. The Government is playing the classic part of catalyst, subsidizing fringe areas such as the indigent, assisting in capital financing of hospitals and now moving into assisting medical education, but staying out of payments for day-to-day services [except for the aged].

Europeans are aghast at the cost occasionally incurred by families in an incomplete health-insurance system, but they are similarly intrigued by some of the methods of organizing services. Group practice is supposed to be an American invention, but its creation required capital and a concept that has not existed to the same degree in other countries.

One can learn that the problem of the aged is not peculiar to the United States. In Sweden and Great Britain the financing of care for the aged has been solved in principle because they are included in the total system, but not necessarily in practice. It has not been solved in practice because the health-services system in all countries is still largely one designed for acute short-term-illness episodes.

One can learn that in different systems the medical profession retains the right to treat patients as it sees fit within the established system. The medical profession and medicine appear to have enough prestige so that there is little lay and governmental interference with how physicians diagnose and treat patients. Within a governmental system professional advice has determined the physician-patient relation. In fact, there is little talk of quality controls, tissue committees, pathological reports and so on that are becoming common here in an essentially non-governmental system. In the governmental systems, however, I have the impression of chronic complaining regarding methods and amounts of payment and working conditions that are regarded as not intrinsic to professional freedom.

In this country, on the other hand, the profession appears to believe that professional freedom also includes the physicians' prerogative to determine the source, amount and method of payment, as well as the freedom to choose methods of diagnosing and treating patients. One is then left with the intriguing impression that the medical profession in this country is coming under greater scrutiny regarding methods and quality of care than its colleagues in other countries, although in a largely non-governmental system.

It seems that, in large part, the fee-for-service method of paying physicians is workable. The tenacity of this method of payment is, indeed, awesome and forces me to conclude that it is an inherent aspect of a professional service in the majority of situations. In Western countries it is the prevailing method of paying physicians outside hospitals.

Finally, it seems that there is no way to determine how much an adequate health service should cost because of lack of solid criteria. Consequently, sources of funds need to be diffused so that no single group has final power of determination. In each country careful attention must be paid to the proper balance between the recipients of services, the providers of service and those who raise and allocate the funds. There is no blueprint for this balance, but it does seem that in the United States the present diversity in responsibilities and sources of funds permits latitude in methods of organization and provision of services, with no dominant and small group of decision makers. In the United States, when voluntary health insurance begins to pay for 80 per cent of costs of all services to families above a certain magnitude, when a public-assistance program takes care of the major medical needs of the 20 per cent of the population in the lower-income group and when the Government continues to assist in capital expenditures for facilities and costs of education, and continues its responsibilities for special problems and groups, a balance not possible in the same way in other countries

will be attained. However, as the standard of living rises in other countries, the private sector will grow to the limits that each country finds congenial. Countries can learn from each other; none has a monopoly on what is a good health-services system. But to learn from each other, they must do more than pore over official reports, make quick junkets abroad and listen to "authorities." Research technics that can probe into use and expenditure patterns on the part of the general population are now available; methods to analyze the operation of organizations beyond the organizational charts are being devised; one is beginning to probe problems of how a professional service like medical care can best be provided so that the physician has the necessary freedom, and the patient has maximum access to services within the tolerances of cost, quality and quantity.

Bibliography

Eckstein, H., *The English Health Service: Its Origins, Structure, and Achievements*, Cambridge, Mass.: Harvard Univ. Press, 1958.

Evang, K., *Health Service, Society, and Medicine: Present Day Health Services in Their Relation to Medical Science and Social Structure*, London: Oxford Univ. Press, 1960.

Great Britain, Medical Services Review Committee, *A Review of the Medical Services of Great Britain* (Porritt Report), London: Social Assay, 1963.

International Labour Office, *The Cost of Medical Care*, Geneva: The Office, no. 51, New Series, 1959.

Jewkes, J., and S. Jewkes, *The Genesis of the British Health Service*, Oxford: Blackwell, 1961.

Page, E., *What Price Medical Care? A Preventive Prescription for Private Medicine*, Philadelphia: Lippincott, 1960.

U.S. Social Security Administration, Div. of Program Research, *Social Security Programs Throughout the World, 1961*, Washington, D.C.: U.S. Government Printing Office, 1961.

21

Formal Connections of Community Leadership to the Health System

*Ray H. Elling
and
Ollie J. Lee*

A CRUCIAL PROBLEM facing voluntary community organizations and the planners who wish to provide more adequate health services is the extent to which the community leaders become involved in that particular area of community life and the forms this involvement takes. Any organization which assumes the responsibility of planning and coordinating the activities of others presumably requires sufficient power resources to accomplish the task. The community health system provides an excellent setting for the exploration of this problem and the influence of community leaders on it. This is because a public awareness of the need for planning and coordination in this area. is growing and, consequently, top local leaders are becoming more involved.[1] This paper is based on an exploratory study of some forms of leadership involvement in health planning bodies and other organizations of the health system in a metropolitan community.

The relationship between community influentials and voluntary and official health and welfare associations, and the decisions affecting these associations, have been the object of a wide range of studies. Some of the studies have explored the importance of financial support resulting from connections between organizations and outstanding individuals who occupy positions of community leadership.[2] Organizations providing health and welfare services which require large amounts of support other than client fees must maintain relationships with key influentials. This ensures the availability of volunteers and clientele.

This paper will identify the top leaders of a metropolitan community in terms of their social characteristics, and will report on their membership on the governing and advisory boards of health planning and service organizations.

Some aspects discussed here include:

1. What are the social characteristics of top community influentials as located in this study?
2. What types of leaders have the most connections to the health system as a whole?[3]

---

[1] An expression of the need for planning and coordination is found in a policy statement by the American Public Health Association adopted in 1950. See "Local Health Department—Services and Responsibilities," *Amer. J. Pub. Health*, 41:302–307, March, 1951. For a businessman's viewpoint, see C. Hood, "Industry's Stake in Regional Hospital Planning," *Trustee*, 15:18–22, January, 1962. For a discussion of various community planning efforts in the hospital field, see

H. Sibley, "Patient Care Planning as Experienced by Hospital Councils," *Amer. J. Public Health*, 52:1918–1924, November, 1962.

[2] A few examples include: L. V. Blankenship, and R. H. Elling, "Organizational Support and Community Power Structure: The Hospital," *J. Health and Human Behavior*, 3:257–269, Winter, 1962; R. H. Elling, "The Hospital-Support Game in Urban Center," in E. Freidson (ed.), *The Hospital in Modern Society*, New York: Free Press, 1963; R. G. Holloway, J. W. Artis, and W. E. Freeman, "The Participation Patterns of Economic Influentials and Their Control of a Hospital Board of Trustees," *J. Health and Human Behavior*, 4:88–99, Summer, 1963; I. Belknap, and J. G. Steinle, *The Community and its Hospitals: A Comparative Analysis*, Syracuse: Syracuse Univ. Press, 1963.

[3] The reader may wonder how the complex, usually fractionated set of health agencies in communities can be conceived of as a system. By system is meant a set of units having an impact

---

From *Milbank Memorial Fund Quarterly, Vol. 44: 294–306, July, 1966; by permission of the authors and publisher.*

3. What types of leaders have board connections with various kinds of health agencies?

**Formal Connections 287
of Community Leadership
to the Health System**

Community leaders are defined as individuals chosen by informed citizens as being the most influential persons in the community. Such perception of power on the part of local citizens does not measure power directly, but does reflect the social reality of the past exercise of power, particularly in a relatively stable social situation. As used here, the term power refers to a person's potential for realizing his will in interactions with others.[4] This potential has various bases, such as wealth, symbolic manipulation, expertise, political popularity, and status in formal organizations, but it is always an aspect of a social system.[5] Social systems possess two kinds of structures: structures of action involving the use of means to attain ends or goals, and structures of power or potential means based on resources.

One of the key elements in power structures is the manner in which others assess this potential and react to it. The evaluation of an individual's potential by others will bring him many of the perquisites of power, e.g., deference, compliance and strategic roles in organizations, where decisions are made and implemented and where resources are utilized. Top community leaders occupy key positions in the community power structure.

Given the above considerations, the theoretical propositions on which this research hypothesis is based may be outlined:

1. The functions of a "power structure," whatever form it may take, are to channel resources and influence decisions. Resources may include financial support, technical knowledge, etc.

2. Organizations in a community seek to preserve themselves and to gain autonomy, support and control.[6]

3. Organizations will better establish themselves by developing connections with community leaders. Although a number of types of connections may be seen, the principal form is membership on a governing or advisory board.

4. Through association with a given organization, leaders are likely to identify with it and to support it in preference to others. Such identification may lead to orientations and interests which are not based on rational assessments of needs, merit or resource supply. This causes problems for the over-all planning function where the community and not the organization is the unit.

5. Some organizations will be more successful than others in recruiting top community leaders. A number of factors affect the manner in which community influentials become involved. Community and family traditions, organizational prestige, the extent to which various organizations' services are considered essential and other background factors are undoubtedly very important. Certain key families may develop traditions of *noblesse oblige* toward certain kinds of institutions. An institution with great prestige, because of its past attraction for leaders, may become the place for a new business executive to "fulfill his community obligations." This leads to a circular chain of influence, because success breeds success, and to distinguish cause from effect may prove difficult.

Two important factors, however, are based on more objective data. They are the leaders'

(for good or ill) on some common purpose. In this case the common purpose is the prevention and alleviation of disability in a geographically bounded population. All health agencies in a community may be assumed to have some actual or potential effect on this matter of common concern.

[4] Weber, M., *The Theory of Social and Economic Organization*, New York: Oxford Univ. Press, 1947, p. 152.

[5] Bierstedt, R., "An Analysis of Social Power," *Amer. Sociol. Rev.*, 15:730–738, December, 1950.

[6] Various organizational imperatives are outlined by P. Selznick, "Foundations of the Theory of Organization," in A. Etzioni (ed.), *Complex Organizations: A Sociological Reader*, New York: Holt, Rinehart & Winston, 1962, p. 26.

position in the power structure and the different functions of the organizations in the health system.

The specific research hypothesis is that community leaders tend to associate with health organizations according to the leaders' position in the community and according to the major functions of the health organizations.

The identified leaders may be divided into three occupational types. Business executives and men of wealth are called *economic dominants*; elected labor officials, politicians, and government officials (all of whom depend for their position on some kind of popular support) are grouped together as *elective leaders*; professionals and executives of community organizations (religious, civic, educational, law, etc.) are called *knowledge specialists*.

Five categories of health organizations, based on their major functions, include: (1) Voluntary organizations which assume planning, funding, or coordinating functions for the health system (e.g., United Fund). (2) Governmental agencies (e.g., the county health department). (3) General hospitals. (4) All other voluntary agencies whose primary functions are within the health field (e.g., the American Cancer Society). (5) Those organizations which provide health-related services, but which are not primarily health oriented (e.g., some private philanthropic foundations). Occupational groups, such as the American Medical Association, are not included.

Certain findings may be predicted, based on the hypothesis above. Economic dominants are more likely to be connected with those health organizations which require large amounts of financial resources and which involve making major decisions regarding such resources. Organizations of this description include hospitals and voluntary coordinating bodies. Since most health agencies are voluntary and require financial contributions, and since the role of top businessmen involves skill and responsibility for major economic allocation, economic dominants will, in general, have more connections with health agencies than will other leaders.

The Study

Pittsburgh was chosen as the setting for this research because of its easy access. Also certain local developments in the health field over the past ten years presented especially interesting examples of a community power system in the coordination and planning of health facilities. Pittsburgh is an old industrial center with a city population of approximately 600,000 and a surrounding population of another one million in Allegheny County. Defining the concept of community and drawing specific community boundaries for a large urban area presents a number of theoretical problems.[7] Therefore, the county was used as the geographical unit.[8]

Research involved several procedures. Exploratory discussions with various health professionals and executives of health planning agencies were conducted to develop an overall picture of the system of health organizations and to identify significant community decisions and developments in health planning. Mailed questionnaires, hospital association files, personal interviews, published sources and state records were used to compile membership lists of health organization boards.

One of the major tasks was to identify community leaders or top influentials. The general controversy over the various procedures for identifying community leadership or power structures is presumably quite well known.[9] A variation of the reputational

7 Warren, R. L., "Toward a Reformulation of Community Theory," *Human Organization*, 15:8–11, Summer, 1956; I. T. Sanders, "Public Health in the Community, in H. E. Freeman, *et al.* (eds.), *Handbook of Medical Sociology*, Englewood Cliffs, N.J.: Prentice-Hall, 1963.

8 Most health services and organizations in Pittsburgh are organized on a county-wide basis. Sanders points out that treating the community as a place is an important consideration where health services are concerned, for epidemiological, organizational and environmental reasons. Sanders, *op. cit.*, pp. 370–371.

9 For discussion, see R. A. Dahl, "A Critique of the Ruling Elite Model," *Amer. Pol. Sci. Rev.*, 52:463–468, June, 1958; R. Wolfinger, "Reputation and Reality in the Study of Community Power," *Amer. Sociol. Rev.*, 25:636–644, October, 1960; L. J. Herson, "In the Footsteps of Community Power," *Amer. Pol. Sci. Rev.*, 55:817–

technique was used not only because of its relative economy, but also because of the results which have been obtained by the use of this method in other communities.[10]

A panel was formed of 23 informants who were generally knowledgeable about the community. The following criteria guided their selection: (1) the panel should represent all major institutional areas of the community; (2) each informant should occupy or have occupied a position which would provide him with an extensive knowledge about one institutional sector of the community; (3) the panel should exhibit some distribution of relevant personal social characteristics such as sex, age, race, religious affiliation, area of residence in the community, etc.

These knowledgeable citizens were asked to name the top 20 influentials in the county. Some named many more than 20, some named less. Using a cut-off point of four mentions as the basis for inclusion gave a total of 47 community leaders in the study population.

Once community influentials were identified, semi-structured interviews were conducted to gather information concerning their awareness of the system of community health facilities, their evaluation of the existing system, their orientations toward general trends and specific changes in the future, and their participation in and knowledge about certain specific recent decisions relating to the problems of coordination and planning. Subjects were asked to list all of their connections with health organizations of all types in the community. Information on both formal and informal connections was solicited. In

addition to interview data, information was obtained from secondary sources such as the standard biographical references and directories.

Results

SOCIAL CHARACTERISTICS OF COMMUNITY LEADERS

Some of the personal and social attributes of top community leaders in Pittsburgh are presented in Table 21–1. These findings are similar to those of other studies. D. C. Miller,[11] W. V. D'Antonio[12] and others have found, in various American and Mexican cities, that businessmen predominate among community influentials. Robert Presthus, on the basis of a comparative study in two small New York communities, hypothesized that "in communities with limited leadership and economic resources the power structure will be more likely to be dominated by political leaders, whereas in those with more fulsome internal resources it will probably be dominated by economic leaders."[13] Linton C. Freeman and associates outline 15 characteristics which set apart top influentials from others in the population.[14] Data were gathered on seven of these characteristics—age, sex, politics, religion, education, birthplace and occupational position. Sex and race are not included in Table 21–1 because these leaders were all white males.

These influentials are predominantly businessmen, Republicans and Protestants. Almost half were born in the local area, and half currently reside in the city.

830, December, 1961; W. V. D'Antonio and E. C. Erickson, "The Reputational Techniques As a Measure of Community Power," *Amer. Sociol. Rev.*, 27:363–376, June, 1962; L. C. Freeman, *et al.*, *Local Community Leadership*, Syracuse: Syracuse Univ. Press, 1960.

[10] Blankenship, L. V., "Community Power and Decision-Making: A Comparative Evaluation of Measurement Techniques," *Social Forces*, 43:207–216, December, 1964; D. Booth and C. Adrian, "Simplifying the Discovery of Elites," *Amer. Behavioral Scientist*, vol. 4, October, 1961. Booth and Adrian defend the reputational technique as both economically practical and theoretically sound.

[11] Miller, D. C., "Industry and Community Power Structure," *Amer. Sociol. Rev.*, 23:9–15, February, 1958.

[12] D'Antonio, W. V., *et al.*, "Institutional and Occupational Representations in Eleven Community Influence Systems," *Amer. Sociol. Rev.*, 26:440–446, June, 1961.

[13] Presthus, R., *Men at the Top: A Study in Community Power*, New York: Oxford Univ. Press, 1964, pp. 410–411.

[14] Freeman, *op. cit.*, p. 16.

The only surprising characteristic is the age distribution. Three out of five are over 60 years old (based on 1964 data). Freeman, *et al.*, found in Syracuse that influentials came mainly from the 35–60 category.[15] Examination of previous studies and other descriptions of Pittsburgh[16] reveals that for the past 20 years the same group of top businessmen, (spearheaded by the Mellon interests and organized into a formal voluntary power mechanism called the Allegheny Conference on Community Development) has been influential in major community redevelopment. At the time many of these men came to the forefront

among them seem to have produced an aging group of top influentials.

PATTERNS OF BOARD CONNECTIONS

Data on board memberships of community leaders in the health field are summarized in Tables 21–2 and 21–3. Although the number of cases is too small to employ statistical techniques such as tests of significance, an inspection of these tables reveals differences which seem to support the hypothesis.

In the first place, community leaders as a group do prefer certain types of health organizations. Out of the total of approximately 130 health organizations in the

Table 21–1—Social characteristics of top influentials in Pittsburgh

Occupation	Age	Birthplace	Religion	Political Affiliation	Area of Residence
Businessmen 65%	45–49 4%	Allegheny County 45%	Episcopalian 21%	Republican 76%	Pittsburgh 50%
Government Officials 6%	50–59 36%	Other Pennsylvania 11%	Presbyterian 29%	Democratic 11%	Other Allegheny County 34%
Labor Leaders 4%	60–65 30%	Other United States 38%	Other Protestant 13%	Independent 2%	Outside County 11%
Professionals and Community Organisation Executives 23%	66–75 23%	Foreign 2%	Catholic 19%	No Information 11%	No Information 4%
	Over 75 6%	No Information 4%	Jewish 6% No Information 11%		

Total Number = 47.
Columns may not add to exactly 100% because of rounding of figures.

during and after World War II, they were two decades younger. The effectiveness of this group in the "Pittsburgh Renaissance" and the relationships which developed

15 *Ibid.*
16 Some of the relevant works include: "Pittsburgh's New Powers," *Fortune*, 35:77, February, 1947; S. Lorant, *Pittsburgh: The Story of an American City*, Garden City, N.Y.: Doubleday, 1964; E. F. Cooke, "Research: An Instrument of Political Power," *Pol. Sci. Quart.*, 76:69–87, March, 1961; A. J. Auerbach, "Power and Philanthropy in Pittsburgh, *Trans-Action*, October, 1965.

community, only 46 had at least one of these top influentials on their boards during the period defined as "current" (1962–1964). The classification of these 46 organizations by function yields this breakdown: voluntary coordinating (7); governmental coordinating (1); hospitals (15); other voluntary agencies (11); and peripheral (12).

As shown in Table 21–2, 77 per cent of all leaders are connected with voluntary coordinating bodies, and the same proportion are on hospital boards. Much smaller proportions are involved in other kinds of health agencies. Table 21-3 shows that leaders are more often associated with voluntary coordinating boards than with other kinds of organizations.

A comparison among types of leaders confirms that economic dominants are much more heavily concentrated on the boards of voluntary coordinating agencies and hospitals than on other types. Ninety per cent of these 31 businessmen are on at least one of the major decision-making boards in the health system concerned with raising resources and allocating them to various agencies. Also, economic dominants are concentrated on these coordinating bodies in about the same ratio as are others on hospital boards. (The fourth row in Tables 21-2 and 21-3 combines the two categories

of non-businessmen for easier comparison with the businessmen.)

The expectation that economic leaders would be connected with more health agencies in general than would the other types of leaders was not supported. The 31 businessmen had an average of 3.38 such board memberships while elective leaders had 3.40 and knowledge specialists 2.91.

As Table 21-2 shows, the county health department has very few formal connections with the top influentials (e.g., through its advisory boards). This suggests that the health department as now constituted has

Table 21-2—Community leaders on health boards, by type of leader and type of health organization

	N	HEALTH SYSTEM PLANNING, COORDINATING AND FUNDING ORGANIZATIONS Voluntary	Governmental	General Hospital	Other Voluntary Health Organizations	Organizations Providing Related Services (Includes Foundations)
		%	%	%	%	%
Economic Dominants	31	90	7	77	36	26
Elective Leaders (Labor and Political)	5	60	20	60	80	60
Knowledge Specialists (Professionals and Agency Executives)	11	46	9	82	64	27
Combination of Elective Leaders and Professionals	16	50	13	75	69	38
Total Set of Leaders	47	77	9	77	47	30

Table 21-3—Average number of health board memberships by leadership type

Type of Health Organization

Type of Leader	N	HEALTH SYSTEM PLANNING, COORDINATING AND FUNDING ORGANIZATIONS Voluntary	Governmental	General Hospitals	Other Voluntary Health Organizations	Peripheral Organizations	Average Number of Positions on All Health Boards
Economic Dominants	31	1.64	0.10	0.87	0.39	0.42	3.38
Elective Leaders (Labor and Political)	5	0.80	0.20	0.60	1.00	0.80	3.40
Knowledge Specialists (Professionals and Agency Executives)	11	0.63	0.09	0.63	1.09	0.45	2.91
Combination of Elective Leaders and Professionals	16	0.69	0.12	0.62	1.06	0.56	3.06
Average for All Leaders	47	1.29	0.10	0.78	0.62	0.46	3.27

nothing like the power budget necessary to pursue the goals of a recent policy statement by the American Public Health Association calling for health departments to coordinate all health services in the community.[17]

Discussion and Implications

The composition and functioning of the largely non-elected system of government may disturb those who would like to see a greater reality behind the theory of this democratic society. Someone no doubt must rule, but today top leadership is in no sense representative of the population, as Table 21–1 reveals.

This situation may not be bad if the leadership, for whatever reason (out of love for fellow community residents or as a matter of protecting and enhancing the value of local investments), has pursued a benevolent policy and sought to raise the level of living in the community.

This is a matter of personal judgment. Extensive benefits have apparently derived from the leadership's decision to focus on and rejuvenate the local community. Those who have not fared well in the process and those who have not yet had their turn at "the table"—for example, the deprived negro and other families in Pittsburgh's notorious "Hill District"—will perhaps judge otherwise.

The problem of democratic government would need no discussion in this paper provided no implications were made for the functioning of the health system. The analysis is not yet complete—the interviews must be completed and qualitative comments categorized and examined—but at this time the involvement of community leaders in segments of the health system is apparently not motivated primarily by understanding and pursuit of the most efficient and effective delivery of all health services to all elements of the population. Why?

First, planning is primarily oriented

[17] "Local Health Departments—Services and Responsibilities," *Amer. J. Pub. Health*, 41:302–307, March, 1951.

toward saving money and eliminating the bother of numerous appeals. One can sympathize with these concerns, but they lead to a concentration on the bricks-and-mortar plans of only a few prestige organizations. Other organizations which have, or should have, an important impact on the level of human functioning in the community are not taken much into account.

Organizations differentiate themselves by orienting their services to different elements of the population. Therefore, some important segments are, relatively speaking, ignored when the leaders attach themselves to a few predominant organizations.

Even more important than the capital expansion plans of a few preferred organizations is the problem of leaders who regard health services as hallowed "professional" ground. These people believe they can influence health services only by upgrading elements of the teaching center in the hope that the "experts" will influence practice in the community. This approach overlooks the separations between "town" and "gown." This division between capital investments and operations would never occur in the minds of these financial and industrial leaders as they consider the development of their own industrial complexes. Yet, in their decision-making in the health sphere they do compartmentalize. Why?

The answers cannot be readily determined. This question will be pursued with particular attention to the following factors: why community leaders become involved in one agency rather than another, experiences with and conceptions of the health system, the role of key professionals and other facets of the interview.

What has already been said has implications for the processes of planning and coordination, however inadequate and limited in conception such implications may be. Certain organizations probably develop boards powerful enough to sway the plans of the planning agency itself.

Can an improved mechanism be instituted which would more adequately stimulate the concern of community leaders for the personal and mass health services in the community? The matter is deserving of much more study and thought. Competition among planning organizations themselves could be eliminated by involving all in an organization which would develop a conscious division of labor among them. An organization with legal authority also seems necessary. Thus a public or quasi-public organization is in order. This too would help focus attention on adequate health services for all segments of the population and would bring the political component of the power structure directly into the policy-making, planning process. The university health center may have a key planning–coordinating role if it is willing to assume responsibility with others for the delivery of health services in an area. In any case an effective power system must be behind the organization. This means that community leaders and others must become involved in such an effort. This type of involvement, in spite of differences among leaders, is not new in Pittsburgh. If the enlightened concerns of some of these men for "more adequate coordination of all health services" become a matter of more general interest, Pittsburgh may serve in the future as a crucible of planning for total community health services.

22

The Hospital as an Organization

Basil S. Georgopoulos
and
Floyd C. Mann

THE COMMUNITY general hospital is an organization that mobilizes the skills and efforts of a number of widely divergent groups of professional, semi-professional, and nonprofessional personnel to provide a highly personalized service to individual patients. Like other large-scale organizations, it is established and designed to pursue certain objectives through collaborative activity. The chief objective of the hospital is, of course, to provide adequate care and treatment to its patients (within the limits of present-day technical–medical knowledge, and knowledge of organizing human activity effectively, as well as within limits that may be imposed by the relative scarcity of appropriate organizational resources or by extraorganizational forces). Its principal product is medical, surgical, and nursing service to the patient, and its central concern is the life and health of the patient. A hospital may, of course, have additional objectives, including its own maintenance and survival, organizational stability and growth, financial solvency, medical and nursing education and research, and various employee-related objectives. But, all these are subsidiary to the key objective of service to the patient, which constitutes the basic organizing principle that underlies all activities in the community general hospital.

There is little ambiguity, if any, about the main organizational objective of the community general hospital. Unlike many organizations, the hospital is able to make the role it performs in the larger community psychologically meaningful to its members. And most of its members try to give unstintingly of their energies to perform the tasks assigned to them. Many doctors and nurses look upon their profession as a sacred calling. Others find working in the hospital deeply satisfying of needs that they cannot easily express in words. They see the hospital as a nonprofit institution dedicated to works of mercy, and they sense that their mission in life is to give of themselves in order to help others. Immediate personal comfort and satisfactions, and even material rewards, are defined by most members as less important than giving good care to the patient and meeting a higher order of obligation to mankind. Serious conflicts regarding material rewards, such as those found in organizations where profit is the chief motive, are virtually nonexistent in the hospital. For all these reasons, motivating organizational members toward the objectives of the organization is much less of a problem for the hospital in comparison to other large-scale organizations. The goals of individual members and the objectives of the organization are considerably more congruent in the case of the hospital.

To do its work, the hospital relies upon an extensive division of labor among its members, upon a complex organizational structure which encompasses many different departments, staffs, offices, and positions, and upon an elaborate system of coordination of tasks, functions, and social interaction.

Work in the hospital is greatly differentiated and specialized, and of a highly interactional character. It is carried out by a large number of cooperating people whose backgrounds, education, training, skills, and functions are as diverse and heterogeneous as can be found in any of the most complex organizations in existence. And much of the work is not only specialized but also performed by highly trained professionals—the doctors—who require the collaboration, assistance, and services of many

From The Community General Hospital, *New York: Macmillan, 1962, pp. 5–15; by permission of the authors and publisher.*

other professional and nonprofessional personnel. In addition to the medical staff, which is highly specialized and departmentalized, there is the nursing staff, which includes graduate professional nurses in various supervisory and nonsupervisory positions, practical nurses, and untrained nurse's aids. In addition to the nursing staff and the medical staff, which are the two largest groups in the community general hospital, there are the hospital administrator and a number of administrative–supervisory personnel who head various departments or services (e.g., nursing, dietary, admissions, maintenance, pharmacy, medical records, housekeeping, laundry) and are in charge of the employees in these departments. There are also a number of medical technologists and technicians who work in the laboratory and x-ray departments of the hospital, as well as a number of miscellaneous clerical and secretarial personnel. And apart from all these staffs and professional–occupational groups, there is a board of trustees which has the overall formal responsibility for the organization, and which consists of a number of prominent people from the outside community. The trustees offer their services to the hospital without remuneration and are not employees of the organization. In short, professionalization and specialization are two of the hallmarks of the hospital.

Because of this extensive division of labor and accompanying specialization of work, practically every person working in the hospital depends upon some other person or persons for the performance of his own organizational role. Specialists and professionals can perform their functions only when a considerable array of supportive personnel and auxiliary services is put at their disposal at all times. Doctors, nurses, and others in the hospital do not, and cannot, function separately or independently of one another. Their work is mutually supplementary, interlocking, and interdependent. In turn, such a high interdependence requires that the various specialized functions and activities of the many departments, groups, and individual members of the organization be sufficiently coordinated, if the organization is to function effectively and attain its objectives. Consequently, the hospital has developed a rather intricate and elaborate system of internal coordination. Without coordination, concerted effort on the part of its different members and continuity in organizational operations could not be ensured.

It is also interesting and important to note here that, unlike industrial and other large-scale organizations, the hospital relies very heavily on the skills, motivations, and behaviors of its members for the attainment and maintenance of adequate coordination. The flow of work is too variable and irregular to permit coordination through mechanical standardization. And the product of the organization—patient care—is itself individualized rather than uniform or invariant. Because the work is neither mechanized nor uniform or standardized, and because it cannot be planned in advance with the automatic precision of an assembly line, the organization must depend a good deal upon its various members to make the day-to-day adjustments which the situation may demand, but which cannot possibly be completely detailed or prescribed by formal organizational rules and regulations. This is all the more essential, moreover, if one takes into account the fact that the patient, who is the center of all activity in the hospital, is a transient rather than a stable element in the system—in the short-stay hospital, he comes and goes very rapidly.

Fundamentally, then, the hospital is a human rather than a machine system. And even though it may possess elaborate and impressive-looking equipment, or a great variety of physical and material facilities, it has no integrated mechanical–physical systems for the handling and processing of its work. The patient is not a chunk of raw material that passively goes through an ordered progression of machines and assembly-line operators. At every stage of his short stay in the hospital, he is mainly dependent upon his interaction with the people who are entrusted with his care, and upon the skills, actions, and interactions of these different people. All of these factors necessitate heavy reliance upon the members of the organization to coordinate their activities on a voluntary, informal, and expedient basis.

Paradoxical as it may seem, however, the hospital is also a highly formal, quasi-bureaucratic organization which, like all task-oriented organizations, relies a great deal upon formal policies, formal written rules and regulations, and formal authority for controlling much of the behavior and work relationships of its members. The emphasis on formal organizational mechanisms and procedures and on directive rather than "democratic" controls, along with a number of other factors, gives the hospital its much talked about "authoritarian" character, which manifests itself in relatively sharp patterns of superordination–subordination, in expectations of strict discipline and obedience, and in distinct status differences among organizational members.

The authoritarian character of the hospital is partly the result of historical forces having their origins at a time when professionalization and specialization were at a primordial stage, and when nursing, medicine, and the hospital were all closely associated with the work of religious orders and military institutions. The absence of substantial professionalization and specialization characteristic of hospital personnel at those times, along with the emphasis of religious and military institutions on social arrangements in which the occupant of every position in the organization presumably knew "his place," and kept to his place by strictly adhering to specified rights, duties, and obligations, had much to do with the hospital's adopting a strict hierarchical and authoritarian system of work arrangements. But, the advent of professionalization and specialization, the gradual independence of hospitals from religious and military institutions, and the impact of an increasingly secular culture have greatly reduced the authoritarian character of the hospital. As Lentz[1] suggests, within the last 50 years the

[1] Lentz, E. M., "The American Voluntary Hospital As an Example of Institutional Change," doctoral dissertation, Cornell University, 1956.

hospital has undergone marked changes, dropping some of its authoritarian and paternalistic characteristics and taking on those of a bureaucratic, functionally rational organization.

Today's community general hospital, however, still has some of its traditional authoritarian characteristics along with its emphasis on rational organization. Moreover, it is unlikely that it will rid itself of all authoritarianism in the near future. There are several major counterforces at work in this connection. First, there is the fact that the hospital constantly deals with critical matters of life and death—matters which place a heavy burden of both secular and moral responsibility on the organization and its members. When human life is at stake, there is little tolerance for error or negligence. And, if error and negligence can be prevented by adherence to strict formal rules and quasi-authoritarian discipline, such rules are important to have and obedience cannot very well be questioned (although blind obedience is mitigated because the hospital increasingly relies on the expertness, judgment, and ethics of professionals who, while abhorring regimentation, are presumably capable of a good deal of self-discipline). Second, there is the great concern of the hospital for maximum efficiency and predictability of performance. In the absence of mechanically regulated workflows, this concern virtually forces the organization to use many quasi-authoritarian means of control (including rigid rules and procedures, directive supervision, rigorous discipline, etc.), in the hope of: (1) attaining some uniformity in the behavior of its members, (2) regulating their interaction and checking deviance within known limits of accountability, and (3) appraising their performance. Third, there is the temptation to adhere to traditional, familiar ways of doing things which, coupled with the lack of apparently equivalent or superior alternatives that could be employed to ensure clarity of responsibility and efficiency and predictability of performance, also serves to perpetuate organizational reliance upon customary directive means of control.[2]

[2] Incidentally, the apparent unavailability of equivalent or superior organizational alterna-

In brief, while historical forces might account for the origins of the authoritarian characteristics of the hospital, it is not likely that some of these characteristics would continue to persist (especially within the context of a highly secular culture) unless they were more functional than not. And this clearly appears to be the case. In the first place, as in any organization designed to mobilize resources quickly in order to meet crises and emergencies successfully, a good deal of regimented behavior is required in the hospital. Lines of authority and responsibility have to be clearly drawn, basic acceptance of authority has to be assured, and discipline has to be maintained. In the second place, the hospital is expected to be able to provide adequate care to its patients at all times, with the precision of a machine system and with minimum error, even though it is a human rather than a machine system. It is expected to perform well continuously and to produce a machinelike response toward the patient, regardless of such things as turnover, absenteeism, and feelings of friendship or hostility among its personnel, or other organizational problems that it may be experiencing. It is also expected to be responsive to the health-related needs and demands of its community, and to meet a variety of medicolegal requirements. Because of these expectations, the hospital places high premium on being able to count upon and predict the outcome of the performances of its members. And predictability of performance can be partly attained through directive, quasi-authoritarian controls which, in the absence of apparently superior alternatives, are rather tempting to the organization.

Coupled with this great concern for predictability of performance, moreover, there is an increasing concern that the hospital operate as efficiently and economically as possible. As the hospital has become a resource for all members of the community, and not just the indigent and the impover-

ished, the public has come to expect of it the best medical and nursing services that can be offered. These services, however, are quite costly, as are the facilities, equipment, supplies, and medicines that are required. And while the public may be willing (though not necessarily able to afford) to pay for these essential costs of hospital care, it also expects the best care possible at reasonable cost or even at least cost. At the same time, it is neither willing to tolerate nor prepared to pay any costs that may result from inefficient operations, poor administration, duplication of services, waste, negligence, and the like. It expects its hospitals to reduce to a minimum or eliminate altogether costs of this latter type and to operate with maximum economy. The hospitals themselves are quite aware of these and other pressures for efficiency, and have come to place very high emphasis on greater efficiency. Great emphasis on economic efficiency, however, is not entirely compatible with the hospital's traditional humanitarian orientation and objective of best service to the patient; the "best" service is not always or necessarily the most economical. Furthermore, this concern for efficiency results both in progressive rationalization of hospital operations and in the institution of more rigid controls within the organization. Such controls, incidentally, serve to maintain the remaining authoritarian characteristics of the community general hospital.

But, efficiency of operations and predictability of performance in the hospital could not possibly be attained only through quasi-authoritatian and directive controls. In fact, if carried to extremes, such controls would in the long run be inimical both to efficiency and to predictability. Efficiency and predictability of performance are also, and perhaps primarily, attained through a number of other factors, which are essential to effective organizational functioning. Probably the most prominent of these factors in the case of the community general hospital are organizational coordination and professionalization.

---

tives is partly the result of our inadequate knowledge about how best to organize and manage human activity in a situation such as that of the community general hospital, and partly the result of the inability of hospitals to utilize the findings of modern research to best advantage.

Because of the high degrees of specialization and functional interdependence found in the hospital, coordination of skills, tasks, and activities is indispensable to effective organizational performance and its predictability. The different specialized, but interacting and interdependent, parts of the organization must fit well together; they must not work at cross purposes or in their own separate directions. If the organization is to attain its objectives, its different parts and members must function according to each other's needs and the needs and expectations of the total organization. In short, they must be well coordinated. But, as we have already pointed out, the hospital is dependent very greatly upon the motivations and voluntary, informal adjustments of its members for the attainment and maintenance of good coordination. Formal organizational plans, rules, regulations, and controls may ensure some minimum coordination but of themselves are incapable of producing adequate coordination, for only a fraction of all the coordinative activities required in this organization can be programed in advance. We shall have much more to say about organizational coordination in subsequent chapters.

The other relevant factor that we wish to consider here, in addition to coordination, is that of professionalization—professionalization being one of the major distinctive features of the community general hospital. The majority of those who hold the principal therapeutic and nontherapeutic positions in the hospital are trained as professionals. The doctors, through their training, have been schooled in certain professional obligations, ethics, and standards of appropriate behavior and have acquired a number of common attitudes, shared values, and mutual understandings about their work and work relations with others. The same is true about the registered nurses. Other groups in the organization are also on the road to professionalization: the administrators, the medical librarians, the medical technologists, the dietitians, and others in paramedical positions.

This high degree of professionalization among those entrusted with the care of the patient has developed along lines of rational, functional specialization, and has had the effect of inculcating many complementary expectations and common norms and values in the members of the principal groups of the hospital—values, expectations, and norms that are essential to the integration of the organization. These include the norms of giving good care, devotion to duty, loyalty, selflessness and altruism, discipline, and hard work. This normative structure underpins the formal rational structure of the organization, and enables the hospital to attain a level of coordination and integration that could never be accomplished through administrative edict, through hierarchical directives, or through explicitly formulated and carefully specified organizational plans and impersonal rules, regulations, and procedures. However, increased professionalization and specialization have also had the effect of sharpening some of the status differences among the people working in the hospital—and sharp status distinctions bespeak of some authoritarianism.

Among other things, increased professionalization in the hospital has helped guarantee that certain minimum levels of competence and skill will exist in the organization, thus having a direct impact upon performance and organizational effectiveness. Similarly, professionalization and specialization have contributed to greater public confidence in the hospital, and to a wider acceptance of the hospital as a resource for the health needs of all people, for high professionalization and specialization imply expertness and knowledge. Increased professionalization has undoubtedly resulted in improved patient care and, in so doing, it has also raised the expectations of the public for both high-quality care and high efficiency in hospital operations. More and more of us go to the hospital for our various health needs nowadays, but, because of improved service, we stay there for a shorter and shorter period of time. In the last 30 years, the average length of stay for adult patients in general hospitals has decreased by about a third, from 12.6 to 8.6 days[3]—making it increasingly appropriate to refer to the community general hospital as the short-stay hospital.

Another of the distinctive characteristics of the community general hospital, closely related to professionalization and specialization, is the absence of a single line of authority in the organization. This feature has already been the subject of considerable discussion by Smith[4] and others, but is important enough to warrant some brief observations here. Essentially, authority in the hospital is shared (not equally) by the board of trustees, the doctors, and the administrator—the three centers of power in the organization—and, to some extent, also by the director of nursing. In the hospital, authority does not emanate from a single source and does not flow along a single line of command as it does in most formal organizations.

A formal organizational chart of the hospital shows the board of trustees as having ultimate authority and overall responsibility for the institution. The board delegates the day-to-day management of the organization to the hospital administrator. In turn, the administrator delegates authority to the heads of the various nonmedical departments (including the director of nursing, who also wields a different kind of authority that originates in her professional expertness). The heads of these departments, in turn, have varying degrees of authority over the affairs of their respective departments and personnel. In the formal organizational chart, the medical staff, its officers, and its members are not shown as having any direct-line responsibility; they are outside of the lay–administrative line of authority. Yet, as is well known both within and outside the hospital, the doctors exercise substantial influence throughout the hospital structure at nearly all organizational levels, enjoy very high autonomy in their work, and have a good deal of professional authority over others in the organization.

[3] Health Insurance Institute, *Source Book of Health Insurance Data*, New York: Health Insurance Institute, 1959.
[4] Smith, H. L., "Two Lines of Authority: The Hospital's Dilemma," *Modern Hospital*, 84:59–64, March, 1955.

Over the nursing staff and over the patients, their professional authority is dominant. And although the board of trustees is in theory shown as the ultimate source of authority, the board actually has very limited *de facto* authority over the medical staff. Partly because the doctors are not employees of the hospital (they are "guests" who are granted practice privileges), partly because they enjoy high status and great prestige, partly because they have almost supreme authority in professional–medical matters, and partly for other reasons, they are subject to very little lay–organizational authority.

Professionals in staff capacities in business corporations—lawyers, doctors, accountants, and others—have little or no authority to be involved in the activities of the line; they mainly serve as consultants and advisors. But this is not so in the case of the hospital. The absence of a single line of authority in the hospital, of course, creates various administrative and operational problems, as well as psychological problems having to do with the relative power and influence on organizational functioning on the part of doctors, trustees, administrators, and others. For one thing, it makes formal organizational coordination rather difficult. For another thing, it allows for instances in which it is not clear where authority, responsibility, and accountability reside. Similarly, it allows for a situation wherein a large number of organizational members, particularly members of the nursing staff, must be responsible to and take orders not only from their supervisors but also from the doctors. The lay authority and the professional authority to which nurses are subject, of course, are not always consistent. The absence of a single line of authority also makes for difficulties in communication, difficulties in the area of discipline, and difficulties in resolving problems that must be resolved through cooperative efforts on the part of both the lay–administrative and the medical–professional sides. Frequently, the administrator, feeling that the responsibility for the overall management of the organization is his, and feeling that doctors through their power and pressures interfere in the discharge of his responsibilities, is motivated or actively attempts to circumvent the medical staff on various matters, and this too is apt to lead to problems. (The doctors, in turn, are likely to try to circumvent the administrator.) For the same reasons, the administrator is likely to be prone toward more and more bureaucratization in the hospital. And increased bureaucratization of organizational operations is likely to be fought and resented by the doctors, for it eventually means a reduction in their influence.

In general, multiple lines of authority require the maintenance of a very delicate balance of power in the organization—a balance of power that is rather precarious. On the positive side, multiple lines of authority may serve as a system of "checks and balances," which may prevent other kinds of possible problems, such as organizational inflexibility and authoritarianism, or may serve to lighten the burden of responsibility in situations where responsibility may be too great for any single group or individual to shoulder. Regardless of the advantages and disadvantages of a system of multiple lines of authority, such a system is an integral part of the community general hospital. Not only is it an integral part, moreover, but also a part that is virtually inevitable for an organization such as this. This is because much of the work in the hospital is performed by influential professionals and not by low-status workers, and because of the high degrees of both professionalization and specialization characteristic of the organization. As Parsons has aptly observed, "The multiplication of technical fields, and their differentiation from each other . . . leads to an essential element of decentralization in the organizations which must employ them."[5] For this reason, he goes on to explain that, unlike

business and military organizations, "A university cannot be organized mainly on a 'line' principle. . . ."[6] In this respect, the community general hospital is very similar to a university. (Hospitals and universities have a number of other interesting characteristics in common, but here we are only interested in hospitals.)

Summary

In summary, the community general hospital is an extremely complex social organization that differs from business and other large-scale organizations on a number of important characteristics. Among its main distinguishing characteristics, the following are worth re-emphasizing:

1. The main objective of the organization is to render personalized service—care and treatment—to individual patients, rather than the manufacture of some uniform material object. And the economic value of the organization's products and objectives is secondary to their social and humanitarian value.

2. By comparison to industrial organizations, the hospital is much more directly dependent upon, and responsive to, its surrounding community, and its work is much more closely integrated with the needs and demands of its consumers and potential customers. To the hospital and its members, the patient's needs are always of supreme and paramount importance. Moreover, there is high agreement about the principal objective of the hospital among the members of the organization, and the personal needs and goals of the different members conflict little with the objectives of the organization.

3. The demands of much of the work at the hospital are of an emergency nature and nondeferrable. They place a heavy burden of both moral and secular–functional responsibility upon the organization and its members. Correspondingly, the organization shows great concern for clarity of responsibility and accountability among its different members and very little tolerance for either ambiguity or error.

[5] Parsons, T., "Suggestions for a Sociological Approach to the Theory of Organizations: II," *Admin. Science Quart.*, 1:225–239, September, 1956, (especially p. 236).

[6] *Ibid.*

4. The nature and volume of work are variable and diverse, and subject to relatively little standardization. The hospital cannot lend itself to mass production techniques, to assembly-line operations, or to automated functioning. It is a human rather than a machine system, with all the attributes this entails. Both the raw materials and end products of the organization are human. And, being human, they participate actively in the production process, thus having a good deal of control over it.

5. The principal workers in the hospital —doctors and nurses—are professionals, and this entails various administrative and operational problems for the organization.

6. By comparison to industrial organizations, the hospital has relatively little control over its workload and over many of its key members. In particular, it has little direct control over the doctors and over the patients —two of its most essential components. In the short-stay hospital, the patients are not only a very heterogeneous and very transient group, but are also, mainly and ultimately, in the hands of their doctors, who are not employees of the organization.

7. The administrator has much less authority, power, and discretion than his managerial counterparts in industry, because the hospital is not and cannot very well be organized on the basis of a single line of authority. The simultaneous presence of lay, professional, and mixed lay–professional lines of authority in the hospital creates a number of administrative and other problems, which business organizations are largely spared.

8. The hospital is a formal, quasi-bureaucratic, and quasi-authoritarian organization which, like most organizations of this kind, relies greatly on conventional hierarchical work arrangements and on rather rigid impersonal rules, regulations and procedures. But, more importantly, it is a highly departmentalized, highly professionalized, and highly specialized organization that could not possibly function effectively without relying heavily for its internal coordination on the motivations, actions, self-discipline, and voluntary, informal adjustments of its many members. Coordination of efforts and activities in the hospital is indispensable to organizational functioning, because the work is of a highly interactional character—the activities of organizational members are highly interlocking and interdependent, and the various members can perform their role only by working in close association with each other.

9. The hospital shows a very great concern for efficiency and predictability of performance among its members and for overall organizational effectiveness.

10. Finally, the community general hospital is an organization which is important to us all, and which is becoming increasingly important. Several basic social trends tend to ensure this: the accelerating accumulation of new medical knowledge, new medical, surgical, and nursing procedures, and new drugs and medicines; rising levels of family income in the nation; increased use of the general hospital for numerous different diseases and health needs; and a growing demand by the general public for the best possible quality of medical–surgical and nursing care.

23

The Participation Patterns of "Economic Influentials" and Their Control of a Hospital Board of Trustees

Robert G. Holloway,
Jay W. Artis
and
Walter E. Freeman

SOCIOLOGISTS have commonly assumed that important economic status occupants are also key people in the community influence and decision-making process—an assumption not without empirical support.[1]

[1] See, for example: F. Hunter, *Community Power Structure*, Chapel Hill: Univ. of North Carolina Press, 1953; D. C. Miller, "Decision-Making Cliques in Community Power Structures: A Comparative Study of an American and an English City," *Am. J. of Soc.*, 54:299–310, November, 1958; D. C. Miller, "Decision-making Cliques in Community Power Structures: A Comparative Study of an American and an English City," *Am. Soc. Rev.*, 23:9–15, February, 1958; W. H. Form and D. C. Miller, *Industry, Labor, and Community*, New York: Harper and Bros., 1960, chaps. 14–15; W. V. D'Antonio and E. C. Erickson, "The Reputational Technique As a Measure of Community Power: An Evaluation Study Based on Comparative and Longitudinal Studies," *Am. Soc. Rev.*, 27:362–376, June, 1962. However, both the

If this assumption is correct, and if we can assume that a hospital board is an important decision-making structure in the community,[2] then it follows that occupants of important economic statuses (hereafter designated "economic influentials"[3]) will also attempt to influence or control the actions of a hospital board. Obviously such attempts could be manifested in a variety of ways: directly by membership and participation in decision-making boards and committees, or indirectly by influencing the behavior of the members of such boards and committees.

As a part of a research project concerned with the ways in which a hospital is structurally linked with the community in which it is situated, an extensive investigation was made of the ways in which boards of trustees reconcile and transform community demands for changes in hospital service. Included in the latter was an investigation of historical

findings and the methodological procedures utilized in these studies have been severely criticized. See, for example: R. A. Dahl, "A Critique of the Ruling Elite Model," *Am. Pol. Sc. Rev.*, 52:463–468, June, 1958; N. W. Polsby, "Community Power: Three Problems," *Am. Soc. Rev.*, 24:796–803, December, 1959; R. E. Wolfinger, "Reputation and Reality in the Study of 'Community Power,'" *Am. Soc. Rev.*, 25:636–644, October, 1960.

[2] The role of the hospital as a significant community unit should be noted. In many communities the local hospital or hospitals are among the largest economic units in the community with regard to total annual budget, number of persons employed, annual payroll, and so on. Hence, positions on the board may be among the most "strategic" in the community from the point of view of the control of community resources. The hospital investigated in the research reported here, although not exceptionally large as hospitals run, employs over 800 persons and operates on an annual budget exceeding four million dollars.

[3] The literature provides many roughly equivalent terms for designating the occupants of such statuses. We have chosen to use "economic influentials," but the term is synonymous with "economic dominant."

From Journal of Health & Human Behavior, *Vol. 4: 88–99, Summer, 1963; by permission of the authors and publisher.*

This report is one of a series of reports on hospital–community relations sponsored under a grant from the National Institute of Health (Research Grant no. RG 4949-C3) through the Social Research Service, Department of Sociology and Anthropology, Michigan State Univ. The writers also wish to acknowledge their debt to D. A. Clelland for sharing his data on economic influentials in the community in which this research was carried out (See D. A. Clelland, "The Role of Economic Dominants in the Power Structure of a Mid-Western Community," unpublished Master's thesis, Michigan State Univ., 1961), and to the helpful criticisms of A. O. Haller and E. C. Erickson.

changes in the participation patterns of economic influentials on a board of trustees and a study of the extent to which they are able to influence the present day operation of a 345 bed non-profit community general hospital in a middle-sized midwestern community.[4]

This paper presents the findings of these investigations and is divided into two parts: the first section reports the results of an examination of the historical pattern of economic influentials' participation on the board of trustees of a hospital; and the second section presents the results of an attempt to empirically measure the degree of influence or control they exert in a board meeting primarily concerned with hospital expansion.

Historical Pattern of Participation of Economic Influentials

The following kinds of evidence of changes in participation patterns were used: (1) membership on the board; (2) board offices held; (3) committee memberships and chairmanships held; and (4) attendance at board meetings. The data were taken from the minutes of 168 meetings of the hospital board covering the time span from its first organizational meeting in April, 1910, to November, 1959.[5] From these minutes a list of board members was constructed tracing

[4] This city had a population of about 170,000 in 1960. The automobile and metal manufacturing industries, and government provide the economic base to this community. Three other hospitals are located in the city: a Catholic general hospital, an osteopathic hospital, and a county chest hospital. Clelland's study (*op. cit.*) examines the historical pattern for this city for other organizations and institutional areas of the community.

[5] It seems unnecessary to set forth all of the serious limitations or advantages involved in utilizing institutional data versus sociological field data at this time. Obviously, little can be said about the *actual* influence or role played by any single individual or category of status occupants by the historical analysis undertaken here. Nevertheless, historical "inventories" of the social composition of community organizations have great relevance to the understanding of community growth and change, and hence for community theory.

each replacement of the 18 founding trustees. One third of the entire 18-man board was elected each year for a three-year term. The board was a self-perpetuating board in that nominations were made by a committee within the membership, and election was by vote of the board. The stability of membership achieved by this replacement procedure is illustrated by the fact that the average replacement rate was only one new member per year (out of a possible 6) since the board's founding. Vacancies occurred for various reasons: death, resignations due to ill health or to "pressing personal or business demands." On such occasions a new member was nominated and elected by the board to fill out an unexpired term. A further index of stability of membership on the board is represented by the length of service of its members. The average length of service per board member was 13.2 years.[6]

In order to rule out the possibility that random variation might account for any differences found, wherever possible the null hypothesis of "no change" in the participation of economic influentials was assumed for each type of evidence, and statistical tests were applied to the data. An "economic influential" was operationally defined by Clelland as one of the largest property owners, the top executives (owner, president, or manager) of business units having assessed evaluation of property ranging from $250,000 to $750,000 and financial units (banks, savings and loans, and insurance companies) with resources ranging from $1,000,000 to $6,000,000 over the 1910–1959 period. Overlapping directorships and number of em-

[6] Economic influentials had a slightly higher length of service as board members (14.4 years) than non-influentials (12.1 years), but the difference is not statistically significant. The hypothesis tested here was that these two populations (influentials and non-influentials) have the same mean, and was tested by the t test. In this case, t = 0.87, which was not significant at the 0.05 level and the hypothesis was supported. See W. J. Dixon and F. J. Massey, Jr., *Introduction to Statistical Analysis*, New York: McGraw-Hill, 1957, pp. 123–124.

ployees (ranging from 150 to 250) were
criteria also used.[7]

Findings on Historical Participation

In order to examine the data for changes
in the representation of economic influentials
for the 50-year period, the data in Table 23–1

50-year period, the absolute number of
influentials on the board.

Table 23–1 shows, in the form of percentage of positions per year occupied by
economic influentials, that influentials were
very uniformly represented on the hospital
board of trustees during the 1910–1949
period. The percentage of influentials on the
board ranged from 54 per cent to 58 per cent
during this period, but dropped to 39 per
cent in the following decade.

The average percentage of influentials over

**Table 23–1—Representation of economic influentials and non-influentials on a
community hospital board of trustees from 1910–1959, by position per year* and total
number****

Time Period	POSSIBLE BOARD POSITIONS (18 per Year) N	POSITIONS OCCUPIED BY ECONOMIC INFLUENTIALS	
		N*	Per Cent of Possible
1910–1919	180	97	54
1920–1929	180	105	58
1930–1939	180	105	58
1940–1949	181***	99	55
1950–1959	180	71	39
Totals	901	477	53

Total Number** of Men on Board　69
Total Number Influentials　35　Per Cent 51

*"Position per year" means the number of persons who are influentials on the 18-man board *each* year, thus making
18 "positions per year" or 180 per decade.
**"Total number" means the absolute number of persons who were on the board and who were influentials for the
entire 50-year period.
***The additional board member was elected for 1943.

are presented in two ways. First, by examining the percentage of influentials on the
board each year (disregarding the fact that
a member might be on the board for several
years) and second, by examining for the total

[7] For the complete list of criteria, the specific
cutting points of assessed evaluation or capital
for each time period used, and the complete
procedure of identification of economic influentials, see Clelland, *op. cit.*, pp. 29–30. Such
sources as the city directories, directory of the
state manufacturers, Dunn and Bradstreet's
Directory of Million Dollar Companies, city and
county histories, newspapers, Poor's Register of
Directors and Executives, Moody's Industrials
and Investments Guides, Rand McNally International Bankers Directory, annual reports of the
state banking department and the commissioner
of insurance, the state building and loan association reports, and reports of the largest economic
units themselves were utilized by Clelland as
sources of identifying the influentials and determining the value of the economic units themselves.

the entire history of the board was 53 per
cent. The same representation is found for
the *total* absolute number of persons on
the board. There were 69 men on the board
during the 50-year period and 35 of them
(51 per cent) were influentials. It is quite
apparent that, except for the last decade,
there was an even balance of influentials and
non-influentials on the board.[8]

[8] The term "non-influentials" is a misleading
one. Individuals are classified as such merely because they do not meet the criteria listed above
for classification as "influentials." The relative
control of members within these two classifications, rather than being assumed, will be examined in the second section of this paper. From the
standpoint of their positions, most of the non-
influentials are "second level" corporate and
company officers, board members, etc. It is
interesting to note that at no time has a person
occupying a "health-oriented" status (e.g., public
health official, nurse, physician, hospital administrator, etc.) been a *voting* member of the board.

This decline in the last decade could have merely reflected a general decline in the number of economic influentials in the community for that period. However, Clelland's data, presented in Table 23–2, show a general increase in the absolute number of economic influentials in the community under analysis.[9] There appears to be no corresponding increase in the absolute number of economic influentials on the board.

In order to test for the possibility of a trend or change in representation, the total period was divided into two equal time

"accepted" on the basis of this statistical test. (See Table 23–3.)

The second set of evidence with which to examine the "no change" hypothesis is contained in Table 23–4, which traces the historical pattern of offices on the board, and committee memberships and chairmanships. Like most organizations, the hospital board changed its executive structure over the

Table 23–2—Number of economic influentials in a midwestern community and on a hospital board of trustees, 1910–1959

	ABSOLUTE NUMBER OF ECONOMIC INFLUENTIALS	
	In Community*	On Board**
Time Period	N	N
1910–1919	30	14
1920–1939	57	24
1940–1959	73	18
Total	160	56

*Data on community influentials were taken from D. Clelland, "The Role of Economic Dominants in the Power Structure of a Mid-Western Community," unpublished Master's thesis, Michigan State Univ., 1961.
**The unit of analysis for this table is the *absolute number* of persons who were influentials for *each* specified time period. Thus, there is an overlap of 21 persons *between* time periods.

periods of 25 years each (1910–1934 and 1935–1959), and a sign test was performed *between* periods *for each board position*. It would be expected, under the "no change" hypothesis, that the first period would not exhibit a significantly greater number of economic influentials on the board than would period two. This hypothesis was

9 Clelland points out that there are no objective standards which one may employ to assess the increase or decrease of economic dominants in the community. Obviously, the number of influentials in any one period will be a reflection of the cutting points of the criteria utilized. These points shift for each time period (decade) to compensate for shifts in increased property evaluation and the growth of industries. It is conceivable that one could set the cutting points to maintain a constant number of influentials for each period. Only on the basis of the limits used by Clelland is an increase demonstrated. It is an open question as to whether utilization of different cutting points would affect the analytical relationship between the number of influentials *on the board* and *in the community*, but there are no reasons apparent to the writers that would lead them to suspect that different points would affect this relationship.

years. For the first decade the executive structure had an average of 5 officers: president, first and second vice-presidents, secretary, and treasurer. During the 1920's and 1930's the number was reduced to 3 on the average, and from 1943 to 1959 the average number increased to 7 including a chairman and vice-chairman—both primarily honorary positions. Inspection of Table 23–4 shows that for *all board offices* held there was a general decline in the percentage of available offices which were held by influentials, although the trend leveled off somewhat after 1930. The percentage of influential representation dropped from 50 per cent for the 1910–1919 period to 31 per cent for the 1950–1959 period with some fluctuation in between. (See column 1.)

Comparing the percentage totals for Columns 1–5, it can be seen that although influentials are less frequently represented in *all board offices held and all committee memberships held*, they are well represented in key positions of *president, executive com-*

mittee memberships, and *committee chairmanships*. Since the committee members were generally appointed by the president of the board, it is important to establish what association, if any, exists between the president's status and the status of the committee members he selected. By comparing the number of economic influential presidents by "office per year" for each decade with the number of influentials who were selected as committee members, a definite association was found (particularly for the most legally powerful of all committees—the executive committee). When the time period was characterized by a high percentage of presidents who were influentials, there was a high percentage of committee members who were influentials. Conversely, when the time period was characterized by a high percentage of presidents who were not economic influentials, a marked reduction in the percentage of committee members who were influentials was found (compare Columns 2 with 3, 4, 5). This association may be accentuated by pointing out that for *all* those years in which the president of the board was an economic influential, 78 per cent of the executive committee was composed of influentials. Finally, although the balance of influentials to non-influentials has been fairly even on the board, there has been a definite increase in influential representation on the executive

Table 23–3—Number of economic influentials by 25 year periods and by board positions per year

Board Position	NUMBER OF INFLUENTIALS** Period I 1910–1934	NUMBER OF INFLUENTIALS** Period II 1935–1959	Sign* If I > II = + If I < II = − If I = II = 0
1	13	0	+
2	13	0	+
3	25	25	0
4	17	25	−
5	6	25	−
6	25	11	+
7	12	25	−
8	0	0	0
9	13	25	−
10	24	20	+
11	17	0	+
12	7	0	+
13	0	0	0
14	12	0	+
15	11	21	−
16	19	13	+
17	25	9	+
18	13	25	−
Totals	252	225	+ = 9 − = 6 = x 0 = 3 N = 15

Sign Test: (a) $H_0 : I = II$
  (b) p (x is less than or equal to 4, or x is more than or equal to 10, N = 15) = 0.059, two-tailed test
  (c) x = 6
  (d) Accept H_0 since p (x) = 6 = 0.61 > 0.059 level of significance

*A nonparametric sign test was used because assumptions necessary for a parametric test for related samples could not be met. For the procedure, see: Sidney Siegel, *Nonparametric Statistics for the Behavioral Sciences*, New York: McGraw-Hill, 1956, pp. 68–71 and Table D, p. 250.
**The 50-year period was divided into two equal time periods in order to equalize the number of possible board positions per period. However, since the data in Table 24–1 indicate a slight decline for the last decade only, a sign test was computed on the average influential representation for the first 40-year period and the last 10-year period. Again the null hypothesis ($H_0 : I = II$) was accepted [p (x) = 5 = 0.30, two-tailed test], since 0.30 > 0.05 level of significance.

Table 23-4—Representation of economic influentials as office holders, committee memberships and chairmanships on a hospital board of trustees by positions per year,* 1910-1959

| | Economic Influentials Holding Office | | | | | | | | | Economic Influentials on Committee | | | | | |
| | ALL OFFICES | | | PRESIDENT | | | ALL COMMITTEE MEMBERSHIPS | | | EXECUTIVE COMMITTEE | | | CHAIRMEN | | |
Time Period	N Possible	N Held	% Held (1)	N Possible	N Held	% Held (2)	N Possible	N Held	% Held (3)	N Possible	N Held	% Held (4)	N Possible	N Held	% Held (5)
1910-1919	50	25	50	10	8	80	55	28	51	19	13	68	16	8	50
1920-1929	33	14	42	10	3	30	43	20	47	14	8	57	16	6	38
1930-1939	31	10	32	10	0	00	52	12	23	28	3	11	16	6	38
1940-1949	58	23	40	10	6	60	48	30	63	32	21	64	15	10	67
1950-1959	70	22	31	10	10	100	73	35	48	27	20	74	22	13	59
Total	242	94	39	50	27	54	271	125	46	120	65	54	85	43	51

* Since every position in this table is "filled" annually—by either election or appointment—the analysis is in the form of "position per year." As we mentioned above, individuals will occupy their positions for varying lengths of time. For example, there have only been 9 men who have been board presidents in the history of the board, yet, for purposes of analysis, there are 50 board president positions—one for each year.

Table 23–5—Number and percentage of hospital board meetings attended by economic influentials and non-influentials, 1910–1959

	I NON-INFLUENTIALS MEETINGS			II ECONOMIC INFLUENTIALS MEETINGS			SIGN If I > II = + If I < II = − If I = II = 0
Time Period	N Eligible To Attend	N Attended	Per Cent Attended	N Eligible to Attend	N Attended	Per Cent Attended	Sign Between Percentages
1910–1919	315	150	48	351	191	54	−
1920–1929	247	106	43	324	107	33	+
1930–1939	128	72	56	166	49	30	+
1940–1949	304	169	56	386	149	39	+
1950–1959	517	324	63	322	157	49	+
Totals:	1477	821	56	1549	653	42	+ = 4 − = 1 = x N = 5

Sign Test: (a) H_0: I = II
      (b) p (x is less than or equal to 0, or x is more than or equal to 4, N = 5) = 0.031, two-tailed test
      (c) x = 1
      (d) Accept H_0 since p (x) = 1 = 0.38 > 0.031 level of significance

committee and committee chairmanships over the last 30 years (see Columns 4 and 5).[10]

Data in Table 23–5 provide the third set of evidence with which to examine the "no change" hypothesis, and also allow a comparison of the attendance at board meetings of influentials with non-influentials. The attendance of each board member was tabulated up to his time of separation from the board. No evidence of economic influentials declining in participation as measured by attendance (or a decline in interest *if* attendance can be taken as an index of this attribute) was found. In fact, attendance increased for both economic influentials and non-influentials for the last 30 years. When the attendance of influentials is compared with non-influentials by means of the sign test, the hypothesis of no difference was accepted, although the non-influentials attended 14 per cent more meetings on the average than did the influentials.

Interpretation of the Historical Pattern

A review of the recent literature concerning changes in the community power structure reveals two sources which are concerned with current changes in the community participation patterns of economic influentials.

[10] This is contrary to Clelland's findings for other organizations in this community. See Clelland, *op. cit.*, pp. 47–67.

The first source is a study by Schulze. As a part of the interpretation of the findings reported in his paper, Schulze hypothesizes a withdrawal of economic influentials from local, civic, and political participation—partly due to a declining interest in and a decline in the functional importance of such activities, and partly due to a lack of effective contact between the new corporate managers and the local leaders with longer community tenure. Schulze concludes from his data that:

The historical drift has been characterized by the withdrawal of the economic dominants from active and overt participation in the public life of Cibola . . . (and). . . . Consequently, the overt direction of the political and civic life of Cibola has passed almost wholly into the hands of a group of middle-class business and professional men, almost none of whom occupies a position of economic dominance in the community.[11]

A hypothesis complementary to the above hypothesis is put forth by Form and Miller. They suggest that, as community life becomes increasingly bureaucratized, economic influentials only appear to be "withdrawing" from active community decision-making participation. They withdraw from the more formal and visible statuses such as public offices, but manage to maintain

[11] Schulze, R. O., "The Role of Economic Dominants in Community Power Structure," *Am. Soc. Rev.*, 23:3–9, February, 1959. The notion of corporate officials (and their families) having minimum contact with local elites has been expressed also by C. W. Mills, *The Power Elite*, New York: Oxford University Press, 1951, 4th printing, chap. 11, but especially pp. 39ff.

effective community relations by occupying positions in important fiduciary committees, leaving their "second-level" managers and the community businessmen to the more formal offices. This trend, they suggest, is a specific adjunct of a general trend of community participation without visible community "accountability" of top executives of large corporations.[12]

Our data bear directly on the "withdrawal" aspects of the above two hypotheses but they do not, of course, allow any testing of hypotheses concerning the subsequent community role or roles of economic influentials who may have withdrawn from membership and participation in the other organizations in the community.

An examination of our data with respect to the hypothesis of withdrawal shows no statistically significant decline in the representation of economic influentials in the 50 years that this hospital board has been in existence. In the last decade we found economic influentials declined *slightly* in representation on the board of trustees but the decline was not statistically significant. For the last 30 years a small decline in influential representation in all board offices combined was noted. It should be pointed out that these declines in representation were more gradual than for any organizational trend found in Cibola by Schulze as well as for any found by Clelland in the present midwestern city. This pattern suggests that perhaps hospitals as well as other organizations involved in community service will remain the last organizations of influential participation. In other words, the rate of withdrawal is not uniform for all community organizations, and of course may not be complete for any given community.

By examining other intra-organizations statuses such as the office of president, committee chairmanships and memberships, and also attendance patterns, evidence was found to support the Form and Miller thesis (i.e., in the office of president, executive committee membership and committee chairmanships). However, the representation of influentials in "non-strategic" positions on the board has continued to be substantial. This suggests, if the hypothesis

[12] Form and Miller, *op. cit.*

of Form and Miller is correct, that this hospital is a strategic community organization for those who wish to maintain effective power relationships in the community.

Perhaps of most importance to people in the hospital field is the implication of such findings for the dynamics of decision-making in the hospital. We would expect that by virtue of the kind of representation on such a board (about half are economic elite in a corporation and financial sense) their primary concern would be centered on finances and legitimately so. We might also suspect that economic influentials more actively control the top-level decisions of the hospital. The next section of this paper reports one attempt to measure such control.

Measurement of Control of Influentials

The Board of Trustees of the hospital is composed of 18 lay members of the community as we mentioned above. During the period of this study, seven of these were economic influentials; however, only four of these were in attendance at the meeting analyzed in this paper (A, B, C and D). The members of the board, the individuals present at the meeting, their code letter, their "primary" occupation and economic units are all presented in Table 23–6. Verbatim electrical recordings of the board meeting (semi-annual) and several committee meetings of the hospital were made after a three- to six-months period of non-participant observation on the part of the senior author. The meetings were recorded and the interaction was unitized and categorized by means of Bales' "interaction process analysis."[13]

[13] Bales, R. F., *Interaction Process Analysis: A Method for the Study of Small Groups*, Cambridge: Addison–Wesley Press, 1951. The 12 categories are: (1) shows solidarity, (2) shows tension release, (3) agrees, (4) gives orientation, (5) gives opinion, (6) gives orientation, (7) asks orientation, (8) asks opinion, (9) asks for suggestion, (10) disagrees, (11) shows tension, (12) shows antagonism.

Table 23–6—Board members and individuals in attendance at meetings by tabled codes, primary occupation and economic influential classification

BOARD MEMBERS IN ATTENDANCE

ECONOMIC INFLUENTIALS

Table Code	Occupation and Economic Unit*
A	President and General Manager of "W" Corporation (1959 Assessed Evaluation : $12 million, 3,700 employees)
B	Publisher, Editor and General Manager of Newspaper (1959 Assessed Evaluation : $1 million)
C	Chairman of Bank Board (1957 Capital : $250,000)
D	President, Insurance Company (1955 Capital : $31 million ; 1959 Assessed Evaluation : $783,000, 625 employees)

Non-Influentials

e	Vice President, Savings and Loan Company (1958 Capital : $42 million)
f	Vice President, Bank (1958 Capital : $1 million)
g	Realtor
h	Vice President, "S" Company (1950 Assessed Evaluation : $217,000 estimated)

Non-Members of the Board— Non-Influentials

i	Director of the Hospital
j	Consultant, Hospital Construction
k	Architect

BOARD MEMBERS NOT IN ATTENDANCE

ECONOMIC INFLUENTIALS

Table Code	Occupation and Economic Unit
None	Vice President and General Manager "G" Corporation (1959 Assessed Evaluation : $61 million, 12,000 employees)
None	President, University

Non-Influentials

None	President and General Manager "D" Company (1959 Assessed Evaluation : $549,000, 152 employees)
None	Attorney
None	Director of Industrial Relations, "G" Corporation (1959 Assessed Evaluation : $61 million)
None	President, Haberdashery
None	Vice President, Secretary, Sales Manager, "S" Company (1959 Assessed Evaluation : $611,000)
None	President, Insurance Company
None	Retired Industrialist, Financier, Banker
None	Vice President, Labor Council

* The information about the economic units above comes from a variety of sources. See footnote 7 for the list of sources.

However, only the 898 unit acts of the board meeting will be analyzed in this paper.

The measurement of control of influence we shall be using is the Index of Directiveness of Control.[14] Of the 12 categories, three categories—6, 5 and 4—are most concerned with directing the activity of actors in the group and are used in the index. Of the three, category 6—"giving orientation, information, repeating information, clarification of a point or confirming a fact"—is the most

[14] *Ibid.*, p. 145.

non-directive. An example would be an actor who says, "There are two points I would like to make. The first one concerns our hospital charge-offs." Both of these would be scored as category 6. The second category, number 5, is more directive than number 6, and is composed of the "giving of opinions, evaluations, analyses of the situation, the expression of feelings, wishes, desires," etc. For example, if an actor says, "I wish we could beat this Blue Cross formula," this would be scored in category 5.

The third category in the index is the most directive of the three and is comprised of the process of "giving suggestions or directions." For example, if an actor says, "The first thing we should do is to provide a new parking lot for our patients," we would score this activity as category 4.

The Index of Directiveness of Control is based on the preponderance of 4 and 5 in the total process as compared to 6. The more an actor makes direct attempts to control the decisions of the group, category 4, the higher the index value. The formula is presented at the bottom of Table 24–7. The index (IDC) may vary from 0 to 1.0, from no control to maximum control. It should be pointed out that the index does not differentiate between two actors who have no interaction and actors who interact but have no frequencies in categories 4 and 5. In both cases their IDC value would be 0. Since means will be computed for each role group, the IDC values which contain any interaction in any of the three categories but which yield a 0.00 value will be asterisked and included in computation of the mean.

Findings on Influential Control

IDC values are presented in Table 23–7 for board members as well as for the three individuals ("i," "j," and "k") who were present but were not board members. The latter included the director of the hospital, an architect, and a hospital construction consultant. The board members were classified as economic influentials (EI's) or noninfluentials (NI's), and their index values computed. Tables 23–8 and 23–9 contain the mean values for these scores.

It can be seen in Table 23–8 that the degree of control increases in every cell as one moves across the table. That is, the EI's exert the least control over their counterparts with a mean of 0.24; they exert more control over the NI's who are members of the board with a mean of 0.35; and they exert the most control over the NI's who are *not* members of the board with a mean of 0.42. The same pattern holds true for the NI's who are members of the board (mean values of 0.17, 0.22, and 0.35, respectively),

and the NI's who are not members of the board (mean values of 0.12, 0.24, and 0.50, respectively).

Table 24–9 contains the simple relationships between EI's and NI's disregarding board membership. EI's as a group have a higher control index over NI's (0.38) than the converse (0.15), a mean difference of 0.23 in favor of the EI's.

Interpretation of Influential Control

There is obviously a definite "pecking order" in terms of the attempts to control the actions of members of the hospital organization at its highest level of authority—the board meeting. In each case, the NI's who are not board members receive the greatest direction or suggestions as to how and what decision are to be made in the operation of the hospital. This finding is logical in terms of who the NI "non-members" are in the management structure of the organization. The director is the general manager and is directly responsible to the board. The architect is hired by the board, and the consultant, although occupying no official hospital status, is also in a subordinate position. Perhaps of more interest is the finding that the remaining members of the board, the NI's who occupy theoretically a position of equal footing with the other board members —at least as far as membership and activity on the board is concerned—also receive more control from the EI's on the board than they in turn attempt with the EI's. This finding, in connection with the above discussion of the trend for influentials to occupy key positions in the decision-making structure of the hospital, would suggest that decisions in the hospital operation, in this organization at least, will increasingly conform to the suggestions of the economic influentials of the board. Whether or not the NI's are able to "out-maneuver" the EI's in the smaller sub-committee meetings or whether they conform to the pattern found above for the board as a whole (at least for the one meeting analyzed) we cannot say at this time. One limitation of the index must also be acknowledged. As we have inferred, the index is a measure of the extent of "attempts" at control rather than "actual" control, since it contains no measure of the acceptance of the directions or suggestions or whether the suggestions were ever put into effect or not.

Summary

In summary then, an examination of the historical pattern of economic influential representation on a hospital board of trustees over a 50-year period revealed: (1) With the exception of 1950–1959 decade, there is no evidence that economic influentials are occupying a changing proportion of board positions and even the decline in the 1950–1959 decade was not statistically significant. (2) A comparison of board

Table 23–7—Index of directiveness of control for economic influentials and non-influentials on a hospital board of trustees

| | | | BOARD MEMBERS | | | | | | | | NON-MEMBERS | | |
| | | | Economic Influentials | | | | Non-influentials | | | | Non-influentials | | |
	Actor		A	B	C	D	e	f	g	h	i	j	k
Board Members	EI's	A	—	0.00	0.00	0.00	0.50	0.00	0.00	0.00	0.00	0.00	0.00
		B	0.00	—	0.50	0.00*	0.00*	0.25	0.00	0.50	0.50	0.17	0.00
		C	0.13	0.34	—	0.00	0.00	0.50	0.00	0.00	0.50	0.00	0.00
		D	0.00	0.00	0.00	—	0.00	0.00	0.00	0.00	0.00	0.50	0.00
	NI's	e	0.00*	0.51	0.00*	0.00	—	0.00*	0.00	0.09	0.00	0.49	0.00
		f	0.00	0.00	0.00	0.00	0.50	—	0.00	0.00	0.00	0.00	0.00
		g	0.00	0.00*	0.00	0.00	0.00	0.50	—	0.00	0.00*	0.00	0.00
		h	0.34	0.00	0.00	0.00	0.00*	0.00	0.00	—	0.25	0.50	0.50
Non-members	NI's	i	0.34	0.00	0.13	0.00	0.00*	0.00*	0.00*	0.17	—	0.00	0.00
		j	0.00*	0.00	0.00	0.00	0.25	0.00	0.00	0.00	0.50	—	0.50
		k	0.00*	0.00	0.00	0.00	1.00	0.00	0.00	0.00	0.00	0.50	—

* 0.00 Value, but index contains interaction. Values are computed according to the following formula:

$$IDC_{x,y} = \left\{ \frac{\dfrac{4}{4+6} + \dfrac{5}{5+6}}{2} \right\} = \frac{(Bales\ Categories)}{2}$$

Table 23–8—Mean IDC value* for EI's and NI's by hospital board membership

| | | BOARD MEMBERS | | NON-MEMBERS |
	Actors	EI's (A,B,C,D)	NI's (e,f,g,h)	NI's (i,j,k)
Board Member	EI's	0.24	0.35	0.42
	NI's	0.17	0.22	0.35
Non-member	NI's	0.12	0.24	0.50

* Means are computed on indexes with any interaction.

Table 23–9—Mean IDC values for EI's and NI's

Actor	EI's	NI's
EI's	0.24	0.38
NI's	0.15	0.30

position per year by decades yields no statistically significant changes in the representation of economic influentials. (3) A comparison of participation of economic influentials on the board during the first half and second half of the board's existence, by board position, likewise shows no significant differences. (4) There is an increasing tendency in the last two decades for economic influentials to occupy the office of president and other executive positions on the board. (5) There is some evidence that economic influentials have, over the last four decades, consistently attended a smaller proportion of hospital board meetings than have the "non-influentials"; however, the difference is not statistically significant at the 0.05 level, and attendance is increasing for both categories.

Keeping in mind the limitations imposed by the fact that the data here presented deal with a single institution in a specific community, it appears that the data do not support the Schulze hypothesis that economic influentials are withdrawing from all local decision-making bodies; however, they appear to offer some support to Form and Miller's hypothesis that economic influentials are moving to strategic positions within this local decision making organization.

An index of the attempts at control of economic influentials *vis à vis* their participants in a board meeting by the use of Bales' Index of Directiveness of Control demonstrated a clear hierarchy of control on the board. The most control is exerted on the NI's who are management and consulting personnel, followed by NI's who are members of the board and "second level" corporate officers, and the least amount of control is exerted over the EI's who occupy the highest corporate positions. This finding appears to add to an accumulation of research evidence that influentials are actively engaged in the decision-making process of the community and, at least for this one case, within one organization in the community—a general hospital.[15]

[15] For a related approach see: L. V. Blankenship and R. H. Elling, "Organizational Support and Community Power Structure: The Hospital," *J. Health and Human Behavior*, 3:257–269, Winter, 1962.

Both positive and negative implications of our findings have been insightfully developed by Blankenship and Elling.[16] To the extent a hospital board does have economic influential representatives, they will tend to link the hospital to the wider community system of control over the allocation of financial resources within the community as a whole.[17] To the extent that large capital expenditures are needed for expansion ("survival" or "modernization") purposes, as was indeed the case in both this and the Blankenship–Elling studies, the success of the community general hospital in such endeavors rests upon its representation of economic influentials and their control.[18]

Although Blankenship and Elling did not

[16] *Ibid.*, pp. 267–269.
[17] On the point also see: T. Parsons, *Structure and Process in Modern Societies*, New York: Free Press, 1960, pp. 22–27; M. Weber, *The Theory of Social and Economic Organization*, New York: Free Press, 1947, chap. 3; C. P. Loomis, "Social Systems for Health," *Social Systems: Essays on Their Persistence and Change*, Princeton, N.J.: D. Van Nostrand, 1960, essay 7, especially pp. 324–327; F. Hunter, R. C. Schaffer and C. C. Sheps, *Community Organization: Action and Inaction*, Chapel Hill: Univ. of North Carolina Press, 1956, p. 90ff; and R. C. Hanson, "The Systematic Linkage Hypothesis and Role Consensus Patterns in Hospital–Community Relations," *Am. Soc. Rev.*, 27:304–313, June, 1962; and B. S. Georgopoulos and F. C. Mann, "The Value Orientations of the Topechelon Groups in the Hospital," *The Community General Hospital*, New York: Macmillan, 1962, pp. 559–566.
[18] Further support for this point is found in: J. P. Harkness, "Hospital Organization in Transition: A Sociological Analysis of Interlocking Social Systems," unpublished doctoral dissertation, Michigan State Univ., 1961; A. J. Muntean, "Community Change and Hospital Development: A Case Study of Community Power Structure," unpublished Master's thesis, Michigan State Univ., 1959; L. V. Blankenship, "Organizational Support and Community Leadership in Two New York State Communities," unpublished doctoral dissertation, Cornell Univ., 1962. Such representation may be increasingly strategic in view of Loomis's observation that hospitals tend to be developing regional cooperation (and presumably support), *op. cit.*, p. 325.

have the data on internal control by influentials, they correctly suggested:

> To the extent that this [organizational integrity, maintenance, and survival] requires drawing upon centers of power external to the organization [i.e., community influentials] there is always the possibility that the "tail will wag the dog."[19]

Our data on the internal control by economic influentials clearly supports their thesis.

The negative implication drawn by Blankenship and Elling that the organization loses flexibility through "commitment to" the community influentials in exchange for survival power (or in our terms, control by and conformity to the norms of the economic influentials), was neither supported nor confirmed. One might postulate that even though the economic influentials control major economic decisions on the board, this does not guarantee they will also control non-economic decisions, particularly those related to health. There are many possible structural arrangements which may offset the influential representation and control at the board level.[20] A few of these which deserve further research (each of which has both negative and positive consequences for the hospital) are:

1. Norms among board members that they should leave all health-related decisions to lower echelons of the organization which possess more expertise in the area, e.g., the administrative, medical and nursing staff and committees.

2. The relative effectiveness of lay, hospital administration trained, or medical-nursing administrators to "guide" (or even circumvent control by) the board.

3. The influence of health-oriented individuals external to the community on the board's decisions, e.g., hospital consulting firms, those who administer Hill–Burton funds, hospital survey and construction representatives, governor's committees and representatives, etc.

4. The relative influence and effectiveness of the medical, nursing and administrative staffs to operate independently of the board in order to maximize their sub-systems' goals.

5. Finally, comparative studies of hospitals with boards of "mixed" representation versus boards predominantly represented by economic interests by *both* external and internal analyses.

Having analyzed the participation patterns of economic influentials and their control over the board, we must await further research on questions such as those listed above before we can make a more definitive statement about the consequences of such patterns.

[19] Blankenship and Elling, *op. cit.*, p. 268.
[20] See R. G. Holloway, "Systematic Linkage, Influence and Control in a Hospital Decision-making Structure: A Cross Validation Study," unpublished doctoral dissertation, Michigan State Univ., 1962, especially chaps. 3–4; and Georgopoulos and Mann, *op. cit.*, "The Influence of Key Groups in the Hospital," pp. 566–575.

A MODERN HOSPITAL requires a large number of highly trained individuals for the provision of adequate patient care. Their efforts must be supported by the ministrations of many others, perhaps less well trained. If the care of individual patients is not to be unduly fragmented, the efforts of all these people must be well coordinated. If the members of the ward "team" work together in reasonable harmony and with full efficiency, there must be a certain degree of "give and take in hospitals."[1]

At least three factors appear to be essential if adequate coordination or integration of any human group is to take place. *First*, there must be adequate channels for communication between all group members. *Second*, there must be some agreement between members concerning common purposes and presuppositions. And *third*, there must be clearly defined allocations of role and authority.[2] It is the purpose of this paper to examine certain aspects of the social structure of the general hospital in light of these requisites of organizational effectiveness. It will be argued that the rigidity of the institutional status system and certain imperfectly assimilated changes in ward organization have created barriers to free communication among hospital personnel. Moreover, differences in institutional ideology will be shown to be related to these factors.

Although it is believed that the evidence

24

Hospital Ideology and Communication Between Ward Personnel

Albert F. Wessen

to be presented is generally applicable to all general hospitals, what follows is a case study of one large, voluntary, general hospital of eight hundred beds, situated in a metropolitan New England city. This institution will here be called "Yankee Hospital." Data for the study were drawn from intensive observations on the wards of this hospital, from informal interviews with members of the staff, employees, and administration, and from detailed formal interviews concerning role relationships and attitudes toward the hospital held with a sample of seventy-five doctors, nurses, dietitians, laboratory technicians, and nonprofessional ward personnel.[3]

1. The Hospital Ward as a Social System

The "heart" of any hospital is the patient ward. Here, the basic work of the hospital is done: patients are received, cared for, diagnosed, treated, discharged. Practically all of the other facilities of the institution—ranging from technical services such as operating room, laboratory, or social service department to "hotel" or administrative

---

[1] The fullest sociological analysis (at this writing) of the general hospital is T. Burling, E. Lentz and R. N. Wilson, *The Give and Take in Hospitals*, New York, G. P. Putnam & Sons, 1956. A very full description of the hospital from the administrative point of view is M. T. MacEachern, *Hospital Organization and Management*, 2nd Edition, Chicago, 1947. For a sociologist's views on hospital administration, see E. Lentz, "Hospital Administration—One of a Species," *Administrative Science Quarterly*, 1:444–463, 1957. And for a concise exposition of the historical development of the modern hospital, see E. D. Churchill, "The Development of the Hospital," in N. Faxon (ed.), *The Hospital in Contemporary Life*, Cambridge, 1949, pp. 1–69.

[2] Some of the sources of this formulation include C. I. Barnard, *The Functions of the Executive*, Cambridge, 1938; Bronislaw Malinowski, *A Scientific Theory of Culture and Other Essays*, Chapel Hill, 1944, and E. W. Bakke, *Bonds of Organization*, New York, 1950.

[3] This material is drawn from the author's dissertation, *The Social Structure of a Modern Hospital*. (Unpublished Ph.D. dissertation, Yale University Library).

315

services such as laundry, kitchen or business office—exist to support the needs of patients and personnel on the wards. And in the bustle or stillness of each ward, both life and death dramas and the tedious routines of therapeutics, training, and research are consummated each day.

How may a sociologist conceptualize the culture of a typical medical or surgical ward?[4] A full delineation would require a monograph. Here, it will be possible simply to identify the main actors in the ward social system and to indicate some of the principal features of the social structure which orders their interaction.

In the typical general hospital ward, the patient is less an actor than a passive observer of the ward social system.[5] This fact differentiates the general hospital from such institutions for long-term care as mental hospitals and tuberculosis sanitaria; it also distinguishes the contemporary hospital from its forebear of a half-century and more ago.

Dependent upon ward personnel for the satisfaction of his simplest needs, the average medical or surgical patient tends to focus his attention upon himself, his condition, and his anxieties. Although he may carry on an active social interaction with patients in nearby beds, in most cases he has little inclination to participate in, or to discuss, the life of the ward except as it directly impinges upon him. Replacement of the old-fashioned open wards by private or semi-private rooms in modern hospitals has further acted to restrict the patient's potential involvement in ward affairs.

From the point of view of ward personnel

the patient is not considered to be part of the ward social life. He is assumed to be neither interested in nor informed about the complicated medical culture which is ministering to him (except, of course, as it affects him directly.) He is believed to have little interest in the problems of hospital organization and management beyond seeing that he gets the most service for the least price. This was the unanimous opinion of ward personnel—doctors, nurses, and auxiliary workers—with whom we discussed this matter. As one physician put it, "The patients? All they are interested in is getting themselves out of the hospital. They take our word for what must be done, and they don't care what happens, or how, so long as it helps them." A similar attitude on a different level was expressed by a janitor who said that although he liked to talk with the patients, "I never talk about my job; they've got enough troubles of their own to worry about."

Thus, for hospital people, the patients are not so much a part of their social system as a vital *reference group* in the midst of which the personnel operate, which they serve, and toward which they orient many of their actions and attitudes. Because the hospital's dominant purpose is to serve patients, it is only natural that explanations of the behavior of all groups of personnel tend to be formulated in terms of its relationship to patient welfare. As we shall see, many of the ideological differences found between the various occupational strata in the hospital come from the fact that these tend to conceptualize patients' needs in different ways.

Representatives of at least twenty-three different occupational status groups are represented on a typical ward at Yankee Hospital or have frequent business there. These are the following:[6]

Physicians:
1. Visiting staff physicians (of various ranks)
2. Residents (and assistant residents)

[4] Medical and surgical wards, as well as those assigned to other specialty services, have of course quite different characteristics. Likewise, private, semi-private, and charity ward units have their typical pecularities. In the final analysis, each ward unit has an individual identity all its own. Here, however, we wish to discuss certain features which all ward units have in common.

[5] This generalization obviously does not apply to all patients. In particular, it does not apply to those who remain in the hospital for more than a fortnight and who during a substantial share of this time are able to observe and participate in events other than those having to do with their own care.

[6] The order of listing these occupations within the subgroups is not necessarily according to rank. Moreover, in various hospitals the terminology for some of these jobs is variable. We utilize those in force at Yankee Hospital.

3. Internes
Nurses
4. Clinical supervisors and/or instructors
5. Head nurses
6. Staff nurses
7. Student nurses
Paramedical professionals and technicians:
8. Dietitians
9. Laboratory technicians
10. X-ray technicians
11. Social workers
12. Occupational therapists
13. Physical therapists
Semi-skilled workers:
14. Trained attendants (licensed practical nurses)
15. Medical technicians
16. Dietitian's aides
17. Ward receptionists and clerks
Unskilled workers:
18. Nurse's Aids
19. Male Aids
20. Ward Helpers ("Pinkies")
21. Floor service maids
22. Cleaning maids
23. Janitors

Like all of its kind, Yankee Hospital organizes these classes of personnel according to a relatively rigid status hierarchy in which doctors are accorded highest prestige, followed by nurses and the several groupings of paramedical and "non-professional" workers. This hierarchy is popularly justified in terms of the necessity for quick, precise, and responsible action in the medical crises which are almost routine in the hospital setting. It is sanctioned by the practice of generations, and presently reflects the very considerable social distance which exists between the various groupings of hospital personnel as members of the larger society. Within the past few years, this hierarchy has been transformed into a full-blown bureaucratic organization patterned after the example of business management. Yet in many respects, the observer is tempted to describe the hospital social structure as almost castelike.

These sharp status-distinctions are manifested both upon the ward and throughout other areas of Yankee Hospital. Their maintenance is simplified and facilitated by

the distinctive uniforms worn by the various categories of personnel. Thus at least twelve different uniforms can be found on a typical ward—and, as in the case of nurses, small variations in the basic uniform often signify further status differences. Although the basic purpose of uniforms in the hospital is without doubt the validation of the status of the various types of personnel who care for patients, they undoubtedly facilitate the maintenance of rigid status distinctions between the various occupational groups.

These status lines are further sharpened by the fact that separate dining rooms are provided for three major groups of personnel —doctors, nurses, and all other employees. The exclusiveness of dining rooms is enhanced by the fact that there are two cafeteria serving lines, one of which is patronized by doctors and nurses, the other by non-professional personnel. Habitual seating arrangements within the dining-rooms themselves further underline the status differences. Thus it is rather unusual to see full-fledged staff nurses eating at the same table with trainees. It was observed, too, that at a typical meal the doctors' dining room may be roughly divided into four sectors. Along one side of the room may be found the surgeons, while the other side is largely filled with practitioners following the medical specialties. These groups both divide themselves so that the section of the room nearer the window is largely reserved for visiting staff members, while internes and residents occupy the opposite half of the room. Within the non-professional employees' dining room, moreover, there is a marked tendency for employees of the different departments to lunch with others in their own category. Commensality—that principal setting for informal conversations in our society—thus tends to be restricted in the hospital to those who belong to the same occupational group.[7]

[7] This form of status distinction is more marked at Yankee Hospital than in many other institutions of its kind. It should also be stated that what is here described is not prescribed by formal rules but is habitual practice.

Segregation between the three major classes of personnel is not rigid. Nurses who desire to do so frequently eat in the general employees' dining room. Physicians and surgeons sometimes bring individuals other than doctors into their dining room as guests. On the other hand, it is quite unusual for nurses to bring non-nurses into their dining room, and doctors rarely lunch outside their own room. These distinctions are to be seen in full force only at luncheon and at dinner. At snack hours, at breakfast, and during the midnight lunch, occupational distinctions tend to break down. In fact, as a general rule it may be observed that occupational segregation is most marked during the day shift, is seen to a lesser degree on the evening shift, and to a minimal extent at night when the smallest numbers of personnel—and practically no wakeful patients or visitors—are active on the ward.[8]

The implications of these occupational status distinctions for the social structure of the ward can be fully understood only when two other characteristics of ward organization are noted. *First*, on every ward there are dual lines of authority and responsibility.[9] One of these "chains of command" governs the care of patients. In over-simplified form it may be represented as passing from doctor to nurse to non-professional personnel. The other deals with matters of hospital management and administration. Here the staff physician is typically completely outside the chain of command. He is not directly responsible to hospital administration; technically he has the status of a "volunteer" who is accorded the privileges of membership in the hospital's medical staff. Rather, authority passes from the hospital administrator through various departments heads and supervisors to members of specific occupational categories. Thus, while each individual staff-nurse into whose hands care of a patient is assigned is responsible for executing the orders of the patient's physician, she is also responsible to her head nurse, her supervisor, and to the upper levels of the nursing administration for matters concerning ward management, technical procedures, and discipline. Similarly, a male aid, like other auxiliary personnel, is responsible not only to the head nurse—and through her to doctors—on the unit to which he is assigned, but also to the supervisor of male aids. That ward personnel appreciate the possibility of playing off one authority against the other is indicated in the comment of one male aid who said "It sure makes me feel good sometimes to know that Mr. ——— is down there to stand behind me if the nurses get unreasonable." The same dual system of authority holds for housekeeping personnel and for most of the other personnel having business on the ward.[10] Thus, communication and loyalty of personnel tend to be channeled within the major occupational lines by this "administrative" chain of command, while at the same time clinical authority tends to move *across* these lines.

Second, as has been implied, the personnel of a ward differ markedly in the extent to which they become a part of a given unit. Some persons are assigned permanently to a "floor." Of these the most important is the Head Nurse, who is responsible for its administration; in large part, according to our informants, she is able to "set the tone" of work and interaction in her unit. Ideally, the full complement of staff nurses, auxiliary nursing personnel, and dietary and house-

8 Along with separate dining rooms, there are special locker rooms and wash-rooms for doctors as distinguished from all other men, and for nurses as distinguished from all other women.

9 See also R. Coser, "Authority and Decision Making in a Hospital," *American Sociological Review*, 23:56–63, February, 1958.

10 Exceptions include dietary department employees, who are responsible directly to the floor dietitians, and paramedical professionals such as social workers who operate on a "referral" basis. There exists a continuum along which the relative power of ward authorities varies as contrasted to that of the administrative supervisors. Thus, the relations of the trained attendants and the nurses' aides to their supervisors approaches the minimum; nursing supervisors and the male aids' supervisor exert somewhat more direct authority and the housekeeping department supervisors exert much more authority over their employees than does the head nurse. This establishment of a dual hierarchy of authority is, of course, a product of the trend toward rationalization and business management in hospital administration.

keeping employees will be assigned permanently to a given ward unit. But shortages and high turnover of personnel, unpredictable changes in work load, and the necessity to set up work schedules to assure full around-the-clock coverage of essential skills, combine to create a situation in which the make-up of the "permanent" personnel of a ward is constantly changing.

Other types of personnel are expected on the ward only sporadically. Most staff physicians appear on the ward only for such regular exercises as rounds or according to the particular needs of their patients. Similarly, laboratory and X-ray technicians, social workers and occupational therapists are apt to come to the ward only when a referral makes necessary their presence there. And the identity of these part-time actors in the ward social system is also subject to change from day to day. The educational purposes of the hospital tend to intensify the instability of the ward social group. Student nurses and physicians-in-training must be given experience with all kinds of patients. The organization of modern hospitals into discrete ward units serving patients of a given type therefore forces the development of a system of rotation of trainees from unit to unit, usually for short periods of time on each.[11]

All this makes for a situation in which it becomes difficult for primary group associations to develop on the wards of a large hospital. New faces appear too constantly. Moreover, since many of these persons constantly face situations in which their responsibility is not only to ward authorities but to superiors of their own occupational category, normal formal mechanisms for developing an integrated group are weakened. Structural pressures in the hospital thus seem to accentuate rather than to minimize occupational difference among personnel.

Contemporary hospital administration makes much of the idea that those who

work on a ward comprise a single therapeutic "team." In many quarters, emphasis is placed upon the necessity for free participation on the part of all concerned if the most effective planning of ward activities is to take place. The application of "group dynamics" has become an important part of recent blueprints for better ward administration.[12] It may perhaps be suggested that these emphases indicate that hospital people are trying to recover the integration and order of a simpler social system which modern hospitals have outgrown.

2. Communication Between Ward Personnel

What are the patterns of communication between personnel as they work on a given ward? To what extent does interaction encompass all the members of a therapeutic team?

Answers to these questions were sought through systematic observation. Personnel on two units—one semi-private and one "charity" ward—were observed over a period of thirty hours (scattered through various parts of the day and over a period of several days). Each time two individuals were seen in conversation, it was noted who was speaking with whom. If there were more than two individuals in the conversation, the members of the group were divided into pairs. Thus, if two nurses and one doctor talked together, it was assumed that three conversations were taking place: one between the two nurses and two between a doctor and a nurse. Each conversation observed was designated as a single unit except that if it was observed to last more than three minutes, a second unit was scored—and so on every three minutes. Because some conversations may not have been seen by the observer, the results to be reported below must be considered as suggestive rather than rigorous. Personnel were divided into three

---

[11] Mention should also be made of a rather evanescent group of volunteers who come to the ward on a part-time basis, usually to perform such specifically defined tasks as offering library books to patients or serving them mid-afternoon "nourishment."

[12] This concept is especially in evidence among nursing administrators.

categories—doctors, nurses, and all others. The numbers of conversations held between members of one of these groups or between members of different groups are summarized in Table 24–1 below.

The fact which stands out in this table is that ward personnel tend to interact mostly with others in their own group. Thus the doctor is three times as apt to speak to another doctor while on the ward as he is to a nurse, and he almost never talks with other personnel. Likewise, the nurse is more than twice as likely to speak with another nurse than to other workers, while her in-group communication is almost seven times as frequent as is her interaction with medical men. The other personnel rarely speak with doctors but do interact with nurses about sixty per cent as often as with others of their own group. These facts may be stated in another way: the greater the social distance between occupational groupings on the hospital ward the less interaction is observed between groups. Moreover, the highest status group—the doctors—are more apt to interact within their own group than are

tendency for those of high social rank to be freed from the obligation to interact with those of lower degree except on their own terms; or as Homans phrases it "a person of higher social rank than another originates interaction for the latter more often than the latter originates interaction for him."[13] The data in Table 24–1 can provide only indirect evidence on this point. This table shows, however, that physicians tend both to interact within their own group to a greater extent than other ward personnel and also to allocate a relatively higher percentage of their conversation to nurses and other (non-professional) personnel than do the latter groups to them; these differences are consistent with Homans' hypothesis.

This tendency for interaction across status differences to move from above downward is in part a result of the necessity for authority to move along a chain of command. It is also a result of the respect accorded to higher status. Within the hospital, this is to be seen most clearly in behavior toward physicians. Respect for the doctor's prestige—already a very strong element in general American culture—is systematically indoctrinated in hospital per-

Table 24–1—Distribution of conversations between members of various occupational groups on two "Yankee Hospital" wards

Group with Which Interaction Was Observed:	Doctors (N = 228)	Nurses (N = 562)	Others (N = 441)
Interaction Within Own Group:	74.12%	61.57%	61.68%
With the Remaining Groups of Relatively Higher Status:	23.24A	9.43C	1.36C
With the Remaining Group of Relatively Lower Status:	2.64B	29.00B	36.96A

A = Nurses   B = "Others"   C = Doctors

(N's refer to the total number of conversations observed involving members of each group.)

the nurses or other personnel (mostly non-professional workers). It would seem that insofar as these data are valid it strongly supports the impression that communication on the hospital ward is channelized along occupational lines.

The hospital status system was described as involving an almost caste-like set of segregatory patterns which quite effectively limit informal interaction between hospital personnel of different ranks. One would naturally expect these barriers to interaction to carry over into the work situation. Moreover, there seems to be a well nigh universal

sonnel. Deference patterns are most marked, interestingly enough, among the group whose status is second only to the doctors—the nurses. They are painstakingly taught at Yankee Hospital to fledgling student nurses in their "Professional Adjustments" course. The manner in which this is done is made clear in the following excerpt from an interview:

"Insofar as possible, we try to utilize the technique of 'role playing' in teaching our course. And in teaching the girls how to get

13 Homans, G. C., The Human Group, New York, 1950, p. 145.

along in the ward situation, we do little more than help them to apply ordinary rules of common courtesy. For example, at one of our sessions, the girls were acting out what a nurse should do in case of meeting various people at a doorway. And they correctly showed that a nurse should step back to allow a visitor or a doctor to pass through the door first. After class, one of the students came up to me and said, 'Miss ———, I can see why I should stop to let someone like you go through a door ahead of me, but I can't understand why doctors should go first. I was taught that gentlemen should wait for ladies.' So I had to explain to her that not only do men show their respect for ladies in this way, but also that we show respect for other people in similar ways. I explained to her that not only are the doctors older than she and entitled to respect on that account, but that they *contribute more to the community* than she will and hence deserve respect for this reason, too."

Of special interest in our present discussion is the deference which makes nurses "bow out of the picture" when physicians are present. In its most typical form, it involves the nurse stepping back out of the picture if a doctor enters into the conversation which may be going on between a third party and herself. It also is seen in a tendency for nurses to speak only when called upon in formal sessions (such as ward rounds) in which physicians are present.[14]

The average nurse expresses a strong sense of mingled respect and fear of the doctor. This was spontaneously reported by ten of the twenty-two graduate nurses interviewed. As one nurse put it, "You have to be pretty 'Yes sirrish' to the Visiting Staff—they demand a lot of respect." And another pointed out that practically "everyone doesn't like some of the doctors and are afraid of those they don't like." This attitude is most marked among the students, although as one senior pointed out, fear of the physician tends to pass away as increased experience is gained. Nonetheless, six of the

seven students interviewed reported that their relations with doctors tended to be tense and fear-laden. As one put it, "You have so much respect for them that you watch yourself and listen for what they say to get it right."

What may be said of the nurse's relationship to the doctor may be said—in somewhat attenuated form—of the nonprofessional personnel. As one old janitor put it, "I just keep out of their way . . . I wish they'd put a sign on those doc's backs so I'd know when they're coming my way." On a somewhat more sophisticated level, a male aide, in explaining that in his contacts with the doctors he never initiates conversation unless he has to ask for information, said, "We have respect for the doctors and realize that they are in a different circle than we are." At the same time, many of the menial employees express their respect for the doctors in their almost pathetic pride that "the doctors are real nice and speak to me when they see me in the hall."

Paramedical professionals—and particularly the laboratory technicians—fail to show this general deference for physicians to the same degree. This independence seems to be based both on the fact that these people are removed from the ward and its line of clinical authority for much of each working day and upon their status as technical specialists to whom physicians refer particular problems or tests for analysis and solution. As one technician put it, "Technicians can talk to them straighter; they will talk back to the doctors and not let them browbeat them." Another explained the situation by the fact that "the doctors are more polite to us and take our word more than on the floor where they rule supreme." This lack of deference to the doctor allows the technicians to "take them for what they are." As one put it, "Eighty-five to ninety per cent of the doctors are in a cloud. They walk around in another world of medicine alone and are absent-minded about other things. 'Oh, he's a bird' is a favorite expression of ours that more or less sums up how

[14] This enforced deference to the status of the physician continues to be observed—and expected—despite a marked decrease in the formality of the doctor-nurse relationship during the past few years.

we feel about them." It is perhaps not surprising that several of the physicians interviewed spoke spontaneously of the "snippiness" and "impertinence" of the technicians.

While the doctor may walk in splendid isolation behind the walls of deference his superior knowledge and authority have built up, the position of the nurse as supervisor of non-professional ward workers means that she must be in interaction with them to some degree; the testimony of several nurses to the effect that they have to "talk and talk" to these workers in order to make them perform effectively indicates that this purely "supervisory" interaction accounts for a substantial proportion of the on-the-job conversations between the groups. Most nurses, moreover, consider auxiliary nursing personnel as part of the ward family, and a good deal of chit-chat certainly goes on between the groups. The comment of one male aide, however, throws light on what may motivate some of this informal conversation: "When they want something done, they consider you as an equal; at other times, no."

There is evidence, furthermore, that the amount of informal interaction which takes place between nurses and non-professional personnel tends to vary according to the status of the nurse involved. Thus almost all the non-professional ward employees interviewed agreed that a head nurse is more difficult to speak with than are other nurses. As one male aide put it, "The head nurses make you jump through the hoop. I wouldn't have the confidence to talk to them as I would to the other nurses on the ward."

In any case, there is little doubt that the higher status of the nurse affects both the content and quality of her informal conversation with non-professional personnel. Jealous of professional properties, she may sometimes be somewhat abrupt in her insistence that everything "be in apple-pie order." The effect of this is to make nonprofessional people shy away from her. As one supervisor put it, "The nurses and head nurses are not inclined to have much to do with our people. They feel above them. And our folks, once rebuffed, do not try to make

friends again." And one of the auxiliary personnel spoke for himself in saying "You don't like to be dirt under people's feet. Working with the nurses isn't too pleasant, and I avoid them when they act that way."

The status differences just discussed involve both those set up by the hospital as an institution and those of the larger society. Typical differences in education and socio–economic background differentiate doctors from nurses, other paramedical professionals, and from non-professional workers. These differences—between upper-middle, lower-middle and lower class persons—in themselves are apt to minimize communication. Moreover, there are a series of age and sex differentials which complicate the situation as well. Thus, for example, while free and easy communication might be difficult for a student nurse and a senior Visiting Staff physician, it might be both easy and attractive to the same student and an interne.

While such differences may either reinforce or mitigate the effects of the hospital status system, two other factors act to reinforce them. One of these lies at the very basis of the status system itself. This depends upon differential kinds of training for various groups of personnel. And these various levels of training involve both jargons of their own and differences of emphasis which seriously inhibit communication between groups. Naturally, this tendency to difficulty on the part of one group in understanding others is most marked among those of lower status categories. Most non-professional workers cannot understand much of what the doctor says when he is speaking on his own technical level. And even though nurses may understand the gist of what physicians say, they miss many of the fine points. They very frequently report their contacts with a doctor in terms of his explaining something to them. But what is true with respect to understanding of the doctor by other groups tends to a lesser extent to be true with relation to jargons and special emphases of all other occupational groups. Even though one may understand in general what the other fellow is talking about, it is difficult to grasp its full significance unless one has "seen the system from the inside."

Furthermore, interaction between occupational groups tends to be severely formalized. Doctors and especially nurses feel that their behavior on the ward should be strictly "professional"—an attitude that tends to limit the scope of communication to necessary, job-relevant considerations. Much of the communication necessary to coordinate the work of the therapeutic team takes place in formal conferences of one sort or another—ward rounds, "report" conferences, and the like. And prescriptions of physicians for patient care must normally be written in the "order book" rather than simply being given in the course of conversation. On the one hand, this rule guards against verbal error or misconceptions concerning what the doctor wishes done. On the other, it sometimes acts to relieve the doctor of any necessity for verbal interaction with the nurses. As one nurse put it.

"Too often the doctors simply come in, see their patients, write orders in the order book, and leave without our knowing they have ever been around. This means that we must constantly check through the order book to see if any orders have been written up that we don't know about."

Yet if certain of the activities of the hospital tend sharply to restrict interaction across occupational lines, a few of them tend to break down these barriers. It is likely that younger personnel—and particularly those new to the ward situation—perceive status distinctions less sharply than others. (And, sometimes, as between young physicians and nurses, a romantic interest adds its stimulus to communication!) Moreover, interesting cases—particularly those involving important persons or particularly dramatic medical problems—become a common source of interest to all personnel. It has been suggested that a good index of the degree to which a worker is integrated into the life of a ward might be the extent to which he learns about such cases.

Interestingly enough, the interaction across occupational lines seems to be best developed in surgical units. It is characteristic of surgical procedures that they require intense cooperation between physicians and nurses. It might therefore be expected that operating rooms are thus places in which members of these groups might be especially likely to communicate freely with each other.[15]

According to our informants, the preliminary stages of an operation and the final "sewing up" stage are times in which there is a good deal of joking and chit-chat among surgeons, anesthetists and nurses. On the other hand, during delicate portions of operations or at times of crisis, interaction may either subside to a minimal series of orders—"scalpel . . . sponge . . ."—or explode in fits of anger. It seems to us that the tension involved in surgery accounts for much of this ambivalent character of operating room interaction. On the one hand, much of the horse-play and joking acts as a tension-reducer; on the other, the surgeon who shows his temper during an operation does so largely because of the tension that his concern for his patient and his difficult technique have built up within him. At the same time, the fact that in the operating room the patient is usually unconscious seems of great importance. And Parsons[16] has shrewdly observed that one of the major reasons medical men are loath to allow laymen to witness operations is that they do not wish them to observe the joking and small talk that goes on during an operation which may involve the life of an acquaintance of the observer.

3. The Ideology of Hospital Workers

Thus far, two of the essentials for integration of a group have been discussed with respect to the situation on a typical hospital

[15] This need of the surgeon for assistance from the nurse carries over into the surgical ward, where it is very common for a doctor to ask for a nurse's help in technical procedures, in removing and replacing dressings, etc. These collaborations occur somewhat less frequently on medical wards. The result is that there tends to be more interaction between surgeons and nurses than between internists and nurses.

[16] Parsons, T., *The Social System*. New York: Free Press, 1951, chapter X.

ward. It has been shown that there are real barriers to communication between ward workers which tend to follow occupational and status lines. More briefly, it has been pointed out that lines of authority on the hospital ward tend to overlap because of the existence of both administrative and clinical chains of command. The matter of the extent of agreement between members concerning common purposes and pre-suppositions remains to be discussed.

We may expect that members of any group will develop a body of beliefs which serve as a rationale for their behavior within the group. Insofar as these ideas are directed toward the aim and character of the group itself, they may be called an "institutional ideology."[17] What is the nature of this ideology at Yankee Hospital? Do personnel have similar beliefs about their hospital? Or do their ideologies follow the lines of cleavage manifested in the ward social structure?

It is a sociological truism that barriers to communication within a group tend to foster the development of disparate attitudes and patterns of behavior among members. Homans has formulated this idea positively,[18] "the more frequently persons interact with one another, the more alike in some respects both their activities and their sentiments tend to become." If occupational status differences have the significance indicated above, therefore, each major occupational grouping in the hospital ought to have a distinctive ideology.

We may begin this analysis with an investigation of opinions of Yankee Hospital personnel concerning the aims and purposes of their institution. Study of the operations of the hospital, of its historical development, and of its stated aims revealed *five* broad ends or purposes for which it exists—and for the fulfillment of which its personnel are presumably to work. The oldest and most

[17] On the sociological use of the concept "ideology," see for example, K. Mannheim, *Ideology and Utopia*. (1936), p. 63 *et passim*, and R. T. LaPiere, *Sociology*, (1946), pp. 285 ff. Compare the concept of "charter" in Malinowski, *op. cit.*

[18] Homans, *op. cit.*, p. 120.

basic of these, of course, is the primal purpose of *giving care to its patients*. A second, in which the hospital has been engaged for more than eighty years is the *education of personnel* through formal programs—an aim so comprehensive it now touches at least eight health service occupations. A third purpose, much emphasized in the last twenty-five years and the watchword of the hospital's public relations program, is to be of *service to the community*—to provide health services valuable to all residents of the area whether they be sick or well. The fourth purpose, though a fond hope for years, is still largely programmatic at Yankee Hospital; this is the aim of doing *research*. The fifth purpose is common to all institutions, and may be called *instrumental*; it refers to the hospital's aim of self preservation—its "desire" to maintain the esteem of the community, to provide satisfaction to patients and employees alike, and to remain solvent.

In an effort to determine the extent to which hospital personnel perceived the basic purposes for which they cooperate, the following types of questions were asked of the seventy-five hospital people who were formally interviewed:

1. What is the purpose of Yankee Hospital? What does it exist to do? What are its basic aims?

2. What are the basic policies of the hospital directed toward? What is it aiming to accomplish now?

3. What would the hospital do if it had unlimited funds as its disposal? Why?

Responses of the interviewees to these questions were combined and analyzed according to the basic purposes to which they referred. The results are shown in Tables 24–2, 24–3 and 24–4 opposite.

These tables reveal that there is no unanimity among hospital personnel concerning what the basic aims and purposes of their institution are. It is striking how few of the well-publicized and rather obvious basic purposes could be verbalized by our interviewees—the average for all personnel was but 1.73 out of a possible score of 5.0. As might be expected, the better educated,

Table 24–2—Summary of responses made by hospital personnel concerning institutional purpose and policy

Type of Purpose or Policy	Doctors (N = 16)	Nurses (N = 29)	Other Employees (N = 30)	Total
Patient Care	20	47	37	104
Community Service	26	22	4	52
Education	36	13	7	56
Instrumental Aims	1	13	18	32
Research	2	7	3	12
	85	102	69	256

(Responses re research were omitted in computing chi square.
Chi square = 64.01, p = less than 0.001.)

Table 24–3—Percentage of personnel recognizing various institutional purposes

Type of Purpose	Doctors	Nurses	Skilled "paramedical" Personnel	Unskilled Non-prof's	All Sample
Patient Care	100.00%	82.76%	88.24%	61.54%	84.00
Community Service	43.75	41.38	11.76	0.0	28.00
Education	68.75	37.93	23.53	0.0	34.67
Research	6.25	10.34	0.0	0.0	5.33
Instrumental Aims	0.0	10.34	41.17	46.15	21.33

Table 24–4—Average number of responses of personnel concerning institutional purposes*

Optimum Expected Number	5.00
Doctors	2.19
Nurses	1.83
Other workers	1.40
(Skilled paramedical personnel)	1.64
(Other non-professional workers)	1.08
Average, all personnel	1.73

* (Computed on the basis of Question #1 only.)

higher-status personnel were better informed than their lower-status associates. But of special importance in the present connection are the systematic differences—of statistically significant quality—in the perception of basic hospital aims by the different status groups. Although the primal purpose of patient care was recognized quite universally, the doctors emphasized the highly publicized educational and community service purposes more heavily than any other group. On the other hand, the non-professionals—most dependent on its fulfillment, perhaps—were most insistent upon the importance of the hospital's instrumental aims. One is forced to conclude that status differences in the hospital are associated with diversity in the ideologies of the institutional group.

We may now characterize these ideologies in somewhat greater detail. The members of Yankee Hospital's Medical Staff who were interviewed not only elaborated a more extensive ideology than did members of other groups, but one which was qualitatively different as well.[19]

These doctors' ideology is basically conservative. New trends toward complexity of hospital organization and administration were seen by the doctors as real dangers. As one physician put it, "I guess we've got to have all these business departments, but again, there's a tremendous overgrowth. Their expansion has been terrific and out of

[19] In this and the following analyses, our purpose is to present the majority point-of-view. Not all interviewees agreed with these formulations, and they do not necessarily represent the feelings of doctors, nurses, and other hospital workers at institutions other than Yankee Hospital.

proportion to the increase in beds." Perhaps because he eschews all interest in day-to-day problems of the administration, the doctor's conception of the ideal hospital seems somewhat unrealistic. He is embarrassed by the tremendous costs of medical care, yet at the same time he inveighs against the "dollars and cents attitude" of the administration. He wants his hospital to supply all the technical facilities necessary for the most modern patient care. But though he has gotten these special services and facilities, he sometimes fails to see that it is in large part precisely these services which have complicated the work of the administration he so readily condemns as being too bureaucratic. In his emphasis on the education and community service purposes of the hospital, the average doctor has lost sight of the importance of its instrumental purpose.

Similarly, physicians tended to object to new developments leading to higher standards in the nursing curriculum. Their ideal nurse seemed to be one who faithfully serves patient and doctor without benefit of much more than a thorough practical training. One physician stated this position clearly: "The trouble with our nursing schools is that they give too much theory and too little practice." Another elaborated saying, "They're educating our nurses out of existence; there's too much of a gap between the kind of training the graduate receives and the kind of reality she faces. It has gotten to the point where some of us feel that nurses are practically becoming doctors. So they will do a beautiful technical job, but won't do such necessary things as preparing food, changing linens, and so on." The animus of the doctors is not as a rule directed primarily toward students or staff nurses. These are thought of as "good gals" whose superiors are leading them on a dangerously independent road. The doctors are almost unanimous in their indictment of supervisors and higher nursing administrators, even though they concede that these groups have improved somewhat over the years. One physician was blunt: "Heads of nursing schools are old battle-axes and don't give nurses enough responsibility."

The doctor also sees nursing as becoming unduly bureaucratic. As one physician put it, "a great deal of the brass in the nursing department is unjustified. There is too much inter-office communication and too much writing among the nurses." Or, as another said, "Many times on the ward, the patients' lights are not answered because the floor nurses have to chart, do record work, or maybe are just above nursing. The house staff have to do many procedures without nursing help even though they need it because the Training School Office just won't allow it. Their attitude is 'It's not our job'. "

These attitudes are not just those of a group which is wary of change; they are also motivated by the doctors' concern to maintain what they feel is their rightful power and prestige in the hospital. They seem to interpret much of what goes on in the hospital as directed against them. Thus several physicians remarked that always some staff members feel that "the administration is trying to put something over on us." Nine of the sixteen physicians interviewed believed that the actual center of power in the hospital was rightly in the hands of the Medical Staff. Three others gave this body a measure of authority almost equal to that of trustees and administration. And four reported that "although laymen run Yankee Hospital, this situation is (somewhat unfortunate)." As one of the doctors put it, "We doctors are frightfully fearful of direction by lay-people. But although we want our prerogatives, we don't always accept our responsibilities." Another said that "The doctors are losing their intrinsic influence in the hospital and that's bad." On the other hand, many of the physicians would agree with one who pointed out that "any administration tends to run away on half-baked tangents, but we don't let them get away with it."

The ideology of the physicians is profession-oriented in another sense. They often tend to think of the hospital as the "doctor's workshop." As one explained the basic purpose of the institution, "the hospital should be a place where a doctor can get extra care for his patients which he cannot give them in his office. It should be the place where he can get a combined consultation over and above that which he can obtain by sending them to specialists." This physician was thinking primarily of what Yankee Hospital could do to help him manage his private patients; like others, he felt that "we are lucky that the charity load has not had an enormous part in the hospital's program. The pauper load is handled at the City Hospital and elsewhere. Here, charity is properly pigeon-holed, not an inherent load which overburdens the hospital." Or, as another put it, "this hospital is directed primarily at the middle class—those who can pay their own way and are in the habit of doing it." Still another said "all kinds of people come here, but it is encouraging how many of the very rich do come to Yankee Hospital." No doubt this emphasis upon middle and upper-class patients in the minds of these physicians is related to their strong beliefs in "free enterprise in medicine."

The foregoing feelings about the charity load are carried over into the opinion of physicians about the out-patient clinic—a department of the hospital which has been little developed. In general, physicians oppose much increase in out-patient service because it "would be competing with the G.P.'s." They are frank to say that its principal justification is that it is a necessary part of the program of medical education.

There is a whole-hearted support of this program because it helps raise the standards of the medical profession as a whole. Yet many staff doctors desire a program that is oriented toward practice; there is strong opposition to the approach of "academic medicine." As one doctor put it, "Our contribution to the region lies in our ability to give excellent patient care. We would make a second- or third-rate medical school teaching hospital. I feel this is because our staff wouldn't want to teach; we don't have one iota of the medical school point of view." Or as another said, "we aim to be one of the few hospitals in the country to train good practicing doctors and not professors."

But when the physician talks of education, he refers largely to the program of *medical* education. Thus, 30 out of 36 responses of physicians concerning the hospital's educational aims had to do with training programs

for doctors. When the physician looks at the hospital, he tends to see in it only what is relevant to his own professional needs.

The physician tends also to equate good patient care with the fulfillment of his demands. In terms of clinical criteria, this equation is obvious, but it also carries over into his perceptions of hospital organization as may be seen from his attitude toward nurses and the nursing administration. The opinions of several doctors will bring out the dynamics of these attitudes.

"I feel strongly about the modern attitude of the nurses. It seems as if they've lost sight of their primary purpose—to take care of the sick and help the doctor do a better job."

Another physician saw himself and his colleagues as being at the top of a great pecking order.

"The doctors of the visiting staff want all the prerogatives of doctors—want the nurses to be valets to them and not to the patient. The staff uses the nurses, and the nurses use the trained attendants and technicians and so on."

Still another said,

"The courtesy shown by the nurses toward the doctors is improving. It has been very poor. But you can't raise too much hell about it or you lose nurses."

On the other hand, another point of view was expressed by the doctor who felt that,

"The average doctor considers the good nurse as a co-worker and not a servant. I think nurses have their real function in treating the patients' whole personality—this we can't handle."

Another believed that,

"The average doctor takes nurses as a matter of course. They are supposed to be there and do what he wants. The trouble is that we are not getting nurses who are interested in helping patients. They aren't interested in carrying bed-pans, making beds and so on. They want to be administrators."

A final change on the theme was rung by the doctor who declared that,

"Most doctors here feel that the nurses

should get their orders from the medical team and they resent supervisors and administrators as invaders of the doctor–nurse relationship."

We do not wish to impugn in any way the motives of the doctors. Like other hospital people, they have what they consider to be the best interests of their institution at heart. Their standard of ethics and intention to render good service to their patients is as unquestioned as is their competence. At the same time, as members of a profession whose status entitles them to an influential voice in determining hospital policy, it is only natural that their ideology includes provisos which aim to protect what they consider to be their legitimate interests. And because the doctors honestly seem to feel that what is good for physicians is also good for the hospital, they assert themselves in all good conscience.

The ideologies of the nurses and non-professional workers are by no means as consistent and well-developed as that of the medical staff. They have no need to be, for they perform different functions. The doctor is in a position to influence, if not to dictate, hospital policy and must have an ideology which will guide him in exerting this influence. His platform, therefore, needs to be "political" in nature. The nurses and non-professional workers, on the other hand, are not in position to influence policy to the same degree; for most of them, as hospital employees, institutional life is largely regulated by directives from above. The character of their ideology, therefore, tends to be expressive. Its functions are, on the one hand, to express those attitudes and desires which arise from the work situation and on the other hand, to justify the activities of personnel within the organization.

The status of the nurse, midway between that of the physician and most other hospital employees, is ambiguous. Hers is a professional status; nevertheless, at every turn she finds herself pressed down by the overwhelming authority and prestige of the doctor. And although her upward mobility has been blocked, her status is being more and more invaded by non-professional workers such as trained attendants. It is not surprising, then, that her ideology should cling to and emphasize her special responsibilities in the work of the hospital. In emphasizing the care of the whole patient, the nurse is staking out for herself a field of competence which, for the moment at least, seems secure from invasion.

The ideology of the nurses, moreover, is an outgrowth of the history of their profession. The very basis for the professionalization of nursing was rooted in the necessity for improving the quality of personnel who served hospital patients. In order to improve personnel, it was necessary to implant in them ideals of service of a very exalted sort; the profession of nursing thus became, in the eyes of women like Florence Nightingale, a sacred calling. Their service, from the beginning was conceived of in diffuse terms; the nurse was to minister to all the needs of the patient as ordered by the doctor. Although its verbal expression is a relatively recent development, the idea of treating the whole patient thus goes back to the beginnings of the modern profession of nursing.

This idealistic aim of treating the "whole patient" involves not merely a desire to care for the patient's mental and spiritual condition as well as for his body; it extends also to the nurses' taking full responsibility for all the care which is given to the patient (other than by the doctor). Thus as auxiliary workers increasingly relieve the nurse of the more routine tasks of patient care, the latter feels a need to take charge of their actions and see that everything is done correctly. The holistic element in the nurses' ideology thus affects her relations with other hospital employees. It has been especially noticeable in affecting the relationships between nurses and dietitians. For although the installation of the latter on the wards has relieved the nurses of a very onerous work load, the nurse resents the intrusion of the dietitian into what was originally her own sphere. One nurse justified this attitude on the grounds that "we feel we know more about patients than the dietitians do." The ideology of the nurse will not permit her easily to accept the competence of people other than herself and the doctor to deal with patients.

Because the nurses believe very strongly that the hospital is an institution dedicated to works of mercy, they do not easily accept the hard facts of medical economics. Neither does the expansion of the hospital into an organization which operates on a large scale and in an efficient, impersonal manner accord well with their ideals. As one nurse put it, "There's too much emphasis on making the patients pay. The hospital is money-mad. This makes it hard and un-idealistic." Another noted that, "The need is for supportive nursing. You're a woman, the patient is, too, and you're the liaison between her and the doctor. But we haven't time for anything except vital signs. There's too much emphasis on speed and too much mass production. Things have become too impersonal; with penicillin, much of the personal part of nursing has gone. Someone has to prove to me that all this is progress." Still another nurse noted that "The hospital is no longer the big family it once was. Conveyors and tubes have changed all that and made the hospital an impersonal place. Now, you often don't know anyone except in your own department."

For the nurse, the purpose of patient care is the outstanding aim of the hospital and all other aims are interpreted in terms of how they tie in with this basic purpose. Thus the nurses tended to interpret the community service purpose of the hospital primarily in terms of a ministry of preventive medicine, out-patient clinics, and public health education. Moreover patient care in the eyes of the nurses is not simply a matter of physical treatment. Rather it involves both "getting him well as quickly as possible, ministering to his mental and spiritual welfare as well as to his physical body." In this endeavor the nurses consider that they play the crucial role; as one said, "It is our job to care for the patient. We must try always to be friendly and treat the patient as a personality and not as an 'it' with a disease." Or as another nurse said, "the nurse has the biggest part in the work of the hospital. She has the closest contact with the patient and the first responsibility to him. Without the nurse, I don't believe we could have a hospital, just as we wouldn't have an army without soldiers. Not that the doctor isn't in the picture—he is a very close second." In an institution which has been rendered more and more impersonal by expansion and new techniques, nurses feel that they are the representatives of the human qualities, and as such, the executors of its highest ideals.

Although they consider themselves quite competent to criticize doctors' orders—which they believe are sometimes "crazy" —nurses readily agree that it is the physicians whose knowledge makes possible the healing work of the hospital. Therefore, they are willing to pay them the respect they deserve. It is the hallmark of the professional nurse to be dignified, and to have respect for "those in authority." Nurses believe that the hospital demands the highest standards of conduct on the part of its personnel; sometimes, too, they think that it is the professional employees who must bear the responsibility for maintaining these standards. As one put it, "One and all should uphold the dignity of the profession they are in. I doubt, though, if we can trust the intelligence of the laboring classes to do this."

If the ideology of the nurses is idealistic and altruistic, it is also imbued with a certain missionary zeal. It is a keystone of nursing belief that in teaching lies the way to the fulfillment of the purposes of the hospital. They are enthusiastic about the whole gamut of Yankee Hospital's teaching programs, and are tremendously concerned with the academic standards of their training school. And the nurses feel that teaching should go beyond training of health service personnel; to them, one of the principal ways in which patient care could be improved is by developing more adequate methods of teaching patients to avoid future illnesses and to live with their infirmities. In this endeavor, they feel that their concern for the "whole patient" is crucial.

Perhaps because they believe that their approach is basic to the success of the hospital, nurses are concerned about their status in the institution. As one put it, "The policy toward personnel should change. Some people still think that students should be looked down on and that the nurse is so far below the doctor that she shouldn't even be talked to." And another insisted that "the days of Florence Nightingale are gone. You can still love humanity and get paid— you have that feeling long before you think about wages." After decades of what they believe to have been little short of exploitation, nurses are beginning to feel that the instrumental purposes of the hospital should extend to employees as well as to patients.

It is this kind of thinking which characterizes the average nurse's attitude toward the hospital. She identifies herself extremely closely with it. The institution is, for her, a concrete means of making her ideals come alive in reality. Not only does it actuate her altruistic motives, but it satisfies her desire for prestige and respectability. As one put it, "Yankee Hospital is a very nice place to work, and I'd advise anyone to work here. It gives one prestige in the community to work here because of the very fine doctors who are on the staff, the nurses—who are fine women—and so forth." Yet sometimes the pressure of the work blots out both the nurse's feelings about what the hospital is and ought to be and her sense of identification with it. The work load on an under-staffed floor can make the nurse see in her job nothing but drudgery, fatigue, and techniques, and in her hospital nothing but the insistent white call lights that mean more and more work. As one nurse tiredly protested when we asked her questions concerning her ideology, "The hospital does so many things—and we're too busy to think of them. There are so many departments that you don't have time to think of. And there are so many patients to take care of and so many lights to answer that we don't know what we're doing or why we're doing it."

Thus the ideology of the nurses sometimes is honored more in the breach than in the observance. Because many think of education for their profession as "training," and of their service in terms of performing procedures properly and efficiently, it becomes difficult for these nurses to see in

their work anything but drudgery—or any compensation other than to lean on the stiff, starched proprieties of professional status.[20] And because they feel a real responsibility for the administration of the ward—and, perhaps see in this area opportunity for enhancing their status—they tend very often to emphasize administrative matters, (the execution of which is quickly recognized and controlled from above.) The more intangible matter of care for the whole patient thus sometimes becomes more a theoretical goal than an actual achievement. But all this is simply to say that it is not always possible to live up to high ideals.

The ideology of the other paramedical workers is much more fragmentary than that of the nurses. Two principal facets characterize it. On the one hand, there is a great consciousness of the service orientation which working in a hospital involves and a strong sense of identification with the institution. This generalization applies to ideological statements made by dietitians, laboratory technicians, and housekeeping employees alike. As one put it, "We are working for the patient not just for the boss. Our main object is to make the patient well and comfortable. This is vaguely in the back of all our minds. Don't I sound like I had a halo?" On the other hand, the ideology of these workers seems to be strongly focused on the technical aspects of hospital operation —on how best to do their job, on the physical facilities which characterize the hospital and on how to make it run more efficiently. While the dietitians and technicians and unskilled workers largely tend to see only the problems of their own occupation as needing attention, their overall interest is strongly centered upon the instrumental purpose of the institution. Because they feel proud to be a part of it they want to help it. The non-skilled worker particularly tends to make the more dramatic technical operations of the hospital the symbol of its work. On the other hand, the dietitians tend to think of it in administrative terms.

Most employees wish naturally for better hours and higher pay. However, there is

[20] Devereux, G., and F. R. Wiener, "The Occupational Status of Nurses," *American Sociological, Review* 15:628–634, October, 1950.

little tendency toward a "union" point of view. Even the menial employees are acutely conscious of the financial limitations under which the institution operates. As one put it, "with conditions as they are, they do about as well as they can. If they had more money, they would do more. We read in the paper about their terrible expenses and how they work to overcome them." And they are conscious, too, of the financial plight of hospital patients; "There's one thing I don't like: many patients are injured and keep talking about how the credit office asks for money the first thing they come in. They have to charge enough anyway." For these reasons, there is not a strong feeling among employees that management is exploiting them. There is a general realization on their part that higher wages are available elsewhere. But such intangible advantages as security and the satisfaction of "helping people" mean more to them than the increased salaries they could earn on the "outside."

There are, of course, differences in the ideology of the paramedical and nonprofessional employees. The interesting thing, however, is that the broad outlines of the ideology of the male aid is rather like that of the laboratory technician; and the janitor believes much the same sort of thing as does the dietitian. The skilled employees, of course, have an ideology which possesses greater scope and refinement than that of the unskilled employees, but both groups build upon their identification with the hospital's purpose of patient care and their concern for the achievement of its instrumental aims.

The three basic ideologies which we found among hospital personnel each tends to have its own organizing theme. Thus, the doctors conceive of a hospital as an institution whose basic function is to help the medical profession in its efforts to provide the best possible medical care. And the nurses feel strongly that the hospital is an institution which should minister to the health of an entire community in the spirit of altruistic service; this ministry in their eyes should be directed toward the "whole patient." Finally, other ward workers tend to believe that service to patients subsumes

the whole aim of the hospital; to them, it is a miracle-working institution to which they are willing to dedicate their working hours, and the instrumental aims of which they are greatly concerned to see achieved. There is unity among all groups concerning the tremendous importance of good patient service in the life of the hospital. But there is a great deal of difference among the groups as to the implications of this primal purpose. And the way in which these implications are conceived constitutes the core of the ideology of each group, and helps determine its actions within the institution.

Conclusion—There are in the hospital certain tendencies which appear to set limits upon the degree to which integration of the organization's personnel can take place. It has been shown that communication tends to be for the most part channeled within occupational lines, giving rise to a tendency for those who work together on the wards to know and associate principally with those of their "own kind." Associated with this tendency to isolation on the part of the various occupational status-groups is a set of disparate institutional ideologies. Each group expressed divergent ideas concerning hospital purpose and policy, and these attitudes point up areas of latent conflict between the groups. These tendencies, together with the strain imposed by a dual hierarchy of authority upon the hospital ward, may go far to explain much of the tension which from time to time appears in hospitals.

But one should not dwell solely on the negative implications of hospital social structure. Diversity of opinion can be productive of new approaches which would otherwise be difficult to conceive; each of the institutional ideologies depicted above gives emphasis to an integral part of Yankee Hospital's mission which might otherwise tend to be obscured. Similarly, considerations of efficiency and interest justify much of the tendency of hospital personnel to interact primarily with members of their own group. And it is hard to see how the execution of clinical needs of patients can ever be fully rationalized into the hospital's administrative chain of command without endangering the quality of medical care.

What can be said is that these structural tendencies cannot be taken for granted without risking the snowballing of legitimate differences of interest and approach into major misunderstandings. Moreover, they must not only be recognized and acknowledged but held within limits. Hospital workers—like participants in any other division of labor—do constitute an interdependent team. And teamwork demands the free contribution of all those involved. Rigidity of status, undue limitation of intergroup communication, and unresolved differences of opinion can be disruptive. There is need in the hospital, as in every institution, for tolerance and understanding of why others behave as they do.

25

IT MAY BE ASSUMED that all forms of social participation are the outcome of actions and attitudes directed toward or extracted from an environment of persons, things and symbols. On this assumption three broad principles can be seen to follow: (1) The greater the similarity between the environment of persons, things and symbols and the participant's actions and attitudes, the more likely is he to remain within it. (2) The more constant or enduring the relation between the environment of persons, things and symbols and the participant's actions and attitudes, the more likely is he to remain within it. (3) The closer or more intimate the relation between the environment of persons, things and symbols and the participant's actions and attitudes, the more likely is he to remain within it.

The first principle summarizes the many respects in which participants may be characterized as similar, alike or identical to one another and their environments. It is equivalent to any statement which suggests some form of equity between human beings and their life situations. Thus, if the reality, appearance or style of environmental relationships are such as to lend coherence to participants' activities, they will strive to maintain them. Under these conditions significant elements of comparability and openness obtain. The absence of such elements is best described by social relations which separate or differentiate participants from the dominant features of their environment, including other people. Thus, participants who feel alien, act in devious ways or frequently experience the impact of discordant circumstances are quicker to withdraw from their surroundings. This withdrawal is hastened for those whose capacity to discriminate among disparate aspects of life leads them to view themselves in highly individualistic ways.

The second principle highlights the common notion that change begets change. The more transient the persons, things and symbols in the participant's environment, the more frequently will he seek new associations. Those who have reason for believing

A General Theory of Labor Turnover in Hospitals

Llewellyn Gross,
Elliott H. Grosof
and
Constantine A. Yeracaris

that their environment will not endure, that their relations with surrounding events will not persist, are continually receptive to new possibilities. Unencumbered by ties which hold people to permanent social locales, they manifest strong tendencies to evade or escape their present situation. Since they move about frequently, they seem at all times prepared for physical and social mobility.

The third principle takes as its guideline the spatial metaphor of nearness or closeness. It assumes that participants are encouraged to maintain those relations among persons and things which are central to their worlds of experience. When social contacts are frequent and intense, when participants are in continuous propinquity and not dispersed through a wide region, their impact on the actions of others is sufficiently strong to reinforce mutual attachments. The shift, then, to new worlds beyond current experience is less acceptable.[1]

[1] The three principles of similarity, constancy and closeness (or difference, inconstancy and distance) overlap in meanings and, for this reason, cannot be sharply distinguished. However, some common sense distinctions can be offered. Difference and dissimilarity may be

This report is part of a study sponsored by the Division of Hospital and Medical Facilities of the United States Public Health Service (Grant no. HM-00123). The authors wish to acknowledge the assistance of Mr. Walter C. Hobbs and Miss Nina Pane Pinto.

Though global in their implications, these principles rest upon the simplest perceptual foundation, the elementary capacity to discriminate between things which are alike or different, changing or unchanging and distant or close at hand. Upon such fundamental notions the classic concepts of sociology are grounded. Thus, the early American sociologist Cooley defined primary group by referring to (1) face-to-face association, (2) intimacy, (3) permanence, (4) unspecialized associations and (5) the small number of persons comprising it.[2] Face-to-face association and intimacy are exemplifications of closeness in respect to physical and social distance. Permanence is an exemplification of constancy and absence of specialization an exemplification of similarity or likeness. The size of the group is less clearly an exemplification than a condition of both likeness and nearness. Large groups are bound to be more heterogeneous and less intimate insofar as participants are unable to have repeated contacts with the same persons at similar points.[3]

In Weber's analysis, primary groups consist of social relations based on the subjective feeling of belonging together.[4] They are contrasted to secondary groups based on a rationally motivated balance of interests. The phrase "belonging together" suggests likeness and the spatial metaphor of closeness just as "balance of interests"

suggests the reconciliation of differences. Similarly, Toennies' concepts of *Gemeinschaft* and *Gesellschaft*,[5] the one referring to traditional, face-to-face, intimate group organization, the other to emancipated, contractual and impersonal group organization, place elements of constancy and closeness in opposition to those of distance and difference. Note especially that a contractual relation calls to mind an agreement based on the resolution of diverse interests.

For most sociologists "locality" suggests spatial restrictions and hence the idea of constancy, propinquity or nearness and, on occasion, similarity. Thus, Simmel[6] suggested that the persistence of groups depends upon permanency of locality and common symbols (constancy, likeness and, perhaps, closeness, are combined). Sanderson[7] held that propinquity and physical proximity mean greater interpersonal influence and Ross[8] classified all groups into local, likeness and interest groups. In the present formulation, interest groups may be taken as a possible opposite of local and likeness groups.

Of particular relevance here is the probability that many of the more intangible concepts of sociology are mixed interpretations of those discussed above. Faris,[9] for instance, finds the intimate relations of primary groups manifested in group consciousness, *esprit de corps* and we-feeling (cases of closeness in likeness). And for Sumner,[10] in-groups—typically associated with closeness—are characterized by the likeness of we-feeling, group loyalty, sacrifice and comradeship. These concepts are not comprehensible without assuming certain similarities of thought and feeling among the individual members comprising a group.

present in relatively unchanging societies, as witness, for instance, the diverse positions and roles of those included in the ancient castes of India and in the slave system of the early South. Per contra, similarity and likeness may be present in societies subject to rapid social change. Thus aspirations and patterns of behavior were very similar in the Western regions of the United States during most of the nineteenth century and in Europe between the two great wars. In brief, similarity and difference may arise in either a rapidly changing or relatively stable society.

[2] Cooley, C. H., *Social Organization*, New York: Scribners, 1937.

[3] Chapin, S., *Contemporary American Institutions*, New York: Harper and Brothers, 1935.

[4] Weber, M., *The Theory of Social and Economic Organization*, trans. by A. M. Henderson and T. Parsons, ed. with Introduction by T. Parsons, New York: The Free Press, 1947.

[5] Toennies, F., *Fundamental Concepts of Sociology*, trans. by C. Loomis, Princeton, N.J.: van Nostrand, 1940.

[6] Simmel, G., *The Sociology of Georg Simmel*, trans., ed. and with introduction by K. H. Wolff, New York: Free Press, 1950.

[7] Sanderson, D., "Group Description," *Social Forces*, 16:309–319, March, 1938.

[8] Ross, E. A., *Principles of Sociology*, 3d ed., New York: Appleton-Century, 1938.

[9] Faris, E., "The Primary Group: Essence or Accident," *Amer. J. Sociology*, 38:41–50, July, 1932.

[10] Sumner, W. G., *Folkways*, Boston: Ginn, 1906.

Group consciousness, *esprit de corps*, group loyalty, sacrifice and comradeship suggest a social union based on similar purposes. They depend upon powers of attraction among participants, hence a close association.

It is apparent from the above that many of the most widely used terms in sociology carry within their meanings the connotation of likeness, similarity or identity, of constancy, durability or persistence and of nearness, closeness or proximity. Consider, additionally, the relevance of these connotations for the sociologist's use of "cohesion," "solidarity," "social norms," "collective behavior" and "mass society." Their antonyms include such terms as anomie, alienation, conflict, estrangement, social isolation and social deviance—in brief, ideas which typically emphasize difference, distance and change. Of course, the latent meanings of "similarity," "constancy" and "closeness" extend beyond any simple list of synonyms, antonyms, analogies and contrasting words. Advantageous as such a list is for purposes of "empirical" research it cannot define the precise boundaries of general principles. This is both inevitable and desirable. Unless the scope of principles provides room for the growth of new interpretations, discoveries arising from the latest research cannot be subsumed under them.

Confronted with a lexicon of terms which vary from the indeterminate to the nearly determinate, the meaning of each expression must rest, at least in part, upon linguistic contexts. From the broadest possible perspective, "similarity" means any kind of likeness, uniformity, comparability, analogy or affinity. By contrast, "difference" suggests some kind of departure, divergence or deviation or any noticeable degree of distinction, discrepancy or disparity. Thus, logical inconsistency, the psychological exercise of strong propensities and antipathies and the sociological manifestation of group discord may be included as relevant indexes.

The most prominent synonyms of "constancy" are permanence, persistence and preservation. Their antonyms include impermanence, transience and perishability. That constancy and similarity are not mutually exclusive is apparent in the meanings shared by some of their antonyms. Words like variation, modification, alteration, conversion, revision, transformation and fluctuation connote both inconstancy and difference.

Finally, "closeness" suggests any relationship characterized by frequent or repeated social contact, contiguity, adjacency or near coincidence in physical, psychological or social distance. On some occasions the term suggests compactness or density of social response. When its meaning spreads to the idea of firmness or consolidation of social components, its usage is not unlike that of "constancy." Thus "closeness" seems to be a descriptive term in some contexts and a metaphorical one in others. Contrariwise, "distance" suggests remoteness from the center of reference; by selecting appropriate shifts in synonyms it may be seen to merge into "difference" and then into "inconstancy," with which it has vernacular affinity.

Following is a general summary of the results of a large-scale study of hospital employees designed to test the hypotheses that were generated by the foregoing theories and conceptualizations related to hospital labor turnover. (Space limitations prevent presenting the methodological details of our research.)

Application to Labor Turnover

Our theory of labor turnover holds that those who are quickest to move from job to job are those whose group ties are *different*, *inconstant* and *distant* in one or another of the shifting interpretations of these terms. Our major task, then, is to develop the meaning of such terms within a framework of general principles and empirical findings on labor turnover.

(1) It may be noted, to begin with, that youthful males of single marital status differ from the general population of older married males and females. The institutional constraints against mobility increase for

those who are older with children to support. For the youthful and unmarried, environmental demands are less persistent since they have fewer social responsibilities. Without close ties to family and community they can turn more easily from one job to another. Being physically and socially *mobile* they contribute more than their share to labor turnover. (See Table 25–1 for summarization of data.)

(2) A second set of conditions contributing to labor turnover is evident in the job history of participants. Those participants who differed from the average insofar as they worked for the first time or had a comparatively large number of previous jobs were less likely to find satisfaction in their hospital job. This divergent result not only follows from the statistical data in question but is consistent with the expectation that those of previously short employment and *fluctuating* socio–economic status will be less satisfied than those whose employment status has remained unchanged. (For summarization of data see Table 25–2.)

(3) A third set of conditions favoring labor turnover is the number and size of towns in which participants resided prior to coming to the hospital. It may be assumed that those born in the southern region of the United States lived under circumstances less conducive to mobility than those born in the Northeast or those who lived in western regions of the United States. No doubt, the more mobile group of participants were subject to more variable life conditions, including differentiated social stimuli, than those coming from relatively homogeneous environments. Accustomed to responding to diverse kinds of experiences they are more often isolated from close group and community contacts. Thus, the impact of *difference* and *distance* along with *inconstancy* seems to affect labor turnover (see Table 25–3).

(4) Demographic factors reflecting combinations of the three principles include the relationship of labor turnover to white racial status, to high formal education, to membership in the Catholic church and to homogeneity of birthplace for workers and relatives. In addition to being more mobile, those who are white and of higher formal education are subject to a wider range of social stimuli than are other categories of people. They are more often called upon to express their individuality, a consequence which sometimes leads to feelings of individual separateness, the most extreme forms of which are *alienation*. Generally, membership in the Catholic church is a cohesive factor contributing to personal stability but, in the context of a predominantly Protestant hospital cohesion accentuates the differences between Catholics and others. As members of an out-group they must work with situations and personalities which contrive to keep them at some distance from others. A similar principle seems to be operative for those who have the same birthplace as relatives—an anomalous occurrence in a world where mobile families generally have diverse birthplaces. For religion and homogeneity of birthplace, *closeness* among members of the out-group appears to be correlated with *distance* from members of the in-group. (See Table 25–4 for summarization of data.)

(5) Less easily explained is the empirical discovery that both the absence of hospitalization experience and its failure to influence decisions for hospital employment contribute to labor turnover. This result appears to be further confused when relatives' hospitalization together with incidence of other kinds of hospital employment for relatives and friends is found to contribute to labor turnover. Nevertheless, these associations may, each and all, follow from the unfavorable influence of both absent and indirect hospitalization experiences on participants' responses in their work situation. If, to the inexperienced participant, hospitalization was reputed to be undesirable, he may have entered hospital work with a predisposition to leave. Under these circumstances, personal isolation together with negative responses to relatives' hospitalization and work experience—indices, respectively, of social *distance* and social *difference*—may have combined to produce labor turnover (see Table 25–5).

(6) The preceding interpretation is rein-

Table 25–1—Turnover rates by age, sex, marital status and parental status

Rates (per 100 Participants)

					Sig. Level
Age	Under 24 years	(38.0)	Over 24 years	(18.8)	< 0.001
Sex	Males	(35.1)	Females	(23.2)	< 0.001
Marital Status	Single	(32.2)	Nonsingle	(20.8)	< 0.001
Parental Status	No children	(30.8)	Children	(19.6)	< 0.001

Table 25–2—Turnover rates by number of previous jobs, length of previous employment, previous occupational status and intergenerational mobility

Rates (per 100 Participants)

					Sig. Level
Number of Previous Jobs	None, 3 or more	(26.9)	1–2	(20.4)	< 0.01
Length of Previous Employment	1 yr. or less	(27.4)	1 yr. or more	(20.8)	< 0.05
Previous Occupational Status*	High	(24.8)	Low	(20.3)	< 0.05
Intergenerational Mobility**	Mobile***	(28.3)	Stable	(23.0)	< 0.05

*U.S. Bureau of the Census, *1950 Census of Population, Alphabetical Index of Occupations and Industries*, rev. ed., Washington, D.C., 1950.
**Measured in terms of a comparison between respondent's index of occupational status and father's index of occupational status: Cf. A. Reiss, *et al.*, *Occupations and Social Status*, New York: Free Press, 1: . pp. 263–275.
***Includes both upwardly and downwardly mobile participants.

Table 25–3—Turnover rates by place of birth in U.S., size of town or city, number of towns lived in and prior residence in U.S.

Rates (per 100 Participants)

					Sig. Level
Place of Birth in U.S.	Other Regions	(26.4)	South	(11.0)	< 0.001
Size of Town or City	More than 50,000	(28.3)	Less than 50,000	(20.6)	< 0.001
Number of Towns Lived	Two or more	(27.9)	One	(22.8)	< 0.05
Prior Residence in U.S.	Other Regions	(26.1)	South	(12.0)	< 0.001

Table 25–4—Turnover rates by race, education, spouse education, religion and nativity

Rates (per 100 Participants)

					Sig. Level
Race	White	(27.1)	NonWhite	(12.8)	< 0.001
Education	College or more	(28.6)	H.S. or less	(21.4)	< 0.01
Spouse Education	College or more	(25.7)	H.S. or less	(18.9)	< 0.05
Religion	Catholic	(27.6)	Protestant	(21.0)	< 0.02
Nativity*	Homogeneous	(26.5)	Heterogeneous	(22.4)	< 0.05**

*Place of birth of respondent, parents and spouse's parents.
**One-tailed.

Table 25–5—Turnover rates by participants' hospitalization, influence of participants' or relatives' hospitalization, relatives' hospitalization, employment of distant relatives by other hospitals and employment of friends by other hospitals

Rates (per 100 Participants)

					Sig. Level
Participants' Hospitalization	No	(28.0)	Yes	(22.8)	< 0.05*
Influence of Participants' or Relatives' Hospitalization	High	(14.7)	Low	(25.5)	< 0.02
Relatives' Hospitalization	Yes	(25.0)	No	(18.8)	< 0.05*
Employment of Distant Relatives by Other Hospitals	Yes	(29.3)	No	(22.9)	< 0.05
Employment of Friends by Other Hospitals	Yes	(25.1)	No	(22.6)	ns

*One-tailed.

forced with evidence that participants who feel distant from patients and co-workers are quicker to leave hospital employment. Thus, those who feel their primary obligation is to the job rather than the patient as well as those who deny any relationship between social distance from patients and hospital performance are highest in labor turnover. More surprising is the apparent relationship between greater satisfaction received from attending private patients *vis-à-vis* ward patients and labor turnover. However, on the assumption that this reaction represents the individualized responses of those who lack identification with the broader problems of a common humanity, it accords well with our principles. The more alienated person finds it difficult to embrace within his sympathies the undifferentiated needs and problems of many others. Perhaps this is the reason why he is less able to give personal services to all or to participate in recreation and other forms of entertainment directed to a group in which everyone is similarly included. The factor of particularized envolvement—never fully satisfactory—rather than generalized attachment to others may account for his greater readiness to accept unconditionally extra job orders from supervisors and his greater devotion to organization-centered rather than patient-centered activities. Perhaps some participants are incapable or indisposed to identify strongly with any human response, individual or group. Such a reaction might be expected from those who describe both actual and ideal supervisors as traditional rather than bureaucratic, charismatic or affectional. But this interpretation depends upon the viewpoint taken by hospital employees of the word "traditional." The interpretation follows only if "traditional" means "ritualistic" and not "bureaucratic." (For summarization of data see Table 25–6.)

(7) The combination of *social distance* and *individual difference* suggested by *weak identification* reappears in several sets of responses found among participants who fall in the labor turnover group. This group denies the importance of helping co-workers with personal problems or of protecting co-workers against supervisors. They work harder than their co-workers and take extreme views on the relationship between effective supervision and social distance. They disagree more frequently with their supervisors and deny that people think of nursing as tender, loving care. They have little empathy for persons who are physically handicapped, without friends and a home or saddened by personal loss. However, they appear to have more empathy for persons who are either upset by family relations or dependent upon others for help. Is the latter type of empathy a species of self-pity, a reflection of personalized feelings stemming from social isolation? This questionable speculation is suggested by the inability of the group to empathize with persons who differ markedly from themselves, to exercise the kind of empathy which depends upon "acquaintance" rather than "intimacy." That widespread empathy is probably not a strong characteristic of the turnover group is further evidenced by the fact that they express a preference for certain job activities over others, even an antipathy for some, and see themselves as making sacrifices. Indeed, the fact that they elected hospital employment for rational reasons or for reasons of having been sent there or accepted there and that they found the quality of hospital employment below expectations count against the interpretation of strong empathies for this group (see Table 25–7).

(8) A major expression of the principle of difference is exemplified in the capacity of the turnover group to recognize distinctions not apparent to those more stable. The former show greater discrimination in naming hospital departments, indicate preference for particular jobs and have plans for working elsewhere in five years. Typically, they are in communication with a larger number of hospital departments and take a more relativistic view of sociocultural practices. In addition, there are certain employment conditions which contribute not only to the *difference* and *distance* of this group from others but also to their own *impermanence*. Especially worth mentioning is their relatively short, and

Table 25–6—Turnover rates by obligation to job, primacy of patients, high social distance from patient, preference for private patients, type of previous job, submission to authority, experimental satisfaction, actual supervisor and ideal supervisor

	Rates (per 100 Participants)				Sig. Level
Obligation to Job	Strong	(33.3)	Weak	(23.7)	ns
Primacy of Patient	Weak	(25.7)	Strong	(18.7)	< 0.02
High Social Distance from Patient	Undesirable	(27.6)		(22.4)	< 0.05
Preference for Private Patients	Strong	(24.3)	Weak	(18.3)	ns
Type of Previous Job	Other Types	(24.7)	Personnel, Recreational–Entertainment	(18.6)	< 0.05 *
Submission to Authority	High	(25.0)	Low	(22.0)	ns
Experimental Satisfaction	Organization–centered	(23.6)	Patient-centered	(21.0)	ns
Actual Supervisor	Traditional	(26.8)	Bureaucratic, Charismatic or Affectual	(19.0)	< 0.01
Ideal Supervisor	Traditional	(25.7)	Bureaucratic, Charismatic or Affectual	(18.7)	< 0.01

*One-tailed.

Table 25–7—Turnover rates by aiding co-worker, protecting co-worker, "rate-busting," social distance from supervisor, agreement with supervisor, evaluation of nursing role, empathetic orientation, preference in job, antipathy to job, sacrifices, reasons for choosing hospital work, job evaluation and reasons for choosing a particular hospital

	Rates (per 100 Participants)				Sig. Level
Aiding Co-worker	Negative	(27.0)	Positive–Ambivalent	(22.4)	< 0.05 *
Protecting Co-worker	Non-protective	(28.3)	Protective–Ambivalent	(21.7)	< 0.02
"Rate-busting"	Negative	(25.0)	Positive–Ambivalent	(17.1)	< 0.02
Social Distance from Supervisor	Positive–Negative	(23.9)	Ambivalent	(13.0)	< 0.05 *
Agreement with Supervisor	Disagree	(27.2)	Agree	(22.3)	< 0.05 *
Evaluation of Nursing Role as Maternal	Weak	(24.4)	Strong	(13.9)	< 0.05
Empathetic Orientation					
Physically Handicapped	Non-empathetic	(22.8)	Empathetic	(10.9)	< 0.05 *
Without Real Friends	Non-empathetic	(23.1)	Empathetic	(10.3)	< 0.05
Without a Home	Non-empathetic	(25.2)	Empathetic	(9.3)	< 0.01
Loss of a Loved One	Non-empathetic	(28.9)	Empathetic	(16.7)	< 0.05 *
Upset by Family Relations	Empathetic	(25.5)	Non-empathetic	(8.2)	< 0.01
Dependent on Others	Empathetic	(24.8)	Non-empathetic	(11.8)	< 0.05
Preference for Specific Job Activities	Yes	(28.3)	No	(18.4)	< 0.001
Antipathy to Job Activities	Yes	(30.2)	No	(20.1)	< 0.001
Sacrifices	Present	(26.9)	Absent	(22.3)	< 0.05 *
Reasons for Choosing Hospital Work	Rational Reasons	(26.1)	Other Reasons	(18.6)	< 0.05 *
Job Evaluation	Below Expectations	(39.1)	Above Expectations	(23.4)	< 0.01
Reasons for Choosing a Particular Hospital	Accepted or Sent	(29.3)	Other Reasons	(21.6)	< 0.02

*One-tailed.

often part-time, employment in the hospital and their predominance in, and dissatisfaction with, the later work shifts. As previously suggested, and by his own admission, the turnover participant is not fully satisfied with his hospital job. (For summarization of data see Table 25–8.)

unify rather than divide. The same kind of consideration applies to occupational groups, where, let us say, there may be *similarity* and *constancy* without *closeness*. In such groups, interaction may obtain without a high degree of mutual support (closeness between members may be absent). Again, a strongly democratic organization may be tied together by the kind of unity which *constantly* maintains the right of persons to *differ*

Table 25–8—Turnover rates by departments named, occupational search, five year occupational plans, interdepartmental communication, absolute esthetic and moral standards, self-insight, humanistic values, length of employment in hospital, employment status, preference for night shift and job satisfaction

	Rates (per 100 Participants)				Sig. Level
Naming of Hospital Departments	Unspecified	(26.1)	Specified	(23.9)	ns
Occupational Search Behavior	Different Job Present	(29.8)	Absent	(20.5)	< 0.001
Five-year Occupational Plans	Work Elsewhere	(46.8)	Remain	(14.1)	< 0.001
Interdepartmental Communication	High	(25.8)	Low	(23.6)	ns
Esthetic and Moral Norms	Relativistic	(29.3)	Absolutistic	(14.2)	< 0.02
Length of Employment	Under 1 Year	(38.6)	1 Year and Over	(18.0)	< 0.001
Employment Status	Part Time	(29.0)	Full Time	(22.0)	< 0.02
Preference for Night Shift	Ambivalent–Negative	(24.7)	Positive	(8.8)	< 0.01
Shift	Evening	(29.5)	Morning/Afternoon	(22.3)	< 0.05
Job Satisfaction	Low	(30.3)	High	(14.0)	< 0.01

The Bearing of Hospital Organization on Labor Turnover

The principles of similarity, constancy and closeness are intricately woven. They converge, merge and diverge as successive patterns of interaction are formed. Although it may be assumed that they typically fall in the order of priority presented above, in many instances priorities are altered by those aspects of each principle which qualify, verbally or adjectivally, the meaning of the others. Hence, *similarity* and *difference* will be more or less prominent depending upon how fully *closeness* and *constancy* condition their expression. Family members, for instance, are known to *differ* considerably in age, sex, education, authority, etc., but when members are in *constant* and *close* communication, these *differences* serve to

among themselves in *close* (face-to-face) interactions. It can be said that they manifest "*constancy and closeness amidst difference*" or "*constancy in difference without loss of closeness.*" Of course, other possibilities arise in other kinds of situations. "*Distance in the presence of constant differences*" may arise among various social classes thrown together in an air raid shelter, tornado or major accident, where injuries are randomly distributed.

Granting the thesis that labor stability in hospitals reflects an optimum balance between similarity, constancy and closeness, what are its implications for hospital organization?

A major source of structural stress in large organizations can be described as an antinomy between bureaucratic and democratic processes. Bureaucratic processes contribute heavily to the rigidity and rationality (*constancy*) of organizational structure by virtue of their emphasis upon hierarchy, spheres of authority or competence and schemes of normative regulation (*preservation of difference*). The hallmarks of a typically bureaucratized hospital structure include pre-determined social *distances* between ranks and occupations, authority and rules as keys to organizational effectiveness and externally imposed discipline as an instrument of organizational control and participant reliability (*persistence of differences*). It also includes fixed qualifications for narrowly defined hierarchical positions graded in prestige and authority (*differentiated similarities*), restriction of interpersonal relationships to organizationally determined behaviors and the prohibition of sentiment and spontaneity as relevant features of participants' roles (*constant distances*).

In contrast, democratic or counter-bureaucratic processes contribute to the flexibility and spontaneity (*inconstancy*) of hospital organization. They stress a total conception of individual worth in the division of work, together with themes of equalitarianism, humanism and freedom (*similarity* and *closeness* are compatible with human *differences*). Unlike a fully developed bureaucratic organization, democratic processes do not assess the participant's organizational contribution or utility on his "value-as-a-producer." Democratic processes join his "value-as-a-producer" with his "value-as-a-person." Inasmuch as an individual's prestige is not exclusively or exhaustively bound to his place in the organizational hierarchy, status *distinctions* are reduced. Equalitarianism cutting across organizational rank evokes reasoned justification for the application of organizational authority, sanction and discipline (*enduring principles reduce difference and distance*). Equalitarianism as an expression of democratic tendencies questions the orthodox bureaucratic view that superordinates can make better decisions than subordinates simply by virtue of their superordinate status (*equalitarian similarities oppose hierarchical differences*). If democratic processes weaken hierarchical arbitrariness, then the chances for reciprocity in communication processes are increased.

A fundamental difference between bureaucratic and democratic processes appears in the risks assumed as proposals to the problem of moral worth. The former argues that hierarchical grading of technical accomplishments is equivalent to a hierarchical grading of moral perfectability (*similarity of hierarchical ranks*). The latter questions the validity of the proposition that the higher the organizational rank, the better the person. To this extent, democratic processes are unwilling to assume the risk that moral perfectability is reducible to technical competence (*dissimilarity of hierarchical ranks*).

It would be premature, however, to conclude that bureaucratic organizations are inherently undemocratic and "tough-minded." On the contrary, bureaucratic organizations are democratic in the sense that they attempt to eliminate extra-organizational statuses such as wealth, social position and aristocracy in favor of objective standards of individual accomplishment (*irrelevant differences are displaced by relevant similarities*). Similarly, democratic organizations are bureaucratic in the sense that they attempt to eliminate individual power and self-assertion in favor of the principle that no individual's claim for privilege is absolute. Apart from analytical considerations, real world organizations are never wholly bureaucratized or wholly democratized. The two processes stand in some kind of equilibrium–disequilibrium. Too great an emphasis upon democratic processes leads to normative patterns based upon *similarities* and *closeness* while too great an emphasis upon bureaucratic processes leads to normative patterns based upon *dissimilarities* and *distance*. Where bureaucratic processes outweigh democratic processes, individuals possessing a drive toward dissimilarity and distance may be less inclined to leave the organization.

We have seen that the turnover group in the general hospital is characterized by expectations of dissimilarity and distance, which presumably are not fulfilled in organizational experience. It may be argued, in effect, that the hospital is deficient in providing normative patterns typical of bureaucratic processes. On these grounds the turnover group would seek greater social distance between hierarchical statuses, insist that each person do his defined share, idealize the technically competent supervisor and withhold empathy toward others in the organization. Perhaps this highly competitive atmosphere is illustrative of an organizational situation in which individual success and individual productivity evoke dominant bureaucratic patterns.

The inability of the hospital to meet the claims of its better educated and technically competent personnel is a reflection of imbalances in bureaucratic processes. No other large-scale organization is required to take such a *total* view of its clientele (patients) with the exceptions of prisons or asylums. Asylums and prisons can allow bureaucratic processes to predominate since they can deny the uniqueness of their clientele. They can eradicate individual identity, prior statuses and rights through uniform organizational practices. By treating individuals in a like manner, personality differences are submerged. In contrast, the general hospital must accept a patient's identity, his uniqueness, his rights, his dependency and helplessness and his communal status as legitimate objectives of organizational policy. The principle of bureaucratic impersonality becomes untenable in view of the necessity to treat unlike cases in a uniformly individualized manner. The philosophy of "tender loving care" reflects the hospital's attempt to assimilate the patient's unique identity by getting closer to him.

Moreover, giving substance to a patient's identity creates an inner stress within bureaucratic processes. How can a hospital maintain *dissimilarity* and *distance* as organizational inducements when there is a clear and present need for *closeness* in relation to patients? To achieve organizational effectiveness (service to clientele), the hospital must lessen efforts directed at strengthening bureaucratic norms. The primacy of patients'

needs supports the prescriptive norm of closeness. Every occupational category, from housekeepers to nurses' aides to physicians, is enjoined to consider the patient as an *individual*. That is, all personnel are not only responsible for but responsible to the patient in the performance of their organizational duties.

Responsibility to the patient countervails the bureaucratic principle of responsibility to hierarchical status and technical competence since it creates surplus role opportunities for those less well-trained and bound to narrowly defined organizational positions. Given the climate of activities in modern hospitals (from specialization to the alleviation of suffering), the expectations of those with greater technical competence cannot be easily met. Like the turnover population, they expect difference and dissimilarity to be typical of their position in the organization. They expect to occupy clearly defined positions in the hierarchy of organizational behaviors. They expect to give the organization time and effort in return for wages. A housekeeper, on the other hand, can clean a patient's room, be conversant about his illness, run errands, arrange flowers, window shades and the like. Her surplus roles are expressions of discretion, spontaneity and individuality. The net effect of such freedom lessens her anxieties about bureaucratic regularity, discipline and hierarchical distinctions.

Participants with a "drive" toward *distance* and *difference* support the bureaucratic principle that responsibility should rest exclusively and exhaustively upon hierarchical status. Thus, if patients' gratitude is both reward for services and public recognition of the nurse's ministering role, these rewards should, on the bureaucratic view, be consistent with hierarchical status. However, the prescriptive norm of closeness, expressed as patient-centeredness, provides contexts where "illegitimate" rewards are made, as illustrated in the case of the housekeeper. Evidence of organizational accommodation to those seeking difference and distance may be seen in the variety of uniforms, insignia and nameplates worn by hospital personnel. Nevertheless, externalization of hierarchical differences does not effectively counteract closeness as a prescriptive norm.

There is a subjective side to organizational experience for the bureaucratically inclined group. One of the notable findings concerning this group is the paucity of empathetic attitudes. The absence of empathy may be interpreted as a protest against the organizational emphasis upon democratic processes (i.e., the surplus roles of lower status participants, total conception of patient's uniqueness). To deny empathy in the round of hospital interactions is an alienating experience and provides unstable conditions for sustained participation. It is an extreme mode of adaptation, since it not only denies the participant's own humanity, but denies

primary organization objectives. It is an open question whether or not greater equilibrium between bureaucratic and counter-bureaucratic processes would provide stabilizing conditions of employment for this group. It seems paradoxical that gains in organizational empathy (organizational effectiveness) are correlated with losses of technically competent participants. By hyperbole there appears to be a Gresham's Law operating in hospital organization, where the less educated and less competent drive out the better educated and more competent.

26

Exchange as a Conceptual Framework for the Study of Interorganizational Relationships

Sol Levine
and
Paul E. White

SOCIOLOGISTS have devoted considerable attention to the study of formal organizations, particularly in industry, government, and the trade union field. Their chief focus, however, has been on patterns within rather than between organizations. Studies of interrelationships have largely been confined to units within the same organizational structure or between a pair of complementary organizations such as management and labor. Dimock's study of jurisdictional conflict between two federal agencies is a notable exception.[1] Another is a study of a community reaction to disaster by Form and Nosow in which the authors produce revealing data on the interaction pattern of local health organizations. The authors observe that "organizational cooperation was facilitated among organizations with similar internal structures."[2] March and Simon suggest that interorganizational conflict is very similar to intergroup conflict within organizations but present no supporting data.[3] Blau has commented on the general problems involved in studying multiple organizations.[4] In pointing up the need to study the organization in relation to its environment, Etzioni specifies the area of interorganizational relationships as one of the three meriting further intensive empirical study.[5]

Health and social welfare agencies within a given community offer an excellent opportunity for exploring patterns of relationship among organizations. There are an appreciable number of such organizations in any fairly large urban American community. Most of them are small so that relatively few individuals have to be interviewed to obtain information on their interaction. Within any community setting, varying kinds of relations exist between official and voluntary organizations concerned with health and welfare. Thus welfare agencies may use public health nursing services, or information on the status of families may be shared by such voluntary organizations as the Red Cross and the Tuberculosis and Health Association.

Facilitating communication between local organizations has been a major objective of public health administrators and community organizers. Their writings contain many assertions about the desirability of improving relationships in order to reduce gaps and overlaps of medical services to the citizens, but as yet little effort has been made to appraise objectively the interrelationships that actually exist within the community.

In the following pages we should like to present our own theoretical interpretation of interorganizational relationships together with a discussion of our research approach and a few preliminary findings, pointing up some of the substantive areas in organiza-

[1] Dimock, M. E., "Expanding Jurisdictions: A Case Study in Bureaucratic Conflict," in R. K. Merton, A. P. Gray, B. Hockey, H. C. Selvin (eds.), *Reader in Bureaucracy*, New York: Free Press, 1952.

[2] Form, W. H., and S. Nosow, *Community in Disaster*, New York, 1958, p. 236.

[3] March, J. G., and H. A. Simon, *Organizations*, New York: Wiley, 1958.

[4] Blau, P. M., "Formal Organization: Dimensions of Analysis," *Amer. J. Sociol.*, 63:58, 1957.

[5] Etzioni, A., "New Directions in the Study of Organizations and Society," *Social Research*, 27:223–228, 1960.

From Administrative Science Quarterly, Vol. 5: 583–601, March, 1961; by permission of the authors and publisher.

**Exchange as a Conceptual 345
Framework for the Study of
Interorganizational Relationships**

tional sociology for which our study has relevance. Our present thinking is largely based on the results of an exploratory study of twenty-two health organizations in a New England community with a population of 200,000 and initial impressions of data on a more intensive study, as yet unanalyzed, of some fifty-five health organizations in another New England community of comparable size.[6]

The site of our initial investigation was selected because we found it fairly accessible for study and relatively independent of a large metropolis; moreover, it contained a range of organizations which were of interest—a full-time health department, a welfare department, autonomous local agencies, local chapters or affiliates of major voluntary health and social welfare organizations, and major community hospitals. Of the twenty-two health organizations or agencies studied, fourteen were voluntary agencies, five were hospitals (three with outpatient clinics and two without) and three others were official agencies—health, welfare, and school. Intensive semistructured interviews were conducted with executive directors and supervisory personnel of each organization, and information was obtained from members of the boards through brief semistructured questionnaires. In addition, we used an adaptation of an instrument developed by Irwin T. Sanders to locate the most influential leaders in the community for the purpose of determining their distribution on agency boards.[7] The prestige ratings that the influential leaders assigned to the organizations constituted one of the independent variables of our study.

[6] Project was sponsored by the Social Science Program at the Harvard School of Public Health and supported by Grant 8676–2 from the National Institutes of Health. Professor Sol Levine was principal investigator of the project and Benjamin D. Paul, the director of the Social Science Program, was coinvestigator. We are grateful for the criticisms and suggestions given by Professors Paul, S. M. Miller, I. T. Sanders and H. E. Freeman.

[7] Sanders, I. T., "The Community Social Profile," *Amer. Sociol. Rev.*, 25:75–77, 1960.

Exchange as a Conceptual Framework

The complex of community health organizations may be seen as a system with individual organizations or system parts varying in the kinds and frequency of their relationships with one another. This system is enmeshed in ever larger systems—the community, the state, and so on.

Prevention and cure of disease constitute the ideal orientation of the health agency system, and individual agencies derive their respective goals or objectives from this larger orientation. In order to achieve its specific objectives, however, an agency must possess or control certain elements. It must have clients to serve; it must have resources in the form of equipment, specialized knowledge, or the funds with which to procure them; and it must have the services of people who can direct these resources to the clients. Few, if any, organizations have enough access to all these elements to enable them to attain their objectives fully. Under realistic conditions of element scarcity, organizations must select, on the basis of expediency or efficiency, particular functions that permit them to achieve their ends as fully as possible. By function is meant a set of interrelated services or activities that are instrumental, or believed to be instrumental, for the realization of an organization's objectives.

Although, because of scarcity, an organization limits itself to particular functions, it can seldom carry them out without establishing relationships with other organizations of the health system. The reasons for this are clear. To fulfill its functions without relating to other parts of the health system, an organization must be able to procure the necessary elements—cases, labor services, and other resources—directly from the community or outside it. Certain classes of hospitals treating a specific disease and serving an area larger than the local community probably most nearly approximate this condition. But even in this case other organizations within the system usually control some elements that are necessary or, at least, helpful to the carrying out of its functions. These may be money, equipment, or special personnel, which are conditionally lent or given. Usually agencies are unable to obtain all the elements they need from the community or through their individual efforts and, accordingly, have to turn to other agencies to obtain additional elements. The need for a sufficient number of clients, for example, is often more efficiently met through exchanges with other organizations than through independent case-finding procedures.

Theoretically, then, were all the essential elements in infinite supply there would be little need for organizational interaction and for subscription to co-operation as an ideal. Under actual conditions of scarcity, however, interorganizational exchanges are essential to goal attainment. In sum, organizational goals or objectives are derived from general health values. These goals or objectives may be viewed as defining the organization's ideal need for elements— consumers, labor services, and other resources. The scarcity of elements, however, impels the organization to restrict its activity to limited specific functions. The fulfillment of these limited functions, in turn, requires access to certain kinds of elements, which an organization seeks to obtain by entering into exchanges with other organizations.

Interaction among organizations can be viewed within the framework of an exchange model like that suggested by Homans.[8] However, the few available definitions of exchange are somewhat limited for our purposes because they tend to be bound by economics and because their referents are mainly individual or psychological phenomena and are not intended to encompass interaction between organizational entities or larger systems.[9]

We suggest the following definition of organizational exchange: *Organizational exchange is any voluntary activity between two organizations which has consequences, actual or anticipated, for the realization of their respective goals or objectives.* This definition has several advantages. First, it refers to activity in general and not exclusively to reciprocal activity. The action may be unidirectional and yet involve exchange. If an organization refers a patient to another organization which then treats him, an exchange has taken place if the respective objectives of the two organizations are furthered by the action. Pivoting the definition on goals or objectives provides for an obvious but crucial component of what constitutes an organization. The coordination of activities of a number of individuals toward some objective or goal has been designated as a distinguishing feature of organizations by students in the field.[10] Parsons, for example, has defined an organization as a "special type of social system organized about the primacy of interest in the attainment of a particular type of system goal."[11] That its goals or objectives may be transformed by a variety of factors and that, under some circumstances, mere survival may become primary does not deny

---

formally voluntary agreement involving the offer of any sort of present, continuing, or future utility in exchange for utilities of any sort offered in return." Weber employs the term "utility" in the economic sense. It is the "utility" of the "object of exchange" to the parties concerned that produces exchange. See M. Weber, *The Theory of Social and Economic Organization*, New York: Free Press, 1957, p. 170. Homans, on the other hand, in characterizing interaction between persons as an exchange of goods, material and nonmaterial, sees the impulse to "exchange" in the psychological make-up of the parties to the exchange. He states, "the paradigm of elementary social behavior, and the problem of the elementary sociologist is to state propositions relating the variations in the values and costs of each man to his frequency distribution of behavior among alternatives, where the values (in the mathematical sense) taken by these variables for one man determine in part their values for the other." See Homans, *op. cit.*, p. 598.

[10] Parsons, T., "Suggestions for a Sociological Approach to the Theory of Organizations—I," *Admin. Sci. Quart.*, 1:63–85, 1956.

[11] *Ibid*, p. 64.

---

[8] Homans, G. C., "Social Behavior As Exchange," *Amer. J. Sociol.*, 63:597–606, 1958.

[9] Weber states that "by 'exchange' in the broadest sense will be meant every case of a

that goals or objectives are universal characteristics of organizations.

Second, the definition widens the concept of exchange beyond the transfer of material goods and beyond gratifications in the immediate present. This broad definition of exchange permits us to consider a number of dimensions of organizational interaction that would otherwise be overlooked.

Finally, while the organizations may not be bargaining or interacting on equal terms and may even employ sanctions or pressures (by granting or withholding these elements), it is important to exclude from our definition, relationships involving physical coercion or domination; hence emphasis is on the word "voluntary" in our definition.

The elements that are exchanged by health organizations fall into three main categories: (1) referrals of cases, clients, or patients; (2) the giving or receiving of labor services, including the services of volunteer, clerical, and professional personnel, and (3) the sending or receiving of resources other than labor services, including funds, equipment, and information on cases and technical matters. Organizations have varying needs of these elements, depending on their particular functions. Referrals, for example, may be seen as the delivery of the consumers of services to organizations, labor services as the human means by which the resources of the organization are made available to the consumers, and resources other than labor services as the necessary capital goods.

The Determinants of Exchange

The interdependence of the parts of the exchange system is contingent upon three related factors: (1) the accessibility of each organization to necessary elements from sources outside the health system, (2) the objectives of the organization and particular functions to which it allocates the elements it controls, and (3) the degree to which domain consensus exists among the various organizations. An ideal theory of organizational exchange would describe the interrelationship and relative contribution of each of these factors. For the present, however, we will draw on some of our preliminary

findings to suggest possible relationships among these factors and to indicate that each plays a part in affecting the exchange of elements among organizations.

Gouldner has emphasized the need to differentiate the various parts of a system in terms of their relative dependence upon other parts of the system.[12] In our terms, certain parts are relatively dependent, not having access to elements outside the system, whereas others, which have access to such elements, possess a high degree of independence or functional autonomy. The voluntary organizations of our study (excluding hospitals) can be classified into what Sills calls either corporate or federated organizations.[13] Corporate organizations are those which delegate authority downward from the national or state level to the local level. They contrast with organizations of the federated type which delegate authority upwards—from the local to the state or national level.

It appears that local member units of corporate organizations, because they are less dependent on the local health system and can obtain the necessary elements from the community or their parent organizations, interact less with other local agencies than federated organizations. This is supported by preliminary data presented in Table 26–1. It is also suggested that by carrying out their activities without entering actively into exchange relationships with other organizations, corporate organizations apparently are able to maintain their essential structure and avoid consequences resulting in the displacement of state or national goals. It may be that corporate organizations deliberately choose functions that require minimal involvement with other organiza-

[12] Gouldner, A. W., "Reciprocity and Autonomy in Functional Theory," in L. Gross (ed.), *Symposium on Sociological Theory*, Evanston, Ill., 1959 and A. W. Gouldner, "The Norm of Reciprocity: A Preliminary Statement," *Amer. Sociol. Rev.*, 25:161–178, 1960.

[13] Sills, D. L., *The Volunteers: Means and Ends in a National Organization*, New York: Free Press, 1957.

tions. An examination of the four corporate organizations in our preliminary study reveals that three of them give resources to other agencies to carry out their activities, and the fourth conducts broad educational programs. Such functions are less likely to involve relationships with other organizations than the more direct service organizations, those that render services to individual recipients.

An organization's relative independence from the rest of the local health agency system and greater dependence upon a system outside the community may, at times, produce specific types of disagreements with the other agencies within the local system. This is dramatically demonstrated in the criticisms expressed toward a local community branch of an official state rehabilitation organization. The state organization, to justify its existence, has to present a successful experience to the legislators—that a minimum number of persons have been successfully rehabilitated. This means that by virtue of the services the organization has offered, a certain percentage of its debilitated clients are again returned to self-supporting roles. The rehabilitative goal of the organization cannot be fulfilled unless it is selective in the persons it accepts as clients. Other community agencies dealing with seriously debilitated clients are unable to get the state to accept their clients for rehabilitation. In the eyes of these frustrated agencies the state organization is remiss in fulfilling its public goal. The state agency, on the other hand, cannot commit its limited personnel and resources to the time-consuming task of trying to rehabilitate what seem to be very poor risks. The state agency wants to be accepted and approved by the local community and its health agencies, but the state legislature and the governor, being the primary source of the agency's resources, constitute its significant reference group. Hence, given the existing definition of organizational goals and the state agency's relative independence of the local health system, its interaction with other community agencies is relatively low.

The marked difference in the interaction rank position of hospitals with out-patient clinics and those without suggests other differences between the two classes of hospitals. It may be that the two types of hospitals have different goals and that hospitals with clinics have a greater "community" orientation and are more committed to the concept of "comprehensive" care than are hospitals without clinics. However,

Table 26–1—Weighted rankings* of organizations classified by organizational form on four interaction indices

Interaction Index	Sent by	N	SENT TO VOLUNTARY HOSPITALS					Total Interaction Sent
			Corporate	Federated	Without Clinics	With Clinics	Official	
Referrals	Vol. corporate	4	4.5	5	3.7	4.5	5	5
	Vol. federated	10	3	4	3.7	3	4	3
	Hosps. w/o clinics	2	4.5	3	3.7	4.5	3	4
	Hosps. w. clinics	3	1	1	1.5	2	1	1
	Official	3	2	2	1.5	1	2	2
Resources	Vol. corporate	4	5	2	1	4	5	3.5
	Vol. federated	10	4	3	3	4	4	3.5
	Hosps. w/o clinics	2	2	4.5	4.5	5	3	5
	Hosps. w. clinics	3	1	1	2	1	2	1
	Official	3	3	4.5	4.5	2	1	2
Written and Verbal Communication	Vol. corporate	4	5	3	2	4	5	4
	Vol. federated	10	3	1	3	3	3	2.5
	Hosps. w/o clinics	2	2	5	4.5	5	4	5
	Hosps. w. clinics	3	4	4	4.5	1	1.5	2.5
	Official	3	1	2	1	2	1.5	1
Joint Activities	Vol. corporate	4	4.5	4	3	5	3.5	5
	Vol. federated	10	3	3	5	3	1	3
	Hosps. w/o clinics	2	2	5	1	2	3.5	4
	Hosps. w. clinics	3	4.5	2	2	1	5	1.5
	Official	3	1	1	4	4	2	1.5

* Note: 1 indicates highest interaction; 5 indicates lowest interaction

whether or not the goals of the two types of hospitals do indeed differ, those with out-patient departments deal with population groups similar to those serviced by other agencies of the health system, that is, patients who are largely ambulatory and indigent; thus they serve patients whom other organizations may also be seeking to serve. Moreover, hospitals with out-patients clinics have greater control over their clinic patients than over those in-patients who are the charges of private physicians, and are thereby freer to refer patients to other agencies.

The functions of an organization not only represent the means by which it allocates its elements but, in accordance with our exchange formulation, also determine the degree of dependence on other organizations for specific kinds of elements, as well as its capacity to make certain kinds of elements available to other organizations. The exchange model leads us to explain the flow of elements between organizations largely in terms of the respective functions performed by the participating agencies. Indeed, it is doubtful whether any analysis of exchange of elements among organizations which ignores differences in organizational needs would have much theoretical or practical value.

Exchange as a Conceptual 349
Framework for the Study of
Interorganizational Relationships

In analyzing the data from our pilot community we classified agencies on the basis of their primary health functions: resource, education, prevention, treatment or rehabilitation. Resource organizations attempt to achieve their objectives by providing other agencies with the means to carry out their functions. The four other agency types may be conceived as representing respective steps in the control of disease. We have suggested that the primary function determines an organization's need for exchange elements. Our preliminary data reveal, as expected, that treatment organizations rate highest on number of referrals and amount of resources received and that educational organizations, whose efforts are directed toward the general public, rate low on the number of referrals (see Table 26–2). This finding holds even when the larger organizations—official agencies and hospitals—are excluded and the analysis is based on the remaining voluntary agencies of our sample. As a case in point, let us consider a health organization whose function is to educate the public about a specific disease but which renders no direct service

Table 26–2—Weighted rankings* of organizations, classified by function on four interaction indices

Interaction Index	Received by	N	RECEIVED FROM Education	Resource	Prevention	Treatment	Rehabili-tation	Total Interaction Received
Referrals	Education	3	4.5	5	5	5	5	5
	Resource	5	3	4	2	4	1	3
	Prevention	5	2	1	3	2	2.5	2
	Treatment	7	1	2	1	1	2.5	1
	Rehabilitation	2	4.5	3	4	3	4	4
Resources	Education	3	4.5	5	4	5	4.5	5
	Resource	5	1.5	3	3	4	3	3.5
	Prevention	5	1.5	4	2	3	4.5	3.5
	Treatment	7	3	2	1	2	2	1
	Rehabilitation	2	4.5	1	5	1	1	2
Written and Verbal Communication	Education	3	4	5	4.5	5	5	5
	Resource	5	3	2	2	3	2	2.5
	Prevention	5	2	4	3	4	4	3
	Treatment	7	1	1	1	2	3	1
	Rehabilitation	2	5	3	4.5	1	1	2.5
Joint Activities	Education	3	4	4	1	3	4.5	4
	Resource	5	2	1	3	4	1	3
	Prevention	5	1	2	2	2	3	1
	Treatment	7	3	3	4	1	2	2
	Rehabilitation	2	5	5	5	5	4.5	5

* Note: 1 indicates highest interaction; 5 indicates lowest interaction.

to individual clients. If it carries on an active educational program, it is possible that some people may come to it directly to obtain information and, mistakenly, in the hope of receiving treatment. If this occurs, the organization will temporarily be in possession of potential clients whom it may route or refer to other more appropriate agencies. That such referrals will be frequent is unlikely, however. It is even less likely that the organization will receive many referrals from other organizations. If an organization renders a direct service to a client, however, such as giving X-ray examinations, or polio immunizations, there is greater likelihood that it will send or receive referrals.

An organization is less limited in its function in such interagency activities as discussing general community health problems, attending agency council meetings or co-operating on some aspect of fund raising. Also, with sufficient initiative even a small educational agency can maintain communication with a large treatment organization (for example, a general hospital) through exchanges of periodic reports and telephone calls to obtain various types of information. But precisely because it is an educational agency offering services to the general public and not to individuals, it will be limited in its capacity to maintain other kinds of interaction with the treatment organization. It probably will not be able to lend or give space or equipment, and it is even doubtful that it can offer the kind of instruction that the treatment organization would seek for its staff. That the organization's function establishes the range of possibilities for exchange and that other variables exert influence within the framework established by function is suggested by some other early findings presented in Table 26–3. Organizations were classified as direct or indirect on the basis of whether or not they provided a direct service to the public. They were also classified according to their relative prestige as rated by influential leaders in the community. Organizations high in prestige lead in the number of joint activities, and prestige seems to exert some influence on the amount of verbal and written communication. Yet it is agencies offering direct services—regardless of prestige—which lead in the number of referrals and resources received. In other words, prestige, leadership, and other organizational

Table 26–3—Weighted rankings* of organizations classified by prestige of organization and by general type of service offered on four interaction indices

			Received from				
			HIGH PRESTIGE		LOW PRESTIGE		Total
Interaction Index	Received by	N	Direct Service	Indirect Service	Direct Service	Indirect Service	Interaction Received
	High direct	9	1	1	1	1	1
Referrals	High indirect	3	3	3.5	3	3.5	3
	Low direct	6	2	2	2	2	2
	Low indirect	4	4	3.5	4	3.5	4
	High direct	9	2	2	2	2	2
Resources	High indirect	3	3	3	3	3.5	3
	Low direct	6	1	1	1	1	1
	Low indirect	4	4	4	4	3.5	4
Written	High direct	9	2	2	3	1	2
and Verbal	High indirect	3	3	3	1	3	3
Communication	Low direct	6	1	1	2	2	1
	Low indirect	4	4	4	4	4	4
	High direct	9	1	1.5	2	2	2
Joint Activities	High indirect	3	2	1.5	1	1	1
	Low direct	6	4	3	3	4	3
	Low indirect	4	3	4	4	3	4

* Note: 1 indicates highest interaction; 5 indicates lowest interaction.

Exchange as a Conceptual 351
Framework for the Study of
Interorganizational Relationships

variables seem to affect interaction patterns within limits established by the function variable.

An obvious question is whether organizations with shared or common boards interact more with one another than do agencies with separate boards. Our preliminary data show that the interaction rate is not affected by shared board membership. We have not been able to ascertain if there is any variation in organizational interaction when the shared board positions are occupied by persons with high status or influence. In our pilot community, there was only one instance in which two organizations had the same top community leaders as board members. If board plays an active role in the activities of health organizations, they serve more to link the organization to the community and the elements it possesses than to link the organization to other health and welfare agencies. The board probably also exerts influence on internal organizational operations and on establishing or approving the primary objective of the organization. Once the objective and the implementing functions are established, these functions tend to exert their influence autonomously on organizational interaction.

Organizational Domain

As we have seen, the elements exchanged are cases, labor services, and other resources. All organizational relationships directly or indirectly involve the flow and control of these elements. Within the local health agency system, the flow of elements is not centrally co-ordinated, but rests upon voluntary agreements or understanding. Obviously, there will be no exchange of elements between two organizations that do not know of each other's existence or that are completely unaware of each other's functions. Even more, there can be no exchange of elements without some agreement or understanding, however implicit. These exchange agreements are contingent upon the organization's domain. The domain of an organization consists of the specific goals it wishes to pursue and the functions it undertakes in order to implement its goals.

In operational terms, organizational domain in the health field refers to the claims that an organization stakes out for itself in terms of (1) disease covered, (2) population served, and (3) services rendered. The goals of the organization constitute in effect the organization's claim to future functions and to the elements requisite to these functions, whereas the present or actual functions carried out by the organization constitute *de facto* claims to these elements. Exchange agreements rest upon prior consensus regarding domain. Within the health agency system, consensus regarding an organization's domain must exist to the extent that parts of the system will provide each agency with the elements necessary to attain its ends.

Once an organization's goals are accepted, domain consensus continues as long as the organization fulfills the functions adjudged appropriate to its goals and adheres to certain standards of quality. Our data show that organizations find it more difficult to legitimate themselves before other organizations in the health system than before such outside systems as the community or state. An organization can sometimes obtain sufficient elements from outside the local health system, usually in the form of funds, to continue in operation long after other organizations within the system have challenged its domain. Conversely, if the goals of a specific organization are accepted within the local agency system, other organizations of the system may encourage it to expand its functions and to realize its goals more fully by offering it elements to implement them. Should an organization not respond to this encouragement, it may be forced to forfeit its claim to the unrealized aspect of its domain.

Within the system, delineation of organizational domains is highly desired.[14] For example, intense competition may occur occasionally between two agencies offering the same services, especially when other

[14] In our research a large percentage of our respondents spontaneously referred to the undesirability of overlapping or duplicated services.

agencies have no specific criteria for referring patients to one rather than the other. If both services are operating near capacity, competition between the two tends to be less keen, the choice being governed by the availability of service. If the services are being operated at less than capacity, competition and conflict often occur. Personnel of referring agencies in this case frequently deplore the "duplication of services" in the community. In most cases the conflict situation is eventually resolved by agreement on the part of the competing agencies to specify the criteria for referring patients to them. The agreement may take the form of consecutive handling of the same patients. For example, age may be employed as a criterion. In one case three agencies were involved in giving rehabilitation services: one took preschool children, another school children, and the third adults. In another case, where preventive services were offered, one agency took preschool children and the other took children of school age. The relative accessibility of the agencies to the respective age groups was a partial basis for these divisions. Another criterion— disease stage—also permits consecutive treatment of patients. One agency provided physical therapy to bedridden patients; another handled them when they became ambulatory.

Several other considerations, such as priorities in allocation of elements, may impel an organization to delimit its functions even when no duplication of services exists. The phenomenon of delimiting one's role and consequently of restricting one's domain is well known. It can be seen, for instance, in the resistance of certain universities of high prestige to offer "practical" or vocational courses, or courses to meet the needs of any but high-status professionals, even to the extent of foregoing readily accessible federal grants. It is evidenced in the insistence of certain psychiatric clinics on handling only cases suitable for psychoanalytic treatment, of certain business organizations on selling only to wholesalers, of some retail stores on handling only expensive merchandise.

The flow of elements in the health system is contingent upon solving the problem of "who gets what for what purpose." The clarification of organizational domains and the development of greater domain consensus contributes to the solution of this problem. In short, domain consensus is a prerequisite to exchange. Achieving domain consensus may involve negotiation, orientation, or legitimation. When the functions of the interacting organizations are diffuse, achieving domain consensus becomes a matter of constant readjustment to compromise, a process which may be called negotiation or bargaining. The more specific the functions, however, the more domain consensus is attained merely by orientation (for example, an agency may call an X-ray unit to inquire about the specific procedures for implementing services). A third, less frequent but more formalized, means of attaining domain consensus is the empowering, licensing or "legitimating" of an organization to operate within the community by some other organization. Negotiation, as a means of attaining domain consensus, seems to be related to diffuseness of function, whereas orientation, at the opposite extreme, relates to specificity of function.

These processes of achieving domain consensus constitute much of the interaction between organizations. While they may not involve the immediate flow of elements, they are often necessary preconditions for the exchange of elements, because without at least minimal domain consensus there can be no exchange among organizations. Moreover, to the extent that these processes involve proffering information about the availability of elements as well as about rights and obligations regarding the elements, they constitute a form of interorganizational exchange.

Dimensions of Exchange

We have stated that all relationships among local health agencies may be conceptualized as involving exchange. There are four main dimensions to the actual exchange situation. They are:

1. *The parties to the exchange.* The characteristics we have thus far employed in classifying organizations or the parties to the exchange are: organizational form or affiliation, function, prestige, size, personnel characteristics, and numbers and types of clients served.

2. *The kinds and quantities exchanged.* These involve two main classes: the actual elements exchanged (consumers, labor services, and resources other than labor services), and information on the availability of these organizational elements and on rights and obligations regarding them.

3. *The agreement underlying the exchange.* Every exchange is contingent upon a prior agreement, which may be implicit and informal or fairly explicit and highly formalized. For example, a person may be informally routed or referred to another agency with the implicit awareness or expectation that the other organization will handle the case. On the other hand, the two agencies may enter into arrangements that stipulate the exact conditions and procedures by which patients are referred from one to another. Furthermore, both parties may be actively involved in arriving at the terms of the agreement, or these terms may be explicitly defined by one for all who may wish to conform to them. An example of the latter case is the decision of a single organization to establish a policy of a standard fee for service.

4. *The direction of the exchange.* This refers to the direction of the flow of organizational elements. We have differentiated three types:

(*a*) *Unilateral:* where elements flow from one organization to another and no elements are given in return.

(*b*) *Reciprocal:* where elements flow from one organization to another in return for other elements.

(*c*) *Joint:* where elements flow from two organizations acting in unison toward a third party. This type, although representing a high order of agreement and co-ordination of policy among agencies, does not involve the actual transfer of elements.

As we proceed with our study of relation-

ships among health agencies, we will undoubtedly modify and expand our theoretical model. For example, we will attempt to describe how the larger systems are intertwined with the health agency system. Also, we will give more attention to the effect of interagency competition and conflict regarding the flow of elements among organizations. In this respect we will analyze differences among organizations with respect not only to domain but to fundamental goals as well. As part of this analysis we will examine the orientations of different categories of professionals (for example, nurses and social workers) as well as groups with varying experiences and training within categories of professionals (as nurses with or without graduate education).

In the meantime, we find the exchange framework useful in ordering our data, locating new areas for investigation, and developing designs for studying interorganizational relationships. We feel that the conceptual framework and findings of our study will be helpful in understanding not only health agency interaction but also relationships within other specific systems (such as military, industrial, governmental, educational, and other systems). As in our study of health agencies, organizations within any system may confidently be expected to have need for clients, labor, and other resources. We would also expect that the interaction pattern among organizations within each system will also be affected by (1) organizational function, (2) access to the necessary elements from outside the system, and (3) the degree of domain consensus existing among the organizations of the system. It appears that the framework also shows promise in explaining interaction among organizations belonging to different systems (for example, educational and business systems, educational and governmental, military and industrial, and so forth). Finally, we believe our framework has obvious value in explaining interaction among units or departments within a single large-scale organization.

27

Physicians and Medicare: A Before-After Study of the Effects of Legislation on Attitudes

John Colombotos

SELDOM HAS A LAW been more bitterly opposed by any group than was Medicare by the medical profession (see Harris, 1966; Feingold, 1966; Rose, 1967:400–455). Just before Medicare was passed by Congress in 1965, there was even talk about a "boycott" of the program by physicians. This paper examines how individual physicians reacted, in their behavior and in their thinking, to Medicare after it became law.[1] The more general issue raised by this question is the role of law as an instrument of social change, an old sociological problem.

[1] It is of course necessary to distinguish between the attitudes of individual physicians toward Medicare and official AMA policy. The AMA leadership is commonly regarded as more conservative than the rank-and-file; however, the opposition of the AMA to Medicare before its passage apparently was supported by the majority of its membership. In a national poll of private practitioners in 1961, less than twenty per cent were in favor of the program "to provide hospital and nursing home care for the aged through the Social Security System" (Medical Tribune, May 15, 1961).

Law as an Instrument of Social Change— One view, attributed to early sociologists such as Herbert Spencer and William Graham Sumner, is that law can never move ahead of the customs or mores of the people, that legislation which is not rooted in the folkways is doomed to failure. Social change must be slow, and change in public opinion must precede legislative action. In brief, "stateways cannot change folkways." This view was expressed by Senator Barry Goldwater in the 1964 Presidential campaign (The New York Times, Nov. 1, 1964:1): "I am unalterably opposed to . . . discrimination, but also know that government can provide no lasting solution. . . . The ultimate solution lies in the hearts of men."

Others see law as a positive force in initiating social change (Allport, 1954:471): "It is a well known psychological fact that most people accept the results of an election or legislation gladly enough after the furor has subsided. . . . They allow themselves to be re-educated by the new norm that prevails."[2]

These are oversimplified statements of the role of law as an instrument of social change and miss the complexity of the problem. The question must be specified: under what conditions do laws have what effects?

*Effects: Behavior vs. Attitudes—*Sumner's negative position on law as an instrument of social change has been distorted, according to one reappraisal of his writings (Ball et al., 1962:532–540). Sumner (1906:68), in distinguishing between the effects of law on behavior and on attitudes, did not reject the power of law to influence men's behavior: "Men can always perform the prescribed act, although they cannot always think or feel prescribed thoughts or emotions."

This is in agreement with the views of the majority of contemporary politically liberal social scientists, who see law primarily as a way of changing behavior, not attitudes. For

[2] Allport qualifies this remark elsewhere in his book. It is quoted here to state the issue in its largest form.

From *American Sociological Review, Vol. 34: 318–334, June, 1969; by permission of the author and the American Sociological Association.*

Supported by U.S. Public Health Service Research Grants 5 RO1 CH 00045 and CH 00249. This is a revised version of a paper read at the Annual Meeting of the American Sociological Association, San Francisco, Calif., August 31, 1967. The interviewing for the study was done by the National Opinion Research Center, Univ. of Chicago.

example: "[Legal action] cannot coerce thoughts or instill subjective tolerance. . . . Law is intended only to control the outward expression of intolerance" (Allport, 1954: 477). And according to MacIver (1954: viii), "No law should require men to change their attitudes. . . . In a democracy we do not punish a man because he is opposed to income taxes, or to free school education, or to vaccination, or to minimum wages, but the laws of a democracy insist that he obey the laws that make provisions for these things. . . ."

The distinction between the effects of law on attitudes and on behavior is supported by empirical studies showing a discrepancy between the two (see Deutscher, 1966:235–254). In race relations, for example, study after study has shown that in concrete situations—in hotel accommodations (LaPiere, 1934:230–237), restaurant service (Kutner et al., 1952:649–652), department store shopping (Saenger and Gilbert, 1950:57–76), hospital accommodations, and school desegregation (Clark, 1953:47–50)—expressions of prejudice are not necessarily accompanied by discriminatory behavior. There are undoubtedly instances of the opposite, that is, verbal expressions of tolerance accompanied by discriminatory behavior, but they are not as well documented. The flight of white, liberal, middle-class families from the cities to the suburbs may be such an instance (Scott and Scott, 1968:46 ff.).

But to say that attitudes and behavior are not perfectly correlated is not to say they are unrelated, and there is evidence that change in behavior leads to change in attitudes. Studies of integrated army units, housing projects, and children's camps show that white people in these situations develop more favorable attitudes toward Negroes (Swanson et al., 1952:502; Deutsch and Collins, 1951; Yarrow, 1958). In an analysis of school desegregation, Hyman and Sheatsley (1964:6) describe the process thus: "There is obviously some parallel between public opinion and official action. . . . Close analysis of the current findings . . . leads us to the conclusion that in those parts of the South where some measure of school integration has taken place official action has preceded public sentiment, and *public senti-*

Physicians and Medicare: 355
A Before–After Study of the
Effects of Legislation on Attitudes

ment has then attempted to accommodate itself to the new situation [emphasis added]."

Other studies (Mussen, 1950:423–441; Campbell, 1958:335–340), however, have found that social contact has little effect in reducing prejudice.[3]

If indeed behavioral change does lead to attitudinal change, then law, by first changing behavior, may ultimately lead to changes in attitudes. As Allport says: "Outward action, psychology knows, has an eventual effect upon inner habits of thought and feeling. And for this reason we list legislative action as one of the major methods of reducing, not only public discrimination [behavior], but private prejudice [attitudes] as well" (1954:477). Berger, too, writes: "Law does not change attitudes directly, but by altering the situations in which attitudes and opinions are formed, law can indirectly reach the more private areas of life it cannot touch directly in a democratic society" (Berger, 1954:187). Clark (1953:72), among others, states the issue in more problematic terms: "Situationally determined changes in behavior [as in response to a law] *may or may not* be accompanied by compatible changes in attitudes or motivation of the individuals involved [emphasis added]."

Others, however, see law exerting a *direct* influence on attitudes, without necessarily changing behavior first. Law is conceived as a legitimizing and educational force, supporting one value or set of values against another. For example, according to Dicey (1914:465): "No facts play a more important part in the creation of opinion than laws themselves." And according to Bonfield (1965:111): "Past the change in attitude

[3] In Campbell's study of a desegregating school system, the results were mixed. White students who claimed Negroes as personal friends were more likely to show a reduction of prejudice than those without Negro friends, but the time order of these factors is ambiguous: those who became less prejudiced may then have chosen Negro friends. Also, those who had many classes with Negroes were no more likely to become less prejudiced than those with few classes with Negroes.

which may be caused by legally mandated and enforced nondiscriminatory conduct, *the mere existence of the law itself affects prejudice* [emphasis added]. People usually agree with the law and internalize its values. This is because considerable moral and symbolic weight is added to a principle when it is embedded in legislation."

The results of the few studies done on the effects of law on behavior and attitudes are mixed. Cantril (1947:228) notes: "When an opinion is held by a slight majority or when opinion is not solidly structured, an accomplished fact tends to shift opinion in the direction of acceptance. Poll figures show that immediately after the repeal of the arms embargo, immediately after the passage of the conscription laws, and immediately after favorable Congressional action on lend-lease and on the repeal of the neutrality laws [just before the United States' entry into World War II] there was invariably a rise of around ten per cent in the number of people favorable to these actions." And Muir (1967) found that the Supreme Court decision banning religious exercises in the nation's schools had an over-all positive effect on the attitudes and behavior of 28 officials in one public school system, though there was some evidence of a backlash.

Other studies, however, show that laws and court decisions have negligible effects on relevant attitudes. Hyman and Sheatsley (1964:3) and Schwartz (1967:11–12, 28–41) interpret the increasing acceptance of integration between 1942 and 1964 as a complex of long-term trends that are not easily modified by specific, even highly dramatic events, such as the Supreme Court decision of 1954. The physicians' strike against the province's medical care plan in Saskatchewan, Canada, in 1962 (Badgley and Wolfe, 1967) is an extreme case of noncompliance with a program implemented by a law.[4]

[4] In an experimental study, information that a behavior was illegal did not change the subjects' attitudes toward that behavior (Walker and Argyle, 1964: 570–581). In a follow-up experiment, however, it was found that knowledge of the law and knowledge of peer consensus did

Conditions for Effectiveness of Law—Three commonly cited factors determining the effectiveness of law are: (1) the degree of compatibility of the law with existing values, (2) the enforceability of the law, (3) the clarity of public policy and the diligence of enforcement.[5]

1. To say that a law must be compatible with some major existing values is not to say that it must be compatible with all values. In any society, especially in modern, industrial society, values themselves "are full of inconsistencies and strains, unliberated tendencies in many directions, responsive adjustments to new situations well conceived or ill conceived" (MacIver, 1948:279). A law, then, "maintains one set of values against another" (Pound, 1944:25). Thus desegregation and civil rights laws find support in the democratic creed and due process; Medicare finds support in the principle that adequate medical care is a right, rather than a privilege. This position appears to be in agreement with Sumner's principle of a "strain toward consistency." There is an important difference, however. Whereas Sumner posed the question of compatibility between a new law and existing mores as one of all or nothing, the current view emphasizes

change attitudes, and, furthermore, these effects depended on the authoritarianism of the subjects (Berkowitz and Walker, 1967: 410–422).

[5] These conditions are discussed in the following: Berger, 1954:173–177; Clark, 1953:53–59; Allport, 1954:469–473; Roche and Gordon, 1955:10, 42, 44, 49; Rose, 1959:470–481; Evan, 1965:285–293; Bonfield, 1965:107–122; Mayhew, 1968:258–284. Problems of implementation, specifically, the work and effects of antidiscrimination enforcement agencies, are analyzed by Berger (1954) and Mayhew (1968).

Less commonly cited factors determining the effectiveness of law are: (1) The amount of opposition to the law and the distribution of this opposition. The stronger and the more concentrated the opposition in politically relevant units, along geographical or occupational lines, for example, the more effectively it can oppose the law (Roche and Gordon, 1955:341). (2) The quality of support. A law is more likely to be effective if supported than if it is opposed by community leaders (see Killian, 1958:65–70). (3) The tempo of change. It is argued that the less the transition time, the easier the adaptation to the change enacted by the law (see Clark, 1953:43–47; Evan, 1965:290; Badgley and Wolfe, 1967:45).

conflicts and strains among a system of mores and poses the question of compatibility as a matter of degree (Myrdal, 1944:1045–1057).

2. In order for a law to be enforceable, the behavior to be changed must be observable. It is more difficult to enforce a law against homosexual behavior, for example, than a law against racial discrimination in public transportation.

3. The authorities responsible must be fully committed to enforcing the new law. One reason for the failure of Prohibition was the failure, or disinclination, of law enforcement agents to implement the law. Civil rights legislation runs into the same problem where local authorities, especially in the deep South, look the other way.

The Medicare Law—Medicare, signed into law in July, 1965, is a major piece of social legislation. It is often compared in importance with the original Social Security Act of 1935.

Medicare, Title 18 of the Social Security Amendments Act of 1965 (Public Law 89–97), established a new program of health insurance for people 65 years old or over. It has two parts: hospital insurance (Part A), applying automatically to almost all people 65 or over, which covers inpatient hospital services, outpatient hospital diagnostic services, and posthospital care in the patient's home or in an extended care facility (such as a nursing home); and medical insurance (Part B), a voluntary plan elected by over 90 per cent of those eligible for Part A, which covers physicians' services wherever they are furnished, home health services, and a number of other medical services. Part A is financed by the same method that finances retirement, disability, and death benefits under Social Security, i.e., special Social Security contributions by employees and their employers. Part B is financed by a monthly premium of $3.00, from each participant who elects to pay, matched by $3.00 from the general revenues of the Federal Government.[6]

For twenty years the American Medical

[6] Amendments to the Social Security Act in 1967 made some minor changes in the Medicare program and included an increase in the monthly premium.

Physicians and Medicare: 357
A Before–After Study of the
Effects of Legislation on Attitudes

Association fought bitterly and effectively against such a Federal program of health insurance under Social Security. Now, however, that the program has become law, the question is: How have individual physicians reacted, in their behavior and in their attitudes, to Medicare?

Research Design

Our data come from standardized interviews in 1964 and early 1965, before Medicare was passed, with 1,205 physicians in private practice in New York State (about 80 per cent of a probability sample), and from reinterviews with subsamples of these physicians at two different points in time after Medicare was passed. The interviews were conducted mainly by telephone. An experimental comparison of telephone and personal interviews with small, random subsamples of physicians showed that the responses obtained by the two methods were essentially similar.[7]

The purpose of the first wave of interviews was to study physicians' political attitudes, their attitudes toward issues in the organization of medical practice, and their career values, and to examine the relationship between background characteristics, such as their social origins and specialties, and their attitudes.[8] Among the questions in the first wave of interviews was: "What is your opinion about the bill that would provide for compulsory health insurance through Social Security to cover hospital costs for those over 65—Are you personally in favor of such a plan, or are you opposed to it?"

The bill referred to was passed, as noted

[7] Reported in "The Effects of Personal vs. Telephone Interviews on Socially Acceptable Responses," presented by the author at the annual meeting of the American Association for Public Opinion Research, Groton, Conn., May 14, 1965. [For later reference, see Bibliography, Colombotos, J., 1969c.]

[8] Some of these data are reported in the following papers: Colombotos, 1968; Colombotos, 1969b.

above, in July, 1965, as Part A of Title 18. Part B of Title 18, the voluntary insurance plan that pays for physicians' bills and other services, and Title 19, which provides for Federal matching funds to states for medical care for the "medically indigent," were not covered in the first wave of interviews because they were not introduced in the bill until the spring of 1965. Title 19, as a matter of fact, received little publicity until after the bill was passed. Title 19 is commonly called *Medicaid*; Title 18, parts A and B, *Medicare*.

Thus, before the law was passed, measures were available of physicians' attitudes toward what was generally considered the major feature of the bill, hospital insurance for the elderly, and many related issues, providing a unique opportunity for a natural experiment of the effects of legislation on attitudes.

The 1,205 physicians were stratified on their initial attitude toward Title 18A (i.e., before it was passed) and on geographic area, religious background, and political ideology, all of which were highly correlated with their initial attitude toward Title 18A,[9] and randomly divided into two subsamples, one with 804 and the other with 401 physicians.

The first subsample of 804 physicians was contacted between the middle of May, 1966, and the end of June, 1966, nearly one year after Medicare was passed and just before it was to go into effect. The second subsample of 401 doctors was contacted between the end of January and April, 1967, a little over six months after the main provisions of the Medicare Program had gone into effect. More than 80 per cent of each of these subsamples—676 and 331, respectively—were successfully reinterviewed.

To summarize, 1,205 doctors were interviewed before Medicare was passed (call this Time 1). Of these, 676 were reinter-

viewed about ten months after the law was passed and just before its implementation (call this Time 2),[10] and another 331 were reinterviewed a little over six months after its implementation (call this Time 3).[11] Thus, differences in attitudes between Time 1 and Time 2 would reflect the effects of the Medicare law before actual experience with it; differences between Time 1 and Time 3 would reflect the combined effects of the Medicare law and short-term experience with the program. This design makes it possible to separate the effects on attitudes of the law itself from the effects of its implementation, that is, short-term experience with the program. The design is represented in Figure 27-1.

The Findings

Physicians' Behavior—As the Medicare bill was going through its final stages in Congress in June, 1965, resolutions were introduced at the semiannual meeting of the AMA's House of Delegates calling for a "boycott" or "nonparticipation," when it was passed (The New York Times, June 22,

9 Physicians in New York City were more pro-Medicare than physicians in upstate New York; Jewish physicians were more pro-Medicare than Protestant physicians, with Catholics in between; and those who were Democrats and took a liberal position on economic-welfare issues were more pro-Medicare than those who were Republicans and took a conservative position (see Colombotos, 1968:320–331).

10 Actually, the 676 physicians interviewed at Time 2 include 100 who could not be reached by June 30 and were interviewed between July and October, after Medicare went into effect. Those interviewed after June 30 were a little better informed than those interviewed before June 30 about the services covered by the Medicare program, which is not surprising, but the patterns of change in the attitude toward Title 18A of the two groups were practically the same. The specific month within the Time 2 or Time 3 periods when respondents were interviewed also made no difference in the pattern of change in their attitude toward Title 18A.

11 The original plan of this phase of the study was to reinterview all 1,205 physicians just before Medicare went into effect and again three to four years after it had been in effect. It was decided, however, to set aside a third of this sample (401) to be reinterviewed six months after the law was implemented in order to test the *short-run* effects of implementation. The original sample of 1,205 was not reinterviewed both before and immediately after Medicare's implementation because of the financial cost and because, with the two interviews coming so close together, of a concern about a high refusal rate in the third interview. Reinterviews with all 1,007 (676 plus 331) physicians, interviewed both before and after Medicare, are planned for 1970.

1965:1). Immediately after the law was passed, the president of the AMA predicted that "quite a few" physicians throughout the country would refuse to participate in the program (The New York Times, August 18, 1965:55). By the following March, however, it was reported that "threats of a boycott, if not dead, are at least moot" (The New York Times, March 28, 1966:1). When the AMA House of Delegates met in June, 1966, a month before Medicare was to go into effect, there was little, if any, talk of a boycott.

There has been no boycott, that is, no concerted noncooperation on a large scale, to date.

Physicians and Medicare: 359
A Before-After Study of the
Effects of Legislation on Attitudes

review committee for Medicare patients had agreed to serve; and of those not asked, 66 per cent said they would serve if asked. Slightly higher proportions indicated willingness to serve at Time 3. Furthermore, a physician's refusal to serve on such a committee does not necessarily indicate protest against Medicare. He may refuse for other reasons (see footnote 12, below).

At Time 2, less than 5 per cent said they would not accept patients who get benefits under Medicare. At Time 3, 6 per cent of

FIGURE 27-1   Research design

Medicare Becomes Law (July 30, 1965)		Medicare Program Is Implemented (July 1, 1966)
Time 1	*Time 2*	*Time 3*
January to April, 1964; November, 1964, to March, 1965	May to June, 1966	January to April, 1967
Interviews with 1,205 physicians in private practice	Reinterviews with 676 of a stratified subsample of 804 from 1,205 interviewed at Time 1 [330 of a control sample of 472 also interviewed]	Reinterviews with 331 of remaining stratified subsample of 401 from 1,205 interviewed at Time 1

Responses from the New York State private practitioners interviewed in this study are consistent with the evidence of nationwide compliance by physicians. In the fall of 1965, just a few months after the law was passed, the New York State Medical Society issued a statement that "now that 'Medicare' is an accomplished fact, [the Society] will cooperate in every way possible with the government. . . . As citizens and as physicians, the members of the State Society will obey, and assist in the implementation of the law of the land . . ." (New York State Journal of Medicine, 1965:2779).

The physicians interviewed were asked if they agreed or disagreed with their Society's policy of cooperation. (Note that the answers to this question indicate physicians' *attitudes* toward cooperation with Medicare. They are not reports of actual cooperation.) Ninety per cent agreed at Time 2; 91 per cent agreed at Time 3 (see Table 27–1).

At Time 2, 87 per cent of those who had been asked to serve on a hospital utilization

those who had any patients 65 or over had not treated any patients under Title 18B, but only one of the 331 physicians interviewed at that time had actually *refused* to treat any patients under Title 18B. That doctor explained he was in "semi-retirement" (he was 73 years old), and he wasn't "going to bother with this." The remainder of the 6 per cent indicated that none of their elderly patients had come to them for treatment yet.

To sum up, despite what appeared to be threats of a boycott before Medicare was passed, practically all physicians complied after it became "the law of the land."[12]

12 Our measures of compliance, apart from being reports of own behavior rather than observations of actual behavior, are admittedly simple measures of a complex variable. Consider the following: (1) A physician may provide some services under Medicare, but refuse to provide other services; (2) he may provide services to some patients, but refuse to provide them to other patients; (3) he may cooperate at one point in time after the program goes into effect, and not cooperate at another; (4) he may sabotage

	Time 2	Time 3
Last fall the New York State Medical Society said it would cooperate with the government on Medicare—do you agree or disagree with this policy?**		
Agree	90%	91%
Disagree	8	8
Don't know, no answer	2	1
	100%	100%
Weighted totals	(10,214)	(4,954)
Unweighted totals	(676)	(331)
(If the physician had been asked to serve on a utilization review committee under Title 18): Have you agreed to serve?		
Yes	87%	94%
No	10	6
Not decided	4	0
	101%	100%
Weighted totals	(1,810)	(1,441)
Unweighted totals	(156)	(123)
(If the physician had not been asked to serve on a utilization review committee under Title 18): If you were asked, would you agree to be a member of such a committee?		
Yes	66%	71%
No	27	26
Don't know	7	3
	100%	100%
Weighted totals	(8,323)	(3,513)
Unweighted totals	(516)	(208)
According to your present thinking, do you plan to accept patients who get benefits under Medicare, or not?***		
Accept (have treated)	93%	93%
Will not accept (have not treated)	4	6
Don't know, no answer	4	1
	101%	100%
Weighted totals	(8,941)	(4,345)
Unweighted totals	(609)	(299)

*"Time 1" in these tables refers to interviews conducted before the passage of Medicare, from January to April, 1964, and from November, 1964, to March, 1965; "Time 2," to interviews done after the passage of Medicare but before its implementation, from May to June, 1966; "Time 3," to interviews done after the implementation of Medicare, from January to April, 1967.

All percentages in these tables are based on the weighted figures, which estimate the total number of private practitioners in New York State. The weighted figures do not add up to the actual number of private practitioners in the State because of noninterviews. The sampling design was stratified on geographic area, size of city, and part-time participation in a health department. The unweighted totals represent the number of physicians in a given category actually interviewed.

**This is the Time 2 question. The Time 3 question was: "The New York State Medical Society has said it would cooperate with the government on both Titles 18 and 19. Regarding Title 18, do you agree or disagree with this policy?".

***This is the Time 2 question. The Time 3 question was: "Have you treated any patients who get benefits under Part B of Title 18, or not?" The figures for both questions exclude those physicians who indicated in a previous question that they had no patients 65 years of age or over.

Of the 18 physicians with patients 65 or over who had not treated any of these patients under Title 18B at Time 3, only one had actually refused. The others reported that no elderly patients had come to them for treatment since Medicare.

Physicians and Medicare: **361**
course, for physicians to comply with Medi- **A Before–After Study of the**
care without changing their minds about it. **Effects of Legislation on Attitudes**
What effects has Medicare had on physicians'
attitudes toward the program? In 1964 and
early 1965, before Medicare was passed
(Time 1), 38 per cent of the private practitioners in New York State were "in favor" of
"the bill that would provide for compulsory
health insurance through Social Security to
cover hospital costs for those over 65," the
bill that became Title 18A. This is a sizable
number, but nevertheless, a minority.

At Time 2, ten months after the law was
passed, even before it went into effect, the
proportion "in favor" jumped to 70 per cent.
At Time 3, a little over six months after the
program went into effect, the proportion "in
favor" again jumped, to 81 per cent. At both
Time 2 and Time 3, more than half of those

in favor felt "strongly," rather than only
"somewhat" in favor (see Table 27–2).

Table 27–3 shows that of those opposed to
Title 18A at Time 1, more than half (59 per
cent) had switched by Time 2; 70 per cent
had switched by Time 3.[13] Very few switched
from favoring it to opposing it.

Although the absolute percentage increase
favoring Title 18A of Medicare is greater
between Time 1 and Time 2 (from 38 to
70 per cent), than between Time 2 and Time 3
(from 70 to 81 per cent), it might be misleading, because of the operation of a "ceiling
effect," to argue that the Medicare law itself
had a stronger impact than experience of the
physicians with the program implemented

the program by "over-complying," that is, by
providing more services than are medically indicated. Also, the question of compliance is irrelevant for physicians without patients 65 or over,
such as pediatricians.

As a matter of fact, when the specific behaviors
required of physicians under Medicare are examined, it is difficult to conceive what form a physicians' boycott of Medicare could have taken.
What is a physician asked to do under Medicare?

(1) He must certify that the diagnostic or
therapeutic services for which payment is claimed
are "medically necessary." Such certification can
be entered on a form or order or prescription
the physician ordinarily signs.

(2) Under Title 18, Part B, the physician can
choose between two methods of payment for his
services: he can accept an assignment and bill a
designated carrier (such as Blue Shield, or another private insurance company, depending on
the geographic area), or he can bill the patient
directly. If he takes an assignment, he agrees that
the "reasonable charge" determined by the carrier will be his full charge and that his charge to
the patient will be no more than twenty per cent
of that reasonable charge. If the physician refuses to take an assignment and bills the patient
directly, the patient pays the physician, and then
applies to the carrier for payment. Under this
method, a physician is not restricted by the
"reasonable charge" for a given service. The
patient, however, will be reimbursed only eighty
per cent of the reasonable charge by the carrier.
Although the Social Security Administration had
hoped for wide use of the assignment method,
the AMA's House of Delegates adopted a resolution at its 1966 meeting recommending the use of
the direct billing method (*The New York Times*,
June 30, 1966, p. 1). Use of the direct billing

method cannot be called "noncooperation,"
however, since the law provides for either
method.

(3) In order to promote the most efficient use
of facilities, each participating hospital and extended care facility is required to have a utilization review plan. A committee set up for such a
purpose must include at least two physicians.
Many hospitals already had such review procedures before Medicare went into effect. One
way in which a physician can protest against
Medicare is to refuse to serve on such a committee if asked. But refusal to serve does not
necessarily mean a protest against Medicare,
anymore than unwillingness to run for a local
Board of Education is an indication of protest
against the public school system.

To sum up, the direct and immediate effects of
Medicare on a physician's day-to-day practice
are minimal. For the vast majority of services
under Medicare, the physician is not required to
do anything more or differently in treating patients than he did before Medicare was passed. One
form a boycott on Medicare could have taken
would be for physicians to have refused to treat
patients sixty-five or over, most of whom are
eligible for benefits under both Part A and Part B
of Medicare. This, apparently, few physicians
chose to do. Furthermore, it would be difficult to
interpret such acts as "noncooperation," unless
the physician himself said so. A physician's refusal to admit an elderly patient to the hospital,
for example, could mean that, in his medical
judgment, hospitalization was not necessary.

[13] Physicians' attitudes toward Title 18B,
highly correlated with their attitudes toward
Title 18A, were also very favorable. Seventy-
eight per cent were "in favor" at Time 2 and
eighty-three per cent at Time 3.

Table 27–2—Attitudes of physicians toward medicare (Title 18A) at time 1, time 2, and time 3*

	Time 1	Time 2	Time 3
Favor	38%	70%	81%
Strongly		38	45
Somewhat		31	33
Don't Know, No Answer		1	3
Oppose	54	26	19
Strongly		14	10
Somewhat		11	9
Don't Know, No Answer		1	**
Don't Know, No Answer	8	5	**
	100%	101%	100%
Weighted totals	(18,044)	(10,214)	(4,954)
Unweighted Totals	(1,205)	(676)	(331)

*At Time 1, the question was: "What is your opinion about the bill that would provide for compulsory health insurance through Social Security to cover hospital costs for those over 65—are you personally in favor of such a plan, or are you opposed to it?" Respondents were not asked whether they were "strongly" or "somewhat" in favor or opposed at Time 1.

At Time 2, the questions were: "What is your opinion of Part A of Medicare—the part that provides for compulsory health insurance through Social Security to cover hospital costs for those over 65—are you personally in favor of this plan, or opposed to it?" "Would you say strongly (in favor) (opposed) or somewhat (in favor) (opposed)?" At Time 3 the words "Part A of Title 18" were substituted for the words "Part A of Medicare."

** Less than 0.5 per cent.

Table 27–3—Attitudes of physicians toward medicare (Title 18A) at time 2 and time 3 by their attitudes at time 1

	TIME 1 ATTITUDE TOWARD MEDICARE	
	Favor	Oppose
Time 2 Attitude Toward Medicare		
Favor	90%	59%
Strongly	59	25
Somewhat	30	33
Don't Know, No Answer	1	1
Oppose	11	40
Strongly	5	22
Somewhat	6	16
Don't Know, No Answer	0	2
	101%	99%
Weighted Totals	(3,757)	(5,098)
Unweighted Totals	(193)	(411)
Time 3 Attitude Toward Medicare		
Favor	98%	70%
Strongly	84	19
Somewhat	10	48
Don't Know, No Answer	4	3
Oppose	2	30
Strongly	*	17
Somewhat	2	13
Don't Know, No Answer	0	*
	100%	100%
Weighted Totals	(1,877)	(2,787)
Unweighted Totals	(95)	(213)

* Less than 0.5 per cent.

by the law.[14] What can be asserted, however, is that the law itself had a large effect on physicians' attitudes toward Medicare even before it was implemented.

The Effects of Implementation on Attitudes—
Consistent with the increase in the level of physicians' support for Medicare between Time 2 and Time 3 is the fact that they were less worried about the consequences of Medicare at Time 3 than at Time 2. Their earlier fears simply did not materialize.[15]

For example, the proportion who thought that the quality of care physicians give their elderly patients would be "not as good" under Medicare dropped from 28 per cent at Time 2 to 8 per cent at Time 3 (see Table

[14] The effect of an experimental variable on a group is limited by the initial frequency giving a certain response before exposure to that variable. Since the percentage in favor of Medicare is higher at Time 2 than at Time 1, there is "less room" for an increase in the percentage in favor between Time 2 and Time 3 than between Time 1 and Time 2. The statistical effect of this "ceiling" may be "corrected" by dividing the actual percentage difference by the maximum possible increase. Hovland et al. (1949:285–289) call such a measure the "effectiveness index." Such an index for the Time 1–Time 2 change is $0.52[(70-38)/(100-38) = 0.52]$. For the Time 2–Time 3 change it is $0.37[81-70)/(100-70) = 0.37]$. The fact that the Time 1–Time 2 index is larger than the Time 2–Time 3 measure indicates that the larger increase in the percentage of those in favor of Medicare between Time 1 and Time 2 than between Time 2 and Time 3 cannot be explained away as being entirely due to a statistical ceiling effect.

There is another type of ceiling effect, this one due to *selection*. Those still opposed to Medicare at Time 2 are likely to include a higher proportion of "hard-core" opponents of Medicare than those opposed at Time 1. We found, however, that the Time 2 opponents of Medicare were no more conservative on other measures of political ideology at Time 1 than the Time 1 opponents.

The study design has a limitation, too. Since it provides for only one measure of the physicians' attitudes after the law was passed and before its implementation, it is not possible to assess the effect of time alone. It is possible that the change in attitude toward Medicare between Time 2 and Time 3 is a function of time alone and has nothing to do with the implementation of the program. As a matter of fact, the "transition probabilities" between Time 2 and Time 3 are the same as those between Time 1 and Time 2.

[15] Clark (1953:47–50) reports a similar pattern in cases of desegregation.

Physicians and Medicare: 363
A Before–After Study of the
Effects of Legislation on Attitudes

27–4). The proportion who thought there would be "a great deal" or "a fair amount" of unnecessary hospitalization under Medicare dropped from 69 per cent at Time 2 to 38 per cent at Time 3 (27 per cent thought there had actually been "a great deal" or "a fair amount" of unnecessary hospitalization up to Time 3). The proportion who thought there would be "a great deal" or "a fair amount" of unnecessary utilization of physicians' services under Medicare also dropped from 77 per cent to 36 per cent (25 per cent thought there had actually been "a great deal" or "a fair amount" up to Time 3). It is only in the questions about government interference under Medicare and its effects on physicians' income that there were not significant changes, but only 12 per cent at Time 2 and 11 per cent at Time 3 thought that they would earn less money under Medicare than before, compared with more than a third who thought they would earn more money.[16]

Alternative Interpretations

Let us consider some alternative explanations of the large shifts in attitude toward Title 18A:

1. It could be argued that the changes described above could have taken place without the Medicare law and its implementation; that the shift in physicians' attitudes toward Medicare is part of a general, long-term liberal trend in their thinking. Obviously, there is not available a control group of physicians from whom the facts of the passage of the Medicare law and its implementation could be withheld. The argument that the changes in attitude toward Medicare are due to the law, however, is

[16] There is no increase in the level of physicians' knowledge about the details of Medicare between Time 2 and 3—they are poorly informed at both times—and there is no association between their level of knowledge and the amount of experience with Medicare, on the one hand, and change in their attitude toward Medicare, on the other.

Table 27–4—Perceived effects of medicare (Title 18A) at time 2 and at time 3

	Time 2	Time 3
Weighted Totals	(10,214)	(4,954)
Unweighted Totals	(676)	(331)

In your opinion, how will Medicare (Title 18) affect the *quality* of care doctors give their elderly patients—in general, will doctors give *better* medical care, or *not as good* care, or won't Medicare (Title 18) make any difference?

	Time 2	Time 3
Better	14	30
Not as good	28	8
No difference	54	60
Don't know	5	2
	100%	100%

In your opinion, will there be a great deal of *unnecessary hospitalization* under Medicare (Title 18), or a fair amount, or very little, or none at all?

	Time 2	Time 3
Great deal	32	12
Fair amount	37	26
Very little	18	38
None at all	9	20
Don't know	4	4
	100%	100%

Will there be a great deal of *unnecessary* utilization of *doctors' services* under Medicare (Title 18), or a fair amount, or very little, or none at all?

	Time 2	Time 3
Great deal	39	8
Fair amount	38	28
Very little	15	39
None at all	4	20
Don't know	4	5
	100%	100%

In your opinion, will doctors *earn more* money under Medicare (Title 18) than before, or less money, or won't Medicare (Title 18) make any difference?

	Time 2	Time 3
More	35	42
Less	12	11
No difference	41	38
Don't know	12	9
	100%	100%

In your opinion, will the Federal government, under Medicare (Title 18), interfere with the individual doctor's professional freedom—Would you say a great deal, or a fair amount, or very little, or not at all?

	Time 2	Time 3
Great deal	17	21
Fair amount	37	26
Very little	25	31
Not at all	15	16
Don't know	6	6
	100%	100%

Physicians and Medicare: 365
A Before–After Study of the
Effects of Legislation on Attitudes

supported by the following observations:

a. The change in attitude toward Title 18A is a large change—from 38 per cent in favor to 70 to 81 per cent in a period of no longer than three years. It is not plausible to argue that this is due to a general ideological trend unrelated to the passage and implementation of Medicare.

b. The attitudes that do change are highly specific to Medicare. Physicians' responses to questions indicating their position on economic-welfare issues, political party preference, group practice, and colleague controls, all of which strongly related to their attitudes toward Title 18A at Time 1 (Colombotos, 1968), are relatively stable at Time 1, Time 2, and Time 3 compared with their responses to the question on Medicare. If the change in attitudes toward Medicare was part of a more general trend in physicians' thinking and unrelated to the passage of Medicare, then one would expect changes in attitudes toward these other issues as well.

2. It could be argued that the increasingly favorable medical opinion about Medicare and the passage of the Medicare law were both the result or part of a third factor occurring immediately before Medicare was passed. Strong public support for Medicare, for example, could have influenced both medical and legislative opinion. Data in the present study from two independent samples of Manhattan doctors who were interviewed at two different times before Medicare was passed are inconsistent with such an argument. The first sample of 70 physicians was interviewed from January to April in 1964, about 18 months before Medicare was passed. The second sample of 61 physicians was interviewed from November, 1964, to March, 1965, scarcely six months before the law was passed. There was essentially no difference in the proportion in favor of Title 18A in the two samples—53 per cent in the first sample, 57 per cent in the second.

3. It is possible that New York State physicians' acceptance of Medicare after the enactment of the law was influenced by their opposition to the State's Medicaid program. The New York State implementation of Medicaid was one of the most liberal in the country. The first version of the New York State program was signed into law on April 30, 1966. The program was amended and curtailed two months later after strong opposition in upstate New York and threatened boycotts by county medical societies.

At Time 2, just after the first version of Medicaid was passed by the state legislature, 42 per cent of the doctors interviewed said they were in favor of the law. At Time 3, despite, or perhaps because of, the fact the program had been curtailed six months earlier, it was still only 42 per cent.

On all other questions about Medicaid asked at Time 3, it was less well received than Medicare:

a. Forty-six per cent thought that the government would interfere "a great deal" with the individual physicians' professional freedom under Medicaid, compared with twenty-one per cent for Medicare.
b. Fifty-nine per cent thought that the State Medical Society should cooperate with the Government on Medicaid, compared with ninety-one per cent on Medicare.
c. Fifty-five per cent said they planned to accept (or had already accepted) patients under Title 19, compared with all but one physician under Title 18B.

It could be argued that the opposition to Medicaid in New York State had a "contrast" effect on physicians' responses to Medicare; that Medicare looked better to physicians than it would have looked had Medicaid not been passed, and that this "contrast" inflated the size of the oppose–favor switchers on Medicare. For example, at the height of the furor over Medicaid in the state, one county medical society in an advertisement in *The New York Times* agreed to "cooperate" with the "Federal Medicare Law, which provides a sensible and reasonable plan of medical care for all people over 65 . . . ," but found it "impossible to cooperate with the implementation of this State law [Medicaid] . . . as it is presently proposed. . . ." (June 10, 1966:36). It called Medicaid "socialized medicine."

There is no evidence of such a contrast effect in our data. Rather, among those physicians who opposed Title 18A at Time 1, those who were in favor of Medicaid at Time 2 and Time 3 were much more likely to switch and favor Title 18A than those who opposed Medicaid.[17]

4. It could be argued that the physicians' attitudes toward Medicare expressed at Time 1, before its passage, were superficial and equivocal, and merely reflected official AMA policy, and that once the program became law, physicians felt freer to express their "real" attitudes toward Medicare. But this argument misses the point that law may "legitimate" opinion. The fact that the Medicare program was not law is as significant a part of the social situation at Time 1 as the fact that it had become law at Time 2 and Time 3. One could just as plausibly argue for the superficiality of attitudes expressed after the law, because of a "bandwagon effect," as for the superficiality of attitudes expressed before the law.

As a matter of fact, neither the attitudes toward Medicare at Time 1, nor at Time 2 and Time 3 appear superficial. The sub-question on intensity of feeling was not asked at Time 1. In the Time 1 measure, however, less than 8 per cent were "don't knows." Also, attitude toward Medicare at Time 1 was strongly related to other political questions and issues in the organization of medical practice, as noted above (Colombotos, 1968), which argues against its being superficial. In the Time 2 and 3 measures, the number of "don't knows" was even smaller than at Time 1: at Time 2, it was 5 per cent, and at Time 3, it was less than 0.5 per cent. Also, of those in favor more than half responded they felt "strongly" in favor, rather than only "somewhat" in favor.

5. Finally, a number of methodological problems in panel surveys may be involved:

a. *Reinterview Effect.* It could be argued that the Time 1 interview generated an interest in Medicare, thus influencing physicians' responses in the Time 2 interview. We found no difference between the responses to selected questions, including the one on Medicare, obtained from the reinterviewed sample at Time 2 and from a control sample of 330 physicians not interviewed before.

b. *Change in the Interview Instrument,* specifically in the sequence of the questions. The items preceding the question on Medicare in the Time 2 interview were different from those in the Time 1 interview. We found no difference between the responses obtained in two different versions of the interview at Time 2: one in which the repeat (retest) questions were mixed with new questions and one in which the repeat (retest) questions were asked first, followed by the new questions.

c. *Mortality Effect.* It could be argued that physicians in the panel not interviewed at Time 2 and Time 3 were less likely to be pro-Medicare than those who were interviewed. We found that physicians who could not be reinterviewed at Time 2 and Time 3 did not differ from those who were reinterviewed in either background characteristics or attitudes, including their attitude toward Medicare, expressed at Time 1.

Summary and Conclusions

Despite their opposition to Medicare before the law was passed in 1965, physicians are complying with the program. There may be individual instances of noncooperation, but they are rare, at least in New York State, and there has been no boycott in the sense of concerted noncompliance.

Consistent with their compliance with Medicare, a large number of physicians who were opposed to Medicare before it became law switched and accepted it after it became law. In New York State, the proportion in favor rose from 38 per cent before the law was passed to 70 per cent less than a year after it was passed, even before it was implemented, and once again to 81 per cent six months after the program went into effect.[18]

---

[17] Another test of the effects of Medicaid on attitude change toward Title 18A would be to examine the problem in a state where physicians' attitudes toward Title 18A were similar to those in New York State, but where the Medicaid program did not arouse as much opposition as the one in New York State. Unfortunately, such data were not available.

[18] The proportion of private practitioners in favor of Medicare was higher in New York State than in the country as a whole before

The first increase, from 38 to 70 per cent, argues that for law to influence attitudes it does not necessarily have to change relevant behavior first. We have in physicians' response to Medicare a case in which attitudes adapted to the law even before it went into effect.

The ready accommodation, both in deed and in mind, of these physicians to Medicare contrasts sharply with their continuing opposition to Medicaid and, to take a more extreme example, with physician strikes, such as the one in Saskatchewan, Canada, in 1962, against the province's medical care program.

What accounts for such differences in response to a law? The following differences between Medicare and the New York State Medicaid law illustrate some of the conditions listed above and suggest others that promote the effectiveness of a law:

1. *The Content of the Program*—The direct impact on physicians' practice of Medicaid in New York State is much greater than that of Medicare.

a. The number of people covered under Medicare in the state (those 65 or over) is less than two million. Estimates in May, 1966, of the number eligible under Medicaid ranged from 3.5 to 7 million. Furthermore, the number covered by Medicaid could be increased by liberalizing the definition of eligibility.

b. The clients of Medicare are the aged and the program is based on the insurance principle. The clients of Medicaid are the "medically indigent" and the program is based on the welfare principle. Physicians may be more sympathetic to a program serving the medical needs of the aged through insurance than to a program serving the "(medically) indigent," classified with "welfare cases."

c. Medicaid provides more services than

Medicare, including drugs, dental bills, and other services not covered by Medicare.

d. New York State's Medicaid affects the physicians' practice more directly than Medicare. Medicaid attempts to control the quality and cost of medical care: the quality, by establishing criteria for determining who can render care, thus limiting the free choice of physicians; and the cost, by paying physicians fixed fees rather than "usual and customary" charges. Medicare has attempted neither. The direct effects of Medicare on physicians' practice, as a matter of fact, are minimal. Somers and Somers (1967:1) put it this way:

The 1965 enactment of Medicare was heralded as "revolutionary." But, in fact, it was neither a sudden nor radical departure from the march of events in the organization and financing of medical care and government's growing participation. No existing institutions were overturned or seriously threatened by the new legislation. On the contrary, Medicare responded to the needs of the providers of care as well as those of the consumers. It was primarily a financial underpinning of the existing health care industry—with all that implies in terms of strengths and weaknesses.

As a matter of fact, Medicare supports the stability of physicians' income under Title 18B, without controlling their fees. As noted above, more than a third of New York State physicians interviewed thought that under Medicare physicians would earn more money than before, and only about 10 per cent thought they would earn less; the remainder thought it would not make any difference.

Both in terms of consistency with their ideology and in terms of their self-interest, then, Medicare is more acceptable to New York State physicians than Medicaid.

2. *Degree of Popular Support*—Medicare was passed with overwhelming popular support. Two-thirds of the public were in favor of Medicare, according to a nationwide Gallup poll in January, 1965, six months before it was passed. The percentage was probably higher in New York State. In con-

Physicians and Medicare: 367
A Before–After Study of the
Effects of Legislation on Attitudes

Medicare was passed (see Footnote 1). No post-Medicare data from a national sample of physicians are available, however. Note also that our New York State study sample excludes physicians on full-time salary, who are more likely to be politically liberal and in favor of Medicare than private practitioners. (For data supporting the latter point, see Lipset and Schwartz, 1966: 304).

trast, there was little awareness about Medicaid before it was passed, and there was strong opposition, particularly in upstate New York, from industry, farm organizations, and in the press, after the first version of the New York Medicaid law was passed in April, 1966.

3. *Medicare Is the Same throughout the Country, Whereas Medicaid Varies Greatly from State to State*—It is possible that the opposition of New York physicians to their state's Medicaid program, the most liberal in the country, is reinforced by their feeling "worse off" than their colleagues in other states where the Medicaid programs are not as ambitious. A plausible hypothesis, setting aside regional and local differences in values that may or may not be congruent with a given law, is that a national law is more "legitimate" and more likely to be effectively complied with than a state or local law.[19]

Outside the area of medical care, public response in many parts of the country to statutes and judicial decisions requiring the desegregation of schools and other institutions contrasts sharply with physicians' response to Medicare. The issues of desegregation and civil rights will not be taken up here in any detail, but some obvious differences between them and Medicare come to mind:

a. Despite the "American creed" and trends showing a reduction of prejudice and discrimination, at least up to 1964, "white racism" may be more firmly entrenched among large segments of the American public than the fear of government participation in health care among physicians.

b. The distributions of opposition to desegregation and to Medicare are different. Social supports to segregationists are more

widely available than social supports to physicians opposed to Medicare. The general public strongly supported Medicare, and it was the medical profession that was out of step.

c. Desegregation, like Medicaid, runs into a hodgepodge of inconsistent and contradictory local, state, and Federal laws concerning different facilities and institutions—schools, transportation, recreation, housing, employment, marriage. Some of these laws actually *prescribe* segregation. Consider a hypothetical situation in which some states had laws that made it illegal to provide hospitalization and medical care under the terms ultimately provided by the Federal Medicare law![20]

Having established in this paper the fact that the passage and implementation of Medicare had a sharp effect in changing the attitudes of physicians toward the program, the next steps will be (1) to examine the *conditions* under which physicians make both short-term and long-term changes in their attitudes toward Medicare, (2) to examine the long-term effects of Medicare on physicians' attitudes toward the program and toward other related political and health care issues, and (3) to compare the long-term and short-term responses of physicians to Medicare and Medicaid. A fourth wave of inter-

---

[19] In terms of these conditions, the prospects of the plan that physicians struck against in Saskatchewan in 1962 were, in retrospect, not good: (1) the plan's impact on physicians' practice was much greater than Medicare's, providing for universal coverage for all residents in the province and a comprehensive range of services; (2) public opposition to the plan appeared to be stronger and better organized than the opposition to Medicare; and (3) it was a provincial, not a national, plan.

[20] The effects of law on behavior and attitudes are interpretable in terms of cognitive dissonance theory. According to this theory, the greater the dissonance between an individual's continued opposition to a program, behaviorally and attitudinally, and other elements in his cognitive structure, the greater is the probability of his complying and accepting the program. If we conceive as elements in an individual's cognitive structures the passage of a law and the specific conditions for its effectiveness, then it follows that the more of these conditions that apply, the greater the dissonance and the greater the probability of compliance and attitudinal acceptance.

That part of the theory that focuses on the effects of compliance on attitude change and the conditions under which dissonance between these two elements is aroused, however, is not particularly relevant to our case, since we found a large shift in attitudes toward Medicare even before physicians had an opportunity to comply (unless planning to comply is seen as equivalent to complying). The effects of compliance on attitude change in terms of dissonance theory is explicitly applied to desegregation in Brehm and Cohen (1962:269–285).

**Physicians and Medicare: 369
A Before–After Study of the
Effects of Legislation on Attitudes**

views with our physician panel is being planned in 1970—five years after the passage of Medicare—to answer these questions.

1. The two major sets of conditions of individual change in attitudes toward Medicare we shall examine are attitude–structural and social–structural variables. The general assumption is that there is pressure toward both intrapersonal and interpersonal consistency. For example, among those opposed to Medicare before the law was passed, it is predicted that Democrats are more likely to change their attitudes toward Medicare than Republicans; that physicians in areas where support for Medicare was initially strong are more likely to change than those in areas where support was weak; and that physicians who perceive themselves as having different opinions from their colleagues are more likely to change than those who see themselves as being in agreement. Other variables such as physicians' knowledge about Medicare, their experience with it, and their perceptions of its effects on their practice will also be studied as conditions of change in their attitudes toward Medicare.

2. a. The short-term effects of the Medicare law and program on physicians' attitudes toward it were indeed dramatic. What will be the long-term effects—five years later? Will opposition to Medicare continue to wither away, or will it stiffen?

b. We have found that the Medicare law had little short-term effect on physicians' attitudes toward other related political and health care issues. The stability of these attitudes, as a matter of fact, was offered to support the argument that the change in attitude toward Medicare was indeed an effect of the Medicare law and program rather than a part of a more general liberal trend in physicians' thinking. Katz observes that "it is puzzling that attitude change seems to have slight generalization effects, when the evidence indicates considerable generalization in the organization of a person's beliefs and values" (Katz, 1960:199). But our results and Katz' observation, refer to the short-run. It is plausible to expect that a change in one part of an attitude structure will produce changes in other parts of the structure, but the generalization of change *may not take place immediately*. It may

take some time for the structure to become reintegrated. Will physicians' acceptance of Medicare make them more liberal in the longer run in their thinking about political issues and about changes in the organization of medical practice, or will it make them more conservative and resistant to such changes, or will it simply have no effects?[21]

3. In contrast to the ready acceptance of Medicare, physicians continued to oppose Medicaid in New York State nearly a year after it was implemented. How will they feel four years later? What will be the conditions under which physicians make long-term changes in their attitudes toward Medicaid, and how will these conditions differ from those that distinguish changers and non-changers on Medicare? A comparison of the dynamics of the short-term and long-term responses of physicians to Medicare and Medicaid represents a modest test of the conditions under which laws influence behavior and attitudes.

Bibliography

Allport, G. W., *The Nature of Prejudice*, Cambridge, Mass.: Addison-Wesley, 1954.

Badgley, R. F. and S. Wolfe, *Doctors' Strike, Medical Care and Conflict in Saskatchewan*, New York: Atherton Press, 1967.

Ball, H. V., G. E. Simpson and K. Ideda, "Law and Social Change: Sumner Reconsidered," *Amer. J. Sociol.*, 67:532–540, March, 1962.

Berger, M., *Equality by Statute*, New York: Columbia Univ. Press, 1954.

Berkowitz, L. and N. Walker, "Laws and Moral Judgments," *Sociometry*, 30:410–422, December, 1967.

Bonfield, A. E., "The Role of Legislation in Eliminating Racial Discrimination," *Race*, 7:108–109, October, 1965.

[21] Note that "short-term" and "long-term" in attitude change research mean quite different things depending on the perspective of the investigator and the design used. In experimental studies, "short-term" effects are measured within minutes, hours, or at most, a few days after the introduction of the experimental variable; "long-term" effects usually mean no more than a few weeks later. In panel surveys, the time intervals are longer.

Brehm, J. W., and A. R. Cohen, *Explorations in Cognitive Dissonance*, New York: Wiley, 1962.

Campbell, E. Q., "Some Social Psychological Correlates of Direction in Attitude Change," *Social Forces*, 36:335–340, May, 1958.

Cantril, H., *Gauging Public Opinion*, Princeton: Princeton Univ. Press, 1947.

Clark, K. (issue ed.), "Desegregation: An Appraisal of the Evidence," *J. Soc. Issues*, 9:47–50, 1953.

Colombotos, J., "Physicians' Attitudes Toward Medicare," *Medical Care*, 6:320–331, July–August, 1968.

———, "Physicians' Attitudes Toward a County Health Department," *Amer. J. Pub. Hlth.*, 59:53–59, January, 1969.

———, "Social Origins and Ideology of Physicians: A Study of the Effects of Early Socialization," *J. Hlth. Soc. Behav.*, 10:16–29, March, 1969.

———, "Personal Versus Telephone Interviews: Effect on Responses," *Public Health Reports*, 84:773–782, September, 1969.

Deutsch, M., and M. E. Collins, *Interracial Housing: A Psychological Evaluation of a Social Experiment*, Minneapolis: Univ. of Minnesota Press, 1951.

Deutscher, I., "Words and Deeds," *Social Problems*, 13:235–254, Winter, 1966.

Dicey, A. V., *Law and Opinion in England During the Nineteenth Century*, 2nd ed., London: Macmillan, 1963.

Evans, W. M., "Law As an Instrument of Social Change," in A. W. Gouldner and S. M. Miller (eds.), *Applied Sociology*, New York: Free Press, 1965, pp. 291–292.

Feingold, E., *Medicare: Policy and Politics*, San Francisco, Cal.: Chandler, 1966.

Harris, R., *A Sacred Trust*, New York: New American Library, 1966.

Hovland, C. I., A. A. Lumsdaine and F. D. Sheffield, *Experiments on Mass Communication*, in *Studies in Social Psychology in World War II*, Princeton: Princeton Univ. Press, vol. III, 1949.

Hyman, H. H., and P. B. Sheatsley, "Attitudes Toward Desegregation," *Scientific American*, 211:6, July, 1964.

Katz, D., "The Functional Approach to the Study of Attitudes," *Public Opinion Quarterly*, 24:163–204, Summer, 1960.

Killian, L. M., *The Negro in American Society*, Florida State Univ. Studies, 28:65–70, 1958.

Kutner, B., C. Wilkins and P. B. Yarrow, "Verbal Attitudes and Overt Behavior Involving Racial Prejudice," *J. Abn. Soc. Psych.*, 47:649–652, 1952.

LaPiere, R. T., "Attitudes vs. Actions," *Social Forces*, 13:230–237, March, 1934.

Lipset, S. M., and M. A. Schwartz, "The Politics of Professionals," in H. M. Vollmer and D. L. Mills (eds.), *Professionalization*, Englewood Cliffs, N.J.: Prentice-Hall, 1966, pp. 299–310.

MacIver, R. M., *The More Perfect Union*, New York: Macmillan, 1948.

———, "Forward," in Berger, *op. cit.*, p. viii.

Mayhew, L. H., *Law and Equal Opportunity*, Cambridge, Mass.: Harvard Univ. Press, 1968.

Muir, W. K., Jr., *Prayer in the Public Schools: Law and Attitude Change*, Chicago: Univ. of Chicago Press, 1967.

Mussen, P. H., "Some Personality and Social Factors Related to Changes in Children's Attitudes Toward Negroes," *J. Abn. Soc. Psych.*, 45:423–441, July, 1950.

Myrdal, G., *An American Dilemma*, New York: Harper and Row, 1944.

New York State Journal of Medicine, editorial, 62:2779, Nov. 15, 1965.

"Opinions About Negro Infantry Platoons in White Companies of Seven Divisions," in G. E. Swanson, *et al.* (eds.), *Readings in Social Psychology*, New York: Holt, 1952.

Pound, R., *The Task of Law*, Lancaster, Pa.: Franklin and Marshall College, 1944.

Roche, J. P., and M. M. Gordon, "Can Morality Be Legislated?" *New York Times Magazine*, May 22, 1955, pp. 10, 42, 44, 49. In K. Young and R. W. Mack (eds.), *Principles of Sociology: A Reader in Theory and Research*, New York: American Book Co., 1966.

Rose, A. M., "Sociological Factors in the Effectiveness of Projected Legislative Remedies," *J. Legal Ed.*, 11:470–481, 1959.

———, "The Passage of Legislation: The Politics of Financing Medical Care for the Aging," *The Power Structure: Political Processes in American Society*, New York: Oxford Univ. Press, chap. xii, pp. 400–455, 1967.

Saenger, G., and E. Gilbert, "Customer Reactions to the Integration of Negro Sales Personnel," *Internat. J. Opin. Attit. Res.*, 4:57–76, Spring, 1950.

Schwartz, M. A., *Trends in White Attitudes Toward Negroes*, Chicago: National Opinion Research Center, Univ. of Chicago, 1967.

Scott, J. F., and L. H. Scott, "They Are Not So Much Anti-Negro As Pro-Middle Class," *New York Times Magazine*, March 24, 1968, pp. 46 ff.

Somers, H. M., and A. R. Somers, *Medicare and the Hospitals: Issues and Prospects*, Washington, D.C.: The Brookings Institution, 1967.

Sumner, W. G., *Folkways*, New York: New American Library, 1960.

Swanson, G. E., *et al.*, *op. cit.*

Walker, N. and M. Argyle, "Does the Law Affect Moral Judgments?" *Brit. J. Crimin.*, 5:570–581, 1964.

Yarrow, M. R., "Interpersonal Dynamics in a Desegregation Process," (special issue), *J. Social Issue*, 1958, p. 14.

Young and Mack, *op. cit.*

IN [A] BUDGET MESSAGE to Congress, [President Johnson] proposed a quadrupling of federal spending on health care and medical assistance for the poor to $4.2 billion in fiscal 1968:

> The 1968 budget maintains the forward thrust of federal programs designed to improve health care in the nation, to combat poverty, and assist the needy. . . . The rise reflects the federal government's role in bringing quality medical care, particularly to aged and indigent persons.

Three years earlier in a special message to Congress the President had prefaced re-introduction of the medicare bill by saying:

> We can—and must—strive now to assure the availability of and accessibility to the best health care for all Americans, regardless of age or geography or economic status. . . . Nowhere are the needs greater than for the 15 million children of families who live in poverty.

Then, after decades of debate and massive professional and political opposition, the medicare program was passed. It promised to lift the poorest of our aged out of the medical ghetto of charity and into private and voluntary hospital care. In addition, legislation for heart disease and cancer centers was quickly enacted. It was said that such facilities would increase life expectancy by five years and bring a 20 per cent reduction in heart disease and cancer by 1975.

Is the medical millenium, then, on its way? The President, on the day before sending the 1968 budget to Congress, said: "Medicare is an unqualified success."

"Nevertheless," he added, "there are improvements which can be made and shortcomings which need prompt attention." The message also noted that there might be some obstacles on the highroad to health. The rising cost of medical care, President Johnson stated, "requires an expanded and better organized effort by the federal government in research and studies of the organization and delivery of health care." If the President's proposals are adopted, the states will spend $1.9 billion and the federal government $1 billion in a "Partnership for Health" under the Medicaid program.

28

Medical Ghettos

Anselm L. Strauss

Considering the costs to the poor—and to the taxpayers—why don't the disadvantaged get better care? In all the lively debate on that matter, it is striking how little attention is paid to the mismatch between the current organization of American medicine and the life styles of the lower class. The major emphasis is always on how the *present* systems can be a little better supported or a trifle altered to produce better results.

I contend that the poor will never have anything approaching equal care until our present medical organization undergoes profound reform. Nothing in current legislation or planning will accomplish this. My arguments, in brief, are these:

The emphasis in all current legislation is on extending and improving a basically sound system of medical organization.

This assumes that all those without adequate medical services—especially the poor—can be reached with minor reforms, without radical transformation of the systems of care.

This assumption is false. The reason the medical systems have not reached the poor is because they were never designed to do so. The way the poor think and respond, the way they live and operate, has hardly ever (if ever) been considered in the scheduling, paperwork, organization, and mores of clinics, hospitals, and doctors' offices. The life styles of the poor are different; they must be specifically taken into account. Professionals have not been trained and are

From Trans-Action, Vol. 4: 7–15, 62; May, 1967. Copyright © by Trans-Action Magazine, New Brunswick, New Jersey; by permission of the author and publisher.

not now being trained in the special skills and procedures necessary to do this.

These faults result in a vicious cycle which drives the poor away from the medical care they need.

Major reforms in medical organizations must come, or the current great inequities will continue, and perhaps grow.

I have some recommendations designed specifically to break up that vicious cycle at various points. These recommendations are built directly upon aspects of the life styles of the poor. They do not necessarily require new money or resources, but they do require rearrangement, reorganization, reallocation —the kind of change and reform which are often much harder to attain than new funds or facilities.

How to be Healthy Though Poor

In elaborating these arguments, one point must be nailed down first: *The poor definitely get second-rate medical care.* This is self-evident to anyone who has worked either with them or in public medical facilities; but there is a good deal of folklore to the effect that the very poor share with the very rich the best doctors and services—the poor getting free in the clinics what only the rich can afford to buy.

The documented statistics of the Department of Health, Education, and Welfare tell a very different story. As of 1964, those families with annual incomes under $2,000 average 2.8 visits per person to a physician each year, compared to 3.8 for those above $7,000. (For children during the crucial years under 15, the ratio is 1.6 to 5.7 The poor tend to have larger families; needless to add, their child mortality rate is also higher.) People with higher incomes (and $7,000 per year can hardly be considered wealthy) have a tremendous advantage in the use of medical specialists—27.5 per cent see at least one of them annually, compared to about 13 per cent of the poor. [*Ed. note:* See chapter 17 in this volume.]

Health insurance is supposed to equalize the burden; but here, too, money purchases better care. Hospital or surgical insurance coverage is closely related to family income, ranging from 34 per cent among those with family income of less than $2,000 to almost 90 per cent for persons in families of $7,000 or more annual income. At the same time, the poor, when hospitalized, are much more apt to have more than one disorder—and more apt to exhaust their coverage before discharge.

Among persons who were hospitalized, insurance paid for some part of the bill for about 40 per cent of patients with less than $2,000 family income, for 60 per cent of patients with $2,000–$3,999 family income, and for 80 per cent of patients with higher incomes. Insurance paid three-fourths or more of the bill for approximately 27 per cent, 44 per cent, and 61 per cent of these respective income groups. Preliminary data from the 1964 survey year showed, for surgery or delivery bills paid by insurance, an even more marked association of insurance with income.

Similar figures can be marshaled for chronic illness, dental care, and days of work lost.

Strangely enough, however, *cash* difference (money actually spent for care) is not nearly so great. The under $2,000 per year group spent $112 per person per year, those families earning about three times as much ($4,000–$7,000) paid $119 per person, and those above $7,000, $153. Clearly, the poor not only get poorer health services but less for their money.

As a result, the poor suffer much more chronic illness and many more working days lost—troubles they are peculiarly ill-equipped to endure. Almost 60 per cent of the poor have more than one disabling condition compared to about 24 per cent of other Americans. Poor men lose 10.2 days of work annually compared to 4.9 for the others. Even medical research seems to favor the affluent—its major triumphs have been over acute, not chronic, disorders.

What's Wrong with Medical Organization?

Medical care, as we know it now, is closely linked with the advancing organization, complexity, and maturity of our society and the increasing education, urbanization, and need for care of our people. Among the results: Medicine is increasingly practiced in hospitals in metropolitan areas.

The relatively few dispensaries for the poor of yesteryear have been supplanted by great numbers of outpatient hospital clinics. These clinics and services are still not adequate—which is why the continuing cry for reform is "more and better." But even when medical services *are* readily available to the poor, they are not used as much as they could and should be. The reasons fall into two categories: factors in the present organization of medical care that act as a brake on giving care quality to everyone, [and] the life styles of the poor that present obstacles even when the brakes are released.

The very massiveness of modern medical organization is itself a hindrance to health care for the poor. Large buildings and departments, specialization, division of labor, complexity, and bureaucracy lead to an impersonality and an overpowering and often grim atmosphere of hugeness. The poor, with their meager experience in organizational life, their insecurity in the middle class world, and their dependence on personal contacts, are especially vulnerable to this impersonalization.

Hospitals and clinics are organized for "getting work done" from the staff point of view; only infrequently are they set up to minimize the patient's confusion. He fends for himself and sometimes may even get lost when sent "just down the corridor." Patients are often sent for diagnostic tests from one service to another with no explanations, with inadequate directions, with brusque tones. This may make them exceedingly anxious and affect their symptoms and diagnosis. After sitting for hours in waiting rooms, they become angry to find themselves passed over for latecomers—but nobody explains about emergencies or priorities. They complain they cannot find doctors they really like or trust.

When middle class patients find themselves in similar situations, they can usually work out some methods of "beating the system" or gaining understanding, that may raise staff tempers but will lower their own

anxieties. The poor do not know how to beat the system. And only very seldom do they have that special agent, the private doctor, to smooth their paths.

Another organizational barrier is the increasing professionalism of health workers. The more training and experience it takes to make the various kinds of doctors, nurses, technicians, and social workers, the more they become oriented around professional standards and approaches, and the more the patient must take their knowledge and abilities on trust. The gaps of communications, understanding, and status grow. To the poor, professional procedures may seem senseless or even dangerous—especially when not explained—and professional manners impersonal or brutal, even when professionals are genuinely anxious to help.

Many patients complain about not getting enough information; but the poor are especially helpless. They don't know the ropes. Davis quotes from a typical poor parent, the mother of a polio-stricken child:

Well they don't tell you anything hardly. They don't seem to want to. I mean you start asking questions and they say, "Well, I only have about three minutes to talk to you." And then the things that you ask, they don't seem to want to answer you. So I don't ask them anything any more.[1] . . .

For contrast, we witnessed an instance of a highly educated woman who found her physician evasive. Suddenly she shot a question: "Come now, Doctor, don't I have the same cancerous condition that killed my sister?" His astonished reaction confirmed her suspicion.

Discrimination also expresses itself in subtle ways. As Riessman and Scribner[2] note (for psychiatric care), "Middle class patients are preferred by most treatment agents, and are seen as more treatable. . . . Diagnoses are more hopeful. . . ." Those who understand, follow, respond to, and

[1] Davis, F., *Passage Through Crisis*, Indianapolis: Bobbs–Merrill, 1963, pp. 57–67.
[2] Riessman, F., and S. Scribner, "The Underutilization of Mental Health Services by Workers and Low Income Groups: Causes and Cures," *Amer. J. Psychiatry*, 121:798–800, 1965.

are grateful for treatment are good patients; and that describes the middle class.

Professional health workers are themselves middle class, represent and defend its values, and show its biases. They assume that the poor (like themselves) have regular meals, lead regular lives, try to support families, keep healthy, plan for the future. They prescribe the same treatment for the same diseases to all, not realizing that their words do not mean the same things to all. (What does "take with each meal" mean to a family that eats irregularly, seldom together, and usually less than three times a day?)

And there is, of course, some open bias. A welfare case worker in a large Midwestern city, trying to discover why her clients did not use a large, nearby municipal clinic more, described what she found:

Aside from the long waits (8 a.m. to about 1 p.m. just to make the appointment), which perhaps are unavoidable, there is the treatment of patients by hospital personnel. This is at the clinic level. People are shouted at, ridiculed, abused, pushed around, called "Niggers," told to stand "with the rest of the herd," and in many instances made to feel terribly inferior if not inadequate.... This ... was indulged in by personnel other than doctors and nurses.[3] ...

Even when no bias is intended, the hustle, impersonality, and abstraction of the mostly white staff tend to create this feeling among sensitive and insecure people: "And I do think the treatment would have been different if Albert had been white."

The poor especially suffer in that vague area we call "care," which includes nursing, instructions about regimens, and post-hospital treatment generally. What happens to the lower class patient once released? Middle class patients report regularly to their doctors who check on progress and exert some control. But the poor are far more likely to go to the great, busy clinics where they seldom see the same doctor twice. Once out they are usually on their own.

[3] Quoted from an interview document with a Negro mother, by permission of Professor Hyland Lewis, Howard Univ. (from his study of child-rearing practices in Washington, D.C.).

Will the poor get better care if "more and better" facilities are made available? I doubt it. The fact is that they underutilize those available now. For instance, some 1963 figures from the Director of the Division of Health Services, Children's Bureau:

In Atlanta, 23 per cent of women delivered at the Grady Hospital had had no prenatal care; in Dallas, approximately one-third of low-income patients receive no prenatal care; at the Los Angeles County Hospital in 1958, it was 20 per cent; at the D.C. General Hospital in Washington, it is 45 per cent; and in the Bedford Stuyvesant section of Brooklyn, New York, it is 41 per cent with no or little prenatal care.[4]

Distances are also important. Hospitals and clinics are usually far away. The poor tend to organize their lives around their immediate neighborhoods, to shut out the rest of the city. Some can hardly afford bus fare (much less cab fare for emergencies). Other obstacles include unrealistic eligibility rules and the requirement by some hospitals that clinic patients arrange a blood donation to the blood bank as a prerequisite for prenatal care.

Medical organization tends to assume a patient who is educated and well-motivated, who is interested in ensuring a reasonable level of bodily functioning and generally in preserving his own health. But health professionals themselves complain that the poor come to the clinic or hospital with advanced symptoms, that parents don't pay attention to children's symptoms early enough, that they don't follow up treatments or regimens, and delay too long in returning. But is it really the fault of whole sections of the American population if they don't follow what professionals expect of them?

The Crisis Life of the Poor

What are the poor really like? In our country they are distinctive. They live strictly, and wholeheartedly, in the present; their lives are uncertain, dominated by

[4] Lesser, A. J., "Current Problems of Maternity Care," U.S. Dept. of Health, Education, and Welfare, speech delivered May 10, 1963, p. 10.

recurring crises (as S. M. Miller puts it, theirs "is a crisis-life constantly trying to make do with string where rope is needed"). To them a careful concern about health is unreal—they face more pressing troubles daily, just getting by. Bad health is just one more condition they must try to cope— or live—with.

Their households are understaffed. There are no servants, few reliable adults. There is little time or energy to care for the sick. If the mother is ill, who will care for her or take her to the clinic—or care for the children if she goes? It is easier to live with illness than use up your few resources doing something about it.

As Rosenblatt and Suchman[5] have noted:

The body can be seen as simply another class of objects to be worked out but not repaired. Thus, teeth are left without dental care. . . . Corrective eye examinations, even for those who wear glasses, are often neglected. . . . It is as though . . . blue-collar groups think of the body as having a limited span of utility; to be enjoyed in youth and then to suffer with and to endure stoically with age and decrepitude.

They are characterized by low self-esteem. Rainwater[6] remarks that low-income people develop "a sense of being unworthy; they do not uphold the sacredness of their persons in the same way that middle-class people do. Their tendency to think of themselves as of little account is . . . readily generalized to their bodies." And this attitude is transferred to their children.

They seek medical treatment only when practically forced to it. As Rosenblatt and Suchman[7] put it: "Symptoms that do not incapacitate are often ignored." In clinics and hospitals they are shy, frustrated, passively submissive, prey to brooding, depressed anxiety. They reply with guarded hostility, evasiveness, and withdrawal. They believe, of their treatment, that "what is free is not much good." As a result, the professionals tend to turn away. Roth[8]

describes how the staff in a rehabilitation ward gets discouraged with its apparently unrehabilitatable patients and gives up and concentrates on the few who seem hopeful. The staffs who must deal with the poor in such wards either have rapid turnover or retreat into "enclaves of research, administration, and teaching."

The situation must get worse. More of the poor will come to the hospitals and clinics. Also, with the increasing use of health insurance and programs by unions and employers, more will come as paying patients into the private hospitals, mixing with middle class patients and staff, upsetting routines, perhaps lowering quality— a frightening prospect, as many administrators see it. As things are going now, relations between lower-income patients and hospital staff must become more frequent, intense, and exacerbated.

It is evident that the vicious cycle that characterizes medical care for the poor must be broken before anything can be accomplished.

In the first part of this cycle, the poor come into the hospitals later than they should, often delaying until their disorders are difficult to relieve, until they are actual emergency cases. The experiences they have there encourage them to try to stay out even longer the next time—and to cut the visits necessary for treatment to a minimum.

Second, they require, if anything, even more effective communication, and understanding with the professionals than the middle class patient. They don't get it; and the treatment is often undone once they leave.

What to do? The conventional remedies do help some. More money and insurance will tend to bring the poor to medical help sooner; increased staff and facilities can cut down the waits, the rush, the tenseness, and allow for more individual and efficient treatment and diagnosis.

But much more is required. If the cycle is to be *broken*, the following set of recommendations must be adopted:

[5] Rosenblatt, D., and E. A. Suchman, "The Underutilization of Medical-care Services by Blue Collarites," in A. Shostak and W. Gomberg (eds.), *Blue-collar World*, Englewood Cliffs, N.J.: Prentice–Hall, 1964, pp. 341–349.

[6] Quotation from a memorandum written for this paper.

[7] Rosenblatt and Suchman, *op. cit.*

[8] Roth, J., "Institutions for the Unwanted," unpublished paper presented to the Tufts University Colloquium on Social Science and Medicine, April 8, 1965.

Speed up the initial visit. Get them there sooner.

Improve patient experiences.

Improve communication, given and received, about regimens and treatment to be followed.

Work to make it more likely that the patient or his family will follow through at home.

Make it more likely that the patient will return when necessary.

Decrease the time between necessary visits.

This general list is not meant to be the whole formula. Any experienced doctor or nurse, once he recognizes the need, can add to or modify it. An experience of mine illustrates this well. A physician in charge of an adolescent clinic for lower-income patients, finding that my ideas fitted into his own daily experience, invited me to address his staff. In discussion afterward good ideas quickly emerged:

Since teen-age acne and late teen-age menstrual pain were frequent complaints and the diagnoses and medications not very complicated, why not let nurses make them? Menstruating girls would be more willing to talk to a woman than a man.

Patients spend many hours sitting around waiting. Why not have nursing assistants, trained by the social worker and doctor and drawn from the patients' social class, interview and visit with them during this period, collecting relevant information?

Note two things about these suggestions: Though they do involve some new duties and some shifting around, they do not call for any appreciable increase of money, personnel, or resources; and such recommendations, once the need is pointed out, can arise from the initiative and experience of the staff themselves.

Here in greater detail are my recommendations:

Speeding up the Initial Visit

Increased efforts are needed for early detection of disease among the poor. Existing methods should be increased and improved, and others should be added—for instance, mobile detection units of all kinds, public drives with large-scale educational campaigns against common specific disorders, and so on. The poor themselves should help in planning, and their ideas should be welcomed.

The schools could and should become major detection units with large-scale programs of health inspection. The school nurse, left to her own initiative, is not enough. The poor have more children and are less efficient at noting illness; those children do go to school, where they could be examined. Teachers should also be given elementary training and used more effectively in detection.

Train more sub-professionals, drawn from the poor themselves. They can easily learn to recognize the symptoms of the more common disorders and be especially useful in large concentrations, such as housing projects. They can teach the poor to look for health problems in their own families.

Facilitate the Visit

The large central facilities make for greater administrative and medical efficiency. But fewer people will come to them than to smaller neighborhood dispensaries. Imperfect treatment may be better than little or no treatment; and the total effectiveness for the poor may actually be better with many small facilities than the big ones.

Neighborhood centers can not only treat routine cases and act to follow up hospital outpatients, but they can also discover those needing the more difficult procedures and refer them to the large centers—for example, prenatal diagnosis and treatment in the neighborhoods, with high-risk pregnancies sent to the central facilities. (The Children's Bureau has experimented with this type of organization.)

There must be better methods to get the sick to the clinics. As noted, the poor tend to stick to their own neighborhoods and be fearful outside them, to lack bus fare and domestic help. Even when dental or eye defects *are* discovered in schools, often children still do not get treatment. Sub-professionals and volunteers could follow up, provide transportation, bus fare, information, or baby-sitting and housecare. Block or church organizations could help. The special drives for particular illnesses could also include transportation. (Recent studies show that different ethnic groups respond differently to different pressures and appeals; sub-professionals from the same groups could, therefore, be especially effective.)

Hours should be made more flexible; there should be more evening and night clinics. Working people work, when they have jobs, and cannot afford to lose jobs in order to sit around waiting to be called at a clinic. In short, clinics should adapt to people, not expect the opposite. (A related benefit: Evening clinics should lift the load on emergency services in municipal hospitals, since the poor often use them just that way.)

Neighborhood pharmacists should be explicitly recognized as part of the medical team, and every effort be made to bring them in. The poor are much more apt to consult their neighborhood pharmacist first —and he could play a real role in minor treatment and in referral. He should be rewarded, and given such training as necessary—perhaps by schools of pharmacy. Other "health healers" might also be encouraged to help get the seriously ill to the clinics and hospitals, instead of being considered rivals or quacks.

Lower-income patients who enter treatment early can be *rewarded* for it. This may sound strange, rewarding people for benefiting themselves—but it might bring patients in earlier as well as bring them back, and actually save money for insurance companies and government and public agencies.

Improve Experiences in Medical Facilities

Hospital emergency services must be radically reorganized. Such services are now being used by the poor as clinics and as substitutes for general practitioners. Such use upsets routine and arouses mutual frustrations and resentments. There are good

reasons why the poor use emergency services this way, and the services should be reorganized to face the realities of the situation.

Clinics and hospitals could assign *agents* to their lower-income patients, who can orient them, allay anxieties, listen to complaints, help them cooperate, and help them negotiate with the staff.

Better accountability and communication should be built into the organization of care. Much important information gets to doctors and nurses only fortuitously, if at all. For instance, nurses' aides often have information about cardiac or terminal patients that doctors and nurses could use; but they do not always volunteer the information nor are they often asked, since they are not considered medically qualified. This is another place where the *agent* might be useful.

It is absolutely necessary that medical personnel lessen their class and professional biases. Anti-bias training is virtually nonexistent in medical schools or associations. It must be started, especially in the professional schools.

Medical facilities must carefully consider how to allow and improve the lodging of complaints by the poor against medical services. They have few means and little chance now to make their complaints known, and this adds to their resentment, depression, and helplessness. Perhaps the agent can act as a kind of medical *ombudsman*; perhaps unions, or the other health insurance groups, can lodge the complaints; perhaps neighborhood groups can do it. But it must be done.

Improving Communications about Regimens

Treatment and regimens are supposed to continue in the home. Poor patients seldom do them adequately. Hospitals and clinics usually concentrate on diagnosis and treatment and tend to neglect what occurs after. Sometimes there is even confusion about who is supposed to tell the patient about such things as his diet at home, and there is little attempt to see that he does it. Here again, follow-up by sub-professionals might be useful.

Special training given to professionals will enable them to give better instructions to the poor on regimens. They are seldom trained at interviewing or listening—and the poor are usually deficient in pressing their opinions.

Check on Home Regimens

Clinics and hospitals could organize their services to include checking on ex-patients who have no private physicians. We recommend that hospitals and clinics try to bring physicians in poor neighborhoods into some sort of association. Many of these physicians do not have hospital connections, practice old-fashioned or sub-standard medicine— yet they are in most immediate contact with the poor, especially before hospitalization.

Medical establishments should make special efforts to discover and understand the prevalent life styles of their patients. Since this affects efficiency of treatment, it is an important medical concern.

I strongly recommend greater emphasis on research in medical devices or techniques that are simple to operate and depend as little as possible on patients' judgment and motivation. Present good examples include long-term tranquilizers and the intrauterine birth-control device which requires little of the woman other than her consent. Such developments fit lower class life style much better than those requiring repeated actions, timing, and persistence.

As noted, these recommendations are not basically different from many others— except that they all relate to the idea of the vicious cycle. *A major point of this paper is that equal health care will not come unless all portions of that cycle are attacked simultaneously.*

To assure action sufficiently broad and strong to demolish this cycle, *responsibility must also be broad and strong.*

Medical and professional schools must take vigorous steps to counteract the class bias of their students, to teach them to relate, communicate, and adapt techniques and regimens to the poor, and to learn how to train and instruct sub-professionals.

Specific medical institutions must, in addition to the recommendations above, consider how best to attack *all* segments of the cycle. Partial attacks will not do— medicine has responsibility for the total patient and the total treatment.

Lower class people must themselves be enlisted in the campaign to give them better care. Not to do this would be absolutely foolhardy. The sub-professionals we mention are themselves valuable in large part because they come from the poor, and understand them. Where indigenous organizations exist, they should be used. Where they do not exist, organizations that somehow meet their needs should be aided and encouraged to form.

Finally, governments, at all levels, have an immense responsibility for persuading, inducing, or pressuring medical institutions and personnel toward reforming our system of medical care. If they understand the vicious cycle, their influence will be much greater. This governmental role need not at all interfere with the patient's freedom. Medical influence is shifting rapidly to the elite medical centers; federal and local governments have a responsibility to see that medical influence and care, so much of it financed by public money, accomplishes what it is supposed to.

What of the frequently heard argument that increasing affluence will soon eliminate the need for special programs for the poor?

Most sociologists agree that general affluence may never "trickle down" to the hard-core poverty groups; that only sustained and specialized effort over a long period of time may relieve their poverty.

Increased income does not necessarily change life styles. Some groups deliberately stand outside our mainstream. And there is usually a lag at least of one generation, often more, before life styles respond to changed incomes.

In the long run, no doubt, prosperity for all will minimize the inferiority of medical care for the poor. But in the long run, as the saying goes, we will all be dead. And the disadvantaged sick will probably go first, with much unnecessary suffering.

29

ONE OF THE MOST important concerns about being sick is how to pay for it. But through legislation, and the mass consumption of private insurance, largely financed by industry in exchange for wages on the job, everyone will soon become a paying patient at the doctor's office, the hospital and nursing home and then purely economic barriers to medical care will disappear. In reality, however, financing medical care is only the top portion of an iceberg. As in so many other social, economic, and political problems, money is only a step in the solution of more basic and fundamental problems.

In medical care, even with everyone a paying patient, at least four important problems remain submerged from recognition and debate. (1) Do we want treatment to reach everybody? (2) Does everyone get the best possible treatment? (3) Do we care who treats us? (4) Do we care about the size and location of our hospitals and practices?

After Everyone Can Pay for Medical Care: Some Perspectives on Future Treatment and Practice

John D. Stoeckle
and
Irving K. Zola

Do We Want Treatment to Reach Everybody?

Our treatment institutions, our hospitals, clinics, and medical practices, have traditionally viewed the public who did not seek medical aid as being relatively healthy or certainly not very sick. For, if they really were, they would come to the doctor. Similar views have been expressed about patients who did not regularly keep their appointments, who broke off in the midst of treatment, or who did not wait around in a waiting-room or on a waiting list. Yet many studies and observations of those who are not going to the doctor have revealed a high prevalence of sickness, disease, and disability. In one recent industrial survey some 90 per cent of the workers were found with treatable but untreated disorders. No one knows how large is this population with unmet needs that does not seek medical aid, that is apathetic about getting treatment, that procrastinates in going to the doctor; but it has been estimated at near some 40,000,000 Americans. What is more important is the fact that this population of non-

users, slow users, treatment drop-outs, is found predominantly, but not only, in our lower socio-economic classes. The irony of unmet medical needs in a country of plenty was shown in a recent survey of one of our major cities, where it was noted that those with greatest medical care needs for example, the elderly and other low income, and "minority" groups—have the lowest recognition of their medical needs and the longest duration of care once it is initiated.

REASONS FOR NON-ATTENDANCE

Again and again health surveys have demonstrated that the section of our population that does not participate in immunization campaigns or take preventive action— cancer check-ups, going to the doctor early, mass X-rays—is not a random one. Investigators have emphasized the potential patient's contribution to this problem and have studied the characteristics of this non-attending population. They have pointed out their lack of psychological readiness, their lack of medical knowledge, their fear of seeking medical aid, their negative views of treatment and of the doctor, clinic or

From Medical Care, *Vol. 2: 36–41, January–March, 1964; by permission of the authors and publisher.*

hospital delivering medical services, and finally, their personal (that is, idiosyncratic) and very unscientific ideas about being sick or healthy.

Too often, however, it appears as if this delay or unwillingness to seek help is all the patient's fault. Yet some is fostered, at least indirectly, by the health professions. The reasons, of course, are manifold. One is our activistic over-emphasis on dramatic "cures" fostering unrealistic expectations on the part of much of our population. Either one does not have to worry because the illness can easily be cured, or the condition is hopeless and nothing can be done. These black and white expectations have not only blinded us to the necessity and appreciation of the importance of preventive measures but have also led to considerable unwillingness to embark on any long-term course of treatment which will not lead to a "complete cure." The potential patient is often unenthusiastic about continuing in a course of long-term treatment which guarantees at most only remission, control or relief, and physicians, trained in a framework of specific techniques and skills to cure or remove certain acute conditions, may find the treatment of chronically ill patients unsatisfying and so neglect it.

Another reason treatment may not reach everyone is professional reliance on the lay decision to go to the doctor. The patients who come to see him may not be all the people who can be treated. Medical advances appear more and more capable of detecting disease or its precursors in asymptomatic populations. To rely on testing only those coming to the doctor will not, of course, find all the treatable cases. Large-scale mass testing will be necessary. So often, too, medical seriousness of a patient's symptoms may not be the major factor getting him to the doctor. In fact, he may be unaware or ignore early symptoms of sickness.

Since there may also be a general reluctance to see a doctor, it may be necessary to re-evaluate what aspects of health and illness can truly be left to individual initiative and to what extent the health professions are willing and able to assume more initiative

and responsibility for the initial steps in detection and treatment. Just sitting in the office waiting for the patient will not reach all the public. In the same way as getting alcoholics into treatment, some people will have to be educated, some coaxed, some led, and some sought out.

SOLUTIONS TO THE PROBLEM

Today the social-welfare value of making medical services available to everyone is generally accepted. While removing financial barriers to such services will help to make them more accessible, this will not lead automatically to mass participation. As we have stressed, more attention will have to be paid to the segment of unrecognised treatable illness and the reasons for the lack of action by many of us in seeking medical aid. Such facts will provoke questions about how our treatment institutions can work better and how our population's views of sickness and seeking help might be changed. But easy solutions and answers are not at hand. They will have to encompass (1) realistic health education, particularly of children, which would result in realistic expectations of patients and their families, particularly regarding the more chronic disorders, (2) development of treatment techniques and services acceptable to and able to reach different segments of the population and illness groups who may customarily avoid treatment, and (3) improving the availability of treatment, not just for the individual patient in the doctor's office but for everybody in his group— whether at school, the company office, the factory plant, his housing project, or home —wherever medical resources of detection, prevention, diagnosis, and treatment can practically be brought to bear.

Does Everyone Get the Best Possible Treatment?

Up to this point our concerns have been what illnesses or potential patients do not come to the attention of a doctor when we aim that treatment should reach everyone. But what of those who do come? Does everyone get the best of our services or are there differences in treatment and services unrelated to the patient's diagnosis? We do not have to look very far for objective examples of differential treatment. A walk round our cities will often reveal how marginal are the facilities of many municipal hospitals compared to the superior facilities of private voluntary ones. Even the historical basis of our private voluntary hospitals with their built-in differential service to "charity" patients is only slowly disappearing, hastened a bit by the paying status of the consumer. What confronts the patient here may still run the gamut from shabby surroundings, detailed questioning on his "means" and resources, to delays and inconvenient scheduling of diagnostic and treatment service.

DIFFERENTIAL TREATMENT

Other examples of differential treatment have been documented. In a recent survey of hospital care in New York City, experts rated privately owned, proprietary, profit-making hospitals poorer in standards of care than voluntary or government hospitals. That treatment was not solely related to the patient's need based on psychiatric diagnosis but also to his social class has been documented in Hollingshead and Redlich's much quoted study of psychiatric care. With the same diagnosis higher-class patients received psychotherapy while lower-class patients were given more organic forms of treatment.

Similar observations about bias in the medical diagnosis have been made among patients from different ethnic backgrounds. Among patients seen at three medical clinics, *despite* the same objective degree of psychological difficulties, emotionally caused symptoms were diagnosed more often in Italian as compared to Irish and Anglo-Saxon patients. Such problems of communication between patient and doctor may lead to under-diagnosis of treatable medical diseases. And some observers feel that when patients are treated in any bureaucratic and institutional setting they get less treatment—that is, less personal attention—than when they are treated in a private office. All these studies demonstrate that the quality of

treatment in our country is not only uneven but that it is influenced by important historical and sociological conditions.

SOCIAL–PSYCHOLOGICAL FACTORS

Even our legislation has a narrow orientation toward medical care, in spite of evidence to the contrary that good care and treatment is not just medical. It has become clearer, but often not an acknowledged fact, that the problems of patients presenting at medical institutions and medical practices are social and psychological in important respects. Many recent studies have shown that the patient's decision to see a doctor is rarely based only on his medical symptoms or his knowledge about diseases, but more often on important events and factors in his family situation and social relationships. Other studies have shown similar influences in the decisions to undergo surgery, to re-hospitalize mental patients, and to place old people in nursing homes. Likewise, it is becoming increasingly difficult to ignore the widespread prevalence of emotional and psychological distress and disability. Whether we take the results of national opinion surveys on where people take their acknowledged personal concerns, the mental distress reported from morbidity surveys of residents in mid-town Manhattan, the Jersey suburbs, and rural America, or the experience of doctors in practice, social–psychological factors in illness and patient care are large. When such factors are unrecognized and untreated by the physician it prevents rational diagnosis and handicaps the patient treatment.

The scientific understanding and handling of these aspects of illness, so important for future practice in the community, are still a matter of much debate in the education and training of the doctor. The curriculum and training experiences are already crowded with medical subject matter and medical orientation for practice in the hospital. Since training for practice in the community is not in itself an acknowledged aim and since hospital clinical care and research departments play so large a role in what is taught, curriculum additions dealing with the psychosocial study of illness and patient care are, in spite of their documented need, considered unnecessary.

Solutions to differential treatment (like making sure that everyone receives treatment) will have to encompass the patient, the public, and the professions. Where education contributes to professional treatment skill, there is need not only for upgrading traditional medical teaching in some schools but for greater recognition of their responsibility to the community and of the need for newer programs in the social study of illness and disease. Yet, as G. Silver argues, education alone may not be translated into an improvement of treatment unless an appropriate organization —the family medical team—is developed to apply social skills and preventive medicine.

Do We Care Who Treats Us?

Our nation's professional journals carry endless definitions of professional specializations, of limited and exclusive enclosures of competence, of the role of the doctor, nurse, social worker, and a host of subspecialists within the professions themselves. No role, in turn, is more discussed than that of the doctor, and that of various types of doctors. Much of our thinking and planning of patient care centers on the transfer of the doctor's functions into an institutional setting, a big clinic or a group practice, or the division of his functions among various practitioners in the community. Complaints are frequently made that there is too much division of treatment labor among specialists, that there is no one doctor for everyone in the family, that there is no "personal doctor" to deal with the more intimate problems and concerns, that no one practitioner is available for initial medical aid, advice, and direction to other sources for help, that physicians are too busy to give "physicals" to healthy individuals or to be interested in the early detection and prevention of disease, that the doctor's office is located farther and farther away from the neighborhood and home, or that emergency round-the-clock help is no longer available. These are important care-taking and treatment functions of the family doctor, who has largely disappeared in fact but not in fancy.

To want a family doctor may no longer be a question of choice. The question that needs to be asked is how are his functions being met in our organizations and patterns of specialization. Many of these essential functions are now in several hands. Much of the public, at least in the middle-class suburbs, seems to be using multiple "specialists" for health care needs at different periods of life: the pediatrician for the children and the baby; the obstetrician–gynecologist for delivery and the mother's check–ups; and the internist for the mother's, father's, and grandparents' "medical troubles." Every "specialist" may be expected to take on some of the functions of the family doctor at times, and yet their professional training and orientation does not acknowledge this and their own definition as specialists deals only with technical diagnostic questions about the patient.

This problem becomes exacerbated as medical men increasingly specialize and as the lay population becomes more medically sophisticated and so goes directly to specialists or asks to be referred. This will not be "bad" if the patient's "other problems" and concerns are recognized and he is directed to a suitable source of help. But since there will often be no family physician to whom the specialist can return such patients when these other problems arise, he will have to deal with them himself —a situation for which his medical education may have left him largely unprepared.

ANCILLARY PROFESSIONS

While much debate is centered on how the various medical specialists should be related, a still more fundamental issue concerns the transfer and division of functions among other health professions, who may do diagnostic and therapeutic work. It is in this area that what is truly "team medicine" may develop. The expectation, however, that the doctor, as "the specialist" of the team, will deal only with the complicated medical aspects of the patient, leaving personal concerns to the nurse and social worker, and ordinary diagnostic skills to the technicians, is not a likely possibility. This might seem a rational division of the technical skills of the team, but there will be social limits. For example, the patient, in seeking help, will not always view the professions as they see themselves nor be able to diagnose his illness and choose or accept the right kind of help. Called to see a patient vomiting at night, the doctor may come upon a family quarrel and a crisis over the behavior of a child. Some would argue that the family called the wrong person, that it should have called the psychiatrist or the social worker. But since the call for help was in response to a child's vomiting, it is unlikely that anyone other than a medical man would have been called and expected to cope with such a crisis.

There is, however, another side to this coin: it concerns the limits of competence of the community practitioner. Psychosomatic complaints and physical symptoms of behavior disorders are most likely to come to the attention of physicians and may require some medical surveillance and be subject to rational psychological treatment. Yet there is no evidence that more general behavioral problems are most appropriately treated by "medical men" as they are now trained. Some would even contend than the psychological training of a PhD clinical psychologist is often more extensive than that of many psychiatrists and certainly of most physicians. Whether behavioral problems such as delinquency, malingering, anti-social acts and even much of what is called neurotic should be considered "illness" and therefore under the sole dominion of the medical professions has been questioned by at least one psychiatrist, Thomas Szasz.

PUBLIC HEALTH NURSE

A less noticeable transfer and fractionization of medical duties is taking place in still another sphere. As our professions specialize and centralize—for example, at hospitals

and medical centers—as they limit the hours they work and the calls they make—for example, no house calls—and as we fail to train enough doctors or to organize health personnel for the needs of the population, makeshift solutions in treatment develop. For instance, the public health nurse is filling a doctor-gap for large segments of our lower socio–economic classes, as well as for still larger populations abroad. She has become a sort of second-choice-doctor—giving some emergency treatment, teaching health care and prevention, and doing a considerable amount of family counselling. Since it is rarely recognized or acknowledged that she is engaged in such tasks, she is often without connecting links to any chain of medical practice and lacks the face-to-face communication with colleagues that is important in patient care. One of the dangers of being outside any network of medical practice is the lack of informal supervision of the quality of patient care which ordinarily occurs through mutual consultation and interchange among professional staffs. Whether she will ultimately become the "family doctor" of choice is inextricably entwined with the degree to which doctors will continue to withdraw from and reject such duties.

Thus, who takes care of the patient—the division of labor of medical practice—will ultimately depend on the patients' views of their illness and of the professionals they seek to treat them as well as on the internal needs of professionals themselves. Fractionization of medical care has already and inevitably taken place. Much of the current dissatisfaction is due more to ineffective communication between therapists and their lack of co-ordination and "team-work" than to any inherent "badness" in a division of treatment itself. Unwillingness to recognize this phenomenon has resulted in scant attention being paid to how immediate medical aid can be organized, what treatment can and should be co-ordinated, who can treat personal concerns and behavioral problems, how exclusively "specialistic" should a specialist's training and education be—to what, in fact, is the appropriate use of other professions, whether they be behavioral scientists, human relations experts, or public health nurses. As long as these problems are not even acknowledged, effective planning of treatment work is impossible.

Do We Care about the Size and Location of Our Hospitals and Practices?

Not because of "specialization" but because of rising costs, the work of hospitals has also been scrutinized. Demands are made to restrict the hospital as a sickbed institution only to the performance of technical procedures required in complicated diagnosis and treatment of acute illness. At the same time, the hospital has been taking on other functions besides bed care and maintaining a "sick room away from home." For example, all phases of illness—from the acute attack to convalescence, rehabilitation, chronic care, and terminal stages—have increasingly become hospital functions. There has also been a greater recognition of the care and treatment which can be organized for a patient without hospitalization. Certainly more medical care is possible with ambulant patients, in out-patient clinics and offices, although such functions rarely receive the public, professional, or institutional support which the bed functions do.

All these trends make the hospital a bigger and bigger "center," a diversified organization with more care-taking services on its grounds. However, the mere bringing of all care-taking services to hospital grounds does not guarantee that nursing home, chronic disease treatment, and ambulatory care will, in turn, get better facilities, better professional staff, better organization of treatment and more investment. The hospital as an institution has its own priorities and can just as well neglect certain treatment functions as the community at large.

How the bigger hospitals grow will also determine the future existence of our small local hospitals and local practices where much general care is given and where many patients prefer to attend. It will depend on whether there is merely centralization of facilities and services and practices—witness the private practice office buildings moving to hospital grounds—or whether there is growth through more effective integration and alliance with and among smaller local community institutions and practices. The trend to add and centralize more and more activities on the hospital grounds will certainly make some of our traditional local hospitals and practices less important, but growth by co-operation and integration should not have this effect. "Regionalization" has become the shorthand for this co-operative organization of medical services in a community. Unfortunately, in some situations it has only meant dividing up clientele areas, thus limiting medical competition among big hospitals. It may, however, mean a brake on duplication, on the purchase of expensive equipment by each of several hospitals, and the selected development of expensive therapies. And it can mean even more—such as the development of working relationships among institutions and medical practices for the management of illness and disability in an urban treatment area. An important yet intangible by-product could be the informal supervision of the quality of patient care in the community that can occur through mutual consultation and interchange among professional staffs, managers, and the lay boards alike. Now they so often work in relative isolation.

MENTAL HEALTH CARE

Finally, we might want our hospitals to grow in still another way. For example, a major concern of our hospital staffs, managers, and boards might be whether our traditional medical institutions, whose practices are in reality concerned as much with mental health, should include treatment departments, divisions, and even special hospital units for social and psychiatric care. Such health care has long been an implicit function of the work of the personal doctor or "GP," but as a hospital function it has developed into special mental institutions parallel to but separate from our general medical ones. Large-scale psychiatric services, particularly in in-patient care, is still a comparatively rare phenomenon in a general hospital.

Some would say that to join these traditionally separate systems is too difficult an alliance both ideologically and practically. For example, mental institutions and psychiatric care have been financed through taxes and thus have a history and background different from that of the community's general voluntary hospitals with their history of private financing. However, even these differences are disappearing. As voluntary hospitals rely more and more on patient-care receipts and government programs, they are becoming increasingly like traditional public institutions, at least in financing. Another similarity is administrative management. Mental hospitals are taking on discharge and treatment policies and practices like general hospitals, returning many chronic patients to the community. Recent studies have shown that for many psychiatric patients, hospitalization in a general hospital has distinct treatment advantages and that their care can be managed with minimal disruption of hospital routine. Notwithstanding differences that still exist, if demands and needs for health care are not just medical but also psychosocial, then the integration of these parallel services is a major public concern.

SOLO PRACTICE

The question of centralization of functions in the hospital has its counterpart in the current debates about medical practice. Perhaps in fear of the growing tentacles of the hospital or medical center, there is concern about whether solo *entrepreneurial* practice, a more dominant style of organization in America, is suitable for the complexities of patient care as opposed to group practice where medical specialization is formally organized for treatment. Will the

solo practitioner, the individual firm, the medical small business, like the corner grocer, be swallowed up by or affiliate with a big chain like a group practice or clinic? And, if he does join, will he contract his skills to the group or *entrepreneur* within it?

The alternatives in organization have always been pictured as either one system or another, private practice or "government medicine," solo or contractual practice. For example, it seems clear that even individual solo practice has already done many things which make ideological views outdated—it has remained as an informal network of colleague practices, it has formed into group practice units, and even contracted for medical care of groups. Some have also located on the hospital's grounds as a big private *entrepreneurial* business, alongside more contractual forms of group practice and clinics. Large clinics with contractual practice have also sprung up in response to the needs of the blocks of consumers found in industry, unions, and colleges. Harvard, for example, has organized a pre-paid in-plant medical service for students, faculty, and employees with contractual services of doctors.

This retail view of practice and organization may not appeal to us when we are dealing with such charged transactions as our own health, illness, and treatment. However, it may caution us against too ideological a commitment to one form of practice for everybody. It may also modify views which regard only our own consumer choice as ideal and all others as undesirable, without a real respect for other choices in the domestic scene. When it comes to actual facts about what organization is best, we often adhere to traditional concepts with little evidence as to what actually works best for whom.

But there are many other public concerns about organization of medical practice. Equally important is its location—at the hospital, the school, the plant—in addition to the traditional location in the neighborhood or down-town. Medical practices at these institutional sites, in contrast to the *entrepreneurial* organization of private practice, have usually been contractual, with the doctors as employees. Practitioners at these sites have always been ambivalent about the scope and depth of their medical services to their clientele. Should they provide personal and comprehensive health services or restrict themselves to job-related injuries and employment examinations? The uneasiness in deciding to do the former has been due to the fear of competing with private practice. To add to the dilemma, recent research has documented the importance of the work situation on the individual's physical and psychological health. Surely, if we hope to reach everyone, these on-the-spot sites may be realistic ways of offering personal and preventive medical services, and our traditional ambivalence about competition will have to give way to concern about availability and consumption of services.

Epilogue

Remembering the high prevalence of treated and untreated symptoms and disorders, cited previously, there are those who claim that we cannot treat everything. There are others who note that there is probably a great deal we should not treat such as many self-limiting disorders—for example, minor burns, some communicable childhood diseases, unnecessary tonsillectomies. The task of treatment is indeed monumental, for the very progress and development of man introduces new dangers, new agents of disease. Man experiments with synthetic products and changes his diet; he constructs cities that breed rats and infection; he builds automobiles, factories, and bombs which pollute the air. When one disease or disorder is controlled, its control mechanism may produce the breeding ground for still another disease. As René Dubos contends, the goal of complete freedom from disease and struggle is almost incompatible with the progress of living; so also with medical care. Whether we should strive to provide medical care for everything is impossible to say.

Until we recognise that illness and health is more than the mere presence or absence of symptoms, that seeking medical aid is more than reactive behavior to symptoms, and the health professions' responsibility is more than to wait for patients and then to treat these symptoms, our solutions for providing medical care will only be stopgaps.

With more and more possibilities of therapeutic intervention for everything, a philosophy of medicine is needed to define what is "good medical care," comprehensive care or the "best medical care in the world." While medical care experts can furnish us with measurements of the quality and quantity of treatment, we also need to consider our directions, for example, the other problems produced by the technical capacity to prevent death at any cost in old age, the values of genetic counselling particularly in regard to the problem of treating congenital defects, or the use of the medical services to meet personal needs—that is, as a "refuge in a storm"—as much as we need to consider utilitarian demands of keeping people healthy and on the job.

Finally, it is often complained that the government will set the policies regarding medical care and practice. The basic problems besetting medical care, however, are neither financial nor administrative but the professional and public needs and aspirations. In this commentary specific solutions have not been suggested but several important issues, often submerged from view, have been discussed. Only when such issues are recognized can solutions be found: and only then can we claim to provide not only the best medical care but the best possible medical care.

Bibliography

Dubos, R., *Mirage of Health*, New York: Doubleday, 1959.

Hollingshead, A. B., and F. C. Redlich, *Social Class and Mental Illness*, New York: Wiley, 1958.

Klarman, H. E., *Hospital Care in New York City*, New York: Columbia Univ. Press, 1963.

Silver, G. A., *The Family Health Team*, New York: Columbia Univ. Press, 1962.

Szasz, T. A., *The Myth of Mental Illness*, New York: Hoeber, 1961.

Name Index

This index includes only those names cited in the text proper.

Subject Index